THE SURGICAL TECHNIC

OF

ABDOMINAL OPERATIONS

By

JULIUS L. SPIVACK, M. D.

*Assistant Professor of Surgery, University of Illinois College of Medicine; Professor
of Operative Surgery and Surgical Anatomy, Cook County Graduate School
of Medicine; Attending Surgeon Oak Forest Infirmary,
Columbus Hospital, etc.*

SECOND EDITION
REVISED AND ENLARGED

677 ILLUSTRATIONS ON 362 FIGURES.
MOSTLY ORIGINAL.

CHICAGO
S. B. DEBOUR, PUBLISHERS
1938

TO MY WIFE

PREFACE TO THE SECOND EDITION

The reception accorded the first edition both by the medical profession and reviewers here and abroad was most gratifying. The fact that the first edition was completely exhausted in about six months and that two printings had to be made to satisfy the demand within a year after publication, proves conclusively that there is need for books of this type. This is also supported by the fact that the medical profession in Spanish speaking countries has already shown a profound interest in a Spanish translation which was published recently.

The present edition does not radically differ from the first one, but the author embraced the opportunity to render the diction in some places more lucid. Another feature which enhances the value of the book is an alphabetic subject index in addition to the author's index.

The author expresses his appreciation to the many readers and to his former students for their manifestations of interest in the first edition, and hopes that the second edition will be received as well as the preceding issue.

JULIUS L. SPIVACK.

Chicago, Illinois
January, 1938

PREFACE TO THE FIRST EDITION

This book is an outgrowth of lectures on Operative Surgery as delivered by us for many years to our students, both undergraduate and postgraduate.

No apology is needed for writing a book on Surgical Technic: The great number of books on surgery usually deal with "what to do", and very little emphasis is made as to "how to do", probably because it is taken for granted that the reader knows "how to do it", which knowledge he acquired in the time of apprenticeship. We do not consider for a moment that this book can replace apprenticeship. On the contrary, we believe that a book of this type can render the most service while the beginner is studying the technic of operations on cadavers, living animals, or by actual assistantship. For this reason, we believe this book to be useful for medical students while they study operative technic on cadavers and on living animals, just as well as for a busy practicing surgeon who wishes to review in detail the technic of the operation he is going to perform.

The subject is presented in a didactic manner: At the beginning simple procedures are presented with numerous pictures; farther on, more complicated operations are described, and only such pictures are added which enable the reader to grasp at once the correct sequence of the steps of the operation under discussion.

In many chapters a brief historical review of the evolution of the operation is given. This makes it possible for one to study the mistakes made by our predecessors, thus enabling us to learn how to overcome them. Wherever possible, we have mentioned the name of the originator of the operation, and have tried as well as we could to establish the priority of the man who described this or the other method. More than one technic for each type of operation is described for the reason that we believe that the surgeon should be familiar with more than one method, so that he can choose the type of technic suitable for the particular occasion.

In the title of many operations we have retained the name of the originator, although the text we have used may deviate in some details from the text as written by the originator of the method, and may include some improvements made later by someone else.

Our desire to present only modern methods of operative treatment did not prevent us from describing some appliances which are seldom used now, such as the Murphy button. The reason for this is, that still under definite circumstances some surgeons are using the button even today, and another reason is that many times we have been requested by postgraduate students to demonstrate its use. However, describing its use in detail, we emphasize our belief that suture methods should be given preference to all other methods in which mechanical appliances are used.

The bibliography contains not only references to recent work published, but also "old" literary work. The reason for this is evident. We are giving first of all the references to the original work of the authors who laid the foundation for this or the other operation. The bibliography does not refer only to subjects dealing with the technic; it refers also to all other subjects discussed in the book, such as anatomy, indications, dangers connected with the execution of the operation, etc.

To Dr. W. A. Newman Dorland, of Chicago, we wish to express our deep appreciation for his invaluable suggestions and wise counsel.

To Dr. Karl A. Meyer, of Chicago, we wish to express our thanks for the kindly interest shown throughout the preparation of the book.

The illustrations are, with few exceptions, original. The pictures have been drawn by Miss A. Bartenbach, the medical artist of Cook County Hospital, Miss F. Foy and Messrs. G. Dalstrom, G. Orloff, and G. Vollum. We wish to express our thanks to them for their excellent and painstaking work.

JULIUS L. SPIVACK.

Chicago, Illinois
May, 1936

TABLE OF CONTENTS.

PART I.

THE SURGICAL TECHNIC
OF
ABDOMINAL OPERATIONS
PART I.

CHAPTER I.

GENERAL SURGICAL TECHNIC IN THE ABDOMINAL CAVITY.

GENERAL CONSIDERATIONS PERTAINING TO
ABDOMINAL SURGERY.

Every operation, no matter how complicated and extensive, consists of a combination of two simple procedures, namely, division and union of tissues.

In order to perform a satisfactory operation, from the technical point of view, several factors have to be taken into consideration:

1. **The tissues should not be mutilated and should be handled very gently.**

    This can be accomplished by using sharp knives or scissors and by not mauling the tissues.

2. **The bleeding vessels should be grasped with as little of the surrounding tissues as possible.**

3. **Constant practice by the surgeon of the different essential elements of the operative technic, such as suturing and tying knots.**

    There is hardly any profession in which manual dexterity is of importance, in which its members engage in the development of their technical skill as little as does even the busy surgeon.

4. **Each step of the operation should be familiar to the surgeon before he starts any operation.**

    He should never start an operation that he has never performed before, unless he has done it on a cadaver and on living animals.

5. **Time element is of no great importance provided that it does not overstep a reasonable limit.**

    For the average major operation, 45 minutes up to 1 hour is good time (including opening and closure of the abdomen). Of course, an appendectomy should not take one hour, and certainly one is allowed more than one hour for a gastrectomy. The length of the operation does not depend so much on quick movements as it does on standardized technic. The surgeon should learn to **make each movement accomplish a definite purpose.**

6. **The operative field should always be well exposed and accessible.**
   This means that it should be brought as close to the surface of
   the skin as is possible and be well illuminated. This simplifies
   the performance of the operation.

7. **All bleeding points must be controlled.**

8. **Dead spaces must be avoided.**

9. **The surgeon should not change the posture of his body.** He should
   not lean over the patient's body, compressing the latter's chest.
   He should not push his assistants aside or obscure the operative
   field from his assistants. All these things can be accomplished
   either by changing hands (which means that if the surgeon cannot accomplish a movement with his right hand, then he should
   use the left hand instead and *vice versa*) or instruments (scissors
   instead of knife and *vice versa*).

LIGATURES AND SUTURES.

Suture-material is used for the approximation of the edges of incised
tissues and for the ligation of blood-vessels. If it is used for ligation of
blood-vessels it is called a **ligature,** and if for holding the approximated
tissues together, it is called a **suture.**

Historical.—Ligatures and sutures have been known from remote
antiquity. In the Edwin Smith Papyrus, written about 4,000 years ago,
we learn that the surgeons of Egypt were accustomed to close opened
wounds by adhesive plaster made from strips of linen, and reinforced
by sutures.

Susruta (600 B. C.), who is considered the father of Hindu surgery
and who is the author of Samhitá, taught closure of the open abdomen
with sutures, and as suture-material used cotton, strips of leather, plaited
horse-hair or animal sinews.

Archigenes of Apamea, a great Syrian surgeon who lived about 100
A. D., taught ligation of the large blood-vessels before amputating the
extremity. From the writings of Celsus and Galen we learn that they
knew well the usage of ligatures and sutures.

In the Medieval Period, Rhazes, the great Arabian surgeon of Bag-
dad (860-932), was the first who sutured the open abdomen with harp-
strings which were made from the twisted intestine of the sheep.

In the time of the Renaissance, Guglielmo di Salicetti, the surgeon
who introduced the "glover suture" in intestinal surgery, knew the comparative merits of silk and waxed linen thread as material for the ligation
of blood-vessels.

Leonardo Bertapaglia (XV Century), of the School of Padua, taught
isolation of blood-vessels before their ligation, instead of ligating them
"en masse", as was customary at that time.

However, the ancient and medieval surgeons preferred the cautery
and boiling oil to ligatures as hemostatics, and strips of adhesive plaster

to sutures as suture-material.

The credit for reviving the interest in ligatures belongs to the great French surgeon-barber, Ambroise Paré (1509-1590), formerly prosector for the great anatomist Sylvius, and later court surgeon to the French Kings—Frances II and Charles IX. The ligature was more extensively used in Continental Europe; in England it was not much in use until the beginning of the nineteenth century. To Mr. Sharpe, of Guy's Hospital in London, belongs the credit of popularizing its usage in England.

Suture-material for suturing of wounds came into use much later than the use of ligatures, in fact not until the first half of the nineteenth century. Up to the first quarter of this century, surgeons used strips of adhesive plaster for the closure of wounds, even of the opened abdomen.

All suture-material can be divided into two large classes:

> A.   **Absorbable sutures;**
>
> B.   **Non-absorbable sutures.**

A. Absorbable sutures.— These are so named because when left in the tissues of the body for a short time (1 to 4 weeks) they are dissolved. They are all of animal origin. They are made from the tendons of different animals, such as the kangaroo, or rat; from the aorta of the ox; from the intestinal wall of sheep, etc.

Catgut actually replaced all other kinds of absorbable suture. It is made from the submucous layer of the intestinal wall of the sheep.

Catgut occurs in different forms, depending on the method of its preparation and of the component parts of the chemicals by which it is treated. It is prepared in different sizes. Each size has a definite diameter and is three one-thousandths of an inch (0.0762 mm.) larger, than the next smaller one. Thus, the size of catgut is standardized as follows:

For number 000—the size is 0.2286 mm. (nine one-thousandths of one inch).

For number 00—the size is 0.3048 mm. (twelve one-thousandths of one inch).

For number 0—the size is 0.3810 mm. (fifteen one-thousandths of one inch).

For number 1—the size is 0.4572 mm. (eighteen one-thousandths of one inch).

Catgut is manufactured in sizes 000-00-0-1-2-3-4-5-6-7; the sizes most commonly used are 00-0-1-2-3.

Depending on the method of chemical treatment, catgut is subdivided into:

> a.   **Plain Catgut.** This is catgut which has not been treated with any reagent that would in any way increase its ability to resist absorption.
>
> b.   **Chromic catgut.** This is plain catgut suture which has been treated by chromium trioxide. The object of chromicizing catgut is to render it more resistant to tissue fluids and thus delay its absorp-

tion. It is customary to name chromic catgut as "ten-day," "twenty-day" or "forty-day"—the number of days designating the length of time which is necessary for the catgut to be absorbed in a normal striate muscular tissue.

c. **Iodine catgut.** This is catgut which has been immersed in a solution of iodine and iodide of potassium. The object of using iodine catgut is to have a suture-material which exerts a local germicidal action in the tissues and thus prevents the suture from bacterial invasion, which would hasten absorption of the catgut and also delay the healing process.

d. **Iodochromic catgut.** This is plain catgut which has been treated with a solution of iodine, potassium iodide, and potassium di-chromate.

e. **Silverized catgut.** This is plain catgut which has been treated with silver, which increases its strength and delays its absorption.

The length of time that is needed for the absorption of catgut depends on numerous conditions: it is absorbed more rapidly in infected than in healthy tissues. The absorption period varies in relation to its size, to the morphological type of tissue in which it is buried (peritoneum, muscle, fascia) and to the degree of impregnation with chromium salts.

The tensile strength of catgut depends on its size and whether it is plain or chromicized. It slightly differs with the method of preparation, and for this reason slightly differs with each manufacturer.

The strength of plain catgut is approximately as follows:

For size 000— 3 lbs. is the breaking point.
For size   00— 4 lbs. ” ”   ”   ”
For size   0— 7 lbs. ” ”   ”   ”
For size   1—10 lbs. ” ”   ”   ”
For size   2—14 lbs. ” ”   ”   ”
For size   3—19 lbs. ” ”   ”   ”
For size   4—21 lbs. ” ”   ”   ”

Kangaroo tendon is obtained from the tail of a kangaroo; it is very strong; the fine size has a tensile strength of about 27 pounds; the medium size about 38 pounds; and the coarse about 50 pounds. It absorbs very slowly. It was used quite extensively in former years for the repair of hernias, but is not used much today in abdominal surgery.

Recently other varieties of soluble suture-material have been introduced by different surgeons. Although we give a brief description of them, we believe that their value is not sufficiently established yet and a more prolonged study of them is necessary.

Carnofil is a soluble suture-material prepared by Bost from the muscles of a horse. This suture is even, wiry and flexible. Its tensile strength is great: a strand of 0.5 mm. in diameter withstands a tension of 3.3 lbs. (1.5 kg.) and a strand of 0.8 mm. in diameter withstands a tension of 24.2 lbs. (11 kg.). It may be subjected to unlimited sterilization without impairment of its properties. It absorbs well and it does not produce anaphylaxis, except in sensitized animals.

Nerves as suture material were introduced by Preobrazensky. The nerves are treated with 20 per cent. acetic acid, twisted, dried and sterilized in 2 per cent. brilliant green. Absorption takes place in 12 to 14 days. It is used for intestinal suturing.

To the soluble sutures belong also different types of **"living sutures,"** that is, strips of aponeurosis or tendons which are still connected with the mother-tissue and used for suturing purposes. As examples of this type of suture we may mention repair of hernia by strips of the aponeurosis of the external oblique muscle, fixation of the stomach to the anterior abdominal wall by the round ligament of the liver, fixation of the uterus to the anterior abdominal wall by the round ligaments of the uterus, etc.

B. **Non-absorbable sutures.**—Non-absorbable sutures are those which do not dissolve when left in the body; they stay indefinitely. They are either of:

1. **Inorganic nature**—metallic sutures.

Metallic sutures were used extensively in the pre-antiseptic days; later, they were nearly discarded. However, recently interest in them has been revived, and they are now used by some surgeons in nearly all countries. They have definite advantages and disadvantages over other types of sutures. The advantages are that the abdominal wall can be closed very rapidly, the wires may be loosened if they constrict the wall too much, and are reapplied without destroying the action of the individual suture. The disadvantages of metallic sutures are that occasionally the patients complain of pain until the sutures are removed; occasionally the metallic sutures cut through the skin, thus leaving scars.

   a. **Gold,** in the form of wires. On account of the high cost they were used very little and now not at all.

   b. **Silver,** in the form of silver wire, is now seldom used in abdominal surgery. In pre-aseptic days it was used quite extensively. It finds its application even now in orthopedic surgery.

   c. **Combination of different metals (Alloys).** Michel clips are used for closure of the skin of the abdomen; the Murphy button is occasionally used for anastomosis of two hollow viscera.

Stainless steel wire was recommended by W. Babcock for closure of the skin and also as tension-sutures. According to him, the steel wire is less brittle than silver or bronze wire and is strong, smooth, non-irritating and inexpensive.

Nickeline is an alloy which was introduced by Minine. It is used chiefly in gynecological operations and for the closure of the abdominal wall.

2. **Organic of vegetable nature.**—**Linen** is used now quite extensively. In the form of the **Pagenstecher** celluloid thread, it is an excellent suture-material. It is much stronger than silk of the same diameter and for this

reason it can be used in smaller sizes. It is easily disinfected by boiling, and it is much cheaper.

3. **Organic of animal nature.**

   a. **Silk,** braided or twisted. This is strong, particularly the braided variety. It is easily sterilized. It is pliable, does not swell when placed in the tissues, and does not irritate them; it is easy to tie; the knots are tight and have little tendency to slip. However, its capillarity makes silk unsuitable for skin closure, since it may act as a wick to carry infection into the deeper tissues.

   b. **Silkworm gut** is prepared from the silk-forming glands of the silk-worm. It is easily sterilized by boiling, which softens it and renders the tying easy. It is best used for tension-sutures. It should never be used as a buried suture.

   c. **Horsehair** is obtained from the tail of a horse. It is light and flexible but has great capillarity. It is very breakable, so that it will not stand much tension. For this reason, it is advisable to use it only for skin-suturing in cases in which silkworm-gut tension-sutures are also placed, so that the horsehair is holding only the edges of the skin-wound in approximation. In tying them no great force should be employed, since they will break if the pulling force exceeds $1\frac{1}{4}$ lbs. It should be kept in mind that horsehair requires a thorough sterilization on account of a possibility of the presence in it of the resistant *Actinobacillus mallei*.

   d. **Dermal** is made of pure silk threads carefully spun from selected silk-fibers and finished by special processes. Dermal is characterized by a greater tensile strength than horse-hair. It can be boiled for sterilization purposes. It is twice as strong as horse-hair of the same diameter, and for this reason is preferable to horse-hair for suturing of the skin.

   e. **Kal-dermic** is used for skin and tension-sutures. It is a silk thread which has been subjected to special treatment by chemicals to render it resistant to the action of the body fluids and to capillary action. This suture is strong, flexible and non-irritating.

Selection of suture-material.

In selecting the suture-material, the surgeon is guided by several considerations. The suture-material should be easily sterilized, and while being sterilized it should not lose its properties, such as tensile strength; it should be pliable; it should be of sufficient tensile strength to hold the tissues together until union takes place; it should not be bulky; it should become absorbed as soon as the need for it has passed. There is not a single type of suture-material which satisfies all these requirements, and for this reason it is extremely difficult to decide—which material should be given preference—absorbable or non-absorbable.

The advantage of catgut (soluble material) is in its absorbability. **The disadvantage** of it is that it is difficult to sterilize it; cases have been reported of severe wound infection, such as tetanus or gas-bacillus infection which could be traced to contaminated catgut. Occasionally, there is severe irritation of the tissues by the chemicals used for sterilization of catgut. Cases have been reported of allergic action of catgut in susceptible patients. This action has been manifested by different clinical symptomocomplexes, such as asthma, or by a very quick absorption of the catgut before union of the tissues has taken place, with ensuing evisceration of the abdominal contents after laparotomy. **The advantages of insoluble material are:** it can be easily sterilized by boiling; its tensile strength is greater than that of a corresponding thread of soluble material; it is more pliable; the knots are less bulky.

The disadvantage of insoluble material is that it remains in the tissues as a foreign body. In many cases this is of no importance; however, occasionally it irritates the tissues and if the wound becomes infected, the insoluble material may become infected, harbors the micro-organisms and becomes the main cause which will prevent the healing of the wound.

The majority of surgeons prefer to use absorbable suture-material. However, quite recently several articles appeared from different clinics in which the authors have been advocating the use of non-absorbable suture-material.

In our work we use soluble material (plain and chromic catgut) for suturing the abdominal wall and tying even the largest blood vessels, and also in all gastro-intestinal work when suturing the mucosa only, or when making over-and-over sutures in which all the layers of the gastric or intestinal wall are included.

We use non-absorbable material in suturing the serosa or seromuscular layer of the gastro-intestinal tract, in which case we use the Pagenstecher celluloid linen-thread. The skin should be sutured by non-absorbable material, because skin-sutures cannot be safely removed before from 7 to 9 days. Absorbable suture-material when placed in the skin begins to deteriorate before the 7 to 9 days; therefore it contaminates the wound. **For skin-suturing, we use horsehair, dermal, or Michel clips.**

NEEDLES.

In suturing the anterior abdominal wall, we use both straight and curved needles. For suturing the peritoneum, transversalis fascia and muscles, we use round curved needles; for suturing the fascia, sharp curved needles; for sewing the skin, sharp curved or sharp straight needles.

In sewing the gastro-intestinal tract, we use straight or curved round needles. The essential thing is that the point of the needle should be round; if it is sharp it will cut the tissues. For most purposes, the straight round needles will serve; only in some particular cases, when it is necessary to work deeply, curved needles will be more convenient. When working with straight needles, it is not necessary to use a needle-holder; when working with curved needles, we may or may not use a needle-holder. The work without a needle-holder is more precise because the surgeon can feel exactly how deep he is going into the tissues. Usually, surgeons working with curved needles use a needle-holder, but some use their fingers instead.

KNOTS.

The following are the knots which are most commonly used in surgery:

1. **Square knot (Reef knot, Sailor's knot)** (Fig. 1, a).

This can be recognized from other types of knots by having one **vertical limb** of the loop pass **in front** of and **the other vertical limb**

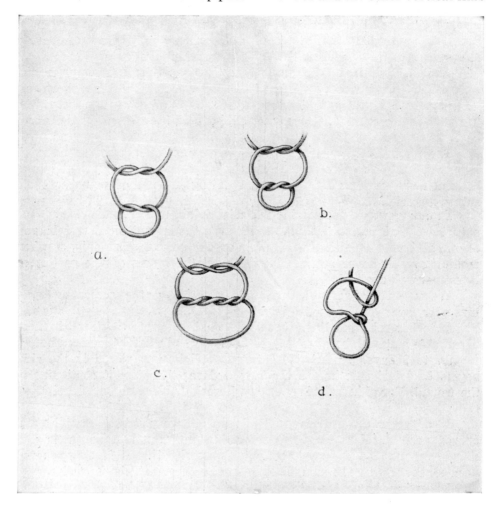

FIG. 1.
a.—Square knot;   b.—Granny knot;   c.—Surgical knot;   d.—Slip knot.

behind the horizontal limbs. This knot is the most reliable; there is no tendency to untie; it resists pressure from inside more than any other knot (with the exception of the surgical knot); however, before it is completed, namely after only the first "half-hitch" is made, it may occasionally slip; for this reason, when working deeply in the abdominal cavity, and especially if the field is not entirely visible, it may be necessary to make a:

2. **Surgeon's knot (Surgical knot)** (Fig. 1, c).

This knot differs from the previous one in this respect only—that when the first half-hitch is made, the ends are not pushed away

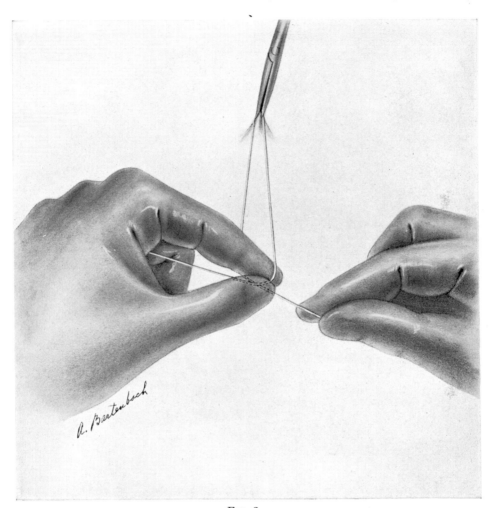

FIG. 2.

Making the first turn of a square or granny knot; the index finger is within and the thumb outside the loop.

from each other, but another half-hitch is made **in the same direction.** Then the ends of the thread are pushed away from each other. This constitutes the first half of the surgeon's knot. The second half of the knot is made by turning the ends in the opposite direction so as to make it a square knot. The details of how to make this knot will be given below. This knot has only one advantage over the square knot, namely, that it does not slip away before it is completed. However, it does not constrict the tissues tighter than a square knot. Its disadvantage is that it is more bulky. In former days it was considered an excellent knot for ligation of blood-vessels. Now, this knot is very seldom used, and even in ligation of large arteries, it is not used very much. **Its**

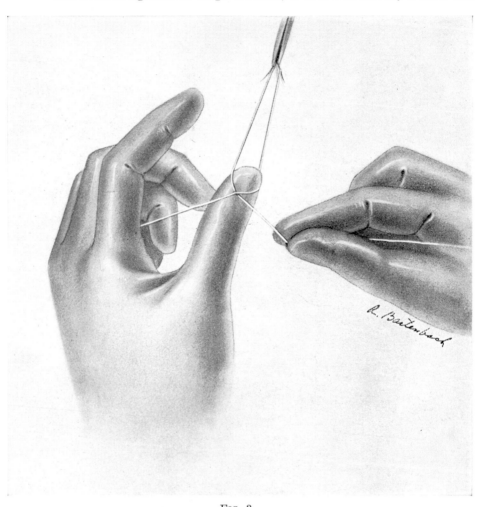

Fig. 3.

Making the first turn of a square or granny knot; the thumb is turned upward and lies in the loop.

usefulness now is only in cases when a blood-vessel has to be tied deep in the field, when even the point of ligation is not well seen.

3. **Granny knot** (Fig. 1, b).

In this knot, each of the **vertical limbs** passes in **front** of one of the horizontal limbs and **behind** the other horizontal limb. This knot is only a little less dependable than the square knot. Its resistance to pressure from within the loop is somewhat less than in the case of the square knot; however, the ends can be more easily untied than can the square knot, probably **because they are not bent so sharply back upon themselves in the same plane as they are in a square knot.** For this reason, if a large artery is tied, it is best to do it by a square knot, and if a granny knot is employed, then it is

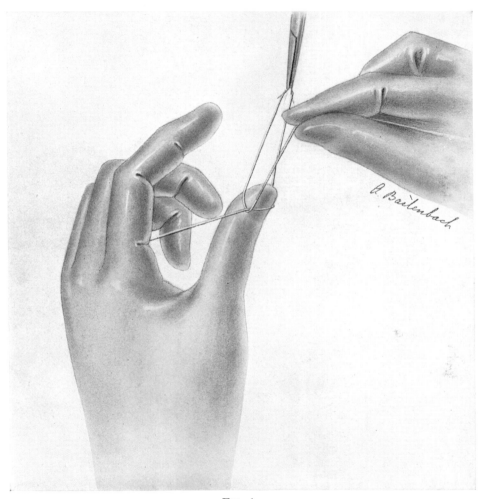

FIG. 4.
Making the first turn of a square or granny knot; the short end of the thread is laid on the thumb of the left hand.

advisable always to make the third "half-hitch" in the same direction.

4. **Slip knot** (Fig. 1, d).

This is produced by pulling tightly on one end of the thread, while making a loop with the other end around the taut end as around an axis, and **failing to cross the ends in the opposite direction when**

each half-hitch of the knot is made. It is a very unreliable knot. It is surprisingly easily produced when the operator makes, as he thinks "a one-finger granny knot". Even if the surgeon adds the third and fourth "half-hitch" in the same way, it will not strengthen the knot. This can be easily verified by making the half-hitches around an artery-forceps and later opening the jaws.

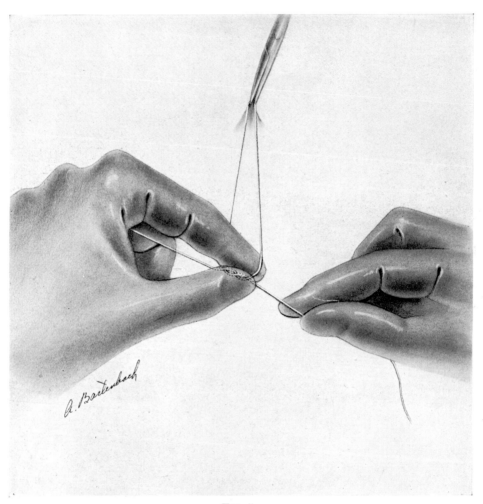

FIG. 5.
Making the first turn of a square or granny knot; the index-finger pushes the thread out of the loop.

In the case of the square and granny knots, the operator will be unable to separate the blades from each other.

THE TECHNIC OF TYING KNOTS WITH TWO HANDS.

Square knot.

In order to make a square knot with both hands, the short end of the thread is held in the right hand between the thumb and the forefinger and the long end in the left hand between the thumb and the forefinger; the short end is placed beneath the long end and so directed that it will cross the long end at the point where the thumb and index-finger of the left hand are situated. With the index-finger and the thumb of the left hand the two threads are grasped at the point of their intersection, so that

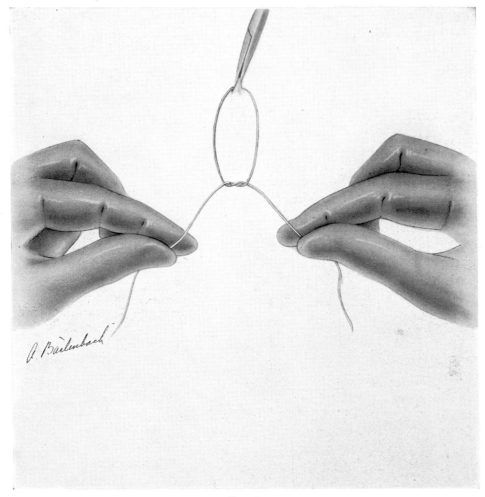

FIG. 6.
Making the first turn of a square or granny knot; the first turn is completed by drawing the ends of the thread apart.

the index-finger will be within the loop and the thumb outside the loop (Fig. 2); the thumb is then turned upward so that it will be in the loop (Fig. 3). With the right hand the short end of the thread is laid on the thumb of the left hand (Fig. 4) and is compressed with the index-finger of the left hand. The index-finger of the left hand is turned downward; it will then push out of the loop the thumb and the short end of the thread which is resting upon it (Fig. 5). This will complete the first "half-hitch" of the knot (Fig. 6). In order to make another "half-hitch" of the square knot, the long end of the thread is held in the left palm and put on the stretch; the dorsum of the first phalanx of the left thumb moves proximally behind the thread (Fig. 7); with the index-finger of the left hand the short end is moved until it crosses the long end and rests on the proximal phalanx of the left thumb (Fig. 7). Then the left index-finger will be inside the loop

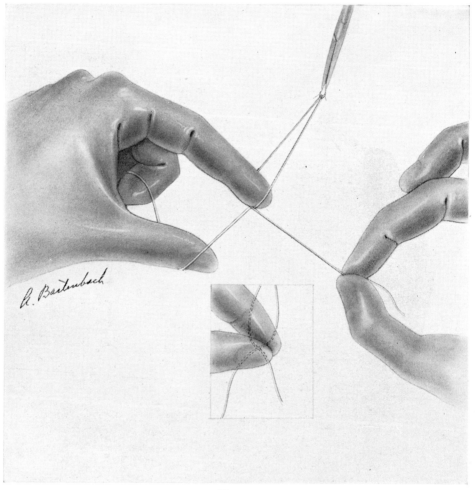

FIG. 7.
Making the second turn of a square knot.

and the left thumb outside (Fig. 7); with the left thumb the point of intersection of both ends is grasped (Fig. 7, insert), and this thumb moves inside the loop (Fig. 8). The short end is then caught by the right hand (Fig. 8), and the second "half-hitch" is thus completed (Fig. 8, insert).

Surgical knot.

The surgical knot consists of two turns in the first "half-hitch", and another "half-hitch" consisting of one turn is made in the opposite direction.

Granny knot. This is made in the following way:

The first "half-hitch" is done exactly as in the first half of a square knot (Figs. 2 to 6) ; this is repeated for the second half.

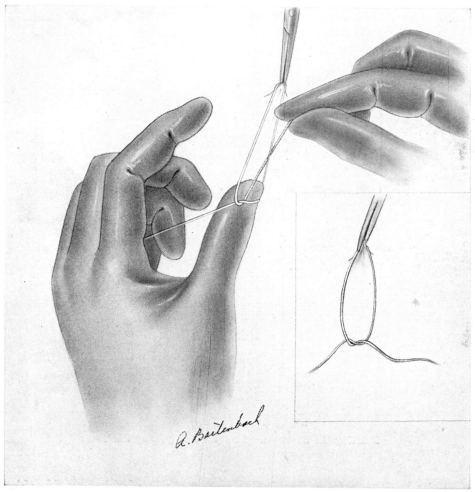

FIG. 8.
Making the second turn of a square knot.

TYING THE KNOTS WITH ONE HAND.

Square knot.

The short end of the thread is grasped between the terminal phalanx of the left index-finger and the thumb about four inches from its end, so that it rests on the palmar surfaces of the second phalanges of the middle

and fourth fingers, while the end of the thread hangs down between the
fourth and the fifth fingers (fig. 9). [The left hand is in a position midway
between pronation and supination]. The long end of the thread, which is
held between the thumb and index finger of the right hand is brought
beneath the ulnar surface of the second phalanx of the fourth finger of the
left hand, so that both ends of the thread touch each other, thus forming a

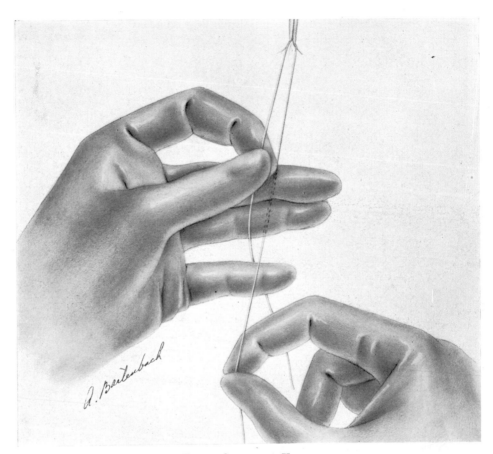

FIG. 9. ONE-HAND KNOT.
Starting the first turn of a square or granny knot.

loop; the middle and the fourth fingers are inside of this loop (fig. 9).
The terminal phalanx of the fourth finger of the left hand is then bent to
such an extent that the short end of the thread rests on the dorsal surface
of the first phalanx of the fourth finger. As a matter of fact, the short end
of the thread lies now between the dorsal surface of the terminal phalanx
of the fourth finger and the volar surface of the terminal phalanx of the
third finger. This short end is now grasped by these two phalanges (Fig.
10) and is carried through the loop (Fig. 11). This will complete the

first half of the square knot. The second half of the knot is done in the following manner: The short end of the thread is grasped between the thumb and the index finger of the left hand and put on the stretch; the third and the fourth fingers of the left hand are held together; the ulnar side of the fourth finger of the left hand is placed upon the short end of the stretched thread, so that these two fingers are in a position midway

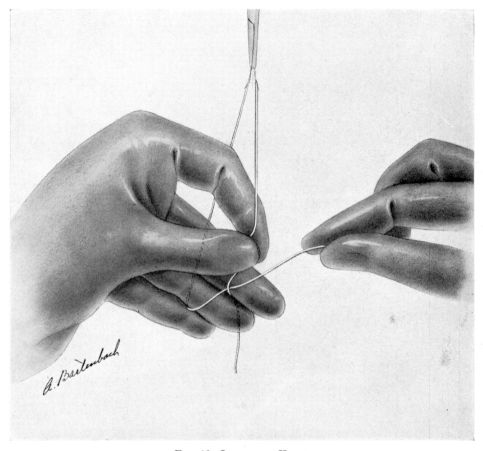

FIG. 10. ONE-HAND KNOT.
The short end of the thread, grasped by the middle and fourth fingers, is ready to be drawn through the loop.

between pronation and supination. The long end of the thread, which is held between the thumb and index-finger of the right hand, is placed on the radial side of the middle finger of the left hand (Fig. 12), so that the ends of the thread cross each other; a loop is thus formed, within which lie the left middle and fourth fingers; the middle finger of the left hand is bent at its terminal joint, so that the thread which is held between the index-finger and thumb of this hand will rest on the dorsum of the terminal phalanx of the middle finger (Fig. 13). Then this terminal phalanx is straightened, so that the thread will be caught between the third and fourth fingers of the left hand, which is carried through the loop.

Granny knot.

The first half of a square knot is twice repeated.

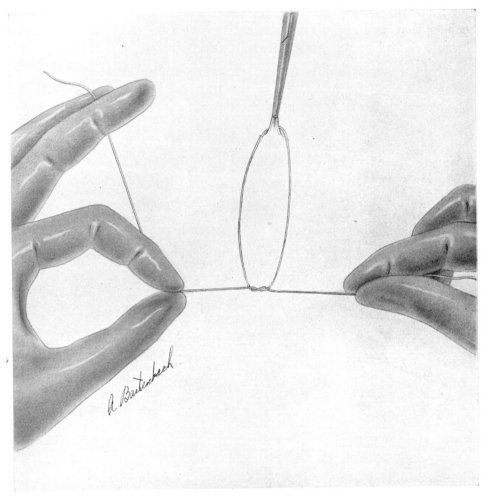

FIG. 11. ONE-HAND KNOT.
The thread drawn out from the loop by the middle and ring-fingers, is grasped between the index-finger and thumb.

OTHER METHODS OF TYING KNOTS WITH ONE HAND.

Square Knot.

The first half of the knot is made in the following manner:

The short end of the thread is grasped by the thumb and middle finger of the left hand; the radial side of the terminal phalanx of the index-finger is placed behind this end of the thread; the long end of the thread is grasped by the right hand, and is put on the stretch close to the ulnar side of the terminal phalanx of the left index-finger so that the two ends form a loop inside of which lies the index-finger. The middle phalanx of the left index-finger is bent so that the volar surface of the terminal phalanx of this finger touches the volar surface of the head of the second metacarpal bone. The terminal phalanx of the index-finger is now moved away from the volar surface of the head of the second metacarpal bone in such a manner that its dorsal surface touches the short end of the thread at some

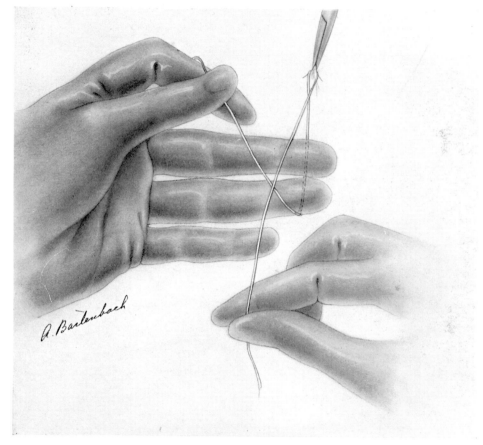

FIG. 12. ONE-HAND KNOT.
Starting the second turn of a square knot.

point between the point of crossing of the two ends of the thread and the point held by the thumb and middle finger (Fig. 14) ; the terminal phalanx of the left index-finger is now completely extended, so that it again enters the loop (Fig. 14, insert). The thread resting on the dorsal surface of the index-finger is now grasped by the left index and middle fingers and the ends of the thread are drawn apart. This is the first "half-hitch" of the knot.

The second half of the knot is made in the following manner:

The short end of the thread is grasped between the thumb and index-finger of the left hand and put on the stretch. The ulnar side of the middle phalanx of the left middle finger is laid on the short end of the thread; the long end of the thread, caught between the thumb and index-finger of the right hand, is carried to the short one until they form a loop, inside

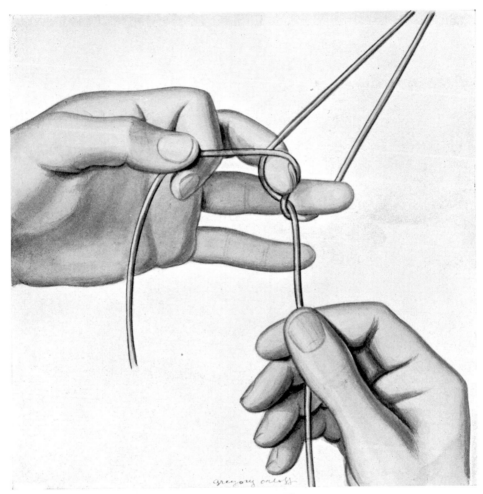

FIG. 13. ONE-HAND KNOT.
The thread is resting on the dorsal surface of the terminal
phalanx of the left middle finger.

of which lies the middle finger. The middle and the distal phalanges of the left middle finger are bent so that the volar surface of the terminal phalanx of the middle finger touches the volar surface of the head of the 3rd metacarpal bone. The terminal phalanx of the middle finger is now moved away from the volar surface of the head of the 3rd metacarpal bone in such a manner that its dorsal surface touches the short end of the thread at some point between the point of crossing of the two ends of the thread and the point held by the thumb and the index-finger (Fig. 15). The middle and the terminal phalanges of the middle finger are now extended so that the middle finger re-enters the loop; the short end of the thread lying on the dorsal surface of the middle finger is now grasped between the middle and the fourth fingers of the left hand and drawn out of the loop (Fig. 13).

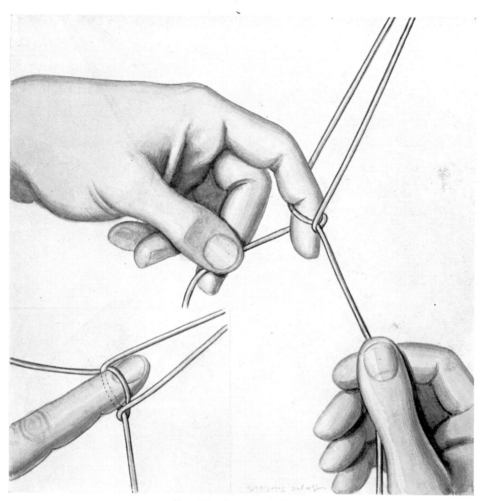

FIG. 14. ONE-HAND KNOT.

Granny Knot.

The first "half-hitch" of the square knot is repeated by one finger (Fig. 14).

TYING KNOTS WITH A THREAD ON ONE END OF WHICH IS
ATTACHED AN ARTERY-FORCEPS.

Square Knot.

The artery-forceps is held in the left hand and the free end of the thread is grasped between the index-finger and thumb of the right hand and is placed to the side of the forceps proximal to the surgeon; thus a triangle is formed. The thread is pressed to the forceps by the left thumb and its free end is turned around the forceps by the right hand. The thread is now pressed to the forceps by the index-finger of the left hand (Fig. 16), and then is pushed downward by this finger and caught by the right hand

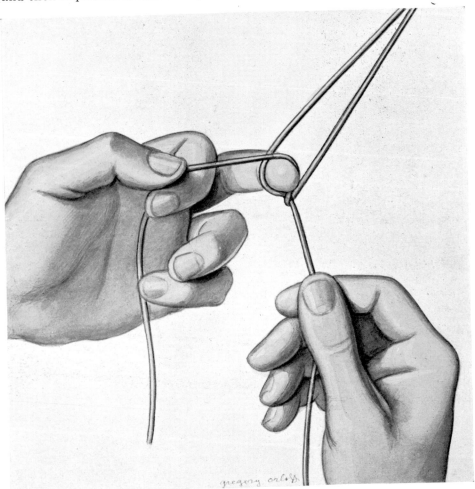

FIG. 15. ONE-HAND KNOT.
The thread is resting on the dorsal surface of the terminal phalanx of the left middle finger.

(Fig. 16). This completes the first half of the square knot. The second half is made in the following way: The free end of the thread is brought to the side of the artery-forceps which is distal to the surgeon. The index-finger presses the thread against the clamp; the thumb pushes the free end of the thread into the triangle where it is caught by the thumb and index-finger of the right hand.

This tying by artery-forceps is very economical; with the same material one can ligate at least four times as many bleeders with the thread and attached forceps as by the "both hands" method.

Granny Knot.

The first half of the square knot is repeated (Fig. 16).

In case one end of the thread is very short, so that it is difficult or

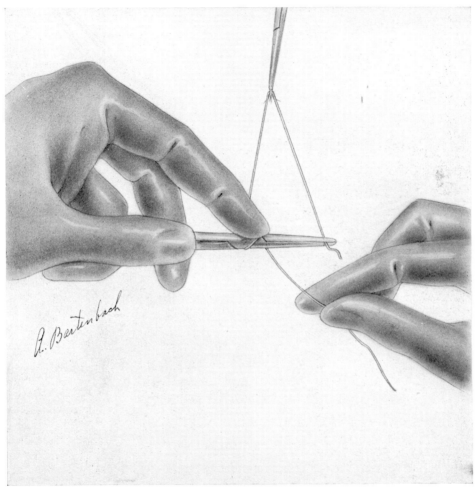

FIG. 16.
Tying knots with a thread on one end of which is attached an artery-forceps.

even impossible to make a knot with two hands, this can be accomplished by the help of tissue-forceps **(Soresi method)** or an artery-forceps **(Grant method).**

TYING A THREAD WITH ONE VERY SHORT END
(GRANT METHOD) (FIG. 17).

The long end of the thread is held in the left hand and the short end is clamped by an artery-forceps; a second artery-forceps is laid across the **long** end of the thread (Fig. 17), and loops this around itself (Fig. 18) ; the short end of the thread is then caught by the forceps and drawn through the loop (Fig. 18, insert) ; this will make **the first half-hitch.** To make the other half of the square knot, the artery-forceps is placed behind the same thread (Fig. 19) and all the steps are repeated. This method is also very economical. Other advantages are that it can be used deep in the

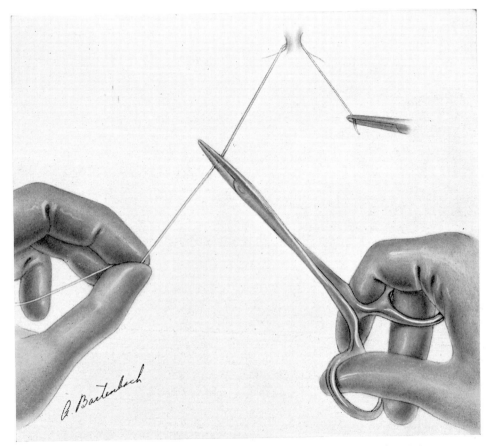

FIG. 17. TYING A SHORT END BY AN ARTERY FORCEPS (First Turn).
The clamp is laid on the thread.

abdominal cavity where there will not be enough room for the hands; and it is also applicable in those cases in which the surgeon does not wish to touch the ligature with his gloved hands at all. Then, it becomes a "No hand touch technic" (Fig. 20).

TYING OF A LIGATURE BY A "NO HAND TOUCH TECHNIC". (FIG. 20).

An artery-forceps clamps each end of the thread; a third clamp is laid in front of the thread; a loop is made with the aid of this clamp as described before and as shown in Fig. 18.

METHOD OF TYING A THREAD ON ONE END OF WHICH IS A CURVED NEEDLE AND ON THE OTHER END AN ARTERY-FORCEPS.

The artery-forceps is held in the left hand and the needle in the right hand so that the thumb rests on the concave surface and the index-finger on the convex surface. The portion of the thread attached to the needle is brought to the surgeon's side of the forceps so as to form a triangle, the

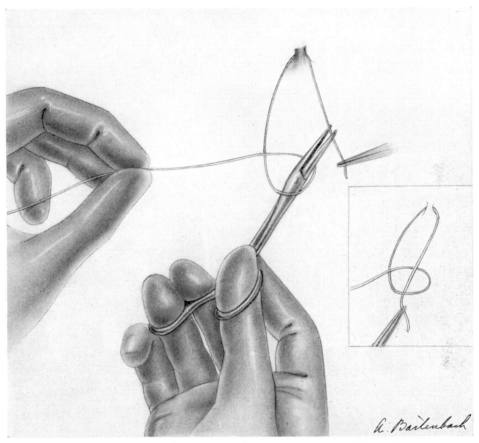

FIG. 18. TYING A SHORT END BY AN ARTERY FORCEPS (First Turn).
The artery forceps forms a loop.
INSERT. The end of thread is drawn from the loop.

sides of which will be each end of the thread and the base the artery-forceps (Fig. 21). The thread is now pressed to the artery-forceps with the left thumb. The needle is passed through the loop with its eye directed toward the surgeon. The eye of the needle is then caught by the left index-finger and pressed to the forceps (Fig. 21). The needle is now caught by the right hand and brought out. The first half of the knot is thus completed.

The second half is done in the following manner:

The thread on the needle is brought to the side of the forceps away from the surgeon and held in position by the index-finger; the needle is brought through the loop with the point looking forward (Fig. 22).

This type of tying is also very economical; with a thread 20 inches long one may easily tie twelve times.

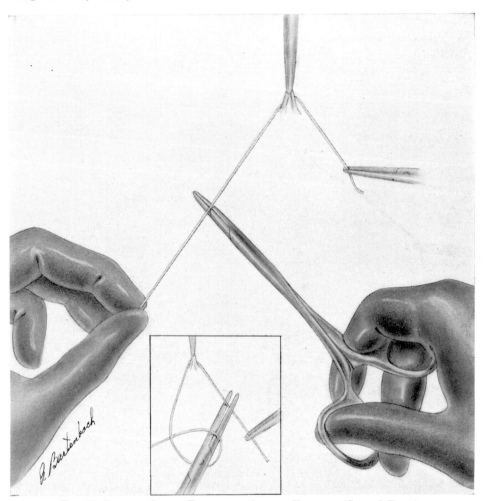

FIG. 19. TYING A SHORT END BY AN ARTERY FORCEPS (Second Turn).

METHOD OF TYING A THREAD ON ONE END OF WHICH IS A STRAIGHT NEEDLE AND ON THE OTHER AN ARTERY-FORCEPS.

The steps are the same as with a curved needle.

METHOD OF TYING AS A SEAMSTRESS (OVIATT METHOD) (FIG. 23).

TRANSFIXED LIGATURES.

Transfixed ligatures are those which pass through the thickness of the tissues and constrict the mass from the center to the periphery. They are usually employed when blood-vessels are situated in a mass of other tissues and when it is either impossible to separate the vessels, or when it is a time-consuming procedure, and when at the same time the mass is too large to permit an ordinary method of applying the ligature on account of the danger of slipping. They are usually applied to the stump of the omentum, to the infundibulopelvic ligament, to the broad ligament, and so forth. There are several methods of placing them.

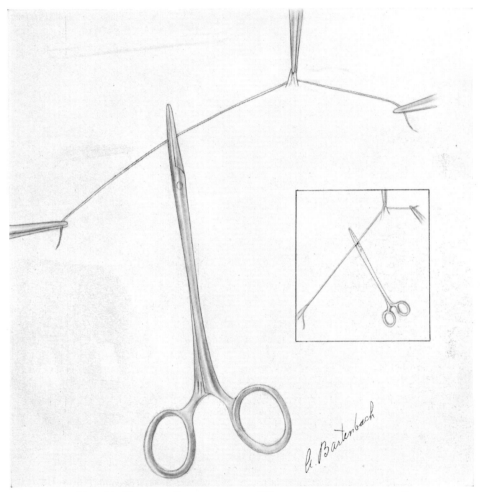

FIG. 20. TYING A LIGATURE BY A "NO HAND TOUCH TECHNIC".
INSERT. Second turn of a square knot.

Method 1.

With the threaded needle the middle of the stump is pierced and that portion of the stump lying to the right (or to the left) of the hole made by the needle is ligated (Fig. 24, a); then both ends of the thread are carried around the entire stump and tied (Fig. 24, b).

Method 2.

A mattress-suture is inserted in the middle third of the stump; the ends are then carried around the entire stump and tied (Fig. 24, c).

Method 3.

Figure-of-8 Transfixion Suture (Fig. 25 a, b).

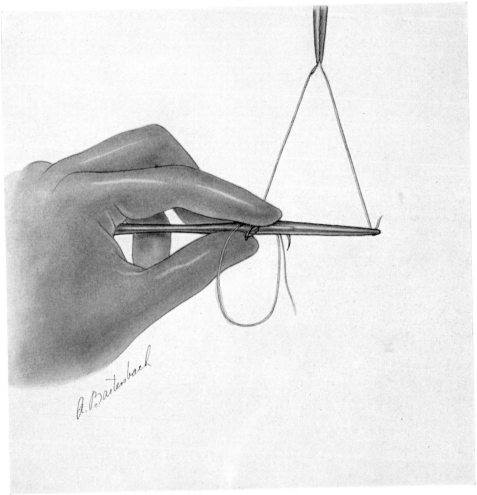

FIG. 21.

Tying a thread on one end of which is a curved needle and on the other end an artery-forceps (first turn).

Method 4.

The Doyen Method of Ligating by Circular Ligation and Transfixion (Fig. 25 c, d, e).

In the aforementioned methods, the stump situated distally to the ligature is entirely deprived of blood-supply. As a result, this stump will become the seat of a dry or white infarct, and this will, in course of time, either become absorbed or be encapsulated as an aseptic foreign body.

However, there are other methods of applying a transfixion ligature which do not shut off the blood-supply completely. It is true that no actual bleeding occurs distal to the ligature immediately after ligation and cutting of the stump; the surgeon believes the ligature to be completely hemostatic; however, a little later collateral circulation is established

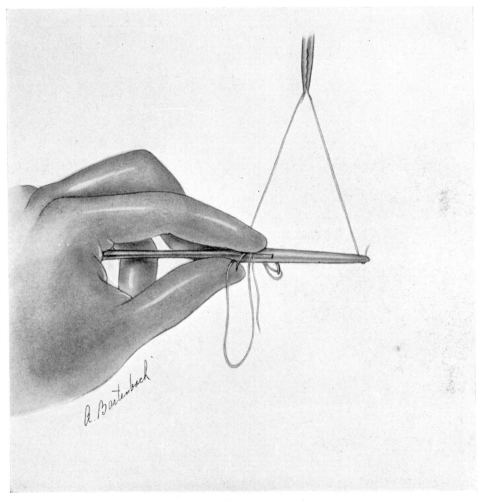

Fig. 22.
Tying a thread on one end of which is a curved needle and on the other end an artery-forceps (second turn).

through the part not caught in the ligature; a red infarct is formed in this distal stump with possible future infection and the formation of adhesions.

The first group of ligatures which completely shut off the blood-supply are known as **occluding** ligatures, and the second type are known as **sub-occluding** ligatures. Below are given a few examples of sub-occluding ligatures **which never should be employed:**

1. A transfixing ligature through the stump leaving part of the stump free; the ligature will not slip but it will be a sub-occluded ligature (Fig. 26, a).
2. Another type of sub-occluded ligature (Fig. 26, b).

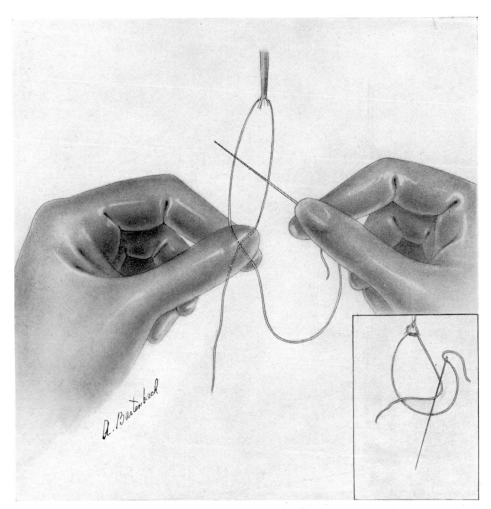

FIG. 23. OVIATT METHOD OF TYING A KNOT (Seamstress Knot).

This however can be transformed into a "chain ligature".

3. Another type of unsatisfactory transfixed ligature:
   A hole in the stump may be formed at point A, due to the pulling of the two threads laterally; bleeding may start from this point (Fig. 26, c).

DIFFERENT METHODS OF SUTURING THE ABDOMINAL WALL.

Suture of the abdominal wall as a routine operative procedure was introduced much later than suture of the abdominal viscera. The number of methods of suturing the abdominal wall is far less than those of suturing the abdominal viscera, and they are in the majority of cases

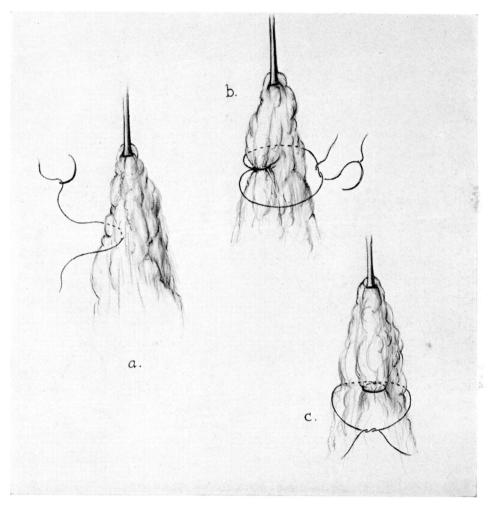

FIG. 24. OCCLUDING LIGATURES.

methods which were already used for suturing the abdominal viscera, especially the intestines. In former days, when surgeons preferred to use non-absorbable material for deep sutures, which were to be removed, many methods were devised for the easy removal of these sutures. Now we very seldom use deep non-absorbable sutures as removable sutures. Another cause of the large number of different methods of suturing in previous years was the desire to suture simultaneously the different layers of the abdominal wall. Now these methods are replaced by the much simpler methods of layer suturing.

1. **Simple Interrupted Suture** (Button-hole Suture) (Fig. 27, a).

This is used for closure of the different layers, namely, peritoneum, muscles, fascia, skin. The advantage of this type of suturing is that each suture is tied separately and therefore breaking or

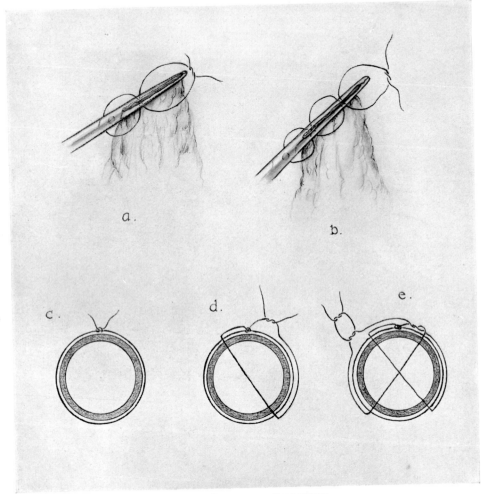

FIG. 25. OCCLUDING LIGATURES.
a and b. Figure-of-8 transfixion suture.
c, d, e. Circular ligation and transfixion suture of Doyen.

removal of one stitch does not weaken the entire length of the suture line. Another advantage is that in case of an irregular skin incision it closes the wound more neatly.

The disadvantages of interrupted sutures are that they require more time for their insertion, and that many knots are made. For all layers with the exception of the skin, it is more convenient to use a curved needle on a needle-holder. For the skin it is more convenient to use a straight needle with a sharp, cutting point. When using a straight needle, a needle-holder is not required. When working with a curved needle on a needle-holder, it is always more convenient to start from the distal lip, and then take a bite on the proximal lip, and from the part of the wound most remote from

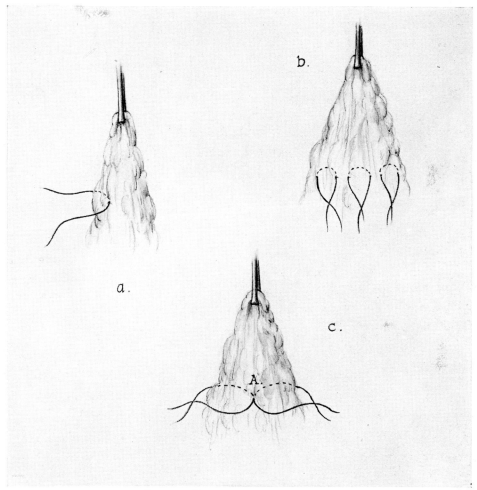

FIG. 26. SUB-OCCLUDING LIGATURES.

the surgeon to the part of the wound closer to him. In working with the straight needle the reverse is true; it is more convenient to catch first the lip proximal to the surgeon and then the distal lip, and from the point closest to the surgeon to the point farthest from him.

2. **Continuous Over-and-over Suture** (Glover Suture) (Fig. 27, b). This is used as the previous one. Its advantage is that it can be

placed more quickly; its disadvantage is, that in case of suppuration or exploration, when it is necessary to remove one suture, the entire suture line is broken.

In order to tie the last stitch, the free end of the thread is made much longer than the other end. When the needle takes the last bite, then on one side of the wound remains the free end of the thread and on the other the needle with a double thread (Fig. 27,

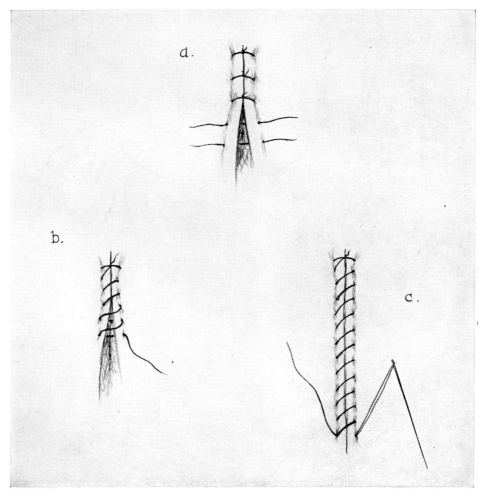

FIG. 27.
a. Buttonhole suture;   b. Glover suture;   c. Glover suture—inserting the last stitch.

c). The free end is now tied to the double thread on the other side of the wound.

3. **Continuous Button-hole Suture** (Fig. 28).

A straight needle is used and the suturing starts from the left side and extends to the right. The lip proximal to the surgeon is first pierced and then that distal to the surgeon, thus making an ordinary button-hole stitch, which is tied by a reef or a granny knot. The thread is held in the left hand, and the needle, held in the right hand, is carried in front of the thread, thus forming a loop through which the needle passes. The last suture is inserted in a reverse direction, thus maintaining the button-hole sutures throughout **(Maunsell suggestion)** (Fig. 28, insert). This suture

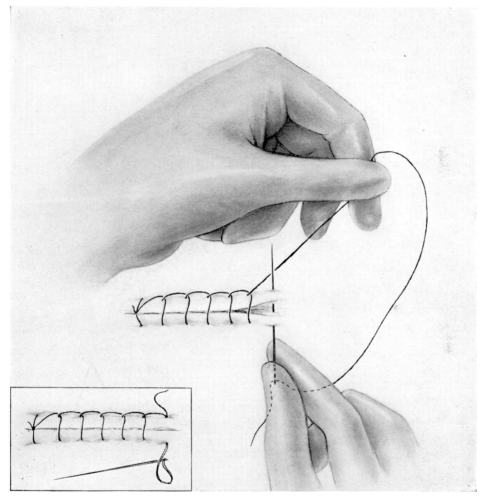

FIG. 28. CONTINUOUS BUTTONHOLE SUTURE.
INSERT. Maunsell method of inserting the last stitch.

nicely approximates the skin edges, but is not a strong one. For this reason it can be used only in those cases in which either tension sutures are used or in which the subcutaneous tissues are sutured before the closure of the skin.

4. **Double-lock Button-hole Suture** (Fig. 29, a).

This has some advantages over an ordinary button-hole suture, in that each link of the chain is less liable to loosen in case one link is cut.

5. **Fig.-of-8 Suture** (Fig. 29, b).

Including the skin, fascia and anterior sheath of the rectus muscle

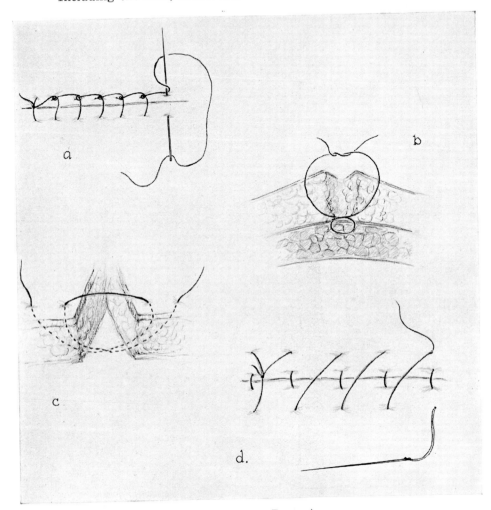

FIG. 29. (AFTER PRINTY).

a. Double-lock continuous button-hole suture.
b. Figure-of-8 suture for skin, fascia and anterior sheath of rectus muscle.
c. Figure-of-8 suture for skin and fascia only.
d. Continuous Figure-of-8 suture.

only. This type of suture was frequently used during the time when the non-absorbable suture was employed not only for suturing the skin, but also the deep layers of the abdominal wall, the surgeon intending later to remove it. But when absorbable suture-material replaced the non-absorbable in suturing the deep layers of the abdominal wall, the employment of this type of suture became infrequent.

6. **Fig.-of-8 Interrupted and Continuous Suture for Skin and Superficial Fascia only** (Fig. 29, c, d).
7. **Horizontal Mattress Suture, Interrupted** (Fig. 30, a).

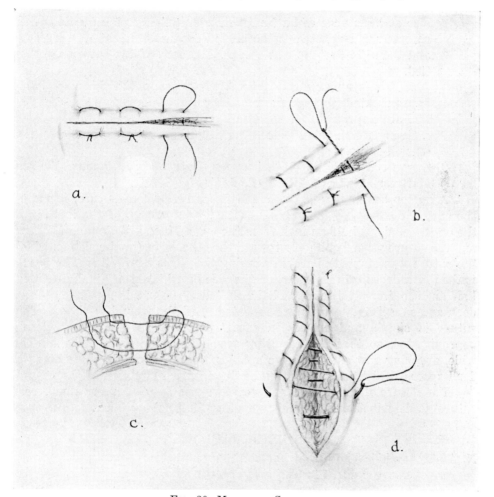

FIG. 30. MATTRESS SUTURES.
a. Horizontal mattress-suture.
b and c. Vertical mattress-sutures.
d. White method of continuous vertical mattress-suture.

This suture was described by the Italian surgeon Lanfranch about the year 1300, and was used for closure of the abdominal wall. **The Continuous Horizontal Mattress Suture** was introduced in the XVIIIth Century by Sabatier and Richerand; it was known under the name of *sutura transgressiva* and it was used up to the middle of the XIX century; it is now obsolete.

8. **Vertical Mattress Suture** (Fig. 30, b, c).

This suture was first described by R. M. McMillen in 1909. The same suture is known under the names of different men, who described it later, evidently being unaware of McMillen's publication. This suture is made in the following manner: A needle penetrates one cutaneous lip at a distance of half an inch from its edge from without inward, then the other lip from within outward also at a distance of half an inch from its edge; the needle is then reversed and penetrates the second cutaneous lip at its very edge and then the first lip at its edge. The ends of the suture are then tied.

This is an excellent suture: the edges of the skin are closely approximated, so that the resulting scar is hardly noticeable. The lips are approximated by broad raw surfaces and for this reason a strong union takes place. The deep limb of the suture acts as a tension-suture.

9. **Superficial and Deep Continuous Suture [Continuous Vertical Mattress-suture (White Method)]** (Fig. 30, d).

A button-hole suture is made and tied; then a deep suture, including the entire thickness of the skin, is carried from one lip of the incision to the opposite, about half an inch from the edge. The needle is then reversed and the suture passed obliquely toward the other side (or the side on which the suture was started) barely engaging the edges of the lips. The needle is then introduced a little lower, on the side on which it originally entered, half an inch from the edge, and the first deep suture is repeated. These deep and superficial sutures are repeated until the wound is closed. This suture is simple and speedy in execution; the edges are very closely approximated, so that the resulting scar will be hardly noticeable. The wide, opposing raw surfaces give a firm union. This suture eliminates the dead spaces, which in itself is conductive to primary union of the wound.

For closure of the skin, in our work, we usually use a vertical mattress suture as described under number 8 (Fig. 30, b, c) or Michel clips.

BIBLIOGRAPHY.

N. Ambrozovskij. The use of horsehair in surgery.
Sovetsk. vrac. gaz. 11: 513-514; y. 1933.

W. D. Anderson. Fascia anchor.
Am. Journ. Surg. 12:282-283; y. 1931.

M. Archdall. The sterilization of catgut and post-operative tetanus.
Med. Journ. Australia, 2:157; y. 1934.

W. W. Babcock. Ligatures and sutures of alloy steel wire.
Journ. Am. Med. Ass. 102:1756; y. 1934.

W. W. Babcock. Catgut allergy. With a note on the use of alloy steel wire for sutures and ligatures.
Americ. Journ. of Surg. 27:67-70; y. 1935.

J. Binnie. Ligatures and sutures.
Tr. M. Ass. Missouri, St. Louis., y. 1892; Pages: 194-202; Discussion —P. 202.

J. Bland-Sutton. On faith in ligatures.
Brit. Med. Journ. II:823-826; y. 1925.

M. Blumberg. Über Verbesserung der Unterbindungs und Nahttechnik und maximale Verbilligung im Catgutgebrauch.
Zbl. für Gynäk. 48:2132-2135; y. 1924.

L. Böhler. Über Catgut sparende Unterbindungen.
Zbl. für Chir. 45:21-22; y. 1918.

V. Bonney. On occluding and suboccluding ligatures.
Lancet. II:455-457; y. 1910.

O. Borchgrevink. Surgical knots.
Surg. Gyn. & Obst. 10:530-536; y. 1910.

G. Bosch Arana & G. E. E. Anschütz. Estudio mecánico de los nudos.
Prensa méd. argent. 21:833-839; y. 1934.

R. D. Bradley. The evolution of the ligature.
West. M. Reporter. XVI:121-122; y. 1894.

W. S. Brindle. The use of fascia lata sutures.
Brit. Med. Journ. II:810-811; y. 1934.

I. Bulinin. Zur Frage der Technik des Schürzens von chirurgischen Knoten.
Arch. f. klin. Chir. 179:526-528; y. 1934.

V. Carabba. A security ligature.
Ann. Surg. 93:1267; y. 1931.

V. Carabba. A modification of the Stewart suture.
Ann. Surg. 94:957-958; y. 1931.

H. S. Chenoweth. The extraction of non-absorbable ligatures.
Med. News, 71:353-355; y. 1897.

R. O. Clock. The fallacy of chemical sterilization of surgical sutures.
Surg. Gyn. & Obst. 56:140; y. 1933.

G. Crile. The cobbler stitch in visceral anastomosis.
Surg. Gyn. & Obst. 4:533; y. 1907.

K. H. Digby. A note on "reef", "granny" and "slip" knots.
Surgery, Gynecology & Obstetrics, 38:695; y. 1924.

L. Drüner. Die Knotenformen.
Deutsche Zietschr. f. Chir. 242:72-75; y. 1933.

L. Drüner. Nachtrag zu meiner Arbeit über das Knupfen.
Deutsche Zeitschr. f. Chir. 242:184-185; y. 1933.

L. Drüner. Unser Knüpfen.
Deutsche Zeitschr. f. Chir. 241:289-293; y. 1933.

A. Edmunds. A continuous "eversion" stitch.
Lancet II:849-850; y. 1930.

E. Erhardt. Die in der Chirurgie gebräuchlichen Nähte und Knoten in historischer Darstellung.
Sammlung Klin. Vortrage, Neue Folge, Chirurgie: No. 580 and 581; y. 1910.

L. Frank. Ligatures and sutures.
Louisville J. of Surg. & Med. 5:310-312; y. 1898.

A. R. Grant. The tying of a surgical knot.
Annals of Surg. 67:439-441; y. 1918.

A. R. Grant. No-hand-touch-technique.
Surg. Gyn. Obst. 36:106-107; y. 1923.

C. M. Gratz. The use of fascia in reconstructive surgery with special reference to operative technic.
Ann. Surg. 99:241-245; y. 1934.

H. F. O. Haberland. Beitrag zur Hautnahttechnik.
Zbl. f. Chir. 56:2515; y. 1929.

K. Von Haefen. Ein Beitrag zur Katgutresorption.
Bruns Beitr. z. klin. Chir. 158:449-456; y. 1933.

F. Härtel. Zur Technik tiefer Unterbindungen.
Zbl. f. Chir. 61:2546-2547; y. 1934.

J. Horgan. An interrupted subcuticular suture.
Med. Annal. Distr. of Columbia, 3:268; y. 1934.

J. W. Kennedy. The supremacy of silk as a ligature and silkworm-gut as a suture.
Am. Journ. Surg. 33:188-189; y. 1919.

F. B. Kilmer, G. S. Mathey & H. J. Dobbs. Ligatures and sutures.
Am. Journ. of Pharm. 95:656-671; y. 1923. 96:6-29; y. 1924.

C. J. Kraissl. Suture Material: A Review of Recent Literature.
Surg. Gyn. & Obst. Intern-Abstr. 62:417-423; y. 1936.

J. LeGrand. Les noeuds rapides d'une seule main.
Journ. de Med. de Paris, 41:183-184; y. 1922.

M. Linnartz. Eine unbekannte Art des Catgutsparens.
Zbl. für Chir. 45:20-21; y. 1918.

T. H. Manley. Some of the uses of the temporary transfixion ligature.
Intern. Journ. of Surg. 2:275-280; y. 1889.

L. Martel. Sur la ligature en chaîne.
Arch. prov. de chir. 6:740-742; y. 1897.

K. Mermingas. Operationen ohne Unterbindungen.
Zbl. f. Chir. 62:23-24; y. 1935.

N. S. Minine. Suture au fil métallique des plaies opératoires.
Rev. franç. de gynéc. et d'obst. 30:201-206; y. 1935.

M. Misch. Einiges über Instrumente, die Nähte, Unterbindungen und Abschnürungen an Stellen ermöglichen sollen die wegen ihrer Tiefe, Enge oder Kleinheit den unbewehrten Finger sich arbeiten Lassen.
Med. Klin. 25:1939-1941; y. 1929.

M. Misch. Zur Vermeidung von Fehlern bei der Anwendung meiner Knüp-fungsinstrumente.
Zbl. f. Chir. 58:2191-2193; y. 1931.

L. Montaz. Une nouvelle ligature en chaîne.
Arch. Prov. de Chir. 3:105-106; y. 1894.

O. Mueller-Meernach. Die neue Drahtlitze.
Zentralbl. f. Chir. 62:310-312; y. 1935.

H. C. W. Nuttall. The selvage stitch.
Brit. Med. Jounr. II:1032-1033; y. 1931.

G. Perthes. Über Catgut sparende Unterbindungen.
Zbl. für Chir. 44:644-645; y. 1917

H. Polano. Ueber die Zug—und Reissfestigkeit chirurgischen Naht-materials.
Zbl. f. Chir. 59:147-148; y. 1932.

P. Preobrazenskij. Nerve as resorbable suture material.
Vestnik khir. 75-76:59-60; y. 1933.

E. P. Quain. A new, quick, and practical surgical knot.
Surg. Gyn. & Obst. 8:300-302; y. 1909.

B. Quarella. Sui vantaggi delle suture profonde temporanee in seta.
Minerva méd. 1:208-210; y. 1931.

M. R. Reid, M. M. Zinninger, and P. Merrell. Closure of the abdomen with through-and-through silver wire sutures in cases of acute abdom-inal emergencies. Ann. Surg. 98:890-896; y. 1933.

J. Sarnoff. A combined superficial and deep continuous suture. A new hemostatic, approximation and tension suture.
Amer. Journ. of Surg. vol. 7:95; July, 1929.

J. Sarnoff. Superficial and deep continuous suture: supplementary report.
Surg. Gyn. & Obs. 53:539-544; y. 1931.

A. Semper. Über Catgutsparen.
Zbl. für Chir. 45:748; y. 1918.

A. R. Smith. Chrome poisoning with manifestations of sensinization.
Journ. Amer. Med. Assn. 97:95-98; y. 1931.

M. Tiegel. Ueber eine neue Methode der Plattennaht (Schraubplattennaht).
Chirurg. 2:882-887; y. 1930.

M. Tomaiuoli. A cuticular suture.
Am. Journ. Surg. 8:770-771; y. 1930.

H. D. Tripp. Catgut allergy.
Journ. Indiana State Med. Assn. 28:383-384; y. 1934.

L. Torraca. Fortlaufende Knopfnaht.
Zbl. f. Chir. 60:1120-1123; y. 1933.

N. V. Voskresenski. Fine nickel wire as suture material.
Sovetsk. Khir. 4:482-485; y. 1933.

A. O. Whipple. The use of silk with repair of clean wounds.
Ann. Surg. 98:662-671; y. 1933.

G. Wolfsohn. Erfahrungen mit dem Fascienfaden.
Chirurg. 2:475-477; y. 1930.

CHAPTER II.

ABDOMINAL INCISIONS.

In making a proper abdominal incision, several prerequisites are necessary:

1. **A good operative field** should be afforded by a properly made incision.

2. **Physiologico-anatomical Considerations.**
   The incisions should be performed in such a manner as to mutilate the abdominal wall as little as possible.

3. **Cosmetic Considerations.**
   The incisions should be made in such direction that they will leave no large and deforming scars.

4. **Psychological Considerations.**

1. That the incision should be made so as to give a good operative field does not require much discussion. Indeed, the recognition of the necessity for a good operative field was one of the most important factors in the development of surgery, and in its importance it stands next to the introduction of anesthesia and antiseptic and, later, aseptic technic in surgery. A good operative field results not only from a properly made incision, but also from the judicious use of retractors, forceps, a proper posture of the patient (as in kidney operations), and a proper elevation of the parts of the body (as in gall-bladder operations).

2. Next in importance to the necessity of a good operative field is the infliction of as little damage as possible to the abdominal wall. Before discussing this in detail, a brief review of the anatomy of the abdominal wall will be of value.

Anteriorly, the abdominal wall consists of the following layers:

Skin.

Examination with a magnifying glass shows quite clearly that numerous fissures cross the skin in a transverse, slightly semicircular direction. They were described by Langer in 1861, and they are known as the **"fissure lines of Langer"** (Fig. 31, a, b). Kocher emphasized the surgical significance of these fissures, and showed that the healing of skin-wounds is much neater when the incisions are made along them; he advocated making such incisions, and these therefore are known as the **"normal incisions of Kocher"** (Fig. 31, a, b).

Superficial Fascia.

This is a layer which is continuous with the superficial layer of the adjoining parts of the body; at a level approximately midway between the umbilicus and symphysis pubis it splits into two layers:

Superficial layer of the superficial fascia **(Camper's fascia)**;

Deep layer of the superficial fascia **(Scarpa's fascia).**

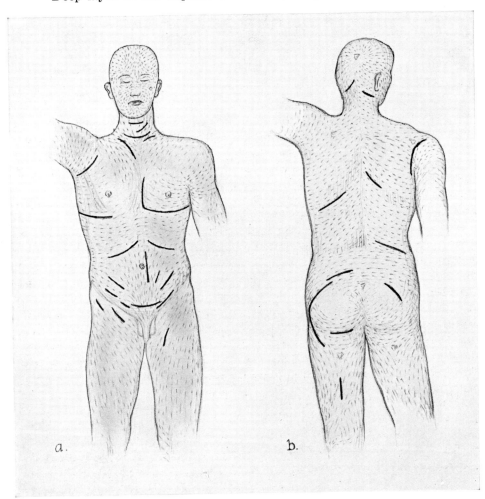

FIG. 31. FISSURE-LINES OF LANGER
NORMAL INCISIONS OF KOCHER (after Kocher).
a. Anterior view.   b. Posterior view.

The superficial layer of the superficial fascia (Camper's fascia) passes downward over the inguinal ligament and becomes directly continuous with the superficial fascia of the front of the thigh.

The deep layer of the superficial fascia (Scarpa's fascia) is carried downwards over the spermatic cord, the penis and scrotum, into the perineum, where it becomes continuous with Colles' fascia. In the region of the groin, the Scarpa's fascia is attached to the fascia lata just a little distal to the inguinal ligament. This line of attachment is known as Holden's line.

The surgical significance of this arrangement is that extravasation of urine from the urethra, ruptured below the urogenital diaphragm, will flow into the scrotum, then over the penis and along the spermatic cord into the anterior abdominal wall. From the abdominal wall it cannot pass downward to the front of the thighs, because Scarpa's fascia is firmly attached to the fascia lata of the thigh.

Deep fascia.

This layer lies behind the superficial fascia. It is not always equally well developed.

Muscles.

Posterior to the deep fascia on both sides of the middle line are situated the rectus abdominis muscles, right and left, and the pyramidalis muscles (the latter being absent in 16 to 25 per cent. of the cases). The direction of their fibers is parallel to the long axis of the body (Fig. 32). On the lateral side of the anterior wall, the muscles are arranged quite differently. They consist here of three layers, external oblique, internal oblique and transversus abdominis muscles. The direction of the fibers of these muscles is such that they cross each other at different angles, in some places at acute angles, in some places nearly perpendicularly, and in other places at obtuse angles. **The exact knowledge of the direction of the fibers and their mutual relationship is of great importance in making a proper abdominal incision.**

The external oblique muscle is a broad flat structure. It takes its origin from the lateral surfaces of the fifth to the twelfth ribs by eight slips. The five upper slips interdigitate with the slips of the anterior serratus muscle and the lower three slips with the latissimus dorsi muscle. These slips join each other and form a thin, flat muscle the fibers of which run downward, inward and forward. The fibers of this muscle do not run everywhere in the same direction; the obliquity increases from before backward, so that in the posterior part of the muscle, the fibers run nearly vertically downward (Fig. 42). The entire muscle, with the exception of the lower posterior portion, ends in a broad aponeurosis. **This aponeurosis which is nothing but the flattened tendon of the muscle,** starts along the entire length of the medial edge of the external oblique muscle, where it helps to form the anterior sheath of the rectus muscle, and also along an imaginary line drawn between the anterior superior iliac spine and the umbilicus. It runs downward, inward and forward and extends between the anterior superior iliac spine and the spine and crest of the pubic bone, forming Poupart's ligament **(inguinal ligament)** (Fig. 32). It is very important to remember this arrangement, because in cases in which the surgeon operates in the region below the imaginary line connecting the anterior superior iliac spine and the umbilicus, the first muscle encountered will be the **internal** oblique and **not** the **external,** which in this region is already aponeurotic. The posterior fibers are attached to the anterior half of the outer lip of the crest of the iliac bone.

The internal oblique muscle is thin and fan-shaped (Fig. 32). It arises from the lumbo-dorsal fascia, the anterior two-thirds of the intermediate lip of the iliac crest, and from the lateral half of Poupart's ligament. The fibers of this muscle run in different directions, forming a wide fan; its

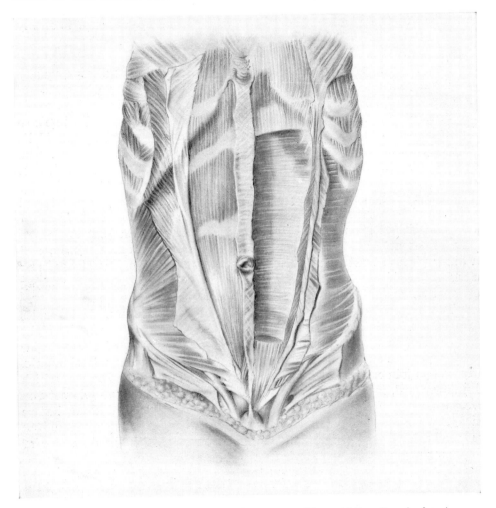

FIG. 32. MUSCLES OF THE ANTERIOR ABDOMINAL WALL (After Cunningham).

posterior fibers run upward and slightly forward and are directly attached to the outer surface of the 10th, 11th, and 12th ribs; the rest of the fibers extend to the lateral border of the rectus muscle and become aponeurotic; this aponeurosis immediately splits into two layers (lamellæ); the anterior lamella fuses with the aponeurosis of the external oblique muscle and forms the anterior sheath of the rectus muscle. The posterior lamella fuses with the aponeurosis of the transverse abdominis muscle and forms the posterior sheath of the rectus muscle (Fig. 33). [The line along which the transversus abdominis muscle becomes aponeurotic is known as the **linea semilunaris (linea Spigelii** in the O. T.)]. This arrangement of the sheath of the rectus muscle persists throughout the length of the muscle with the exception of the uppermost and lowermost portions where the posterior

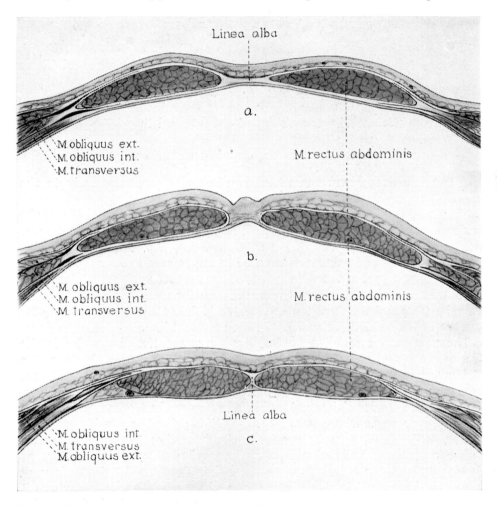

FIG. 33. FORMATION OF THE SHEATHS OF THE RECTI ABDOMINI MUSCLES (After Rauber).

sheath is deficient. In the upper portion it is deficient in that part of the muscle which rests on the chest-wall, and in the lower portion it is deficient beginning approximately from the point midway between the umbilicus and the symphysis pubis.

Beginning at this level, the posterior lamella of the aponeurosis of the internal oblique muscle and the aponeurosis of the transversus abdominis muscle fuse with the anterior lamella of the internal oblique muscle and with the aponeurosis of the external oblique to form the anterior sheath of the rectus muscle. This difference in thickness of the posterior sheath in the upper part and lower quarter of the muscle is clearly shown at the place where their border forms a thickened semi-arcuate line, which is known as the **linea semicircularis** (B. N.) or **semilunar fold of Douglas** (O. T.) (Fig. 32).

The transversus abdominis muscle (Fig. 32) arises:

a. From the posterior surfaces of the cartilages of VII, VIII, IX, X, and the posterior surfaces of the XI and XII ribs by six slips. These interdigitate with the slips of origin of the diaphragm.

b. From the lumbo-dorsal fascia.

c. From the anterior two-thirds of the internal lip of the iliac crest; and

d. From the lateral third of the inguinal ligament.

The muscular fibers run mostly **horizontally** perpendicularly to the midline of the body. The muscle ends in an aponeurosis which participates in the formation of the posterior sheath in the upper three-fourths of the rectus muscle, and in the lower fourth it participates in the formation of the anterior sheath of the rectus muscle. Thus, the aponeurosis of this muscle participates in the formation of the linea alba in its entire length.

The lowest part of the aponeurosis of the transversus abdominis muscle fuses with the aponeurosis of the internal oblique and forms the **falx inguinalis** (B. N.) **(conjoined tendon O.T.),** which is attached to the anterior surface of the pubic bone and to the ilio-pectineal line.

The next structure lying behind the above mentioned muscles is the **transversalis fascia.** This is a continuous layer which surrounds the entire abdominal cavity external to the peritoneum. It is known by different names in different regions, **being at the same time one continuous layer.** Thus, in the anterior abdominal wall it is known as the **transversalis fascia;** in the upper part, where it serves as a lining for the diaphragm, it is known as the **diaphragmatic fascia;** in the fossa iliaca as the **iliac fascia;** in front of the psoas and quadratus lumborum muscles as the **lumbar fascia;** and on the pelvic floor as the **pelvic fascia.** This layer is very important because it is strongly elastic, and according to modern views it **prevents the formation of hernia more than any other single factor.** Its fibers are circular and always **perpendicular to the longitudinal axis of the body** (Fig. 34).

The next layer is the **peritoneum;** however, between the transversalis fascia and peritoneum there is accumulated a definite amount of fat; this fat in some places accumulates in larger quantities (as around the kidneys, suprarenal glands, abdominal aorta, etc.).

The surgical significance of it is that occasionally it misleads an inexperienced operator; after cutting the transversalis fascia he thinks that he is already in the abdominal cavity; he begins to dig into the fat trying to orientate himself instead of going boldly through the fat and the peritoneum and entering the abdominal cavity.

In the midline of the body is found the **linea alba,** which is composed of the fused anterior and posterior sheaths of the recti muscles. This line is not of equal width; in the upper part it is approximately 1 to 2.5 cm. wide and in the lower 1.4 to 1.8 cm.

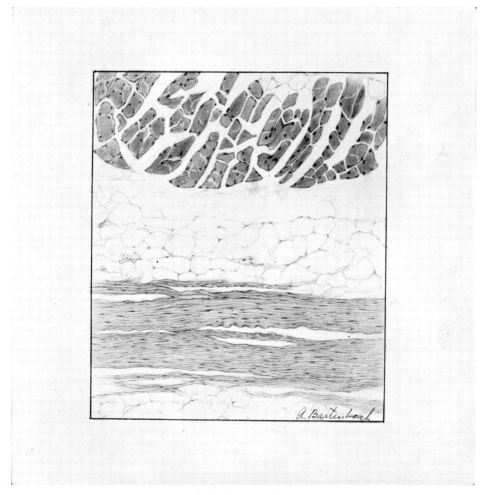

FIG. 34. CROSS SECTION OF THE ANTERIOR ABDOMINAL WALL.
The fibers of the transversalis fascia are running perpendicularly to the midline.

Let us recapitulate the most important features of the arrangement of the anterior abdominal wall in connection with the future discussion of the anterior abdominal incisions.

The linea alba (Figs. 32, 33), which extends between the ensiform process and the symphysis pubis, consists of numerous fibers which are a continuation of the anterior and posterior sheaths of the recti muscles; **the direction of these fibers are horizontal, and when making a midline incision they are cut transversely, perpendicular to the direction of their fibers.** The anterior sheath of the rectus muscle is not a fascia; it is an aponeurosis, i.e. a flattened tendon, formed by a fusion of the aponeurosis of the external oblique muscle with the anterior lamella of the aponeurosis of the internal oblique muscle; its fibers run perpendicularly or obliquely to the long axis of the body, and when incising the anterior sheath of the rectus muscle longitudinally we actually cut transversely the terminal parts of the external oblique muscle and of the anterior lamella of the internal oblique muscle.

Rectus abdominis muscle.

The fibers run longitudinally, and splitting of the fibers gives free access to the abdominal cavity. **However, the accompanying injury to the nerves makes muscle-splitting of the rectus not a desirable feature.**

The oblique muscles of the lateral abdominal wall (external and internal oblique muscles and transversus abdominis muscle) have their fibers running in different directions; for this reason the fibers of the entire thickness of the wall cannot be split in one direction. The **external oblique muscle can be split only in a downward, inward and forward direction, and only after the split parts are retracted can the internal oblique muscle be split according to its location:**

 a. **In the upper part of the lateral abdominal wall,** in an upward, inward and forward direction.

 b. **In the middle part of the lateral abdominal wall,** in an inward and forward direction; and

 c. **In the lower part of the lateral abdominal wall,** in a downward, inward and forward direction.

The transversus abdominis muscle can be split, after the split lips of the external and internal oblique muscles are retracted; they can be split in an inward direction.

The transversalis fascia can be split only in a direction perpendicular to the midline; incision in any other direction will cut its fibers.

The peritoneum can be split in a transverse direction only; incision in any other direction will cut the fibers.

The blood-supply of the anterior abdominal wall is derived from the following arteries (Fig. 35) :

  Superior epigastric;
  Tenth and eleventh intercostal;
  Subcostal;
  All the lumbar arteries (4 or 5 in number) ;
  Inferior epigastric;
  Deep circumflex iliac;
  Superficial epigastric;
  Superficial circumflex iliac; and
  Some branches of the external pudendal artery.

The nerve-supply of the anterior abdominal wall (Fig. 35) is derived from the 7th, 8th, 9th, 10th, 11th, and 12th thoracic nerves, and from the ilio-hypogastric and ilio-inguinal branches of the first lumbar nerve.

If we will analyze the course of the fibers of the recti muscles and the direction of the blood-vessels and nerves, we will notice that the main blood-vessels (superior and inferior epigastric arteries) run in the same

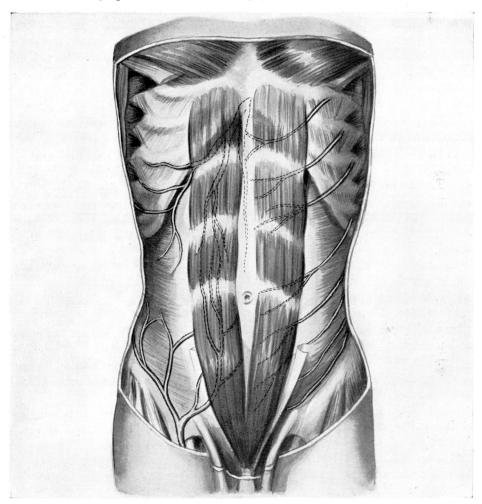

FIG. 35. BLOOD-SUPPLY AND NERVE DISTRIBUTION OF THE ANTERIOR ABDOMINAL WALL.

direction as the fibers of the muscles, and that the intercostal arteries run in a direction perpendicular to these fibers. The nerves run perpendicularly to the fibers of the recti muscle. This means that in opening the abdomen by splitting the fibers of the rectus muscle, we preserve part of the blood-supply (superior and inferior epigastric arteries) and we sacrifice another part of it (abdominal termination of the lower intercostal arteries), and also the fibers of the sheaths. By opening the abdomen through a transverse incision we sacrifice the superior (or inferior) epigastric artery, but preserve the abdominal terminations of the lower intercostal arteries and also the fibers of the sheaths. In either case there will be enough blood-supply left to take care of the nutrition of the abdominal wall.

However, with the nerve-supply things are different. In the case of the longitudinal, muscle-splitting incision, **we preserve the muscle and cut the nerve-supply.** The number of severed nerves depends on the length of the incision. In the case of a longitudinal incision between the ensiform process and the umbilicus, at least three nerves will be sacrificed. In making a longitudinal incision, the farther we go from the median line, the more muscle is left without innervation and the more damage is done to the muscles lying to the inner side of the incision. By cutting the rectus muscle **transversely,** we preserve the nerve-supply.

By making an incision in the anterior abdominal wall lateral to the recti muscles, there is only one way to preserve both the muscles and the nerves, namely, to make a muscle-splitting incision with retraction of the nerves which lie on the transversus abdominis muscle.

The earliest types of abdominal incision were longitudinal. However, in many of these cases post-operative ventral hernias followed. At first it was thought that this was due to frequent suppuration of the wound, to the use of an unsuitable suture-material (some blamed the use of soluble material, some of insoluble), to the method of suturing, some considering that each layer should be sutured separately while others believed that the layers should be sutured together, devising for this purpose the figure-of-eight suture. Some considered that the deep fascia should be carefully sutured, etc. However, in many cases in which no suppuration ensued, where either soluble or insoluble suture-material was used, where the abdomen was sutured either through its entire thickness, or through several layers, or separately through each layer, in a definite number of cases ventral hernia followed the operation sooner or later. In some of the cases the discomfort produced by the post-operative ventral hernia was greater than the discomfort due to the disease which called for the abdominal operation. The inability of the surgeons to prevent the formation of post-operative hernia irrespective of the type of suture-material and the method of closing the abdomen, led some investigators to believe that the cause of post-operative ventral hernia lies in the making of improper incisions.

In 1898, P. Assmy, of Czerny's Heidelberg clinic, carried out, at the suggestion of Czerny, several experiments making longitudinal abdominal incisions in which several nerves were cut, and transverse incisions in which the nerves were preserved. He was able to demonstrate that in the case of the longitudinal incisions the part of the muscle lying to the inner side of the incision became atrophied, whereas the part lying laterally remained normal. The scar that was formed was attached laterally to normal muscle and medially to atrophied muscle. Sprengel, in 1912, emphasized the fact that in cutting the anterior sheath longitudinally the operator **actually severed the aponeurotic continuation of the lateral abdominal muscles (See Anatomy of the Anterior Abdominal Wall), and for this reason the scar sooner or later became wider, thinner and weaker; and if this reached a definite degree, the scar gave way and a ventral hernia ensued.**

After the work of Assmy many surgeons started to use transverse incisions. However, it should be remembered that transverse incisions were made by some surgeons before the work of Assmy. Billroth, when he performed his first gastrectomy in 1881, used a transverse incision. However, these surgeons did this not because of less injury to the nerve-supply but because they considered that such an incision gives better exposure and more convenient drainage. It is used far less frequently than the longitudinal incision; nevertheless, it has been used in such a great number of cases that definite conclusions can be made, and its advantages are quite evident:

1. It is followed far less frequently by post-operative ventral hernia, or by an acute disruption of the wound;

2. The closure of the abdomen is easier because the approximation of the edges is easier and it is not necessary to "fight" with protruding bowels;

3. Due to less tension the patient is not afraid to cough, and for this reason cases of post-operative pneumonia are far less frequent;

4. The time of confinement to bed is shorter;

5. The scar is less visible, and thus cosmetic results are obtained.

It seems to us that transverse incision, not only of the skin but also of the entire thickness of the abdominal wall, will become more and more the choice in the future.

The numerous incisions which have been described may be subdivided into three large categories:

  A. Transverse and gridiron incisions;
  B. Longitudinal incisions;
  C. Flap incisions.

A. TRANSVERSE INCISIONS.

These are characterized by a transverse cutting of the abdominal wall, observing the following prerequisites:

1. The skin is cut along the "fissures of Langer";
2. The anterior sheath is cut perpendicularly to the midline;
3. The muscle is either retracted or cut transversely;
4. The posterior sheath, transversalis fascia, and peritoneum are cut transversely; there is then no injury to the nerves;
5. The blood-vessels should be spared as much as possible, but, as mentioned above, the arrangement of these vessels is such that some of them have to be sacrificed no matter how the incision is made.

1. **Mikulicz-Kausch Incision.** Suggested in 1900. (Fig. 36[1]).

This runs from the lower part of the right costal arch medially and slightly downward until it reaches the midline. It cuts transversely all the structures of the abdominal wall—skin, fascia, anterior sheath of the right rectus muscle, right rectus muscle, posterior sheath of the right rectus muscle, transversalis fascia and peritoneum. It does not injure the

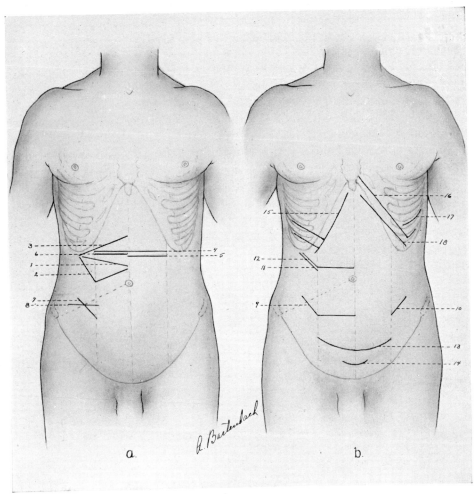

FIG. 36.
a and b. Different transverse and oblique incisions.

nerves, leaves enough blood-supply, and cuts the anterior sheath and posterior sheath of the rectus muscle **along the course of its fibers. It is useful for gall-bladder operations, and for work on the pylorus, duodenum and biliary ducts.**

2. **Sprengel Incision** (Fig. 36[2]).

This incision consists of two limbs, made at right angles to each other;

the short one running obliquely downward and inward until it reaches the lateral border of the rectus muscle; the inner one crossing the rectus muscle **in a medial and slightly upward** direction. The shorter limb cuts through the skin, superficial and deep fascia, and splits the fibers of the external oblique muscle, not going any deeper; the medial limb cuts transversely the rectus muscle and its posterior sheath, the transversalis fascia and the peritoneum—all in a transverse direction. Essentially, it is the same as the Mikulicz-Kausch incision, with additional space for work in case of stout patients. **It is used for work on the gall-bladder, biliary ducts, duodenum and pylorus.** The same type of incision, made only on the left side, is suitable **for all work on the stomach, spleen, splenic flexure of the colon, and the transverse colon.**

3. **Courvoisier Incision** (Fig. 36[3]).

This runs from the lower border of the right costal arch medially and slightly upward until it reaches the midline. In technic of execution, in the merits of the incision, and in the indications for the kind of operations for which it is suitable, it is analogous to the Mikulicz-Kausch incision.

4. **Bilateral Transrectus Transverse Incision** (Fig. 36[4]).

This consists of a transverse incision from the right border of the right rectus muscle to the left border of the left rectus muscle. It cuts through all the structures transversely. After the peritoneum is opened, the falciform ligament is cut between two ligatures. It gives an excellent operative field for work on the stomach. For cases of total gastrectomy it is the best of all "purely abdominal" incisions. It is also excellent for all ordinary work on the **stomach, duodenum, bile-ducts,** and **pancreas.**

5. **Left Transverse Rectus Incision** (Fig. 36[5]).

This incision extends transversely through all the structures from the left margin of the left rectus muscle to the midline. It cuts all the structures transversely, and is **suitable for gastro-enterostomy and gastrostomy operations.**

6. **Right Transverse Rectus Incision** (Fig. 36[6]).

The technic is the same as on the left side. **It is suitable for some cases of gall-bladder work, and for work on the duodenum and the pyloric end of the stomach.**

7. **McBurney Incision** (Fig. 36[7]).

This incision was suggested by Charles McBurney, of New York, in 1894. The incision crosses a point which lies one inch medial from the anterior superior iliac spine on an imaginary line drawn between this spine and the umbilicus. From this point, a line is made perpendicular to the above mentioned line for a distance of two and a-half to four inches; one-third of the incision is situated above this line and two-thirds below. It is a muscle-splitting incision, which does not cut either the muscles or the blood-supply or nerve-supply. The details of the technic will be given below. This incision, although it does not exactly follow the cosmetic requirements, nevertheless is ideal in a physiological sense because it does not injure either the nerves or the muscles, and when correctly made is not followed by post-operative hernia. **It is indicated for appendectomy, appendicostomy, cecostomy, and, in suitable cases, even resection of the cecum is possible.**

8. **Rockey Incision** (Fig. 36[8]).

A transverse incision of one and one-half inches is made, starting from the McBurney point as its center. The skin, superficial and deep fascia are cut, so that the aponeurosis of the external oblique muscle is exposed. The rest of the operation is exactly as in the McBurney "gridiron" incision.

Indication. The same as in the McBurney incision. This operation was suggested by Rockey, in 1905. In Germany, it is known as the **Sonnenburg incision,** and in this country it is also known as the **Davis incision.** Davis suggested it in October, 1905. Although Rockey advocated using a very small incision (1½ inches), we believe that the skin-incision should be larger (2½ inches). This incision satisfies not only the anatomico-physiological, but also the cosmetic requirements.

9. **Harrington Incision** (Fowler Incision, "Weir Extension Incision") (Fig. 36[9]).

This incision was described by F. B. Harrington in August, 1899, by Weir in February, 1900, and by Fowler in March, 1900.

In Germany, it is known as the **Winkelmann incision.** However, Winkelmann did not speak of this incision until 1909, and does not claim originality.

The initial part of this incision is the McBurney "gridiron" incision. When, during the course of operation, it becomes evident, that some other work not contemplated before, is required, and that the "gridiron" incision does not offer enough room, the incision is extended in the following way: The rectus muscle is retracted medially, and the posterior sheath and peritoneum are cut transversely up to the midline. This incision enables the surgeon to work on the appendix, when it is directed medially into the pelvis, and particularly when it is bound down by adhesions, and also on the ovary and the tube on the right side.

10. **Left "Gridiron" Incision** (Fig. 36[10]).

The landmarks and technic of execution are exactly the same as for appendectomy, with the difference only that it is done on the left side. It is used for left inguinal colostomy.

11. **Right Upper "Gridiron" Incision** (Fig. 36[11]).

The technic is exactly the same as in the McBurney incision; the difference is only in locality. The indication is cholecystostomy. However, if in the course of the operation it becomes evident that there is not sufficient room, whether because a cholecystectomy is necessary, or work on the stomach or on the biliary passages, then the incision may be enlarged by transforming it into a:

12. **Right Upper "Gridiron" Incision, with a transverse incision of the posterior sheath of the right rectus muscle up to the midline** (Fig. 36[12]).

In this way, it becomes a "right upper Harrington incision."

13. **Pfannenstiel Incision** (Fig. 36[13]).

Suggested in 1898 and published in 1900.

The skin, superficial and deep fascia are cut transversely (in a slightly semicircular line). The anterior sheath of the rectus muscle is cut transversely. The recti muscles are retracted from each other. The transversalis fascia and peritoneum are cut longitudinally.

This incision is not strictly physiological; however, because in the lower quarter of the abdomen the aponeurosis of the internal oblique and transversus abdominis muscles participates in the formation of the anterior sheath only, the damage caused by this longitudinal incision is confined to the transversalis fascia and peritoneum only. For this reason it is less than if the arrangement of the aponeurosis in this lower quarter was the same as in the other parts of the abdomen. It is of interest to note, that this incision, introduced by a gynecologist for gynecological operations, **was the forerunner of all physiological incisions which were suggested later and introduced in general abdominal surgery.** It is worth mentioning, that arguments were raised by several contemporaries of Pfannenstiel as to whom the priority of the incision belonged. This may be settled by stating that as long ago as 1789, Dr. John Hull in his "A Defense of the Cæsarean Operation with Observations on Embryulcia, and the Section of the Symphysis Pubis", published in Manchester, England, in 1789, advocated the use of a transverse incision for Cesarean section.

14. **Kűstner Incision.** Suggested in 1896 (Fig. 36[14]).

This is a transverse, slightly semicircular incision at the margin of or within the pubic hair, **and extends through the skin only;** all the deeper structures are cut longitudinally through a midline incision. As may be seen, this incision is actually a midline longitudinal incision. It fulfils only cosmetic requirements, because it cuts the skin along the fissure lines of Langer. However, it violates the anatomico-physiological requirements. It is of interest to know, that this incision influenced Pfannenstiel to use his incision, which is considered as a forerunner of all contemporary transverse incisions.

A few other physiological incisions, made by abdomino-thoracic approach (both extrapleural and transpleural) and by lumbar approach, will be given under corresponding headings.

B. LONGITUDINAL INCISIONS.

1. **Midline Incision** (Fig. 37[1]).

This is the oldest type of incision. It may be made either in the epigastric, umbilical or hypogastric regions. The incision has great advantages. The abdomen can be quickly opened and closed; it gives a good view of the entire abdomen, and for this reason it is excellent for exploratory purposes. From the standpoint of a good operative field, it is a very excellent incision, because nearly 80 per cent. of all abdominal work can be done through a midline incision. The objectionable feature of the incision is that it cuts the linea alba, **i. e.** the terminal fibers of the aponeurosis of **all lateral muscles, perpendicular to their course,** and for this reason, under the influence of traction by lateral abdominal muscles, the scar yields, producing a ventral hernia. Another objectionable point is that the linea alba has a very poor blood-supply, and for this reason is not capable of forming a strong scar.

2. Paramedian Incision (Right or Left) (Fig. 37[2]).

This was first described by Hagen-Thorn, in 1884.

It consists of a longitudinal incision through the anterior sheath of the rectus muscle, followed by retraction of this muscle and incision through the posterior sheath of the muscle immediately lateral to the linea alba. The rectus muscle thus lies between the weakened points in the posterior and anterior sheaths, and therefore diminishes the possibility of hernia. However, the objectionable feature of this incision is that it divides the anterior and posterior sheaths longitudinally, *i.e.* in a direction perpendicular to their fibers. In case it is desired to open the abdomen by a longitudinal incision, this should be given preference to a midline incision.

3. Right Midrectus Incision (Riedel Incision) (Fig. 37[3]).

This runs longitudinally midway in the right rectus muscle from the costal arch to the level of the umbilicus. The skin, fascia and anterior sheath of the rectus muscle are incised, the rectus muscle is split longitudinally, and the posterior sheath and peritoneum are divided longitudinally. This incision gives a good operative exposure, but it cuts the sheaths in a non-physiological manner, and also severs at least three intercostal nerves, thereby producing an atrophy of that part of the rectus muscle which is situated medially to the line of the incision. Altogether, we do not recommend this incision on the right side at all, while on the left it may be used occasionally for gastrostomy operations (Fig. 37[13]).

4. Right Upper Pararectus Incision (Fig. 37[4]).

This is used for gall-bladder work.

In Germany, it is known as the **Langenbuch incision,** in English speaking countries, as the **Lawson Tait incision.** It runs along the lateral border of the right rectus muscle. It starts at the point where the lateral border of this muscle crosses the costal arch and runs downward to the level of the umbilicus. It cuts through the skin, superficial and deep fascia and through the anterior sheath of the rectus muscle.

This muscle is retracted medially; then, the posterior sheath and peritoneum are cut longitudinally. It has the same objectionable features as the midrectal incision with this difference only, that instead of a part, the entire rectus muscle may become atrophied.

5. Kocher Incision (Fig. 37[5]).

This runs from the lowermost portion of the right costal arch medially and upward, nearly parallel to the costal arch, until it reaches the midline. This incision cuts the sheaths and muscle obliquely; it injures two or three intercostal nerves. The incision is non-physiological, but it does less harm than other non-physiological incisions.

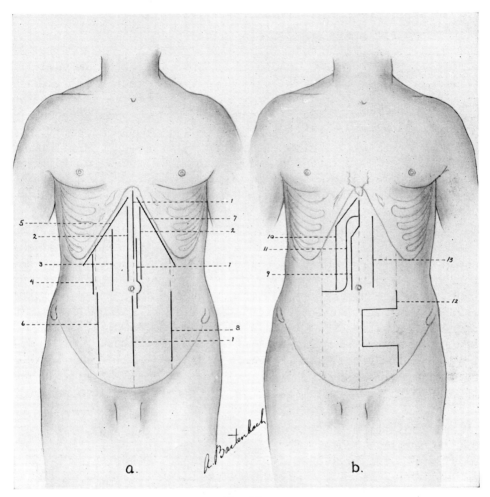

FIG. 37.
a and b. Different longitudinal and some oblique and flap incisions.

6. Right Lower Pararectus Incision (Lennander Incision, Battle-Kammerer Incision, Jalaguier Incision) (Fig. 37[6]).

This incision with slight variations was described by different surgeons: Jalaguier, of Paris described it in 1892, Battle, of London in 1895, F. Kammerer, of New York in 1897, and K. Lennander, of Upsala in 1898.

This incision starts at the level of the umbilicus half an inch medial from the lateral border of the right rectus muscle. It runs downward along the lateral border of this muscle for a distance of four inches. The skin, superficial and deep fascia and the anterior sheath of the rectus muscle are cut longitudinally. The rectus muscle is retracted medially, and the posterior sheath and peritoneum are cut longitudinally. This incision gives a good exposure of the appendix, and can be enlarged upwards if it is decided to work on the gall-bladder. The objectionable feature of it is that the anterior and posterior sheaths are cut in a non-physiological manner.

7. Fenger Incision (Fig. 37[7]).

Suggested in 1854. This is used occasionally for gastrostomy and for work on the splenic flexure of the colon. It preceded the Kocher incision, described above, which is analogous to this incision but is done only on the right side. The remarks concerning the Kocher incision may be repeated for this incision.

8. Left Lower Pararectus Incision (Fig. 37[8]).

This is performed exactly as the right lower pararectal incision. It is used commonly for colostomy operations.

9. Kehr Incision (Fig. 37[9]).

Suggested in 1903. This incision runs from the ensiform process downward for an inch, then it turns to the right obliquely downward and laterally for another inch, and then it turns again downward as a midrectal incision reaching to the level of the umbilicus. Later, Kehr, not being satisfied with this incision, changed the midrectal limb by making it transverse, reaching to the right costal arch. However, in either case the incision is not physiological: in the first instance all the limbs are non-physiological; in the second case, the limbs running vertically and obliquely are non-physiological.

10. Oblique Intrarectus Angular Incision (Fig. 37[10]).

In English speaking countries this is known as the **Mayo Robson incision.** In Germany, it is known as the **Kőrte incision.** It starts at the midline one inch below the ensiform process and runs in an oblique direction downward and laterally until it reaches the lateral third of the rectus muscle, then it turns downward until it reaches the level of the umbilicus.

11. Bevan Incision (Fig. 37[11]).

Suggested in 1897. In its earliest development this was similar to the Mayo Robson incision, with this difference only, that the small upper limb instead of running obliquely ran transversely, and at the lower end there was a horizontal limb. After several modifications, the characteristic feature of which was that the vertical part of the incision was moved closer and closer to the midline, Bevan suggested recently making the vertical part about a quarter of an inch from the medial margin of the right rectus muscle.

12. **Audry-Mixter Incision** (Fig. 37[12]).

This is used by some surgeons when performing colostomy. The incision starts at the level of the umbilicus at the lateral border of the left rectus muscle, and runs downward for two inches; then it turns medially until it reaches the midline; then it turns at a right angle downward and runs for two inches; then it turns at a right angle laterally until it reaches the lateral border of the rectus muscle; then it turns downward along the lateral border of this muscle and extends for two inches. The quadrangular flap thus formed is reflected laterally, and the anterior sheath of the rectus muscle is cut longitudinally for a length of six inches. The rectus muscle is retracted medially and the posterior sheath and peritoneum are incised longitudinally. As may be seen, this is a **longitudinal non-physiological incision.**

C. FLAP INCISIONS.

1. **Czerny-Perthes Incision** (Fig. 38[1]).

This incision was first suggested by Czerny and later advocated by Perthes. It consists of two limbs, a vertical and horizontal. The vertical limb is a midline incision extending from the ensiform process down to one and a half inches above the umbilicus. The horizontal limb extends through the entire width of the rectus muscle. In this way, it cuts through the skin, superficial and deep fascia. The anterior sheath is incised paramedially from the ensiform process toward the umbilicus. The rectus muscle is cut transversely, and the posterior sheath and peritoneum are cut in a semicircular manner. This incision gives an excellent exposure and does not injure the nerves. The objection is that it cuts the anterior and posterior sheaths longitudinally. **It is used in gall-bladder, duodenal and pyloric surgery.**

2. **Kőnig-Perthes Incision** (Fig. 38[2]).

Suggested by F. König, in 1912 and later advocated by Perthes. This is the same as the Czerny-Perthes incision with this difference only, that in the latter the vertical part is shorter than the horizontal portion. It has the same commendable and objectionable features as the Czerny-Perthes incision.

3. **Don Incision** (Fig. 39).

Suggested in 1909. The vertical limb of the incision is made one-half inch to the right of the middle line. It starts from the seventh costochondral junction and ends a little above the umbilicus. The skin, superficial and deep fascia are divided. The anterior sheath of the rectus muscle is divided in the same line, and the medial lip of the anterior sheath is separated from the muscle, which is then retracted laterally and separated from its posterior sheath. The posterior sheath and the peritoneum are divided in the same sagittal plane as the skin, fascia and the anterior sheath. Then, from the lowest point of the vertical incision a semilunar incision is made upward and outward to the lowest point of the right costal arch (10th rib) through the skin and fascia only. The rectus muscle, the posterior sheath and peritoneum are cut transversely. The flap thus formed is reflected upward and outward and gives an excellent operative field. No nerves are injured by this incision; the only objection to the incision is the longitudinal division of the anterior and posterior sheaths.

4. Pochhammer Incision.

Suggested in 1918. The vertical portion of this incision is the same as in the Kőnig-Perthes incision. The rectus muscle is cut transversely.

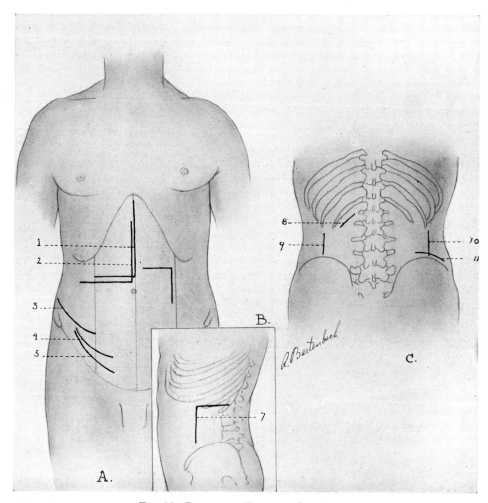

FIG. 38. DIFFERENT TYPES OF INCISIONS.
A.   1. Czerny; 2. Kőnig-Perthes; 3. Albarran;   4. Hartmann; 5. Israel; 6. Schiassi; B.   7. Bardenheuer;   C.   8. For drainage of a pancreatic abscess;   9. Incision for the ascending colon;   10. Incision for the descending colon;   11. Lumbar appendectomy incision.

The posterior sheath of the muscle and the peritoneum are incised in a semicircular line. This incision is very similar to an incision described a few years previously by Don. It has the same commendable and objectionable features as the Don incision.

5. Winkelmann Incision.

Suggested in 1909. As this is described below, it is actually Sprengel's description of Winkelmann's incision. It consists of a longitudinal incision in the midline from the ensiform process to the umbilicus through the skin, superficial and deep fascia (Fig. 40[1], left upper insert). These are retracted

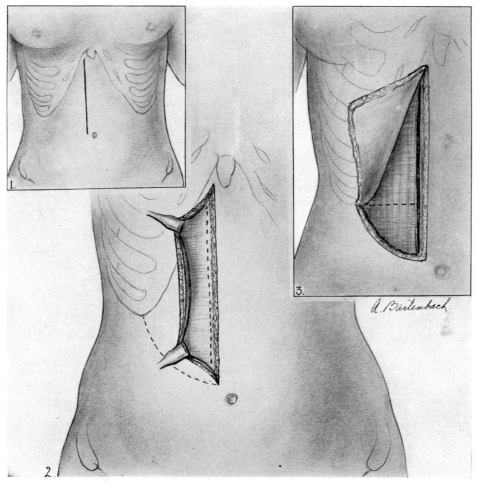

FIG. 39. DON INCISION.

to the right and the anterior sheath of the right rectus muscle is cut longitudinally. The right rectus muscle is retracted laterally and the posterior sheath and peritoneum cut transversely.

This incision gives a good operative field, particularly if it is enlarged in the same manner on the other side (Fig. 40[2] and Fig. 40, main picture).

However, its objectionable feature is that a longitudinal cut is made through the anterior sheath of the rectus muscle. This incision is known in this country as the **Sloan incision.** Sloan described it and brought attention to its merits in 1927.

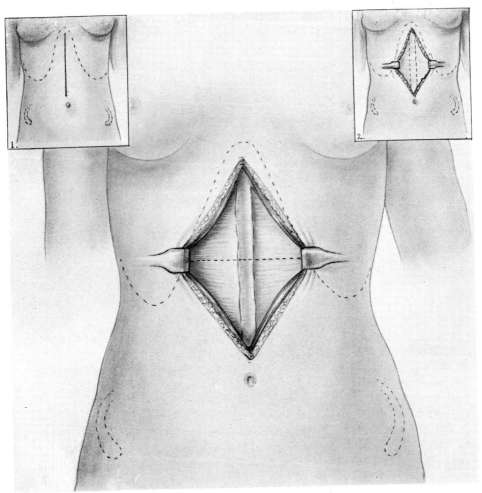

FIG. 40. WINKELMANN INCISION.

LUMBAR INCISIONS.

Recently there has arisen a tendency to approach the abdominal viscera through posterior incisions. As a matter of fact, these incisions were used for some abdominal operations long before the anterior abdominal incisions were employed. For instance, lumbar colostomies were done much earlier than the inguinal type of colostomy. The reason for using a lumbar approach in the pre-antiseptic time was the fear of peritonitis. When aseptic methods were introduced and the fear of peritonitis was lessened, the lumbar and posterior approach in general were abandoned. They were revived only in recent times, not on account of the fear of peritonitis, but because the surgeons felt that the posterior route **lessens the possibility of a post-operative hernia, diminishes the shock** and in some cases gives better access to the diseased organs. These incisions however, find very few followers, and whether they will be widely adopted is questionable. **In many cases, they give a better approach, in some cases they decrease the mortality,** and these may be considered as points of advantage. However, it is far more inconvenient for the patient to take care of a scar placed in the lumbar region than on the anterior abdominal wall. Before describing the abdominal incisions of the lumbar region let us have a brief anatomical review.

ANATOMY OF THE LUMBAR REGION.

Skin (Fig. 31, b).

The fissure lines of Langer run in a semicircular direction and are continuous with the fissure lines of Langer of the anterior abdominal wall.

Superficial Fascia (Fig. 41).

This presents no peculiarities. It is of considerable thickness in which is embedded a considerable amount of fat. Anteriorly, it is continuous with the superficial fascia of the abdomen.

Deep Fascia (Fig. 41).

This layer is attached to the supraspinous ligaments and vertebral spines. Laterally, it is continuous with the deep fascia of the abdomen.

Lumbo-dorsal Fascia (Figs. 41 and 42).

This consists of three fascial layers, called respectively the **posterior,** the **middle** and the **anterior.** These three layers unite at the lateral margin of the sacrospinalis muscle and form a ligament which extends between the last rib and the iliac crest and gives partial origin to the internal oblique and transversus abdominis muscles.

The posterior layer extends from the spines of the lumbar vertebræ laterally until at the lateral border of the sacrospinalis muscle it is joined by the middle layer. In the vertical direction it extends between the last rib and the iliac crest. On the chest, it is continuous with the intercostal aponeurosis. From this layer arises the latissimus dorsi muscle (Fig. 41).

The middle layer extends from the ends of the transverse processes of the lumbar vertebræ in a lateral direction. Posteriorly to it is situated the sacrospinalis group of muscles (semispinalis dorsi, longissimus dorsi and iliocostalis), and anteriorly to it is the quadratus lumborum muscle. Just lateral from the line of fusion of the posterior and middle lamellæ of the lumbo-dorsal fascia the internal oblique muscle takes its origin (Fig. 41).

The anterior layer (Fig. 41) is attached to the anterior surface of the transverse processes of the lumbar vertebræ. It lies in front of the quadratus lumborum muscle and behind the psoas major muscle. It joins the fascia formed by the fusion of the posterior and middle layers just lateral to the point of union of the posterior and middle lamellæ. Laterally from this line of union of these three lamellæ the lumbo-dorsal fascia is continuous with the aponeurosis of the transversus abdominis muscle.

Muscles of the Back (Figs. 41 and 42).

The latissimus dorsi muscle lies superficially; its fibers run upward and laterally; along its lateral side extend the vertical fibers of the rectus

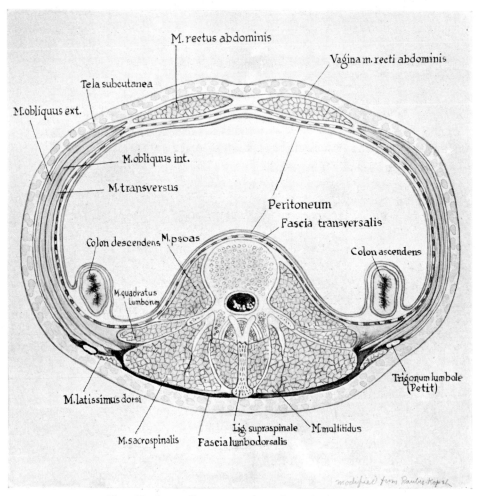

FIG. 41. CROSS SECTION OF THE LUMBAR REGION.

muscle, which run upward and slightly inward. Frequently, the lateral fibers of the latissimus dorsi overlap the medial edge of the external oblique muscle.

The next group of muscles which are exposed after dividing and reflecting the posterior lamellæ of the lumbo-dorsal fascia, latissimus dorsi and external oblique muscles are (enumerating from the median line laterally), the sacrospinalis, the serratus posterior inferior, and the internal oblique muscles. By cutting and reflecting the middle layer of the lumbo-dorsal fascia and the internal oblique muscle the following muscles will be seen (enumerating from the median line laterally), the quadratus

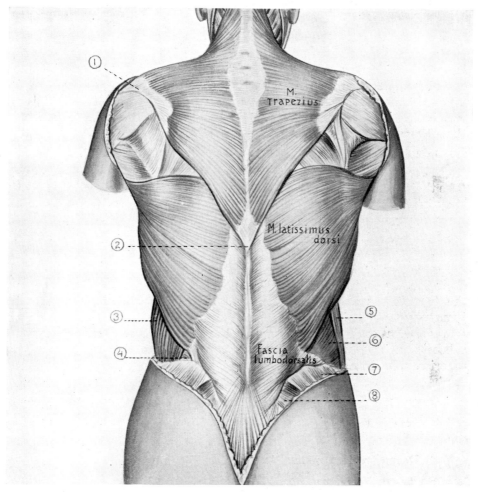

FIG. 42. MUSCLES OF THE BACK (After Rauber).

1. Spina scapulæ.	5. M. obliquus ext. abdominis.
2. Proc. spinosus vertebræ thor. XII.	6. M. obliquus intern. abdominis.
3. M. obliquus ext. abdominis.	7. M. glutaeus medius.
4. Trigonum lumbale.	8. M. glutaeus maximus.

lumborum and transversus abdominis muscles. By cutting the anterior layer of the lumbo-dorsal fascia in the innermost part in front of the trans-verse processes of the lumbar vertebræ there are exposed the psoas major muscle and, more laterally, the transversalis fascia. Cutting through the transversalis fascia, all the retroperitoneal structures, such as kidney, duodenum, parts of the large bowel which have no mesentery, and the large blood-vessels and their branches, will be exposed.

The blood-supply of the posterior abdominal wall is derived from:

a. Subcostal Artery.

This artery, which is actually the twelfth costal artery, takes its origin from the thoracic aorta. It runs laterally, being situated below the last rib. It passes below the lumbo-costal arch to the abdomen, and lies **posterior** to the kidney and colon and **anterior** to the quadratus lumborum muscles. In its further course laterally it pierces the anterior lamella of the lumbo-dorsal fascia and runs between the transversus abdominis muscle and the internal oblique muscle, and anastomoses with the branches of the lower two intercostal arteries, with the lumbar arteries and with branches of the superior epigastric artery.

b. Lumbar Arteries.

There are usually four pairs; occasionally a fifth pair is present. They take their origin from the aorta, run in a lateral direction, lying first on the body of the corresponding lumbar vertebra and then between the transverse processes of each two adjoining vertebræ. At the lateral border of the interval between each two transverse processes each lumbar artery turns laterally and runs posterior to the quadratus lumborum muscle with the exception of the lowest one which passes in front of this muscle. In their further course laterally, they pierce the aponeurosis of the origin of the transversus abdominis muscle, and lie in the interval between the transversus abdominis and the internal oblique muscles. Here they anastomose with each other, with the lower two intercostal arteries, the subcostal artery, with branches of the superior and inferior epigastric arteries, with branches of the deep circumflex iliac artery, and with the lumbar branch of the ilio-lumbar artery.

c. The **lumbar branch** of the ilio-lumbar artery supplies the psoas and quadratus lumborum muscles. It anastomoses with the lumbar and deep circumflex iliac arteries.

d. Deep Circumflex Iliac Artery.

This arises from the lateral side of the external iliac artery immediately above the Poupart ligament. It runs laterally and upward and a little beyond the anterior superior iliac spine. It pierces the transversus abdominis muscle and is continued between this muscle and the internal oblique muscle, where its terminations anastomose with the lumbar branch of the ilio-lumbar artery.

e. Superficial Circumflex Iliac Artery.

This arises from the front of the femoral artery just below the Poupart ligament. It runs laterally and upward as far as the anterior superior iliac spine. It supplies the skin of the groin and anastomoses with branches of the deep circumflex iliac artery.

NERVE-SUPPLY OF THE POSTERIOR ABDOMINAL WALL.

a. Anterior Ramus of the Twelfth Thoracic Nerve. This branch appears below the twelfth rib and passes laterally and downward **behind** the psoas major muscle. In its further course it lies in **front** of the quadratus lumborum muscle and **behind** the kidney and corresponding part of the colon. Then it pierces the transversus abdominis muscle and lies between this muscle and the internal oblique muscle until it reaches the sheath of the rectus muscle. The course of the nerve in the anterior part of the abdominal wall has already been described. It gives off **muscular** branches to the transverse, internal and external oblique muscles and to the rectus muscle, and also cutaneous branches—the **anterior terminal** branch, which, was described in the anatomy of the anterior abdominal wall, and the **lateral cutaneous** branch which, while running through the lateral abdominal wall, is still situated in the muscles and only becomes superficial about two inches behind the anterior superior spine. It supplies the skin of the buttock. The twelfth thoracic nerve receives occasionally a communicating branch from the eleventh nerve, and still more frequently sends a communicating branch to the first lumbar nerve.

b. Lumbar Plexus.

From the first, second, third and fourth lumbar nerves arise **muscular** branches to the quadratus lumborum muscle, and from the second and third lumbar nerves, arise **muscular** branches to the psoas major muscle.

The ilio-hypogastric nerve, which is derived from the first lumbar nerve, traverses the substance of the psoas muscle, and then runs downward and laterally in **front** of the quadratus lumborum muscle and **behind** the kidney and colon. Then it penetrates the transversus abdominis muscle and runs between it and the internal oblique muscle laterally and downward. About one inch in front of the anterior superior iliac spine it pierces the internal oblique muscle and runs between it and the aponeurosis of the external oblique muscle in the same medial and downward direction. It pierces the aponeurosis of the external oblique muscle about one and a half inches above the subcutaneous inguinal ring and becomes cutaneous. In its course it gives off muscular branches to the oblique muscles of the abdominal wall.

The ilio-inguinal nerve is derived from the first lumbar nerve. It runs nearly parallel with the ilio-hypogastric nerve, but **below** it, and traverses the same structures. It runs behind the aponeurosis of the external oblique muscle just above the Poupart ligament and becomes superficial after passing through the subcutaneous inguinal ring.

Its **muscular** branches give innervation to the oblique abdominal muscles. The distribution of its **cutaneous** branches is described in the anatomy of the anterior abdominal wall.

GENERAL REMARKS ON LUMBAR INCISIONS.

From the above description of the direction of the fibers of the skin, fascia and muscles we see that each muscular layer runs in a different direction. If we do not wish to cut the muscle we must make a muscle-splitting incision, and for this reason the opening cannot be very large. Therefore, **operations which require a large operative field are not suitable for a lumbar approach.** Still, it is possible to perform a great number of operations through a lumbar approach. It is also worth noting that incisions leading to the retroperitoneal structures of the abdomen can be

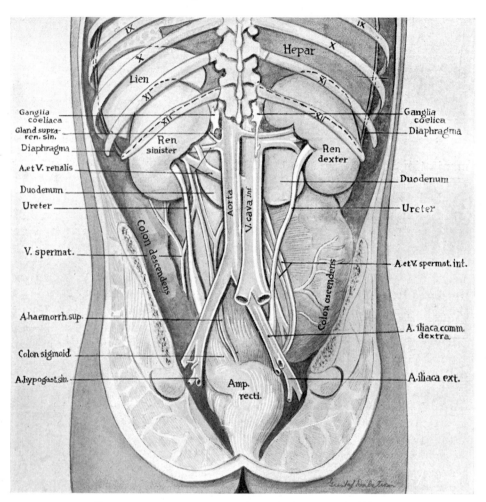

FIG. 43. POSTERIOR VIEW OF THE ABDOMINAL CAVITY.

made only in a comparatively narrow area located laterally to the outer border of the lumbosacral muscle, since in front of this muscle are situated the transverse processes of the lumbar vertebræ which block the entrance into the retroperitoneal space (Fig. 41). It is true that these incisions can be prolonged along the lateral and anterior walls of the abdomen. However, it will hardly be possible then to confine one's-self to strictly muscle-splitting incisions.

1. **Transverse Lumbar Incision for Appendectomy** (Figs. 45 and 46).

The incision starts at the lateral border of the lumbosacral muscle and one-half inch above the crest of the ilium, cutting transversely through the skin up to the posterior axillary line; ordinarily this is about three inches. The skin, superficial and deep fascia are cut transversely. The external oblique muscle is split in the course of its fibers (*i.e.* in an upward

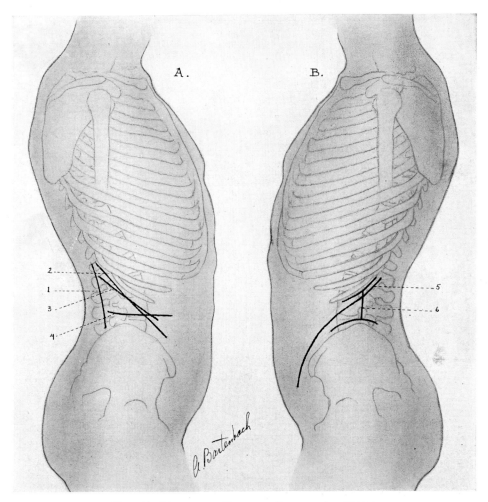

FIG. 44. DIFFERENT TYPES OF LUMBAR INCISIONS.

1. Simon incision.	3. Kocher incision.	5. Israel incision.
2. Bergmann "	4. Péan "	6. Bardenheuer "

direction); the split muscle is retracted, and the internal oblique muscle is split in the course of its fibers (*i.e.* upward and laterally). These fibers are retracted, and the fibers of the transversus abdominis muscle are split in the course of its fibers (*i.e.* transversely). **It is important not to injure the branch of the deep circumflex iliac artery and the ilio-inguinal and ilio-hypogastric nerves.** The ilio-inguinal nerve runs here nearly horizontally very close to the crest of the ilium, and the ilio-hypogastric nerve runs in the same direction, one inch above the ilio-inguinal nerve. The transversalis fascia and peritoneum are cut transversely. This approach is essentially the same as was described by Edebohls as long ago as 1895, and later reappeared under different names, such as the **Sheldon incision,** in 1904, and the **Mermingas incision** in 1931. This incision in some cases may be used even for removal of the cecum.

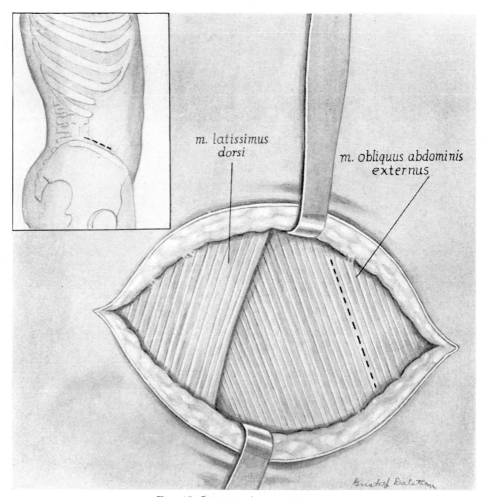

FIG. 45. LUMBAR APPENDECTOMY.
INSERT—Skin incision;
MAIN PICTURE—External oblique muscle is exposed.

2. Lumbar Incision for Excision of the Ascending and Descending Colon (Fig. 38, C, 9 and 10).

This incision, made in the right lumbar region for resection of the ascending colon and in the left side for resection of the descending colon, was suggested quite recently. There is less shock by this method of approach. However, the exposure is not as good as in the case of an anterior approach, and we do not believe that it will replace the anterior approach. **We believe it to be useful only for drainage purposes.**

3. **Lumbar Incision for Removal of the Hepatic and Splenic Flexures.**
What has been said concerning the lumbar incision for excision of the ascending and descending colon is applicable here.

4. **Lumbar Incision for Exposure of the Pancreas, Pancreatic Cysts,**

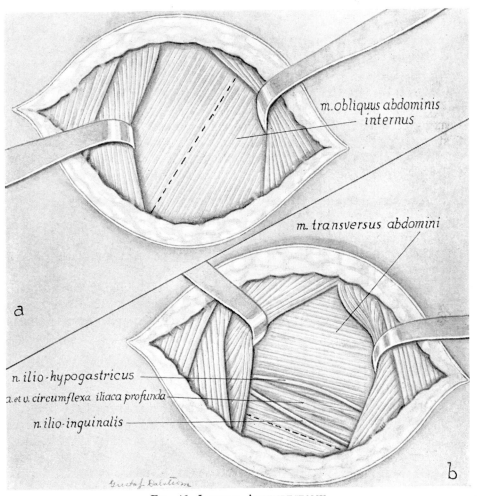

FIG. 46. LUMBAR APPENDECTOMY.
a. Latissimus dorsi and external oblique muscles are retracted; internal oblique muscle is exposed.
b. Transversus abdominis muscle is exposed and ready to be cut.

and Drainage of the Pancreas (Fig. 38, C, 8).

A **left-side** lumbar incision is employed for a posterior approach to the tail of the pancreas, and a **right-side** incision for approach to the head of the pancreas. However, this does not give sufficient room, and for this reason it may be of use for drainage purposes only.

COMBINED ABDOMINO-THORACIC OR LUMBO-THORACIC INCISIONS FOR APPROACH TO THE SPLEEN, LIVER AND SUBPHRENIC SPACE.

There are described a number of incisions through the abdominal and thoracic wall designed to expose the abdominal viscera, both intra-peritoneal and extra-peritoneal. In some of these incisions, both the pleura and the peritoneum are opened; in others, only one cavity is opened—either the pleural or the abdominal. Still in others, the thoraco-abdominal incision does not open either the peritoneal or the pleural cavity, the work being confined to the retro-peritoneal or extrapleural spaces. A few of these types are described below.

I. Transdiaphragmatic Celiotomy with Opening of both the Abdominal and Pleural Cavities.

This is characterized by opening first the pleural cavity and the forming of adhesions between the costal and diaphragmatic pleuræ as the first stage, and by entering the peritoneal cavity as the second stage of the operation. It was first performed by Roser, in 1864, but he did not find followers on account of the dangers connected with it. Volkmann, in 1878, and Israel, in 1879, used this route for the removal of echinococcus. This operation was generally done in two or three stages, in order to prevent infection of the pleural and abdominal cavities. The first stage consisted in **packing** the opened costo-diaphragmatic sinus, so that adhesions should form between the costal and diaphragmatic pleuræ; and later, as the second stage, the diaphragm was opened.

Trendelenburg, in 1883, introduced as the first stage, **suturing** of the diaphragmatic to the costal pleura instead of packing. This approach is used now only by some surgeons to evacuate a **subdiaphragmatic abscess** lying high in the dome of the diaphragm, and **an abscess of the postero-superior surface of the liver or of the spleen.**

Technic.

> **Stage I.**
>
> **Step 1.** The skin-incision starts at the posterior axillary line and passes along the corresponding rib (8th or 9th) for several inches until the cartilage of this rib is reached (Fig. 47, ins.).
>
> **Step 2.** The 8th and 9th ribs are each resected subperiosteally for a length of four inches (Fig. 47).
>
> **Step 3.** The pleural sinus is exposed at the level of the eighth rib and the costal pleura is sutured to the diaphragmatic pleura in a circular manner (Fig. 47).
>
> **Stage II.** This is performed several days later.
>
> **Step 1.** The skin is re-opened.
>
> **Step 2.** The periosteum of the ninth rib, the endothoracic fascia, the pleura costalis, the pleura phrenica, the fascia covering the

thoracic surface of the diaphragm, the muscular part of the
diaphragm, the fascia diaphragmatica (abdominal side), and
the parietal peritoneum are incised.

However, many surgeons advise not to use the transpleural route for
cases in which the pleural cavity is not involved; they suggest using this
method only in cases in which empyema is already present or in which

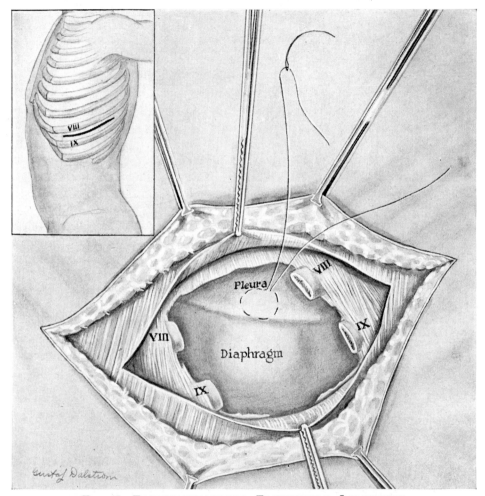

FIG. 47. TRANSDIAPHRAGMATIC, TRANSPLEURAL LAPAROTOMY.
INSERT. Skin incision in the 8th intercostal space.
MAIN PICTURE. The costal pleura is sutured to the diaphragmatic pleura.

there are already present firm old pleural adhesions. For the rest of the
cases (and this constitutes about 70 per cent.) they advise using the
subpleural approach. This approach can be reached either from the **front**
or from **behind.** If it is reached from the front, it can be done either with
the aid of **permanent** resection of some ribs or their cartilages (**method of
Lannelongue, Monod and Vanverts modification of the Lannelongue**

method); or of **temporary** resection (Marwedel, etc.). Or, as suggested by Clairmont and described by his assistant Nather, in 1923, the sub-diaphragmatic space can be reached by incising the anterior abdominal wall parallel to the costal arch, down to the transversalis fascia, then separating this fascia bluntly with a finger in an upward direction until the diaphragm is reached, and then continuing this separation of the

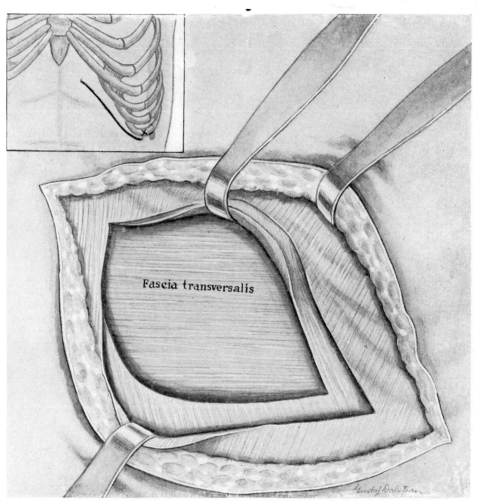

FIG. 48. TRANSDIAPHRAGMATIC LAPAROTOMY BELOW THE COSTO-DIAPHRAGMATIC SINUS.
Canniot modification of the Lannelongue method.

fascia and peritoneum from the muscular portion of the diaphragm until its dome is reached.

II. **Transdiaphragmatic Celiotomy below the Costo-diaphragmatic Sinus.—Anterior Approach** (Figs. 48 and 49).

This method is characterized by opening the peritoneal cavity only.

It was introduced by Lannelongue, in 1887. The technic, somewhat modified by Canniot, in 1891, is as follows:

Step 1. The skin-incision starts three cm. laterally from the ensiform process and two cm. below the costal arch. It is carried laterally as far as the bony portion of the tenth rib (Fig. 48, insert). The skin, superficial and deep fascia, and the external and internal oblique muscles are cut. The costal

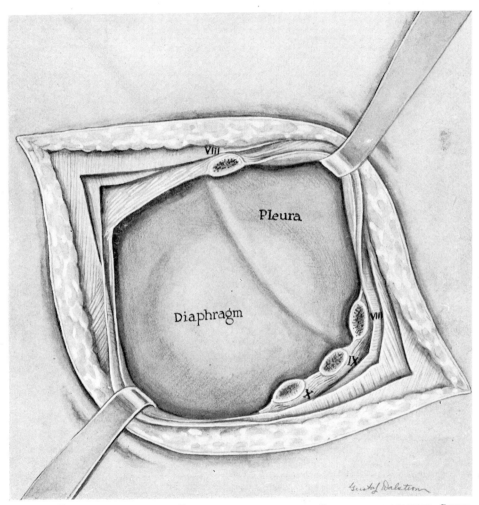

Fig. 49. Transdiaphragmatic Laparotomy below the Costo-diaphragmatic Sinus. Canniot modification of the Lannelongue method.

arch (Fig. 48, main picture) is raised. The attachment of the transverse abdominal muscle and that of the diaphragm are carefully separated from the cartilages of the arch. **The transversus abdominis muscle should not be separated** from the bony portions of the ribs, since the pleura (and the pericardium, if it is the left side) may be opened.

Step 2. The cartilages of the eighth, ninth and tenth ribs are cut through. The cartilage of the eighth rib should actually be resected (cut in two places). This will expose a triangular space in which will be seen the fibers of the internal oblique

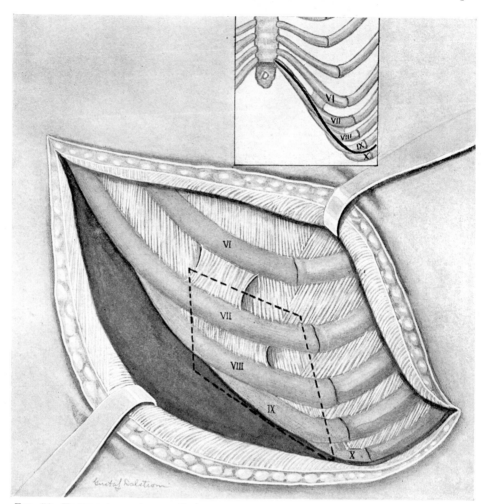

FIG. 50. TRANSDIAPHRAGMATIC LAPAROTOMY BELOW THE COSTO-DIAPHRAGMATIC SINUS. Monod and Vanverts modification of the Lannelongue method.

muscle, the transversus abdominis muscle and the diaphragm.

Step 3. The internal oblique and transversus abdominis muscles are divided. The pleura is now displaced upward and the diaphragm and the peritoneum are divided (Fig. 49).

Another modification of the Lannelongue technic was suggested by Monod and Vanverts:

Monod and Vanverts Modification of the Lannelongue Transdia-phragmatic Celiotomy (Fig. 50).

Technic.

Step 1. The skin-incision starts at the junction of the cartilage of the seventh rib with the sternum, and is continued downward and laterally until the tenth rib is reached. It is then

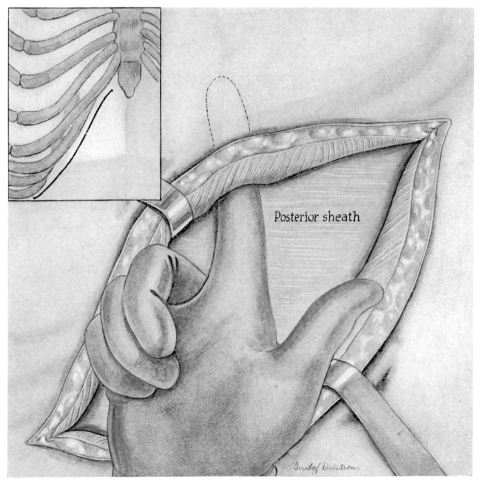

FIG. 51. EXTRAPERITONEAL—EXTRAPLEURAL ANTERIOR SUBDIAPHRAGMATIC APPROACH.
CLAIRMONT TECHNIC.
The finger separates the posterior sheath from the diaphragm.

continued laterally in the ninth intercostal space for another two to three cm. After reflecting the skin with the subjacent soft tissues, the cartilaginous portion of the arch is exposed (Fig. 50).

Step 2. The exposed cartilaginous portion is cut and reflected downward. The attachment of the internal oblique muscle is divided. The transverse abdominal muscle and the diaphragm are separated from the inner surface of the cartilages.

Step 3. The severed cartilages of the eighth, ninth, and tenth ribs are removed, as is also the lower border of the cartilage of the seventh rib.

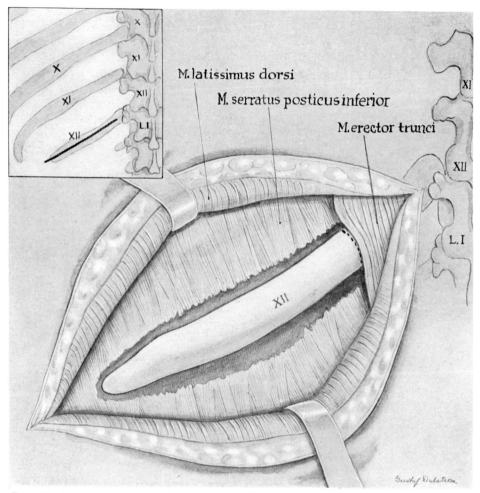

Fig. 52. Extraperitoneal—Extrapleural Subdiaphragmatic Posterior Approach. Clairmont Technic.
Insert.—Skin incision.   Main picture.—The twelfth rib is exposed.

Step 4. The pleura is displaced upward and the diaphragm and peritoneum are opened.

This method gives a better approach than the original Lannelongue procedure.

III. **Extraperitoneal—Extrapleural Anterior Approach to the Dome**

of the Diaphragm or to the Upper Surface of the Liver or Spleen (Clairmont Method).

Technic.

Step 1.   A skin-incision four inches long is made one-half cm. below and parallel to the costal arch. The skin, fascia, external, internal and transverse abdominal muscles are divided.

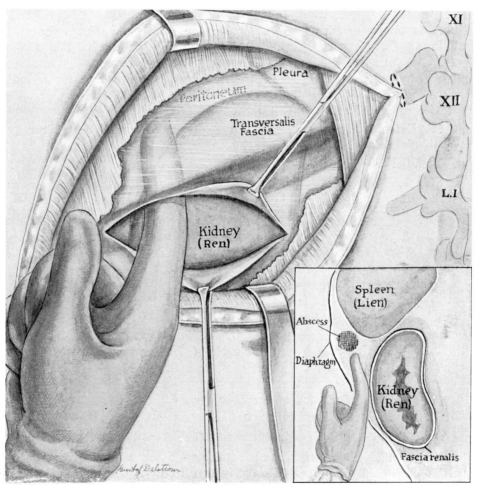

FIG. 53. EXTRAPERITONEAL—EXTRAPLEURAL SUBDIAPHRAGMATIC POSTERIOR APPROACH. CLAIRMONT TECHNIC.
The finger enters through the transversalis fascia and pushes away the peritoneum from the diaphragm.

Step 2.   The finger begins to separate the transversalis fascia and the peritoneum from the superimposed structures in an upward direction until the costal arch is reached; a hook is then placed behind the arch which lifts it, thus facilitating the further separation of the transversalis fascia and peritoneum from the muscular portion of the diaphragm. This is done until the upper surface of the liver or spleen or the dome of the diaphragm is reached (Fig. 51).

This approach is indicated for subphrenic abscess or abscess of the liver or of the spleen.

In case of posterior approach to the dome of the diaphragm this can be done also either by a **transpleural** or **subpleural** method. When it is done below the pleura, the peritoneal cavity may or may not be entered, depending on where the seat of the pathology is located. If it is done for subphrenic abscess or for an abscess of the postero-superior surface of the liver, then the operation may be done not only extrapleurally but also extraperitoneally. It may be done **with resection** of the posterior ribs (subperiosteal resection of the IX or X ribs—**method of Elsberg**), or with resection of the XIIth rib only **(Method of Clairmont).**

IV. **Extraperitoneal, extrapleural Posterior Approach. (Clairmont Method)** (Figs. 52 and 53).

Technic.

Step 1. The skin-incision is made above and along the entire length of the XII rib (Fig. 52, insert).

Step 2. The XII rib is resected subperiosteally.

Step 3. A transverse incision is made through the entire thickness of the muscles at the level of the first lumbar vertebra until the renal fascia is reached (Fig. 53).

[Thus there is no danger, whatsoever, of injuring the pleura].

Step 4. A blunt separation of the renal fascia from the super-imposed structures begins in an upward direction. By going upward the finger separates the transversalis fascia and the peritoneum from the muscle of the diaphragm. This is done until either the dome of the diaphragm is reached, or until the upper surface of the liver is reached, depending on the seat of the pathology (Fig. 53).

METHODS OF OPENING AND CLOSURE OF THE ABDOMEN.

The technic of opening the abdomen varies according to the type of incision employed. We shall describe in detail only a few methods which will serve as examples for the rest.

Right Midrectal Incision.

Step 1. The tip of a sharp-pointed knife is placed at a right angle to the surface of the skin, which is then pierced by pressing the blade downward. As soon as the tip of the knife penetrates the skin, the surgeon immediately feels that the knife is in the fascia. He then changes the direction of the knife to an angle of 45° to the skin, and presses moderately down-

ward cutting through the skin for the desired length of the
incision. Before finishing the incision he turns the knife
again to an angle of 90° to the surface of the skin. [The
reason why we advise starting and finishing the incision
with the knife held perpendicularly to the surface of the
skin is that then **the entire length of the incision is uniformly
deep**; whereas, by keeping the blade constantly at an angle
of 45°, the beginning and end of the incision are not cut deep
enough, and it becomes necessary for the surgeon to deepen
the incision at each end. **This means at least two additional
movements, and it is fundamental in surgical technic not to
make unnecessary movements**].

As soon as the skin-incision is made, this knife is laid aside, and
another is used for the rest of the operation. The reason for doing this is
that it is considered contaminated after cutting through the skin. The
superficial and deep fascia are cut through precisely as described for
incision of the skin.

Step 2.   The bleeding points are clamped with hemostatic forceps,
using small artery-forceps with small jaws, whereby large
masses of tissues will **not** be caught with the blood-vessels.

[**The smaller the amount of tissue which is caught with the blood-
vessel, the less sloughing there will be and the neater the operation**]. In
grasping the blood-vessels we should avoid catching the skin, and this may
be accomplished by keeping the forceps perpendicular to the surface of the
wound.

Step 3.   Towels are attached to the lips of the wound as follows:
The surgeon catches with a tooth of a towel-forceps the skin
of the upper end of the lip on the assistant's side, and with
the other tooth the towel. The towel-forceps is then turned
through 90°, so that it will rest on the assistant's side of
the wound perpendicularly to the length of the wound (Fig.
54, a). The same is done at the lower end of the incision, and
the towel is turned so that it covers the lip of the wound and
the towel-forceps on the assistant's side (Fig. 54, b). The
assistant repeats this procedure on the surgeon's side. When
the towels thus cover the lips of the wound, the surgeon
grasps the two towels at the lower angle of the wound with
a towel-forceps and his assistant does the same at the upper
angle of the wound. The skin should not be caught by these
manipulations; the surgeon covers with a towel the forceps
at the lower end of the wound and the assistant does the
same at the upper end (Fig. 55).

The towels may be attached in a different way: The surgeon attaches the first, and the assistant the second, towel
as described previously; a third towel is then placed so that

it covers the entire wound with its lower edge lying just below the lower end of the wound. With a towel-forceps this end of the towel is attached to the two previously placed towels. Then this towel is lifted from the wound so as to cover the last applied towel-forceps and that portion of the abdomen below the lower end of the wound-incision. The same procedure is repeated with another towel which will

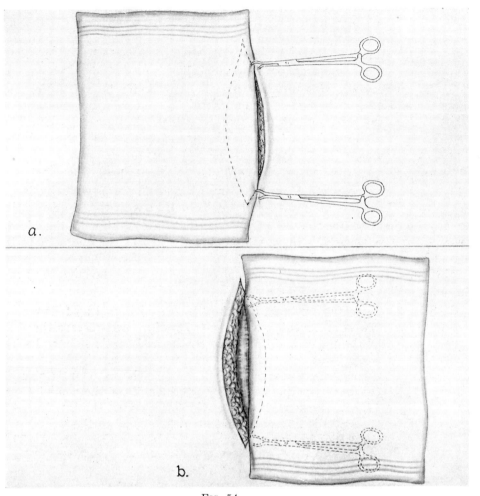

FIG. 54.
a. Fixing the towel on one lip of the wound.
b. The towel covers the towel-clips.

cover the portion of the abdomen above the upper end of the incision. In this way **no instruments are left uncovered** and the wound is walled off from the skin.

Step 4. The anterior sheath of the rectus muscle is incised with a knife for a length of one inch in the center of the intended

incision. This incision is enlarged with **scissors upward and
the knife downward** (Fig. 56).

[The reason why we should **not cut** with the scissors
downward is that in order to do it conveniently, the surgeon
must change the posture of his body and push his assistant,

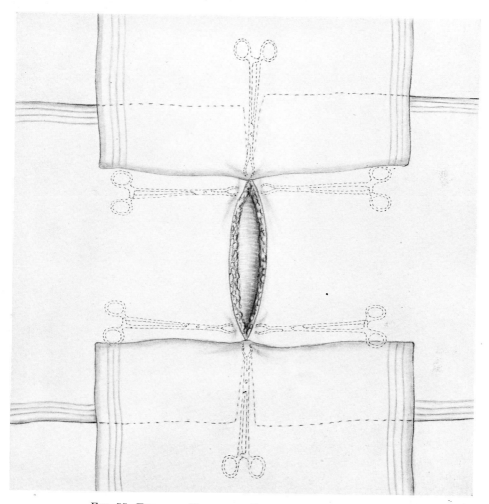

FIG. 55. FIXING A TOWEL ON EACH LIP OF THE WOUND.
Final View.

who is standing at his left hand, aside. As a rule, **the surgeon
should never change the posture of his body.** If he cannot
accomplish a maneuver with his right hand in a normal erect
posture, he should, instead of changing the posture of his
body, either execute this movement by changing hands, that
is, do it with his left hand; or, if he cannot do it with his left

hand, then he should change the instrument]. The length of the anterior sheath-incision should be one quarter of an inch shorter at each end than the skin-incision. After the anterior sheath of the rectus muscle is incised, the muscle-fibers are split with the handle of the knife for a distance which will allow the index-finger of the left hand to enter

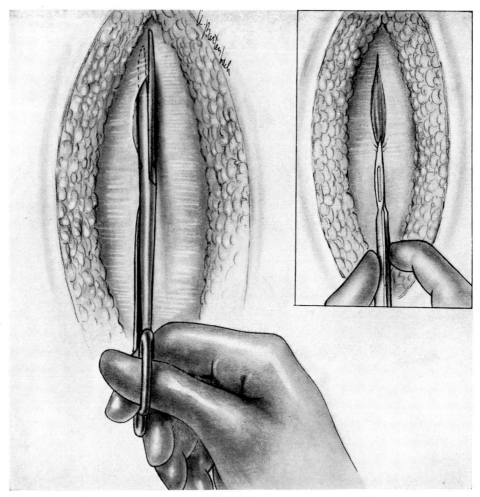

FIG. 56.
MAIN PICTURE. Cutting the anterior sheath of the rectus muscle by scissors in an upward direction.
INSERT. Cutting the anterior sheath by a knife in a downward direction.

the opening made by the split muscle (Fig. 57). This finger is separated from the handle of the knife for a distance of about two inches. The knife is then laid aside and the index-fingers of each hand are then separated from each other, thus splitting the muscles along the entire length of the incision (Fig. 58). All divided blood-vessels are tied.

[We have already spoken of the various methods of tying. There is one suggestion which we would like to offer at this time. Frequently there is a difference of opinion between the surgeon and his assistant as to whether the thread should be cut long or short. In order to avoid these misunderstand-

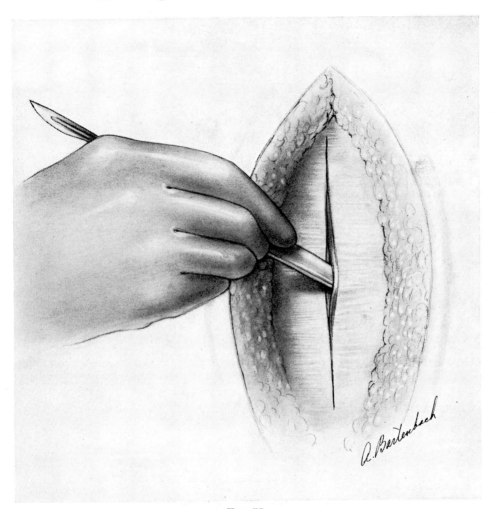

FIG. 57.
The muscle is split by the handle of the knife.

ings in the operating-room, it is well for the surgeon to arrange beforehand with his assistant to cut the thread immediately above the tissue-forceps which are placed by the surgeon at the proper point (Fig. 58, insert)].

Step 5. The surgeon grasps the posterior sheath (with the transversalis fascia and the peritoneum) by surgical tissue-forceps, and the assistant also grasps it one inch away. With the thumb and index-finger the surgeon feels whether any visceral structures are adherent to the peritoneum. If they are not, he then makes with the knife a small opening in it. The edges of this opening are then caught by the

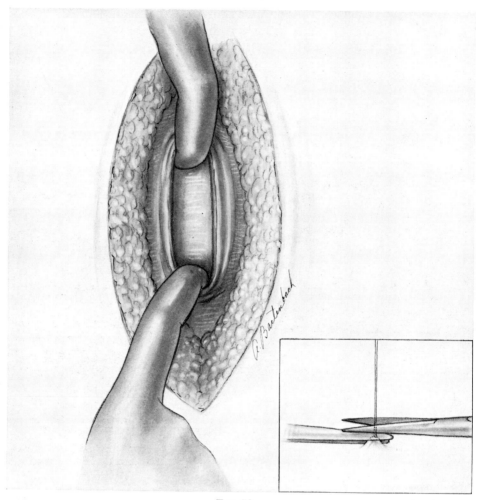

FIG. 58.
MAIN PICTURE. The muscle is split by the index-finger of each hand.
INSERT. Cutting the thread above a tissue-forceps.

surgeon with an artery-forceps on the assistant's side, and by the assistant on the surgeon's side. Stretching the peritoneum with these forceps, **the latter is cut by scissors upward (Fig. 59) and by the knife downward.** The length of the incision should be a quarter of an inch shorter at each end than that in the muscle. To avoid unnecessary trauma-

tism of the peritoneum the artery-forceps which grasp it
are then removed. [**The reason for making the incision in
each subsequent layer a little shorter than in the superim-**

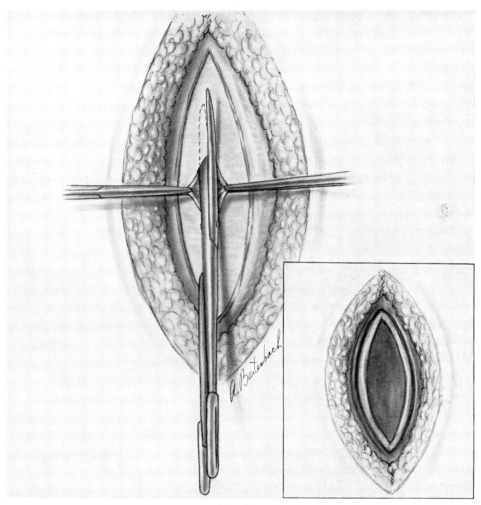

FIG. 59.

MAIN PICTURE. Incising the peritoneum.
INSERT. Showing each deeper layer slightly shorter than the more superficial layer.

posed one is that it is easier then to close the abdomen
(Fig. 59, insert)].

CLOSURE OF THE ABDOMEN.

The closure of the abdomen as practised today is also a process of
surgical evolution. In pre-antiseptic days closure by needle and thread,
although known, was not frequently used. At that time, the surgeons
preferred to use adhesive tape to bind together the lips of the abdominal

wound. None of the layers situated beneath the skin were actually brought together. The reason for this was threefold:

1. The surgeons were afraid to use bloody union methods (needle and thread) because of the danger of piercing the bowel;
2. Adhesive tape could be changed quite frequently; thereby the pus could be evacuated (and in pre-antiseptic days pus was the rule and not the exception);
3. The surgeons believed that in case of increased intra-abdominal pressure, produced by coughing, meteorism, etc., adhesive tape offered greater resistance than suture-material.

However, in the beginning of the Nineteenth Century (1817), Nicolaus Meyer was already teaching closure of the skin by suture and reinforcing this suture by adhesive tape. The peritoneum, muscles and fascia were still not approximated and fixed to each other. Schenk, in 1823, suggested, in the case of a thin abdominal wall, sewing the lips together by a suture penetrating **the entire thickness of the abdominal wall including the peritoneum.** In the fourth decade of the Nineteenth Century, closure by suture was generally employed. Yet the surgeons used a suture penetrating the entire thickness of the abdominal wall except the peritoneum, **which was not sutured at all.** Credé was one of the leading exponents of this type of suturing. The next step in the development of the closure-technic was to close the peritoneum partially and then reinforce this by a suture passing through the entire thickness of the abdominal wall except the peritoneum (Schultze, 1862). About the same time some surgeons began to use the above mentioned suggestion of Schenk by employing sutures which penetrated the entire thickness of the anterior abdominal wall (Spencer Wells, 1859; Gurlt, 1862). For the suture material they used silk, steel-wire (Eisendrahtnahte), silverwire, catgut (plain or chromic), silkworm-gut, or fishgut. The closure was usually done by interrupted sutures.

Czerny, in 1880, was already employing the technic of suturing in two layers:

Deep, which included the peritoneum, transversalis fascia, and the transversus abdominis and internal oblique muscles, and **superficial,** which included the external oblique muscle and the skin.

Billroth, in 1884, introduced suturing of the abdomen in three layers: **Deep,** the peritoneum only, **next,** the muscles, and, **superficially,** a continuous skin-suture.

Bogaewsky, in 1896, introduced three layers of a continuous suture with the same uninterrupted thread, the first layer, the peritoneum, the second, the muscles with their sheaths (or fascia, if suturing the lateral muscles of the abdomen), and the skin. He used only absorbable material.

Koeberlé was the first who emphasized the importance of suturing the fascia. He sutured it as a separate layer. In the United States, W. Gill Wylie, in 1887, emphasized the importance of suturing the fascia.

Hegar, in 1878, suggested the following suture: A bite is taken through the skin at the edge of the incision. Then a bite through the entire thickness of the abdomen, except the skin and peritoneum, half an inch away from the line of the incision on the same side. Then a bite through the peritoneum at the edge of the incision of the same side. The reverse is then done on the other side. In this way the skin and peritoneum of one lip were closely approximated to the skin and peritoneum of the other lip, and the muscles and fascia of the abdominal wall were enveloped between the skin and peritoneum of each lip.

Kehrer, in 1894, used the figure-of-eight stich; a bite was taken through the skin of one side, through the anterior and posterior sheaths and peritoneum of the other side, through the peritoneum, posterior and anterior sheaths of the first side, and through the skin on the other side. No muscles were caught in the suture, and the stitches were later removed.

Edebohls, in 1896, sutured the abdominal wall in four layers:

1. Peritoneum and posterior sheath.
2. Recti muscles.
3. Anterior sheath.
4. Skin.

Kosman, in 1895, emphasized the importance of mere approximation, and not strangulation of the tissues by tight ligation.

Kendal Franks introduced the employment of subdermal sutures, and Pozzi improved the technic of its execution.

Kehrer, in 1887, was the first to spread the omentum over the abdominal cavity after he performed Cesarean section. Jesset, in 1891, advocated this procedure as a routine technic for all abdominal operations.

Laroyenne, in 1895, advocated fixing the omentum by its lower angles to the posterior abdominal wall.

TECHNIC OF CLOSURE.

Today, the essentials of closure are fairly standardized, but there are still many variations in details as used by different surgeons. The method as used in our work is as follows:

We suture the wall in four layers:

1. The **peritoneum** with the posterior sheath are closed with chromic catgut No. 1, by interrupted or continuous suture.
   In case of interrupted sutures, the distance between the successive bites is one-half of an inch.
2. The **muscles** are closed by interrupted sutures (plain catgut No. 1). The distance between the bites is one inch.
3. The **fascia** (anterior sheath) is closed with chromic catgut No. 2, single or No. 1 double thread, interrupted. The distance between the bites is one-half inch.
4. The **skin** is closed by interrupted horsehair or dermal sutures. The distance between the bites is one-half inch.

In fat patients, and in case large incisions have been made, we place three "tension-sutures" of silkwormgut. These sutures penetrate the entire thickness of the abdominal wall except the peritoneum, and are placed immediately after the peritoneum is sutured, but are not tied until the skin-sutures are introduced.

Step 1. The peritoneum and the posterior sheath of the rectus abdominis muscle are caught in four places—at the upper angle, at the middle of the right lip, at the middle of the

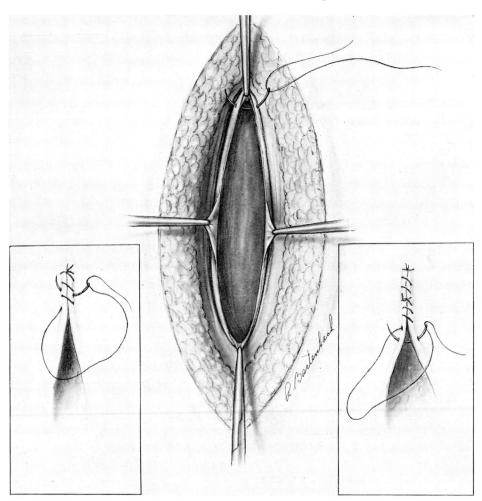

FIG. 60. CLOSURE OF THE PERITONEUM.

left lip, and at the lower angle (Fig. 60). [It is important that the posterior sheath of the rectus muscle be caught with the peritoneum, because, if this sheath is not included, then it is possible, that the most important layer, namely the transversalis fascia which lies between the posterior sheath and the peritoneum, and which is an important factor in the prevention of the development of ventral hernia, will not be

sutured]. The forceps is lifted at the upper end, and with
a curved round needle the suturing is begun from the upper
to the lower end. The bites of the needle should be made
in the direction from the lip of the assistant's side to that
of the surgeon's side. The sutures are continuous or interrupted, and, if continuous, are locked at each third stitch

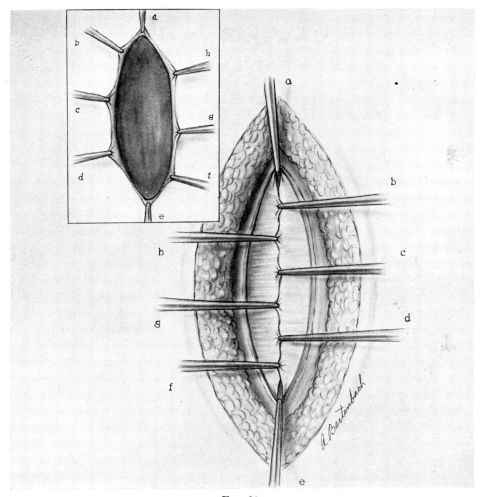

FIG. 61.
INSERT. Grasping the lips of the peritoneum.
MAIN PICTURE. Throwing the clamps across the incision.

(Fig. 60, right lower insert). Each bite is made one-quarter
of an inch away from the other for the first and second
stitches, and one eighth of an inch for each third stitch, which
should be locked. [In this way, we prevent extensive puckering of the peritoneum due to the locking of the stitch].

While suturing, the thread is kept at a moderate tension. The lock-stitch is made by holding the thread in front of the penetrating needle (Fig. 60, right insert), whereby there will be eliminated an extra movement for locking. [Instead of locking each third stitch, we may use each fourth stitch as a **back-stitch**, namely, inserting it just a little

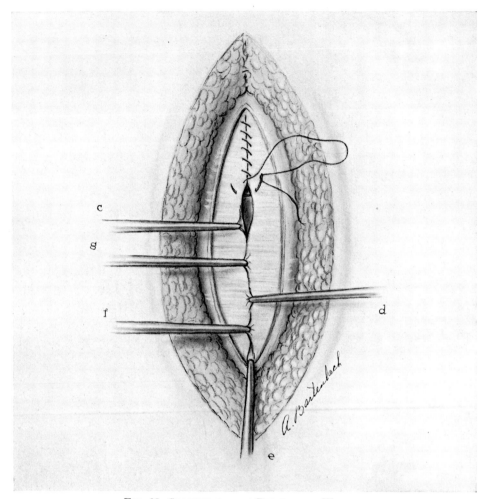

FIG. 62. CLOSURE OF THE PERITONEAL WOUND.

proximal to the point of exit of the third stitch (Fig. 60, left lower insert). **This avoids puckering. We always prefer a back-stitch to a lock-stitch].** When the entire peritoneum is sutured, the free end of the thread is tied to the double thread which is attached to the needle. [N. B. In our discussion, we assume that the surgeon is standing at the lower end of the wound. It is always natural and convenient to

begin suturing from the farthest to the nearest end of the
incision. For this reason, the surgeon begins suturing from
the upper or lower end of the incision depending upon the
place where he stands].

If the bowels protrude and it is difficult to suture the peritoneum, the following maneuvre may be useful: A laparo-

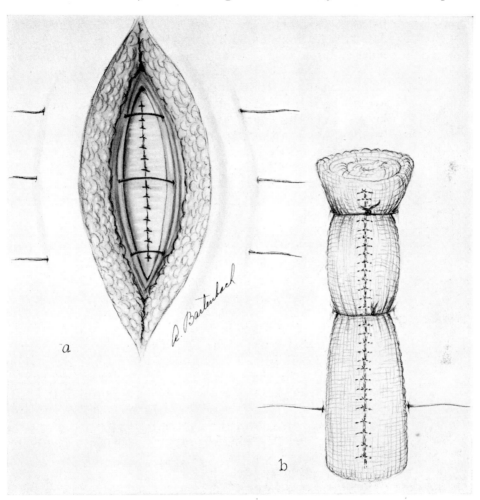

FIG. 63.
a. Tension-sutures are in place.
b. Tying the tension-sutures over a roll of gauze.

tomy sponge is placed in the abdomen. The peritoneum instead of being grasped by four artery-forceps, as previously described, is grasped alternately by six or eight artery-
forceps, depending upon the size of the incision (Fig. 61,
insert). Then, these alternate artery-clamps, are thrown over
the wound (Fig. 61); by this maneuvre the wound is tem-

porarily closed. The suturing begins at one end, and when the part thus temporarily closed, is reached, the forceps closest to the sutured portion is thrown back. This opens a small part of the wound which should be sutured. This procedure of throwing back each clamp as reached is continued until the entire wound is closed (Fig. 62). **[The surgeon must not forget to remove the laparotomy sponge before the peritoneum is closed]**.

Step 2. After the peritoneum, with the posterior sheath of the rectus muscle, is sutured, the split muscles are sewed by interrupted sutures which are placed at a distance of one inch from each other. Only small bites of the muscle are taken and these sutures are not tied tightly **but just enough to keep the muscles approximated.** [In the case of fat or stout persons, or when there is difficulty in suturing the peritoneum, tension-sutures are useful. These act as splints, and are placed before the muscles are sutured together. They are inserted at a distance of two inches apart and also two inches from the skin-edges, and include the entire thickness of the abdominal wall with the exception of the peritoneum and posterior sheath; in this way, the thread includes the **entire width of the rectus muscle.** They are not tied at this time, but artery-forceps are attached to each end (Fig. 63, a). Some surgeons place the tension-sutures in front of, instead of behind, the rectus muscle]. After the muscle is sutured, the skin is well retracted, and the anterior sheath of the rectus muscle is grasped by two forceps, one at the upper and the other at the lower angle. [Occasionally, it may be necessary to add a third and fourth artery-forceps in the middle of each lip]. The sheath is sutured in the same manner as the peritoneum. After the anterior sheath is closed the skin (together with the deep and superficial fascia) is sutured. Occasionally, we suture the superficial and the deep fascia separately from the skin. The latter can be closed either by an over-and-over continuous suture (**Glover suture,** Fig. 27, b), by a continuous buttonhole suture (**Heister suture,** Fig. 28), by plain interrupted sutures (Fig. 27, a), or by metallic clips **(Michel clips).** We usually use a vertical mattress-suture or Michel clips. After the skin is sutured, a strip of gauze is placed on the wound and the tension-sutures are tied (Fig. 63, b).

Opening and Closure of the Paramedian Incision.

This incision was introduced with the intention of having an **unaltered muscle interposed** between the longitudinal incision of the posterior sheath and peritoneum behind the muscle and the anterior sheath in front of the muscle. We will take as an example an incision in the epigastric region. The same technic may be employed in the case of a hypo-gastric incision.

Step 1. A midline incision is made from the ensiform process down to the umbilicus. If it is necessary to enlarge this incision, it is continued downward in a semicircular manner to the left

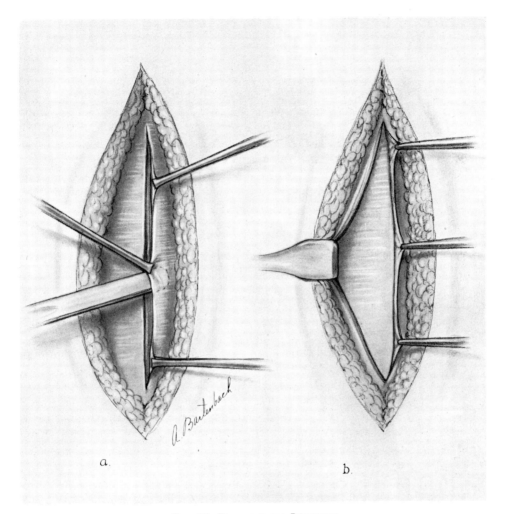

FIG. 64. PARAMEDIAN INCISION.
a. Anterior sheath is incised.
b. The muscle is separated from the sheath and retracted laterally.

of the umbilicus. This incision should pass through the skin, superficial and deep fascia.

Step 2. The skin is reflected laterally for an inch, and the anterior sheath of the rectus muscle is incised.

Step 3. The inner lip of the aponeurosis is grasped by artery-forceps in three places and separated from the rectus muscle (Fig. 64, a).

Step 4. The rectus muscle is retracted laterally (Fig. 64, b).

Step 5. The posterior sheath and peritoneum are cut in the same sagittal plane as the anterior sheath.

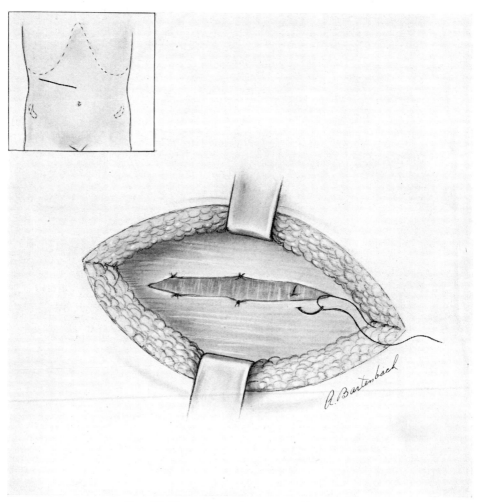

FIG. 65. TRANSVERSE ABDOMINAL INCISION.

INSERT.—Skin incision.

MAIN PICTURE.—Anterior sheath is cut transversely; each lip is sutured to the muscle.

The **closure** of the paramedian incision is the same as has beeen described in closure of the midrectal incision, with this difference only, that in the latter procedure the portions of the split muscle are sutured together. This of course is not done in the case of a paramedian incision.

TRANSVERSE ABDOMINAL INCISIONS.

As an example of a transverse abdominal incision, we will describe one for exposure of the gall-bladder. The skin-incision is made from the lower end of the right costal arch medially to the midline.

Step 1. The skin, superficial and deep fascia are divided (Fig. 65, insert).

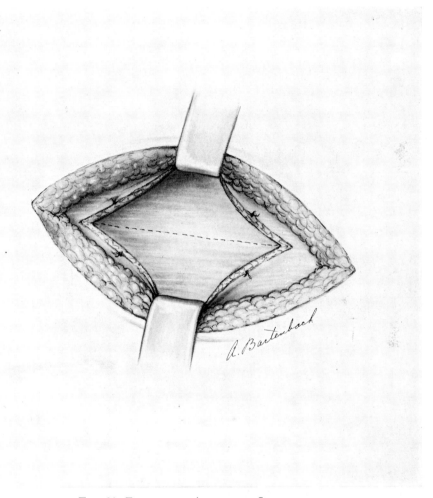

FIG. 66. TRANSVERSE ABDOMINAL INCISION.
The muscle is cut transversely; line of incision in the peritoneum.

Step 2. The anterior sheath of the rectus muscle is cut transversely (Fig. 65).

Step 3. Each lip of the divided anterior sheath is sutured to the muscle at three places (Fig. 65). It is not necessary to include in the bite the entire thickness of the muscle, but just enough to prevent retraction of the fibers after division of the muscle.

[**Alternative Method.**—As soon as Step 1 is completed, a very short longitudinal incision is made along the lateral border of the rectus muscle, two artery-clamps are applied across the muscle, and the latter with its anterior sheath is cut between these forceps].

Step 4. The rectus muscle is cut transversely (Fig. 66).

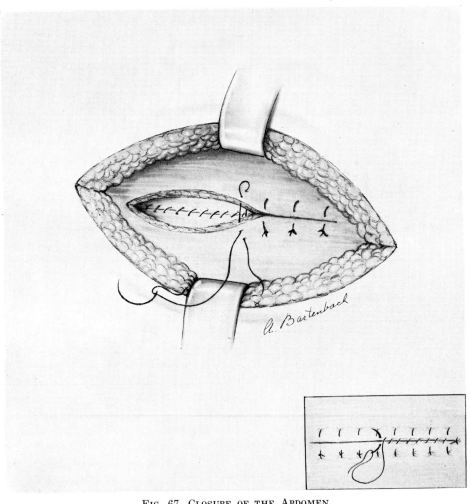

FIG. 67. CLOSURE OF THE ABDOMEN.
MAIN PICTURE.—The peritoneum is closed; suturing of the muscle by interrupted vertical mattress-sutures.
INSERT. Closing of the anterior sheath.

Step 5. The posterior sheath and peritoneum are cut transversely (Fig. 66).

CLOSURE OF THE TRANSVERSE ABDOMINAL INCISION.

Step 1. The peritoneum, with the posterior sheath of the rectus muscle, is grasped at four places with artery-forceps—at the lateral angle, at the medial angle, and at the middle of the upper and lower lips. A continuous suture is made from the medial to the lateral angle (Fig. 67).

Step 2. The upper part of the divided rectus muscle is sutured to the lower part by three interrupted vertical mattress-sutures, as follows: The suture enters the anterior sheath of the rectus muscle and passes through the muscle itself at a distance of one-half inch from the cut edge of the lower lip. Then it penetrates the upper lip in the opposite direction passing through the muscle and the anterior sheath and emerging at a distance of half an inch from the cut edge of the upper lip. Then reversing, it penetrates the upper lip through the edge of the anterior sheath only and then through the edge of the anterior sheath of the lower lip. In this way a **vertical mattress-suture** is placed. Several such vertical mattress-sutures are inserted and tied (Fig. 67). A few superficial sutures are inserted, connecting the lips of the anterior sheath between these mattress-sutures (Fig. 67, lower insert).

Step 3. The skin is sutured by any of the previously described methods.

COMBINATION ABDOMINAL INCISION.

McBurney (Gridiron) Incision.

At the junction of the lateral and middle third of an imaginary line connecting the anterior superior iliac spine and the umbilicus, a perpendicular line is drawn downward and medially for about one and a half inches and upward and laterally for one inch. (Fig. 68, left upper insert). Thus, this incision is about two and a half inches long. Its lower end reaches the lateral border of the rectus muscle. The skin, superficial and deep fascia are divided. The fibers of the external oblique muscle are split and the aponeurosis of this muscle is cut (Fig. 68, a). The fibers of the split muscle and of the incised aponeurosis are retracted. The internal oblique muscle will then come into view (Fig. 68, a). This muscle is split in the direction of its fibers, and the split muscle is separated by retractors (Fig. 68, b). The transversus abdominis muscle will then come into view. Its fibers run horizontally, perpendicularly to the long axis of the body. It is split, and the transversalis fascia and peritoneum are cut as a single layer by the method which is already described for opening the peritoneum at any other place in the body. **The transversalis fascia and peritoneum should be opened in a transverse direction.**

Closure of the Abdomen in a "Gridiron" Incision.

Step 1.   The lateral angle of the peritoneum and transversalis fascia is grasped by one artery-forceps and the medial angle by another. The suturing starts at the medial angle and runs to the lateral angle.

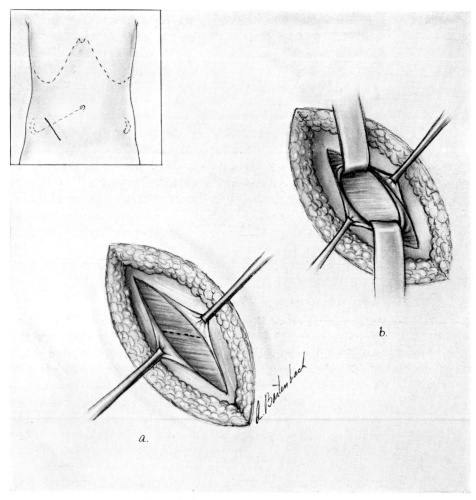

FIG. 68. McBURNEY INCISION.
INSERT. Skin incision.
a. Aponeurosis of the external oblique muscle is cut and retracted.
b. The internal oblique muscle is cut; the transversalis fascia is exposed.

Step 2.   The internal oblique muscle is closed by two or three interrupted sutures.

Step 3.   The external oblique muscle and aponeurosis are closed by a continuous suture or by interrupted sutures.

Step 4.   The skin is closed as described above.

[**Remarks:** In dealing with a "clean case", all the layers may be closed either by a continuous or by interrupted sutures. In the case of a gangrenous appendix or in any "pus case", it is always better to close by series of interrupted sutures.]

For suturing the peritoneum, we use chromic catgut No. 1 single; for suturing the muscles, plain catgut No. 1 single; for suturing the anterior sheath of the rectus muscle, chromic catgut No. 1 double (20-day), or No. 2 single; for suturing the skin, horsehair or dermal; for tension-sutures, we use silkworm gut.

Removal of Sutures.

We remove the tension-sutures on the eighth day and the skin-sutures on the ninth day.

III. COSMETIC CONSIDERATIONS.

Although the cosmetic considerations in making a skin-incision on the abdominal wall are not of such importance as on exposed parts of the body, such as the neck or face, nevertheless it is desirable to make the incision in such a manner that it shall not leave noticeable scars. This can be best accomplished by making the skin-incisions along the fissure-lines of Langer.

IV. PSYCHOLOGICAL CONSIDERATIONS.

In some cases, the surgeon is confronted with a dilemma as to whether he is dealing with a right-sided pelvic condition or with a case of appendicitis. Although, from the surgical standpoint it is best under such circumstances to make a low midline incision, which can be used both for exploratory and for operative purposes, nevertheless **in case of a young unmarried woman,** it will be psychologically more correct to make a right pararectus incision. Cases are known, in which low midline incisions in young unmarried women were the causes of a subsequent marital rift.

BIBLIOGRAPHY.

ABDOMINAL INCISIONS.

G. Abel. Ueber Bauchnaht und Bauchnarbenbrüche.
Arch. für Gynäkologie, 56:656-750; y. 1898.

Amann. Zur Bauchdeckennaht.
Zbl. für Gynäk, 2:894-895; y. 1903.

P. Assmy. Ueber den Einfluss der Durchtrennung motorischer Nerven auf die Narbenbildung bei extramedianen Bauchschnitten.
Bruns Beiträge zur klinischen Chirurgie, 23:109-125; y. 1899.

G. Baggio. La Mc.Burney transformata in incisione a lembi.
Policlinico (sez. prat.) 39:445-447; y. 1932.

W. Bartlett & W. Bartlett. The transverse incision in the upper abdomen.
Surg. Gyn. Obst. 57:93-99; y. 1933.

Battle. Modified incision for removal of the vermiform appendix.
    Brit. Med. Journ. 11:1360; y. 1895.

A. D. Bevan. Abdominal incisions and their closure.
    Annals of Surgery, 96:555-575; y. 1932.

A. D. Bevan. On the surgical anatomy of the bile-ducts and a new incision
    for their exposure.
    Annals of Surg. 30:17-27; y. 1899.

Canniot. De la résection du bord inférieur du thorax pour aborder la face
    convexe du foie.
    Thèse de Paris, 1891.

P. Clairmont & E. Ranzi. Kasuistischer Beitrag zur operativen Behand-
    lung des subphrenischen Absczesses.
    Wien. klin. Wchnschr. 18:653-657; y. 1905.

R. Colp. Disruption of abdominal wounds.
    Ann. of Surg. 99:14-27; y. 1934.

H. Costantini & R. Marill. Sur les avantages de la dissociation musculaire
    élargie dans la chirurgie des flancs.
    Rev. de Chir. 53:497-510; y. 1934.

H. Costantini. La thoraco-phreno-laparotomie sans pneumothorax.
    La Presse Médicale. 33:1107-1108; y. 1925.

R. Danis & R. Loicq. Les incisions transversales franches de l'abdomen.
    Arch. franco-belges de chir. 31:532-537; y. 1928.

L. Dartigues. De l'incision cruciale et de la suture transversale sus-
    pubienne cachée par les poils dans la laparotomie médiane.
    Presse Médicale, 7:202-204; y. 1899.

F. Davies & C. P. G. Wakeley. Abdominal incisions in the light of recent
    work on the intercostal nerves.
    Australian and New Zealand Journ. of Surg. 2:381-391; y. 1933.

J. W. Davies. Abdominal and pelvic fascias with surgical applications.
    Surg. Gyn. & Obst. 54:495-504; y. 1932.

Gwillym G. Davis. A transverse incision for the removal of the appendix.
    Annals of Surg. 43:106-110; y. 1906.

J. S. Davis. The on-end or vertical mattress-suture.
    Ann. Surg. 98:941-951; y. 1933.

C. Davison. The technique of closure of wounds by removable continuous
    suture.
    Surg. Gyn. Obst. 2:92-101; y. 1906.

P. Descomps. L'appendicectomie rétro-colique.
    Rev. de Chir. 59:20-29; y. 1921.

H. L. Devine. Abdominal technique—a system of operative exposures.
    Surg. Gyn. & Obst. 50:455-467; y. 1930.

Don. Incisions for operations on the upper abdominal organs.
Brit. Med. Journ. 1:652-654; y. 1909.

L. Drűner. Der bogenförmige Bauchschnitt in Epigastrium.
Zbl. f. Chir. 41:841-846; y. 1914.

L. Drűner. Studien über die vorderen Bauchwandnerven und über die Bauchschnitte.
Bruns. Beitr. z. Klin. Chir. 124:583-606; y. 1921.

L. Drűner. Ueber die Durchschneidung des Rectus bei Bauchschnitten.
Zbl. f. Chir. 48:404-405; y. 1921.

L. Drűner. Über die pararektale Laparotomie.
Zbl. f. Chir. 61:1880-1883; y. 1934.

J. W. Elliot. A modification of the McBurney incision for appendectomy.
Bost. Med. & Surg. Journ. 135:433-434; y. 1896.

G. Elsberg. A contribution to the pathology, diagnosis, and treatment of subphrenic abscesses after appendicitis.
Ann. Surg. 34:729-752; y. 1901.

Esau. Experimentelle und histologische Beiträge zur Frage der Aponeurosennaht bei Laparotomien.
Deutsch. Zeitschr. f. Chir. 98:487-493; y. 1909.

E. H. Fiske & H. E. Rhame. New incisional approach to the appendix.
Am. Journ. Surg. 25:19-25; y. 1934.

G. R. Fowler. A new improved method of entering the abdominal cavity in the ileocecal region, with special reference to the removal of the vermiform appendix.
The Medical News, 76:321-324; y. 1900.

R. H. Fowler. The modified McBurney incision.
Surg. Gyn. & Obst. 14:190-192; y. 1912.

G. A. Garlucci. Abdominal-wall defects following appendicectomy.
Ann. Surg. 100:1177-1183; y. 1934.

D. T. Gilliam. A coaptation and imbricating suture for closing the abdominal incision.
Surg. Gyn. & Obst. 8:95-96; y. 1909.

R. V. Grace. Disruption of abdominal wounds.
Ann. of Surg. 99:28-33; y. 1934.

O. Hagen-Torn. Zur Frage über die Mittel zur Vorbeugung von Hernien nach Laparotomien.
Zbl. f. Chir. 11:577-578; y. 1884.

F. B. Harrington. Hernia following operations for appendicitis.
Boston Med. & Surg. Jour. 141:105-108; y. 1899.

F. B. Harrington. Choice of method of opening the abdomen in appendicitis.
Boston Med. & Surg Jour. 152:342-344; y. 1905.

H. F. O. Haberland. Versenkte Hautnaht.
   Zbl. f. Chir. 60:2504-2506; y. 1933.

F. Härtel. Retroperitoneale Operationen und hinterer Bauchschnitt.
   Arch. f. klin. Chir. 167:426-437; y. 1931.

Heusner. Ueber die Anlegung der Schnitte bei den Bauchoperationen.
   Münch. med. Wochenschr. 53:693-695; y. 1906.

C. G. Heyd. Disruption of abdominal wounds.
   Ann. Surg. 99:39-46; y. 1934.

John Hull. A defense of the cesarean operation, with observations on embryulcia, and the section of the symphysis pubis.
   Manchester, 1799.

E. Jaeggy. A propos de la taille hypogastrique transversale.
   Arch. des maladies des reins et des organes génito-urinaires. 5:383-387; y. 1930.

Jalaguier. Appendicite à rechute. Excision de l'appendice pendant une periode de calme. Guérison.
   Bull. et Mémoires de la Société de Chirurg. de Paris, 18:349-350:1892.

E. Juvara. L'incision transversale de la paroi abdominale, l'incision de Sprengel, pour les operations dans les hypocondres (foie, voies biliaires, pylore, duodénum, pancréas, rate, etc).
   Bull. et mém. Soc. nat. de Chir. 56:1019-1028; y. 1930.

F. Kammerer. A modified incision at the outer border of the rectus muscle for appendicitis.
   Medical Record, 52:837-839; y. 1897.

W. Kausch. Ueber physiologische Bauchschnitte.
   Arch. f. klin. Chir. 114:969-981; y. 1920.

F. A. Kehrer. Bauchnaht bei Laparotomien.
   Zbl. f. Gyn. 20:1122-1126; y. 1896.

J. W. Kennedy. Tragedies of the abdominal incisions.
   Am. Journ. Surg. 25:512-520; y. 1934.

Kirschner & Melzner. Betrachtungen über die zwei—und dreischichtige Naht des Bauchdeckenschnittes in der Mittellinie.
   Deutsche Zeitschr. f. Chir. 200:410-427; y. 1927.

F. König. Über die Schnittführung bei Operationen an den Gallenwegen.
   Zbl. f. Chir. 39:529-534; y. 1912.

A. Krecke. Seide oder Katgut?
   Münch. Med. Wchnschr. 80:598-600; y. 1933.

O. Küstner. Der suprasymphysäre Kreuzschnitt, eine Methode der Coeliotomie bei wenig umfänglichen Affectionen der weiblichen Beckenorgane.
   Monatsschr. f. Geb. u. Gyn. 2:197; y. 1896.

C. Langer. Zur Anatomie und Physiologie der Haut.
Sitzungsberichte der Kaiserl. Akademie der Wissenschaften (in Wien) ; y. 1861.

Lannelongue. Les abscès tuberculeux périhepatiques et leur traitement.
La Semaine Médicale. 7:235; y. 1887.

P. Lecène. L'incision postérieure sus-iliaque dans certaines formes d'appendicite.
Journ. de Chirurgie. 19:459-468; y. 1922.

F. Léjars. Les suppurations de la zone sous-phrénique.
La Semaine Médicale; 22:97-103; y. 1902.

K. Lennander. Ueber den Bauchschnitt durch eine Rectusscheide mit Verschiebung des medialen oder lateralen Randes des Musculus rectus.
Zbl. f. Chir. 25:90-94; y. 1898.

M. Linnartz. Zur Schnittführung bei Gallenstein und Magenoperationen auf Grund der Erfahrung an 500 Gallensteinfällen.
Zbl. f. Chir. 47:1194-1198; y. 1920.

K. Logothetopulos. Erleichterung der Appendektomie bei Längs—und Querschnitt und Vereinfachung der Eröffnung des Peritoneums.
Zbl. f. Gynäk. 57:878-879; y. 1933.

G. Marwedel. Die Aufklappung des Rippenbogens zur Erleichterung operativer Eingriffe im Hypochondrium und im Zwerchfellkuppelraum.
Zbl. f. Chir. 30:938-941; y. 1903.

T. Mason. A new abdominal incision.
Trans. South. Surg. Assoc. 41:120; y. 1928: also in Arch. of Surg. 19:129-142; y. 1929.

E. Maylard. Direction of abdominal incisions.
Brit. Med. Journ. 11:895-903; y. 1907.

L. L. McArthur. Choice of incisions of abdominal wall; especially for appendicitis.
Chicago Med. Recorder, 7:289-292; y. 1894.

C. McBurney. The incision made in the abdominal wall in cases of appendicitis with a description of a new method of operating.
Annals of Surgery, 20:38-43; y. 1894.

R. M. McMillen. A New Suture.
West Virginia Medic. Journ. vol. 4:90; y. 1909.

R. W. McNealy. Viscera retainer.
Journ. Amer. Med. Assn. 105: 1759-1760; y. 1935.

F. L. Meleney & E. L. Howes. The disruption of abdominal wounds with the protrusion of viscera.
Ann. Surg. 99:5-13; y. 1934.

A. Melnikoff. Die chirurgischen Zugänge durch den unteren Rand des Brustkorbes zu den Organen des Subdiaphragmalen Raumes.
Deutsche Zeitschr. f. Chirurgie 182:83-152; y. 1923.

K. Mermingas. Der Lumbalschnitt bei der Appendektomie.
Zbl. f. Chir. 58:706-708; y. 1931.

K. Mermingas. Ueber ein einfaches Mittel zur Entspannung der Bauchwand bei der Bauchdeckennaht.
Zbl. f. Chir. 58:1771-1772; y. 1931.

Willy Meyer. The additional posterior incision in certain cases of operation for the inflammed retrocecal appendix.
Ann. of Surg. 80:511-518; y. 1924.

A. Moschcowitz. Transverse incisions in the upper abdomen.
Annals of Surg. 64:268-289; y. 1916.

K. Nather. Der prä-oder retroperitoneale Weg zum subphrenischen Abscess als typische Operation.
Arch. f. klin. Chir. 122:24-99; y. 1925.

W. Noetzel. Shonende Bauchschnitte.
Arch. f. klin. Chir. 158:456-471; y. 1930.

A. Ochsner & A. Graves. Subphrenic abscess.
Annals of Surg. 98:961-990; y. 1933.

T. Ohsawa. Über die freie ventro-arco-diaphragmale Thorakolaparotomie bzw. Laparothorakotomie.
Zbl. f. Chir. 57:2467-2472; y. 1930.

G. Perthes. Zur Erleichterung der Naht bei queren Bauchschnitt.
Zbl. f. Chir. 39:1249-1252; y. 1912.

G. Perthes. Zur Schnittführung bei Operationen an den Gallenwegen.
Zbl. f. Chir. 39:1252-1256; y. 1912.

J. Pfannenstiel. Ueber die Vortheile des suprasymphysären Fascienquerschnitts für die gynäkologischen Koeliotomien, zugleich, ein Beitrag zu der Indikationsstellung der Operationswege.
Volkmann's klin. Vorträge, Gynäkologie, Neue Folge, No. 268:1735; y. 1900. (No. 97 Gynäk.).

J. Pfannenstiel. Weitere Erfahrungen über den suprasymphysären Fascienquerschnitt.
Verhandl. d. Deutsch. Gessel. f. Gyn. Zbl. f. Gynäk. 25:731; y. 1901.

C. Pochhammer. Ein physiologischer Bauchdeckenschnitt für die Operationen an der Gallenblase und den Gallenwegen.
Zbl. f. Chir. 45:923-927; y. 1918.

E. H. Pool. The "Zipper stitch" for upper abdominal incisions.
Am. Journ. of Surg. 13:225-226; y. 1931.

V. M. Popovici. L'innervation du muscle grand droit el les incisions de la

paroi abdominale. Les intersections aponévrotiques.
Lyon Chir. 30:145-162; y. 1933.

B. O. Pribram. Zur Technik des Costalschnittes bei Gallenoperationen.
Zbl. f. Chir. 61:1603-1604; y. 1934.

M. R. Reid, M. M. Zinninger & P. Merrell. Closure of the abdomen with through-and-through silver wire sutures in cases of acute abdominal emergencies.
Ann. Surg. 98:890-896; y. 1933.

A. Rockey. Transverse incision in abdominal operations.
Med. Record. 68:779-780; y. 1905.

P. J. Sarma. Anterior abdominal incision.
Intern. Clin. 4:163-196; y. 1929.

E. P. Sloan. Abdominal Incisions.
Am. J. Obst. & Gyn. 23:226-232; y. 1932.

G. A. Sloan. A new upper abdominal incision.
Surg. Gyn. & Obs. 45:678-687; y. 1927.

Sprengel. Kritische Betrachtungen über Bauchdeckennaht und Bauchschnitt.
Arch. f. klin. Chir. 92:536-595; y. 1910.

Ssoson-Jaroschewitsch. Operative Zugänge zur Milz.
Arch. f. klin. Chir. 130:697-735; y. 1924.

L. Stimson. The combined transverse and longitudinal incision in laparotomy.
Annals of Surgery. 40:178-185; y. 1904.

N. P. Trinkler. Zur Bewerthung der modificirten Lumbalmethode der Gallenblasenexstirpation.
Arch. f. klin. Chir. 96:641-656; y. 1911.

K. Vogeler. Der quere bogenförmige Bauchschnitt bei eitrigen Bauchoperationen.
Zbl. f. Chir. 49:163-165; y. 1922.

R. F. Weir. An improved operation for acute appendicitis or for quiescent cases with complications.
The Med. News. 76:241-242; y. 1900.

C. S. White. Closing the skin in abdominal incisions.
Surgery, Gynec. & Obstetrics, 24:373-374; y. 1917.

R. H. Anglin Whitelocke. Appendectomy by a new route.
Brit. Med. Journ. 1:211-213; y. 1920.

K. Winkelmann. Die Laparotomie durch Querschnitt in der hinteren Rectusscheide.
Deutsch. Zeitschr. f. Chir. 98:382-389; y. 1909.

J. L. Yates & F. Raine. Making and closing of abdominal incisions.
Surg. Gyn. & Obs. 52:1020-1027; y. 1931.

CHAPTER III.

ANATOMY OF THE SMALL AND LARGE BOWEL.
INTESTINAL LOCALIZATION.

In order to understand the principles of intestinal suturing it is important to know the structure of the intestinal walls. In order to know what portion of a bowel we are dealing with a knowledge of gross anatomy is essential.

The intestinal tract starts from the pyloric ring of the stomach and ends as the terminal part of the rectum, the anus. It is divided into two large subdivisions, the **small** and **large** bowel. The **small** bowel is subdivided into three portions, the duodenum, the jejunum and the ileum.

Duodenum (Fig. 69).—The length of the duodenum is about ten to eleven inches. It begins at the pylorus and ends in the duodeno-jejunal junction. It forms a horseshoe-shaped curve, the convexity of which is directed to the right and downward, and the concavity is directed to the left and upward. The distance between the two ends of the arch is a little more than two inches. The duodenal arch embraces the head of the pancreas. The duodenum is subdivided into three parts:

a. Pars superior. This is one and a-half to two inches long. It extends from the pylorus to the neck of the gall-bladder. It is more movable than any other part of the duodenum and is situated intraperitoneally.

b. The Pars descendens is three or four inches long. It begins at the neck of the gall-bladder, runs nearly vertically downward to the left of the right kidney and lies on the right side of the second and third lumbar vertebræ. Its anterior surface is covered with peritoneum. **The ampulla** of **Vater** is situated in this part of the duodenum. The common orifice of the common bile-duct and of the pancreatic duct opens in the ampulla **(Papilla major).** Occasionally, one inch above the Papilla major there is situated a separate opening for the accessory pancreatic duct, the **Papilla minor.**

c. Pars inferior. This is the longest and narrowest part of the duodenum. Its length varies from five to seven inches. It runs transversely from the right to the left in front of the inferior vena cava, the aorta and the vertebral column as the **horizontal part,** and then ascends to the inferior surface of the body of the pancreas as the **pars ascendens.** There it bends forward and forms at the level of the first or second lumbar vertebra the **duodeno-jejunal flexure** and continues as the jejunum. From the duodeno-jejunal juncture a band extends upward and laterally to the base of the transverse mesocolon —**the ligament of Treitz.**

The **jejunum** (Fig. 69) starts at the duodeno-jejunal junction. It is attached to the posterior abdominal wall by a peritoneal fold, which contains blood-vessels, lymph-vessels and lymphatic glands and nerves. This fold is known as the **mesojejunum** or the mesentery of the jejunum.

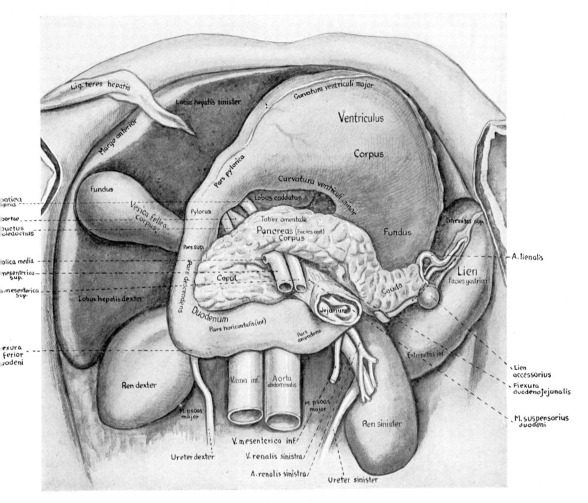

FIG. 69. VIEW OF THE POSTERIOR SURFACE OF THE STOMACH, DUODENUM AND PANCREAS (AFTER RAUBER).

The **ileum** is a continuation of the jejunum. It joins the cecum at the ileo-colic angle. It is attached to the posterior abdominal wall by the **meso-ileum** or mesentery of the ileum. The points of differentiation between the jejunum and the ileum, the length of their respective parts, and their topographical anatomy will be given below under Intestinal Localization.

STRUCTURE OF THE WALL OF THE BOWEL.

a. Tunica serosa (Fig. 70).

This is a peritoneal covering which surrounds the entire circumference of the bowel with the exception of its mesenteric attachment. At that point the tunica serosa is continued as two leaflets of the mesentery, as may

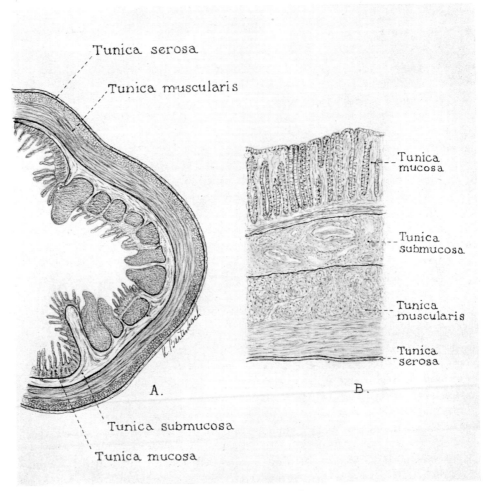

FIG. 70. CROSS-SECTION OF BOWEL.
A. Small bowel.
B. Large bowel.

be seen on a cross section. In the large bowel the tunica serosa is usually absent on the posterior surface of the colon ascendens and descendens.

b. Tunica muscularis (Fig. 70).

This is a muscular coat consisting of unstriped muscle, and is arranged in two layers, the outer or the longitudinal, and the inner or the circular layer. The outer layer is much thinner than the inner. The muscular layer of the bowel diminishes in thickness from above downward. It is the thickest at the beginning of the duodenum and the thinnest at the terminal part of the ileum. **In the large bowel the relations are reversed.** The wall is thinner above and increases in thickness in a downward direction, so that it is the thinnest in the cecum and the thickest in the rectum.

c. Tunica submucosa (Tela submucosa) (Fig. 70).

This is a loose layer of areolar tissue. On its inner side is situated a very thin but strong layer of elastic tissue which some anatomists consider as a separate layer, **the muscularis mucosa.**

The tunica submucosa (and especially the muscularis mucosa) is very important in intestinal suturing, since suturing through this layer gives real strength to the suture-line.

d. Tunica mucosa (Fig. 70).

This is of a reddish color. This layer is the thickest in the upper part of the duodenum and diminishes in a downward direction. It is the thinnest in the distal end of the ileum. It forms circular folds **(plicæ circulares),** which are present in the entire length of the small bowel, with the exception of the upper duodenum and the lowest part of the ileum. These folds run perpendicularly to the long axis of the bowel, and they do not extend through its entire circumference. In the large bowel these circular folds of mucous membrane are called **plicæ semilunares coli.**

BLOOD SUPPLY OF THE SMALL BOWEL.

The blood-supply of the small intestines is derived: (1) from the **hepatic artery** (through its **gastroduodenal** branch which gives off as one of its terminal branches, the **superior pancreatico-duodenal artery,** for the first part of the duodenum) ; and (2) from the branches of the **superior mesenteric** artery **(inferior pancreatico-duodenal artery, rami intestini tenui,** and the **ileal branch** of the **ileo-colic artery).**

All the branches which furnish the blood-supply to the small bowel pass between the two layers of the mesentery. Before reaching the wall of the bowel each branch bifurcates. The bifurcating branches inosculate with each other and form arches with their convexities directed to the bowel. Loops formed in this way are called **"primary loops" (Fig. 71)** ; from such loops small vessels **("vasa recta")** run to the wall of the bowel. If we examine the mesentery at another place, we will find a different arrangement. From the arches of the first loops arise arteries which do not reach the bowel, but bifurcate before reaching it. These bifurcated arteries inosculate with the bifurcated branches of another artery to form another series of loops which are called **"secondary loops" (Fig. 71).** From these secondary loops arise the "vasa recta". In still other places in the mesentery we find **"tertiary loops"**; and, finally, there might be found in the mesentery some places where the arrangement of the blood-vessels is quite irregular, the "primary", "secondary" and "tertiary" loops appearing without any order. The knowledge of the arrangement of the blood-vessels is very important because it helps in defining what part of the bowel we are dealing with.

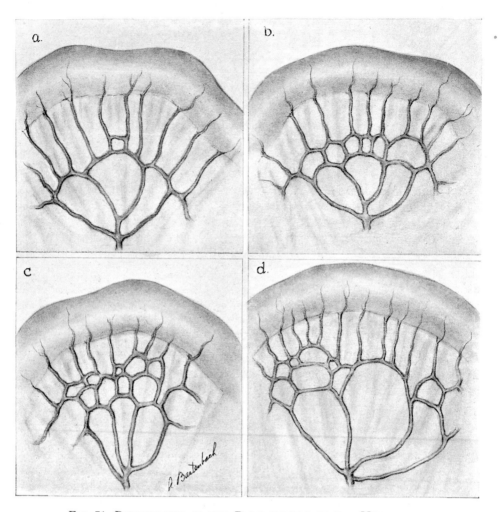

FIG. 71. DISTRIBUTION OF THE BLOOD-VESSELS IN THE MESENTERY.
a. Primary loops;   b. Primary and secondary loops;
c. Primary, secondary and tertiary loops;   d. Irregular arrangement of the vascular loops.

Monks showed that primary loops are usually found in the upper half of the jejunum; primary and secondary, in the lower half of the jejunum; primary, secondary and tertiary, in the upper half of the ileum; and the irregular arrangement in the lower part of the ileum.

The veins are arranged similarly to the arteries.

BLOOD-VESSELS OF THE LARGE BOWEL (FIG. 72).

The blood-supply of the large bowel is derived from:

    I. Superior Mesenteric Artery;

    II. Inferior Mesenteric Artery;

    III. Anterior division of the Hypogastric Artery.

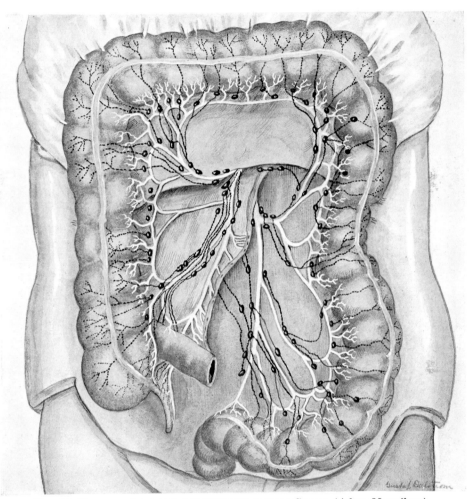

FIG. 72. BLOOD-VESSELS AND LYMPHATICS OF THE COLON (After Moynihan).

I. Superior Mesenteric Artery.

    This vessel gives off:

A. **The ileo-colic artery,** which itself breaks into five terminal branches:

        a. **Ileal.**

        b. **Appendicular.**

        c. **Anterior ileo-cecal.**

        d. **Posterior ileo-cecal.**

        e. **Colic.**

The distribution of these branches can be seen easily from their names.

B. **Right Colic Artery** (Fig. 72).

This artery subdivides into two branches which inosculate with the colic branch of the ileo-colic artery and with the middle colic artery.

C. **Middle Colic Artery** (Fig. 72).

This artery runs in the transverse mesocolon. It bifurcates into right and left branches. The right branch inosculates with the ascending branch of the right colic artery, and the left branch with the ascending branch of the left colic artery. The area of transverse mesocolon surrounded by the loop formed by the inosculation of the left branch of the middle colic and the ascending branch of the left colic arteries (**"Anastomosis Magna" of Riolan**) is of a large size and has comparatively a small amount of blood-vessels traversing it. Hence it is called the **"avascular area of Riolan"**, and in this area of the transverse mesocolon the slit in performing posterior gastro-enterostomy is usually made.

II. **Inferior Mesenteric Artery.**

This vessel gives off:

a. **Left Colic Artery,** which bifurcates, forming an **ascending** branch, which inosculates with the left branch of the middle colic artery; and a **descending** branch, which inosculates with the first sigmoid branch of the inferior mesenteric artery.

b. **Sigmoid Arteries.** These are two or three in number, each of which bifurcates into an **ascending** and **descending** branch. Each ascending branch inosculates with the descending branch of the higher situated artery. Each descending branch inosculates with the ascending branch of the lower situated artery. This is true of the left colic and all the sigmoid arteries except the lowest one, **which does not bifurcate.** It inosculates with the descending branch of the higher situated sigmoid artery, **but it does not inosculate with the superior hemorrhoidal artery.**

All these bifurcated branches appear as one vessel, which is called the **marginal artery.** Through this artery collateral circulation is easily established, if the left colic or any of the sigmoid arteries are ligated. If the ligation of the artery is made at the place where the inferior mesenteric artery breaks into its two terminal branches (namely, the superior hemorrhoidal and last sigmoid), then the superior hemorrhoidal artery will have no blood-supply, and there will be no collateral circulation between it and the marginal artery. The point where the inferior mesenteric artery breaks into its two terminal branches is known as the **"critical point" of Sudeck.** The artery should always be ligated above this point. However, occasionally collateral circulation still may be established between the superior hemorrhoidal and the middle and inferior hemorrhoidal arteries.

III. **Anterior Division of the Hypogastric Artery.**

This vessel gives off:

a. **Middle hemorrhoidal artery,** which takes its origin from the anterior division of the hypogastric artery, and

b. **Inferior hemorrhoidal artery,** a branch of the internal pudendal artery (which is a branch of the anterior division of the hypogastric artery).

LYMPHATICS OF THE SMALL AND LARGE BOWEL.

An exact knowledge of the lymphatic distribution in the small and large bowel is of the greatest practical importance in the surgery of intestinal malignancy. The bowel may be invaded by the malignant growth for only a small distance, but the lymphatics corresponding to a larger area may already be invaded. This would make the excision of only the locally affected part useless; a far wider excision would be required.

The lymph is collected from the walls of the small and large bowel into lymph-vessels, which form four plexuses in the wall of the bowel. Each plexus is situated in a layer of the wall and carries a corresponding name:

1. Mucous plexus.

2. Submucous plexus.

3. Muscular plexus.

4. Subserous plexus.

Each of these plexuses communicates with the others. The lymph from any plexus passes eventually through the subserous plexus on its way to the lymphatic glands.

The lymph-vessels of the duodenum are few in number. It is difficult to inject them. They drain the lymph into the biliary, sub-pyloric and mesenteric lymph-nodes.

The lymph-vessels of the jejunum and ileum, with the exception of the terminal part of the ileum, drain into the mesenteric lymph-nodes.

The lymph-vessels of the terminal part of the ileum drain into the ileo-colic nodes (Fig. 72).

The lymph-vessels of the appendix, cecum and ascending colon drain into the ileo-colic lymph-nodes (Fig. 72).

The lymph-vessels of the right colic flexure and transverse colon drain into the superior mesenteric lymph-nodes (Fig. 72).

The lymph-vessels of the descending colon, iliac colon and sigmoid flexure drain into the inferior mesenteric lymph-nodes (Fig. 72).

Thus, all the lymph-vessels drain into the mesenteric lymphatic nodes. These lie between the leaflets of the mesentery where they form three main groups:

1. Those lying very close to the intestinal wall.

2. **Intermediate nodes** lying along the rami intestini tenui. These nodes are larger than those of the first group.

3. **A terminal group of mesenteric lymph-nodes.**
This group consists of large nodes. They lie around the stem of the superior mesenteric artery. Into them is drained the lymph from the entire small bowel, appendix, cecum, ascending colon, transverse colon and part of the descending colon.

THE NERVE-SUPPLY OF THE INTESTINES.

This is derived from the sympathetic system. The nerves accompany the vessels to the wall of the intestine where they terminate. These nerves spring from the celiac plexus and the superior and inferior mesenteric plexuses of the sympathetic nervous system. Some filaments of the right vagus nerve are also distributed to the upper part of the gastro-intestinal tract.

INTESTINAL LOCALIZATION.

In surgery of the intestinal tract, it is important to know:

a. The position of each part of the intestines in the abdominal cavity.
b. The length of the small and large bowels.
c. How to differentiate between the small and large bowels.
d. How to differentiate between the jejunum and the ileum.
e. Which is the proximal and which is the distal part of a given loop of a bowel.
f. How to find the beginning of the jejunum.
g. How to find the cecum.
h. How to find the appendix.

Among numerous research workers who have contributed to our knowledge in this field, valuable information has been given to us by Monks, Mall, Henke, Sernoff, Stopnitzki, Weinberg, Spivack, etc. Many facts given below are taken from the work of the above mentioned writers.

A.—POSITION OF THE INTESTINES IN THE ABDOMINAL CAVITY.

The position of the intestines in the abdominal cavity can be determined from different points of view as follows:

1. **Holotopic** (surface anatomy) method.
2. **Skeletotopic** method, or the relation of the abdominal structures to the skeleton.
3. **Syntopic** method, or the relation of these structures to other visceral structures.

1. **Holotopic or Surface Anatomy Markings.**
Monks Method:
The external surface of the anterior abdominal wall is marked by a letter "H", the crossbar being directed from the left and above to the right and below, so that the umbilicus will be in the center of this line and the length of the line about six inches. Two perpendicular lines are made, one at either end of the first line (Fig. 73). These lines

of the letter "H" divide the abdomen into three parts—upper, middle and lower. In the **upper** part, which corresponds mainly to the left hypochondrium, is located the upper third of the small bowel. In the **middle** third, which corresponds to the umbilical region, will be situated the lower part of the jejunum and the upper part of the ileum. In the **lower** part, which corresponds to the right iliac region, and

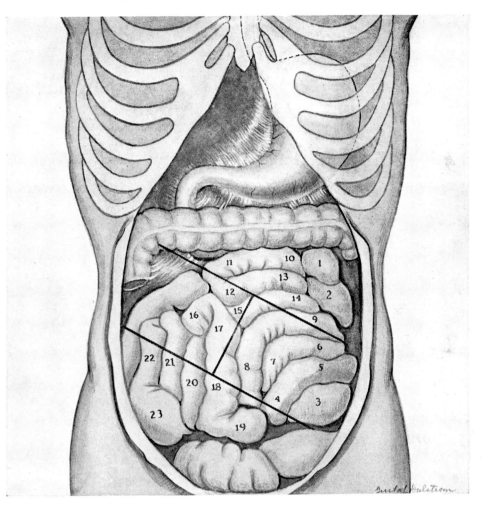

FIG. 73. INTESTINAL LOCALIZATION.

also in the pelvic cavity, is situated the lower portion of the ileum.
Sernoff Method.

As seen from the picture (Fig. 73), all the loops of the small intestines lie either in horizontal or in vertical rows. The horizontal rows are upper and lower. The upper horizontal rows and the left vertical rows, with a part of the middle vertical rows, constitute the jejunum. The lower horizontal rows, with the right vertical rows and all the pelvic loops constitute the ileum.

2.   **Skeletotopic Markings.**

Duodenum.

The **first** part—**pars superior,** starts at the level of the first lumbar

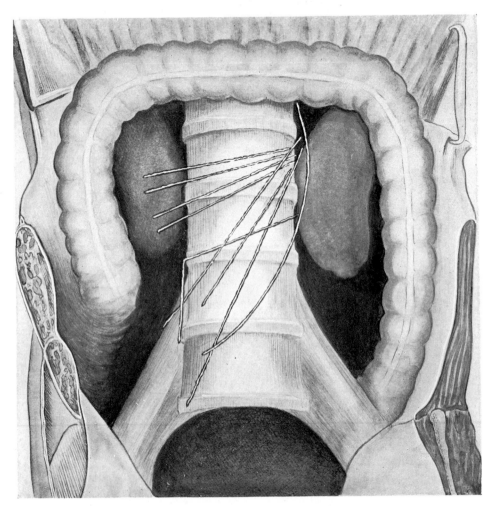

Fig. 74. Different Lines of Attachment of the Mesentery to the Posterior Abdominal Wall (After Stopnitzki).

vertebra and extends laterally to the right, and then backward along the body of the first lumbar vertebra.

The **second** part, **pars descendens,** extends vertically down from the first lumbar to the level of the third or fourth lumbar vertebræ parallel and to the right side of the spine.

The **third** part, **pars inferior,** runs from right to left in front of the spinal column in a slightly oblique direction. It reaches the level of the lower end of the first lumbar vertebra on the left side, where it ends in the duodeno-jejunal junction.

Jejunum and Ileum.

According to Sernoff, about 41 per cent. of the entire length of the small bowel is situated to the left of the spinal column, about 41 per cent. in the pelvis, and 18 per cent. to the right of the spinal column. The bowel is not closely attached to the posterior abdominal wall, but is connected by a mesentery usually along a line which joins the second lumbar vertebra of the left side with the right iliac fossa (Fig. 74) ; the length of this line is 6 inches. However, this line of attachment is not constant. Stopnitzki showed the occurrence of other lines of mesenteric attachment (Fig. 74).

3. Syntopic Considerations.

The **duodenum** is in contact with the liver, gall-bladder, right kidney, right adrenal, and the head of the pancreas. It crosses in front of the inferior vena cava and the abdominal aorta, and is itself crossed anteriorly by the superior mesenteric artery and vein. Behind the first part **(pars superior)** lie the common bile-duct, the portal vein, and the gastro-duodenal artery. The anterior surface of the descending part is crossed by the root of the transverse mesocolon, and the anterior surface of the horizontal part by a part of the root of the mesentery of the small bowel.

The **jejunum** and **ileum** are in contact with the following structures:

Anteriorly, with the anterior abdominal wall, from which they are separated by the great omentum. Not infrequently, however, the omentum is folded in and lies on the right or on the left side. In such cases, the bowel is in contact with the posterior surface of the anterior abdominal wall.

Posteriorly, they rest on the structures which are situated on the posterior abdominal wall, namely, the kidneys, duodenum, and the large blood-vessels (vena cava, abdominal aorta and its branches). **Above,** they are in contact with the transverse colon and transverse mesocolon. **Below,** in the pelvic cavity, in men, they lie between the sigmoid and rectum behind and the bladder in front; in women, between the sigmoid and rectum behind and the uterus and urinary bladder in front. **Laterally,** they come in contact with the cecum and ascending colon on the right side and the descending colon and sigmoid on the left side.

B.   THE LENGTH AND CALIBER OF THE BOWEL.

The length of the bowel varies, according to the height, age and sex of the individual. The taller the person, the longer the bowel. In infants and young children the length of the bowel is relatively larger than in grown persons. **The large bowel** is one-fourth of the length of the small bowel.

Various authors give different estimates of the size of the bowel, thus:
Frederick Treves gives the average length of the small

bowel as								22 ft. 5 in.
Cruveilhier	"	"	"	"	"	"	"	22 ft. 10 in.
Meckel	"	"	"	"	"	"	"	18 ft. 10 in.
Robinson (for a male)			"	"	"	"	"	23 ft. 4 in.
Robinson (for a female)			"	"	"	"	"	19 ft. 4 in.

The length of the entire bowel (from the duodenum to the anus):

Cruveilhier	27 ft. 4 in.
Sappey	32 ft.
Kubo (Japan) (for female)	24 ft. 3 in.
Kubo (Japan) (for male)	26 ft. 2 in.

Some investigators studied the relationship between the length of the bowel and the height of the body. Their findings are listed below:

Jonnesco gives as 4.2:I (the length of the small bowel to the height of the body).

Beneke gives it as $3\frac{7}{8}$:1

The caliber of the bowel is:

Duodenum: Diameter 1.8 to 1.9 inch.

Jejunum (in its upper part): 1.4 to 1.5 inch.

Ileum (terminal part): 1.1 inch.

C. DIFFERENTIATION OF THE SMALL FROM THE LARGE BOWEL.

There are several points of differentiation, only three of which are reliable.

Large Bowel.	**Small Bowel.**
1. Tæniæ longitudinale coli present.	Tæniæ coli absent
2. Appendices epiploicæ " .	Append. epipl. " .
3. Sacculation of the wall " .	Saccul. of the wall " .

D. DIFFERENTIATION OF THE JEJUNUM FROM THE ILEUM.

There is not a marked difference between the end of the jejunum and the beginning of the ileum. The changes come gradually, so that it is impossible to say where the jejunum ends and the ileum starts. However, if the jejunum and ileum are compared in places where their characteristic features are well marked, it is not difficult to differentiate them:

1. **The jejunum is wider than the ileum.** The width of the bowel diminishes from above downward. It is widest at the duodeno-jejunal junction and narrowest at the terminal part of the ileum.

2. **The jejunum has a thicker wall than the ileum.** The thickness of the wall diminishes from above downward.

3. **Color of the bowel.** The color is brighter in the upper jejunum and fades in the downward direction.

4. **Arrangement of the blood-vessels in the mesentery.**

Primary loops with long vasa recta are seen in the upper half of the jejunum.

Primary and secondary loops are seen in the lower half of the jejunum, and the vasa recta are shorter than in the upper part.

Primary and secondary and tertiary loops are seen in the upper half of the ileum, and the vasa recta are still shorter than in any portion of the jejunum.

An irregular arrangement (where, in some places, only primary loops are seen, in other places primary and secondary loops, and in still other places in the same vicinity, primary, secondary and tertiary loops) is usually observed in the lower half of the ileum.

5. **The thickness and transparency of the mesentery.**

The thickness of the mesentery increases from above downward. It is thinnest in the upper mesojejunum and thickest in the lower meso-ileum. In the mesentery which corresponds to the upper seven feet of the jejunum small transparent spots, "lunettes", are found between the vasa recta.

E. WHICH IS THE PROXIMAL AND WHICH IS THE DISTAL END OF A LOOP OF BOWEL?

This is an important point to determine, since in lateral intestinal anastomosis and in case of gastro-enterostomy many surgeons prefer to place the loops of intestines or the stomach and loop of jejunum in an isoperistaltic direction. It is especially important to know this when performing an end-to-side intestinal anastomosis. The simplest and the best method is:

Monks method (Fig. 75).

A loop of bowel is put on the stretch with the palm of the right hand covering the bowel. The index-finger of the right hand slides along one side of the mesentery and the thumb of the same hand along the other side. The mesentery is palpated between the index-finger and the thumb to find whether it is flat or twisted. **A twisted mesentery means that the bowel has changed its direction.** The mesentery should be untwisted. Then, the direction of the bowel will be from above and left to below and right corresponding to the root of the mesentery. **The portion of the bowel directed toward the left shoulder will be the proximal part, and the portion directed to the right hip will be the distal end of the bowel.**

F. HOW TO FIND THE FIRST LOOP OF THE JEJUNUM.

An exact knowledge of the first loop is essential in performing a posterior gastro-enterostomy by the "no-loop method".

In the pioneer days of gastro-intestinal surgery, several methods were suggested for locating the first loop. Some of these, in the light of our modern methods were not only non-scientific but even ridiculous. For instance, one of the earliest methods was to pick up any loop of bowel and follow it in one or the other direction until either the first loop of the jejunum or the terminal part of the ileum was reached. If it was the first loop of the jejunum, all was well. If the terminal end of the ileum was reached, then the surgeon had to follow in the opposite direction until the first loop of the jejunum was finally obtained.

Others used the method of Nothnagel, that is, deciding the direction of the peristaltic wave by placing on the wall of the bowel crystals of sodium or potassium chloride. As soon as the crystals are placed peristaltic contraction occurs, and by following the bowel opposite to the peristaltic wave the first loop of the jejunum is reached.

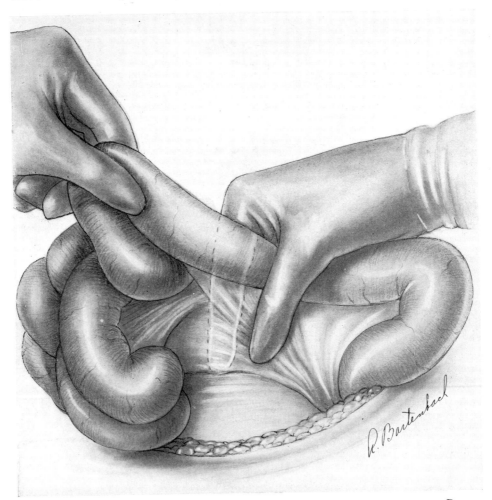

Fig. 75. Monks Method of Differentiation between the Proximal and the Distal End of a Loop of Bowel.

Wölfler, in 1883, and later, Socin, Professor of Surgery in Basel, Switzerland, described an excellent method, which won universal recognition and which in a modified way, is described thus:

Wölfler-Socin Method (Fig. 199).

The omentum is grasped, with the transverse colon, by the left hand.

These are lifted, placing the transverse mesocolon on the stretch. The right hand is then placed on the vertebral column at the base of the transverse mesocolon. This hand then rests on the body of the second lumbar vertebra. The index-finger of the right hand slides to the left side of this vertebra. **The loop which lies between the index-finger and the left side of the second lumbar vertebra is the first loop of the jejunum.** At the duodeno-jejunal junction, which lies close to this point, a more or less developed band will be seen extending obliquely upward and laterally to the base of the transverse mesocolon; this was described by Treitz and is known as the **Treitz ligament.**

G. HOW TO FIND THE CECUM.

Usually, this is easy, especially, when the abdomen is widely open. However, in cases in which the incision is very small, as in the gridiron incision for appendectomy, it may be difficult. The usual method of placing the right index-finger behind the anterior abdominal wall and moving it laterally until the lateral abdominal wall is reached, then posteriorly until the finger strikes the iliac fossa, then medially, keeping the finger constantly in touch with the iliac fossa until the cecum is reached, may be useful in many cases. The most reliable method however is described by Monks.

Monks Method of Locating the Terminal Ileum and the Cecum. (Fig. 76).

The index-finger is placed on the brim of the pelvis, where it feels the pulsation of the external iliac artery; the finger is then moved upward along this artery until the upper margin of the brim of the pelvis is reached, and this movement is continued upward and somewhat laterally until the finger finds a barrier to further upward movement (Fig. 76). The finger then rests on the lower end of the root of the mesentery. The thumb is placed on the side of the structure which rests on the index-finger, and this is brought outside of the abdominal wound. The structure so caught between the thumb and index-finger of the right hand is the terminal part of the ileum, located approximately from 3 to 4 inches away from the ileo-cecal junction. Having located the terminal part of the ileum, it is a simple matter to follow along to the cecum.

Although this is an excellent method, in case of variations in the course of the root of the mesentery, it may prove misleading (Fig. 74).

H. HOW TO FIND THE APPENDIX.

Usually, this is also an easy matter. The base of the appendix is situated on the posterior wall of the cecum, at the point of union of the three tænia longitudinalis. Speaking in geographical terms, it is situated southwest from the ileocecal junction in the normal position of the cecum. However, since we usually, in searching for the appendix, turn the cecum upward, it becomes located in a position northwest from the ileocecal junction.

Difficulty in locating the appendix arises only when that organ is very small—**hypoplasia of the appendix,** or when it lies completely **retrocecal** and the cecum is bound to the iliac fossa and but slightly movable. Cases are described in which the length of the appendix was from 1/10 to 1/12 of an inch. The best guide then is to look for the place of junction of the three tænia. In those cases in which the appendix lies retrocecally and the cecum is bound to the iliac fossa, so that the appendix is entirely covered by the cecum, a real difficulty arises. The appendix cannot be seen at

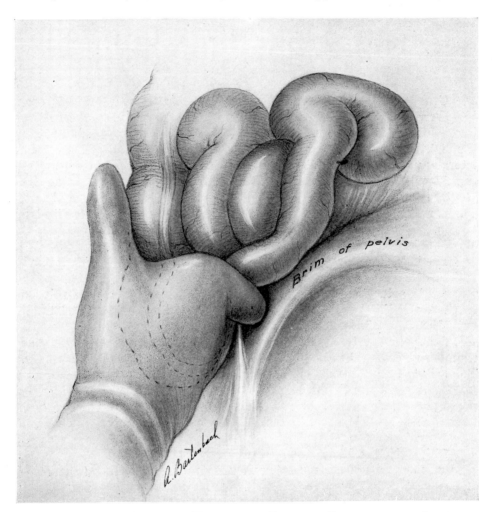

Fig. 76. Monks Method of Finding the Terminal Portion of the Ileum

all, and at the same time the surgeon does not feel justified in mobilizing the cecum with the possible introduction of infection into the retroperitoneal space, since he is not even certain that the appendix is there. Under such circumstances, a very helpful rule has been suggested by Spivack:

Spivack's Rule.

In about 90 to 92 per cent. of these cases, retrocecal appendix is coincidental with attachment of the terminal ileum to the brim of the pelvis. If after careful searching for the appendix, it cannot be found, the surgeon should see whether the terminal part of the ileum is so attached. **If so, then nine times out of ten, the appendix is retrocecal.** In such cases, the cecum should be mobilized and turned medially so that the posterior wall will face anteriorly. Then the appendix will be seen.

BIBLIOGRAPHY.

G. Andreassi. Considerazioni intorno a un caso di atresia congenita del colon ileo-pelvico.
Ricerche di morfol., 11:375-383; y. 1931.

L. Belmonte. Sull'Inversione del ciego.
Rinascenza médica. 10:136-138; y. 1933.

R. J. A. Berry. The anatomy of the vermiform appendix.
Anatom. Anz. 10:761-769; y. 1895.

C. E. Briggs. The extraperitoneal relations of the appendix vermiformis to the posterior surface of the cecum with report of a form hitherto undescribed.
Med. News, 85:116-119; y. 1904.

P. Carnot. Sur le dolicho-colon.
Paris Méd. 1:305-311; y. 1932.

Clado. Appendice caecal; anatomie; embryologie; anatomie comparée; bactériologie normale et pathologique.
Compt. rend. Soc. de biol. Paris, 44:133-172; y. 1892.

Cunningham. Text-book of Anatomy, 5th Ed. pp. 1170-1180 and 1198-1223. y. 1925.

A. Czenes. Mikrocolon congenitum.
Arch. f. klin. Chir. 160:486-498; y. 1930.

A. Dagnino. Dolicocolias.
La Semana méd. 2:1780; y. 1930.

P. Descomps. Les zones accolées du péritoine. Leur décollement opératoire.
Rev. de Chir. 60:451-498; y. 1922.

G. Diliberti-Herbin. Sulle estese resezioni dell'intestino tenue.
Extr. in Zbl. für Chir. 31:105-106; y. 1904.

W. A. N. Dorland. Congenital absence of the vermiform appendix.
Internat.Clinics. 4:44-54; y. 1925.

E. Drost. Beitrag zum Microcolon congenitum.
Deutsch. Zeitsch. f. Chir. 232:764-767; y. 1931.

J. M. Flint. The effect of extensive resections of the small intestine.
Bull. Johns Hopkins Hospit. 23:127-144; y. 1912.

C. E. Gardner Jr. & D. Hart. Anomalies of intestinal rotation as a cause of intestinal obstruction; report of 2 personal observations; review of 103 reported cases.
Arch. of Surg. 29:942-981; y. 1934.

P. Gilis. Situation de l'appendice caecal.
Journ. de l'anat. et la physiol. 36:568-573; y. 1900.

T. M. Green. Surgical significance of derangement of intestinal rotation and distribution.
Surg. Gyn. & Obst. 53:734-741; y. 1931.

L. Grove. Non-rotation of the colon.
Ann. Surg. 91:615-618; y. 1930.

H. E. Haymond & L. R. Dragstedt. Anomalies of intestinal rotation.
Surg. Gyn. & Obst. 53:316-329; y. 1931.

A. Hewson. The anatomy of the vermiform appendix.
Am. Journ. Med. Sc. 106:185-190; y. 1893.

W. C. Hunter. Intersigmoid hernia. Report of a case with a study of anatomy of the fossa.
Northwest Med. 32:138-144; y. 1933.

R. H. Hunter. The ileo-cecal junction.
Journ. of Anat. 68:264-269; y. 1934.

K. Kamniker. Ein Fall von Dünn-und Dickdarm Anomalie bei gleichzeitig bestehenden Ulcus duodeni.
Deutsche Zeitschr. f. Chir. 244:587-590; y. 1935.

J. L. Kantor. Common anomalies of duodenum and colon: Their practical significance.
J. A. M. A. 97:1785-1790; y. 1931.

J. L. Kantor & S. Schechter. Variations in fixation of the ceco-colon; their clinical significance.
Am. J. Roentgen. 31:751-765; y. 1934.

A. J. Labbok. Einige anatomisch-topographische Eigentümlichkeiten der Dickdarmform und—lage.
Anat. Anz. 76:177-194; y. 1933.

B. Lamp. Die Bestimmung der Verlaufsrichtung und der Hohe von Dünn-darmschlingen.
Zbl. f. Chir. 61:853-862; y. 1934.

A. Lucca. Osservazioni sulle dimensioni dell'intestino nell'infanzia.
II Lattante, 2:506-530; y. 1931.

F. Mall. Reversal of the intestine.
Johns Hopkins Hospit. Report. 1:93-110; y. 1896.

F. Mall. Development of the human intestine and its position in the adult.
Johns Hopkins Hospital Bullet. 9:197-208; y. 1898.

F. Mandl. Zur pathologischen Lage des Duodenum und der Flex. duodeno-
jejunalis und ihre klinischen Folgeerscheinungen.
Wien. Med. Wchnsch. 85:289-291; y. 1935.

O. F. Mazzini. Duodeno anormal; sinistrocolia por colon movible. Mesen-
terio común.
Rev. de cirugía de Buenos Aires. 13:40-47; y. 1934.

K. A. Meyer & J. L. Spivack. On the relationship between retrocecal appendix and Lane's kink and its surgical significance.
The Amer. Journ. of Surg. 25:12-13; y. 1934.

G. Monks. Studies in the surgical anatomy of the small intestine and its
mesentery.
Annals of Surg. 42:543-569; y. 1905.

F. Müller. Doppelbildung am Ileum.
Arch. f. klin. Chir. 181:363-373; y. 1934.

P. Nobécourt. Dolicholon et mégacolon chez l'enfant.
Médecine. 11:577-581; y. 1930.

L. Peterson. Ileum terminale fixation and ileus of that portion of intestine; anatomic, clinical and statistical study.
Acta Chir. Scandinav. (supp. 32); 75: Pages 1-487; 1-63; 1-113;
y. 1934.

E. J. Poth. A clean intestinal anastomosis; experimental study.
Arch. Surg. 28:1087-1094; y. 1934.

H. N. Pratt. "Double appendix" associated with other congenital anomalies.
Am. J. Dis. Childr. 45:1263-1276; y. 1933.

Quain. Elements of Anatomy. 11th. Edit.
vol. II, part 2; p. 97-131.

Rauber & Kopsch. Lehrbuch und Atlas der Anatomie des Menschen.
4:112-128; 155-172; y. 1923.

J. A. Reed. Deformities of the colon: Low cecum with absence of ascending colon and hepatic flexure; case report.
Virgin. Med. Monthly, 58:532-535; y. 1931.

C. W. Roberts. Congenital anomalies of the ileocolic region, with special
reference to chronic manifestations.
South. Surgeon. 2:301-312; y. 1933.

I. Schapschal. Zur Kasuistik der Lage des Colon sigmoideum.
Zeitschr. f. Anat. u. Entwickelungsgesch. 102:37-47; 1933.

D. Sernoff. Zur Kenntnis der Lage und Form des mesenterialen Teiles des
Dünndarmes und seines Gekroses.
Internat. Monatschr. für Anatomie u. Physiologie. 11:437; y. 1894.

K. E. Smiley. The relationship of the blood-supply and lymphatic drainage of the sigmoid and rectum to surgical procedures.
West. J. Surg. 41:635-639; y. 1933.

A. Socin. Zur Magenchirurgie.
Korrespondenz-Blatt für Schweizer Aertzte. 14:513-518; y. 1884.

J. L. Spivack. Congenital absence of the appendix vermiformis.
The Americ. Journ. of Surgery, 13:297-300; y. 1931.

J. A. Steward & F. W. Rankin. Blood supply of the large intestine; its surgical considerations.
Arch. Surg. 26:843-891; y. 1933.

A. L. Taylor. Some intestinal malformations and their clinical significance.
Bristol Med.—Chir. Journ. 48:113-134; y. 1931.

Sir Fred. Treves. Lectures on the anatomy of the intestinal canal and peritoneum in man.
Brit. Med. Journ. 1:415-419; y. 1885.

C. H. Webb & O. H. Wangensteen. Congenital intestinal atresia.
Am. J. Dis. Chil. 41:262-284; y. 1931.

R. Weinberg. Topographie der Mesenterien und der Windungen des Jejuno-ileum beim neugeborenen Menschen.
Internat. Monatschr. für Anat. u. Physiol, 13:66; y. 1896.

H. Williams. Normal and surgical anatomy of the vermiform appendix.
Med. News, 66:483-489; y. 1895.

A. Wölfler. Zur Technik der Gastro-Enterostomie und ähnlicher Operationen mit Demonstration von Präparaten.
Verhandl. der Deutsch. Gesellsch. für Chir. XII Kongr. 12:21-25; y. 1883.

CHAPTER IV.

METHODS OF SUTURING THE STOMACH AND BOWEL.

Historical. Suturing of the bowel came into use later than the use of ligatures. However, it too has been known since remote antiquity. In the Hindu Vedas (*e.g.* Susruta's Agur-Veda) are mentioned laparotomy and the suture of wounded intestines. Celsus (30 B.C.-30 A.D.) considered suturing of wounds of the small bowel useless, because it was invariably fatal. However, he advised suturing wounds of the large bowel since they gave some hope for recovery. Galen (129-201 A.D.) did not advise suturing of the bowel at all. He reserved suturing only for wounds of the stomach. Abul-Kasem, the great Arabian surgeon (born in 936 A.D.), used to suture the wounded bowel with a thread made from the gut of animals. He also reports the use, in his time, of the "ant-suture"; this consisted in letting a large-sized ant bite the edges of the intestinal wound, and as soon as the jaw of the ant had caught the two lips of the wound the surgeon immediately severed the head from the body, so that the head **was used as a suture-material.** This "ant-suture" was in vogue among the Arabians. The "ant-suture" was used later by Italian surgeons of the period of the Renaissance. In Dalmatia, even recently (at the end of the nineteenth century), the "ant-suture" was used by the laity for sewing superficial wounds. It is of interest to note that Michel clips, which were first described by Guillemeau in the XVI Century, were actually a mechanical imitation of the jaws of an ant, which were used for the ant-sutures. Further progress in suturing of the intestines was made by the Italian surgeons of the Renaissance period, who introduced a foreign body into the lumen of the bowel and sutured the lips of the wound over it. The foreign body later passed *per viam naturales.* As a foreign body, some used elder wood (*Sambucus nigra*), some, animal gut (Guglielmo di Salicetti). From Italy this method spread to France, where the four celebrated monks (Archimatheus, Petrosellus, Platearius and Ferrarius) employed it, using as a prothesis, the trachea of a goose; this suture is known as the **"Four Masters Suture" (Sutura quatuor magistrorum).**

At first, the surgeons used interrupted sutures, but later they began the use of a continuous suture. To Guglielmo di Salicetti (1210-1280) is given the credit of devising the "glover-suture" (**"furrier's suture"**) (Fig. 27, b and c).

In spite of the fact that surgeons used the intestinal suture for many centuries, their views on suturing were erroneous. Thus, for a long time, they believed that a hole in a small bowel should never be closed for fear of obliterating the lumen of the bowel. A wound of the large bowel, however, could be closed without fear of obliteration of its lumen. Another error

131

which was general even at the end of the eighteenth and the beginning of the nineteenth centuries was that in suturing one bowel to another the mucous layer of one bowel was sutured to the serosa of the other.

The real progress in our knowledge of intestinal suture came with the contributions of Jobert and Lembert. The latter showed that good union will follow **if the serous surfaces of the loops are brought together.** Later experiments, however, have shown that good union of two parts of a stomach or bowel-wall will follow also when the corresponding layers are sutured together namely serosa to serosa, muscularis to muscularis, and mucosa to mucosa, and that the real holding layer, which gives firm strength to the suture line is the **muscularis-mucosa** of each side. This must be included in the suture line. **The serosa in fact serves only as the plastic material which prevents leakage of the gastro-intestinal contents into the free peritoneal cavity.**

DIFFERENT TYPES OF INTESTINAL SUTURE.

The methods of intestinal suturing can be subdivided into **two classes:**

I. APPROXIMATION OF THE SEROUS LAYERS.

This is an approximation of the peritoneal layers of the bowel. The needle penetrates either the serous layer alone, or the sero-muscular layer, or the seromuscular-submucous layer, or the entire thickness of the wall. Several sutures belong to this class:

1. **Lembert Sero-serosa Suture.**
   This is an interrupted suture which includes the serous layer of each lip of the bowel or stomach (Fig. 77, 1, a).
2. **Dupuytren Suture.**
   This is a continuous sero-serosa suture (Fig. 77, 2, b).
3. **Wysler Suture.**
   This is a seromuscular-seromuscular suture (Fig. 77, 1, b).
4. **Wysler-Lembert Suture (Czerny Suture)** (Fig. 77, 3, a and b).
   This consists of two tiers of sutures: the first tier is seromuscular-seromuscular (actually the **Wysler suture**); the second or superficial tier, sero-serosa suture **(Lembert suture).**
5. **Albert Suture** (Fig. 77, 3, c and d).
   This consists of two layers: the first is a through-and-through suture, and the second a sero-serosa suture.
6. **Gély Suture—Interrupted** (Fig. 77, 5).
   This is a suture which embraces the entire thickness of the intestinal wall. The thread armed with two needles first enters at a small distance from the edge of the wound penetrating from without into the lumen, then runs parallel to the edge of the lip within the lumen, and passing through the wall of the bowel emerges on the same side of the lip. The needle on the other end of the thread penetrates from without into the lumen through the other lip; it then runs parallel to the edge of the lip and passing through the bowel-wall emerges on the other

side, when the ends are tied. The edges are thus approximated by their serous surfaces.

7. **Gély Suture—Continuous** (Fig. 77, 4).

The thread is armed with two needles. Each needle penetrates the thickness of the wall from without inward. Then it traverses the lumen for about one-third of an inch parallel to the free edge and emerges by penetrating the entire thickness of the wall. The threads

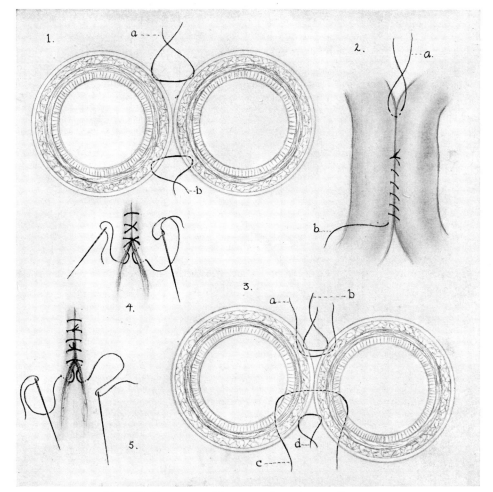

FIG. 77. DIFFERENT TYPES OF INTESTINAL SUTURING.

are then crossed and the needles enter as described before, repeating the previous step. Then the ends are tied.

8. **Appolito Suture** (Fig. 78, a, b).

This is a modification of the Gély suture. It embraces the entire thickness of the wall. It is made with one needle and a double thread. At the end of the thread is a knot.

The technic is as follows:

The needle passes from the inner to the outer side of the lip one-third of an inch away from the edge of the lip. It crosses over the gap of the wound and enters from without into the lumen of the bowel by piercing the opposite lip. Then the needle passes from within outward by piercing the second lip a little distance from its entrance,

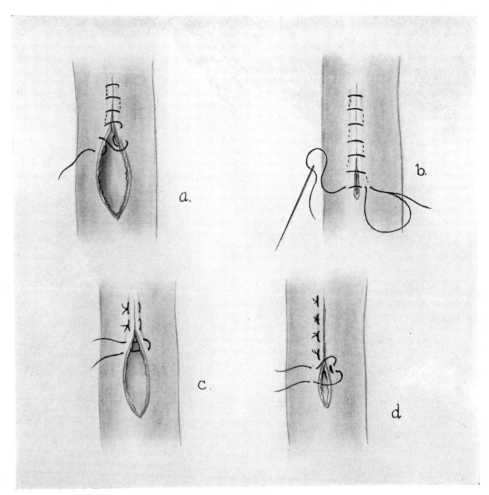

FIG. 78. DIFFERENT TYPES OF INTESTINAL SUTURING.
a, b. Appolito suture;   c. Halsted mattress-suture;   d. Gould reverse mattress-suture.

again crosses the gap of the wound, and pierces the first lip at the distance of one-third of an inch from the edge of the lip from without inward. These steps are repeated until the entire wound is closed. Then, on the side opposite to which the first stitch was inserted, one thread of the double thread is cut. The needle makes a Lembert seromuscular-seromuscular bite, and the two ends are tied. Thus, loops are formed on the inner side of the bowel running parallel to the edges of the lip. This suture closes the wound in folds, whereas Gély's suture closes it in a straight line. It is simpler in execution, but is not as safe.

9. **Halsted Mattress-suture** (Fig. 78, c).
This is a modification of the Emmert suture, including the seromuscular layer only. It is made in the following way:

A sero-muscular bite is taken on one side of the lip one-eighth of an inch away from the edge. Another sero-muscular bite is taken on the other lip, also one-eighth of an inch away from the edge of the lip. Another sero-muscular bite is then taken on the same lip on which the second bite was made, and the fourth bite is taken on the lip on which the first bite was made. There is thus a loop on one lip with the two ends of the thread emerging on the other lip of the bowel.

10. **Gould Reverse Mattress-suture** (Fig. 78, d).
This is a seromuscular suture which has the inverting effect of a Lembert suture and the strength of a mattress-suture. It is done in the following way:

A sero-muscular bite is taken on one lip **toward** the wound. A second sero-muscular bite is taken on the other lip, also **toward** the wound. A third seromuscular bite is taken on the same lip where the second bite was made, but **away** from the wound. A fourth bite is taken on the same lip where the first bite was made, and also **away** from the wound. Each bite should be at a distance of one-eighth of an inch from the edges of the wound and one-eighth of an inch away from each other.

11. **Cushing Right-angle Suture** (Fig. 79, a, b, c).
This is a modification of the Appolito suture, penetrating the seromuscular layer only. It is performed in the following way:

A seromuscular bite is taken one-eighth of an inch away from the edge of the lip in the direction opposite to the intended line of suturing. The thread is crossed at a right angle to the wound, and a seromuscular bite is taken on the other lip parallel to the wound and in the direction of the line of suture (**reversed U-shape suture**). The ends are then tied. The thread again is taken across the wound at a right angle and pierces the seromuscular layer of the first lip parallel to the wound, and so on. The thread must always be drawn along the line of suture **and in the direction of suturing.** Then the line will be smooth and there will be no puckering. To tie the end of the Cushing suture, the thread which is between the next to the last stitch and the last stitch is grasped; this forms a loop, which is drawn tight and tied to the single thread which hangs from the needle (Fig. 79, c).

12. **Purse-string Suture** (Fig. 79, d).
This is a continuous seromuscular suture inserted circularly about one-eighth of an inch from the edge of the wound. The distance be-

tween each two bites is about one-half inch. This suture can be placed before opening the bowel or the stomach.

13. **Maunsell Mesenteric Suture** (Fig. 79, e).

The thread passes through the entire thickness of the inner lip at the mesenteric border of the bowel. It will then lie in the triangular space between the two leaflets of the mesentery. The thread then

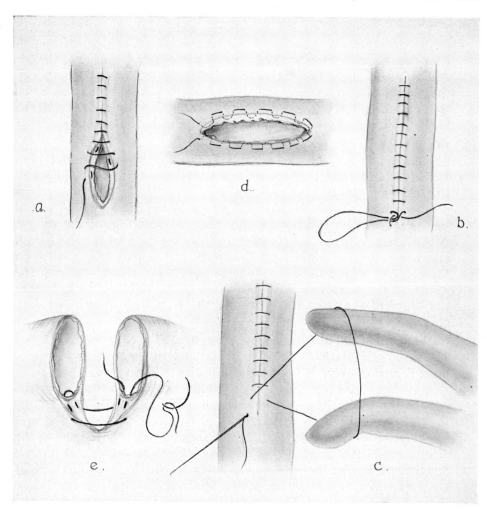

FIG. 79. DIFFERENT TYPES OF INTESTINAL SUTURING.
a, b, c—Cushing suture;   d—Purse-string suture;   e—Maunsell mesenteric stitch.

passes successively through the inner leaflet of the mesentery of this loop, the inner leaflet of the mesentery of the other loop, the inner lip of the second loop, the outer lip of the second loop, the outer leaflet of the mesentery of the second loop, the outer leaflet of the mesentery of the first loop and the outer lip of the first loop. Thus, the ends of the thread will lie in the lumen of one gut and the loop of the thread in the lumen of the other gut. The ends are then tied.

14. **Connell Suture** (Fig. 80, 1).

The thread passes through the entire thickness of the wall of the bowel from within outward in one lip of the wound. Then it crosses the wound and passes through the other lip from without inward. It

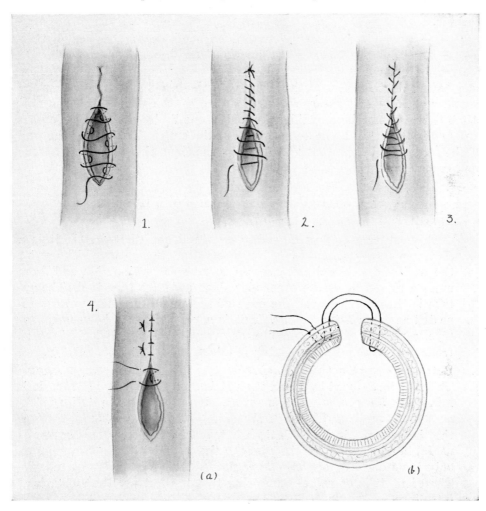

FIG. 80. DIFFERENT TYPES OF INTESTINAL SUTURING.
1. Connell suture;   2. Glover suture;   3. Bell suture;   4. (a, b) Jobert suture.

then emerges by passing through the thickness of the wall from within outward, so that a loop is formed within the lumen of the bowel. Then the thread crosses the wound again, and the process is repeated until the wound is closed. Each bite is at a distance of one-eighth of an inch from the other and about the same distance from the edge of the wound. As may be seen, it includes the entire thickness of the wall, and closely resembles the Gély continuous suture, save that in the latter method two needles are used.

15. **Jobert Suture** (Fig. 80, 4, a, b).
    This suture was described by Jobert (1799-1867) in 1824. Thus, it preceded the Lembert (1802-1851) suture, which was suggested in 1826.

Technic.

It starts as a seromuscular suture on one side of the wound, then crosses the wound and enters the lumen of the bowel by penetrating all the coats from without inward. It then passes from within outward by penetrating the thickness of the same lip of the bowel. Then it crosses the wound and enters as a seromuscular suture of the first lip. When this stitch is tied hemorrhage will be checked in one lip by the penetrating suture and in the other lip by compression of the entire thickness of the wall of the second lip to the first lip. At the same time, there will be a serous approximation of the lips of the wound.

II. APPROXIMATION BY THE MUCOUS LAYERS.

1. **Glover's Suture (Furrier's Suture)** (Fig. 80, 2).
    This suture was first described by Guglielmo di Salicetti. It is a continuous suture. It starts by penetrating the entire thickness of the wall of the bowel from serosa to mucosa on one side and from mucosa to serosa on the other side. The ends are then tied. The suture is then carried over the edge of the wound and the process repeated as often as necessary. This is a very effective hemostatic suture, especially when each bite, or every third bite is locked, or if, from time to time, a back-stitch is taken.

2. **Buttonhole Suture** (Fig. 27, a).
    This was introduced by Laurentius Heister (1683-1758) in 1739. It is a modification of the glover's suture. It penetrates the entire thickness of the wall. The difference between this and the glover's suture is that before crossing a half-stitch is taken in the loop. This suture is useful in approximating the edges of the wound where **approximation only** is needed. Where tension is needed, this suture is not reliable. Therefore, **it is of value in suturing the skin but not the stomach or intestines.**

3. **Bell Modification of the Glover Suture** (Fig. 80, 3).
    This was described by Bell in 1794. The thread passes through the wall from within outward exactly as in lacing a shoe. In the United States this is known as the "baseball suture".

    All the sutures described above are either interrupted or continuous. Both forms have advantages and disadvantages. Thus in:
Interrupted Suture.
1. Breaking of a stitch is not so dangerous.

2. Leakage of contents is more possible in case of an interrupted than of a continuous suture.

3. No purse-string action is possible in this type of suture.

4. It is less rapid than the continuous suture.

Continuous Suture.

1. Breaking of one stitch is dangerous because the entire chain is loosened.

2. Leakage of contents is less possible than in the case of the interrupted suture.

3. Purse-string action might be present if improperly applied.

4. It is more rapid than the interrupted suture.

However, if properly placed, all the advantages and disadvantages of each method can be evenly balanced, so that in most of the cases one method may be substituted for the other.

MECHANICAL DEVICES IN GASTRIC OR INTESTINAL SURGERY.

Today these are very seldom used, but in pre-antiseptic days when fast work was so important since it lessened the chances of contamination of the wound, they were of great importance and more advantageous than the use of sutures. The methods are all based on the same principles:

1. Two serous surfaces brought together form adhesions, *i.e.* unite.

2. Living tissue compressed between two surfaces to a definite degree will slough away.

The first who suggested a mechanical device was Denans, a French surgeon from Marseilles. His device was published in 1826, two years after Jobert published his work on union of serous approximated surfaces. The Denans appliance consisted of three silver rings, two of which had a width of three-tenths of an inch and a **diameter of the lumen of the bowel.** The third had the width of six-tenths of an inch and a **diameter smaller than the other two rings.** A ring of the lesser width was introduced into the lumen of each bowel, leaving about one-third of an inch free, which was turned inside as a cuff, so **that the serous surface** presented in the lumen of the bowel. The third ring was then introduced into the lumen of the two bowels so that the cuff of each bowel was compressed between its own ring and the common ring for the two bowels. Due to compression, the cuffs sloughed away and the rings were expelled *per viam naturales.*

Denans' device was followed by numerous appliances devised by different surgeons, such as the Bobrik method, described in 1850, the Béranger-Ferand method, described in 1870, the Senn bone-plate, described in 1887, the Mayo Robson decalcified bone-bobbin, described in 1892, the Murphy button, described in 1892, and the A. Ramaugé method, described in 1893. The last two methods were described evidently independently at the same time. Murphy described his method in December, 1892, and Adalbert Ramaugé, of Buenos Aires, his method in the early part of 1893. They have a striking resemblance, and at the same time both of them are a clear evolution of Denans and the Béranger-Ferand appliances.

The mechanical devices are little used now. Occasionally a Murphy button is used in the case of ileo-sigmoidostomy. The reason for abandoning the mechanical devices is that occasionally they give way before union takes place, with resulting peritonitis. Secondly, occasionally the mechanical device does not slough away but blocks and obstructs the opening. As the Murphy button is still occasionally used, it will be described in the following chapter.

BIBLIOGRAPHY.

Albert. Zur Kasuistik der Dünndarm—Resektionen.
Wien. med. Presse, 22:517-519 and 597-599; y. 1881.

H. Braun. Zur Technik der Naht bei verschiedenen Operationen am Magen und Darm.
Deutsch. Med. Wochenschr. 17:3-4; y. 1891.

M. E. Connell. An experimental contribution looking to an improved technique in enterorrhaphy, whereby the number of knots is reduced to two, or even one.
Med. Record, 42:335-337; y. 1892.

M. E. Connell. Intestinal anastomosis—by a new method without plates and with but two knots—either silk or catgut sutures may be used.
J. A. M. A. 21:150-154; y. 1893.

F. G. Connell. Intestinal sutures. Some old, some not so old, and a new one.
The Philad. Monthly Med. Journ. 1:37-56; y. 1899.

F. G. Connell. Intestinal suture, perforating and knotted in the lumen.
Surg. Gyn. Obst. 4:534-536; y. 1907.

H. W. Cushing. The "Right angle" continuous intestinal suture.
Med. & Surg. Reports, Boston City Hospital, pp. 83-102, y. 1889.

Czerny. Zur Darmresection.
Berl. klin. Wochenschr. 17:637-642; y. 1880.

Denans. Recueil de la société de méd. de Marseille, y. 1826.

Emmert. Lehrbuch der Chir. III:236; y. 1862.

R. V. Frey. Ueber die Technik der Darmnaht.
Bruns Beiträge zur klinischen Chirurgie. 14:1-136; y. 1895.

M. Gara & F. Mandl. Untersuchungen über die Histologie der Darmnaht und der "Serosaplastik".
Arch. f. klin. Chir. 124:419-434; y. 1923.

Gély. Recherches sur l'emploi d'un nouveau procédé de suture contre le divisions de l'intestin. Paris, 1844.

A. Gould. An improved method of end to lateral intestinal anastomosis. A new mattress stitch.
Boston Medic. & Surg. Journ. 151:707-708; y. 1904.

W. S. Halsted. Circular suture of the intestine. An experimental study.
Amer. Journ. of Medic. Sciences, 94:436-461; y. 1887.

W. S. Halsted. Intestinal Anastomosis.
Bull. Johns Hopkins Hospit. 2:1-4; y. 1891.

Jobert. Méthode de suture par adossement des séreuses.
Arch. générales de médécine; y. 1824.

W. Kausch. Zur Technik der Darmnaht nach Schmieden.
Zbl. f. Chir. 38:761-762; y. 1911.

P. Kuzmik. Zur Kritik der Darmnaht.
Deutsche Zeitschr. f. Chir, 45:301-381; y. 1897.

Lembert. Repertoire d'anatomie et de physiologie pathologiques.
Sur l'enterorrhaphie; y. 1826.

Maunsell. A new method of intestinal surgery.
Am. Journ. Med. Sc. 103:245-257; y. 1892.

J. B. Murphy. Cholecysto-intestinal, gastro-intestinal, entero-intestinal, anastomosis and approximation without sutures—original research.
Chicago Med. Recorder. 3:803-840; y. 1892.

T. A. McGraw. Upon the use of the elastic ligature in the surgery of the intestines.
Journ. Amer. Med. Ass.; 16:685-694; y. 1891.

W. Noetzel. Zu den vorschlägen zur Darmvereinigung von Reich und von Orth.
Zbl. f. Chir., 44:862; y. 1917.

W. Noetzel. Ueber die Technik der mehrreihigen Darmnaht.
Bruns Beiträge zur klin. Chir., 117:155-164; y. 1919.

P. Postnikow. Die zweizeitige Gastroenterostomie.
Zbl. f. Chir. 19:1018-1021; y. 1892.

V. Schmieden. Zur Technik der Darmnaht. Die fortlaufende Einstülpungsnaht bei der Enteroanastomose.
Zbl. f. Chir. 38:531-532; y. 1911.

A. Schubert & Th. Beer. Experimenteller Beitrag zur Technik der Magen-Darmnähte.
Arch. f. klin. Chir.; 133:537-558; y. 1924.

N. Senn. Enterorrhaphy: its history, technic and present status.
Journ. Am. Med. Ass.; 21:215-235; y. 1893.

Sprengel. Geschichte der Chirurgie. Halle; y. 1819.

D. V. Trueblood. Intestinal anastomosis. Using a simplified basting stitch method.
West. J. of Surg. (Obst. & Gyn.); 40:654-658; y. 1932.

P. Walzel. Zur Technik der Darmvereinigung durch Invagination.
Zbl. f. Chir.; 46:20-22; y. 1919.

F. Wysler. Penetrirende Wunde des Unterleibes. Darmvorfall.
Zwei Darmwunden. Neue Darmnaht. Heilung.
Arch. f. klin. Chir.; 6:210-213; y. 1865.

CHAPTER V.

INTESTINAL ANASTOMOSIS.

Intestinal anastomosis is an artificial communication between the lumen of two bowels. There are three possible ways of establishing such communication:

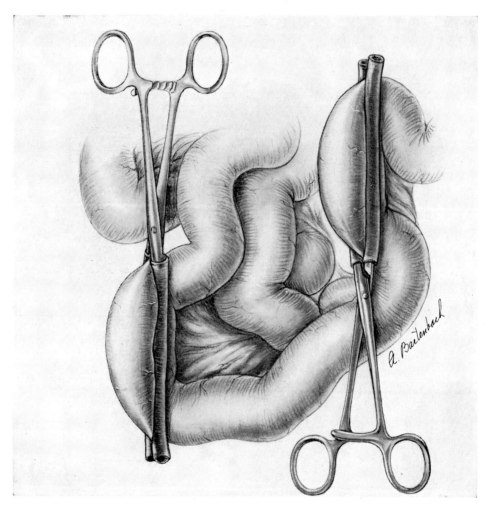

FIG. 81. LATERAL INTESTINAL ANASTOMOSIS.
Loops of the bowel to be anastomosed are clamped.

A. Lateral Intestinal anastomosis.

B. End-to-end anastomosis.

C. End-to-side anastomosis.

A. LATERAL INTESTINAL ANASTOMOSIS.

This was first performed by Maisonneuve (1809-1897), in 1852.

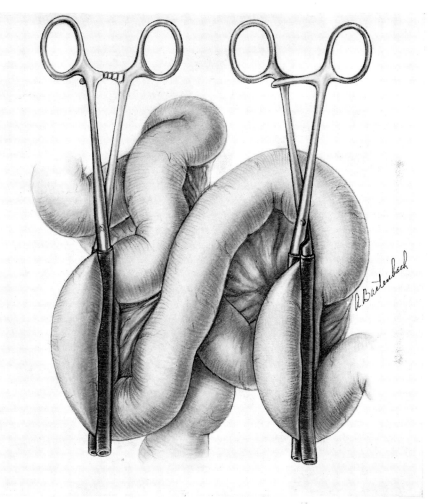

FIG. 82. LATERAL INTESTINAL ANASTOMOSIS.
The loops are placed in an isoperistaltic direction.

Indications—The operation is performed either for short-circuiting a loop of bowel, the lumen of which is narrowed, or as a step in some other operative procedure. Thus, in the case of anterior gastro-enterostomy it is always advisable to supplement the operation by a lateral intestinal anastomosis.

The methods of performing the operation may be subdivided into two groups:

I. Anastomosis by suture methods;

II. Anastomosis by mechanical devices.

With the perfection of suture methods, the mechanical devices are now little used.

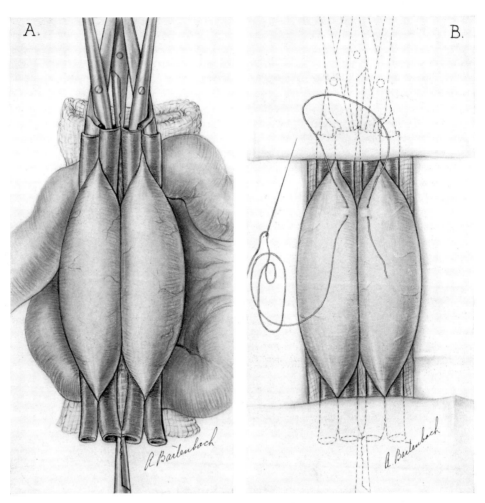

FIG. 83. LATERAL INTESTINAL ANASTOMOSIS.
A. The clamps are fastened to each other;
B. Beginning of the seromuscular suture line.

I. LATERAL INTESTINAL ANASTOMOSIS BY THE SUTURE METHOD.

Step 1. An intestinal loop proximal to the place which should be short-circuited is grasped. The intestinal contents of this portion are squeezed out by the index-finger and thumb of each hand. An

intestinal clamp, the blades of which are covered with rubber
tubing, is placed axially on a fold of the bowel-wall. The handles
of the clamp rest on the assistant's side of the table. The length
of the fold should be about four inches, and the clamp should
compress the wall of the bowel and not the mesentery (Fig. 81).
The blades should not be tightly locked, **only sufficiently to prevent**

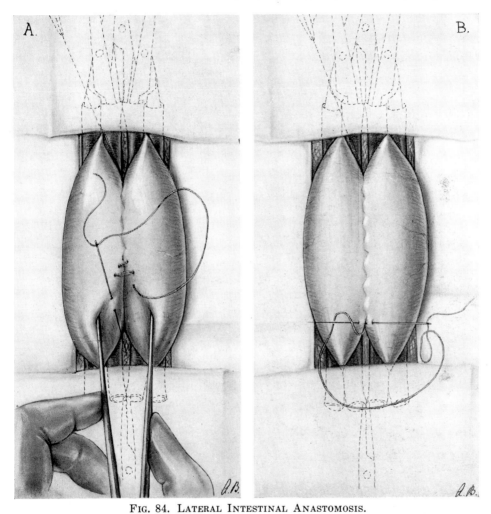

FIG. 84. LATERAL INTESTINAL ANASTOMOSIS.
A. The tissue-forceps is used alternately as a retractor and as a needle-holder;
B. The last seromuscular stitch is locked.

**leakage of the intestinal contents but not to shut off the blood-
supply.** If the wall of the bowel becomes dark, the clamp should
be loosened slightly.

Step 2. Another intestinal clamp is placed distally on a loop of bowel
several inches away from the loop which is to be short-circuited,

with the handles of the clamp resting on the surgeon's side of the table. This clamp, which grasps the distal loop, is rotated in such a manner, that the handles rest also on the assistant's side (Fig 82). Thus, the peristalsis in both loops will move in the same direction (**"isoperistaltic"**) and the clamps will rest side by side with the blades directed toward the surgeon and the handles

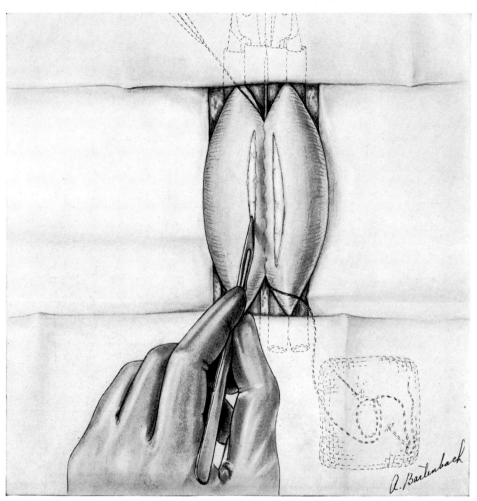

FIG. 85. LATERAL INTESTINAL ANASTOMOSIS.
Cutting the seromuscular layer by the right hand on the right loop and by the left hand on the left loop.

toward the assistant (Fig. 82). A moist sponge is placed between the clamps. This will prevent the contamination of the region between the clamps when the bowel is opened. The rubber tubing on the adjoining blades is grasped by a mosquito forceps (Fig. 83, A). This will keep immobile the relative position of the loops of the bowel. The tubing of the handles of the clamps is also grasped by a mosquito clamp [fastening of the blades is not necessary if the clamps are so constructed that this is done by a mechanical device]. The handles of the clamps, the portions of the blades not engaged in holding the bowel, and the operative field on each side of the clamps are covered by towels moistened in warm normal

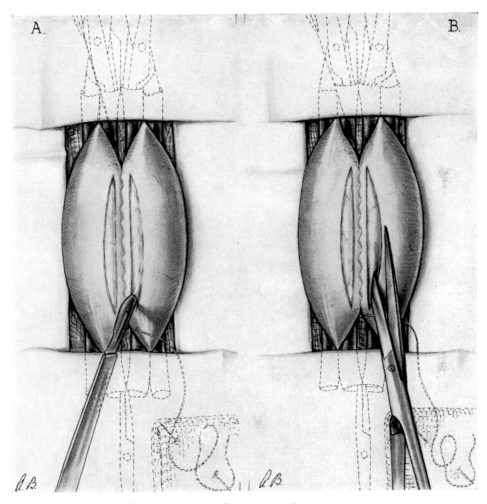

FIG. 86. LATERAL INTESTINAL ANASTOMOSIS.
A. The mucosa is opened by a knife;
B. The incision is enlarged upward by scissors.

salt-solution. After this is done, **the operative field will consist of two loops of bowels surrounded on all sides by towels** (Fig. 83, B).

Step 3. **A seromuscular suture** of the Cushing type is begun from the point most distal to the surgeon. The suture is made with a straight needle and without a needle-holder. The first stitch is a reversed "U" shape stitch (Fig. 83, B). The handle of a tissue-forceps is placed between the adjoining walls of the intestinal loops, and is used as a retractor while inserting the needle into the seromuscular layer, and as a needle-catcher as soon as the point of the needle emerges from the seromuscular layer

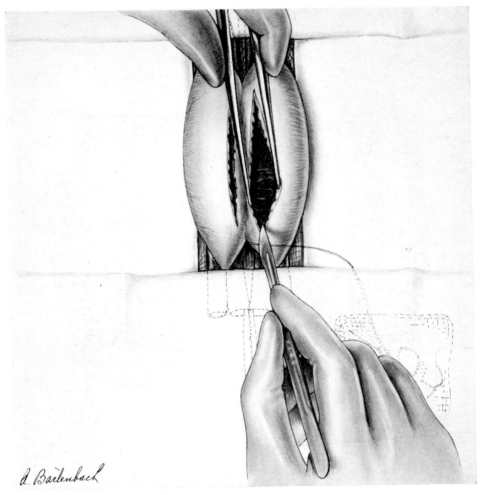

A. Bartenbach

FIG. 87. LATERAL INTESTINAL ANASTOMOSIS.
Cutting the mucosa by a knife in a downward direction. The tissue forceps prevents the knife from injuring the posterior wall.

(Fig. 84, A). The distance of each stitch from the other is one-eighth of an inch. This suturing is continued until the portion of the bowel proximal to the surgeon is reached. Then the last stitch is locked (Fig. 84, B). The needle is then secured to a piece of gauze and laid aside under the towel so that **no instruments,** needles etc. lie uncovered (Fig. 85). **The length of this sero-muscular suture should be about three inches.**

Step 4. The surgeon now puts on the stretch the end of the seromuscular suture closest to himself, and the assistant does the same with the end closest to him. **A seromuscular** incision is then made by a knife for a length of **two and one-half inches** on each loop. **The**

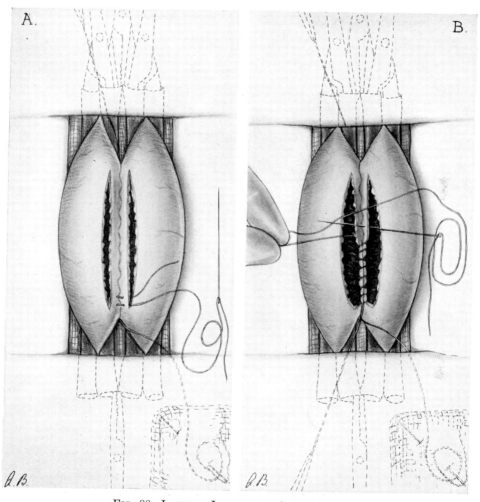

FIG. 88. LATERAL INTESTINAL ANASTOMOSIS.
A. Starting over-and-over suturing of the posterior wall;
B. Suturing of the posterior wall is continued.

knife is held in the right hand while making this incison on the right loop, and in the left hand while making the incision on the left loop (Fig. 85). These incisions should run parallel to the seromuscular line of suture and be at a distance of one-eighth of an inch from it. The incision should start one-fourth of an inch from one end of the suture-line, and should be continued until it reaches a point one-fourth of an inch from the other end of the line (Fig. 85).

The mucosa is now cut at the lower angle by the knife (Fig. 86, A), and the incision is extended upward by scissors throughout the

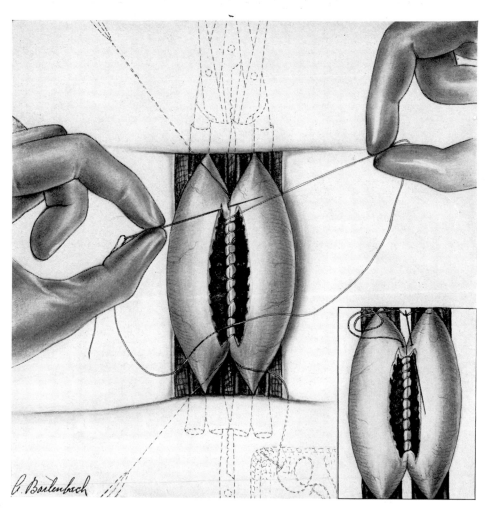

FIG. 89. LATERAL INTESTINAL ANASTOMOSIS.
Closing the angles of the incision.

entire length of the exposed mucosa (Fig. 86, B). If, however, it is necessary to cut the mucosa downward, **it should be done by a knife** (Fig. 87). [The reason for cutting downward by the knife is that the surgeon can do this without changing the position of his body, whereas if scissors were used it would be necessary for him to change his position. **Changing of position is not good**

practice. Frequently, by so doing the surgeon either pushes the assistant aside or obscures the operative field from him. This can be obviated by changing hands or instruments, namely, by using a knife instead of scissors, or by using the left hand instead of the right. Therefore, in order to cut the anterior wall of the

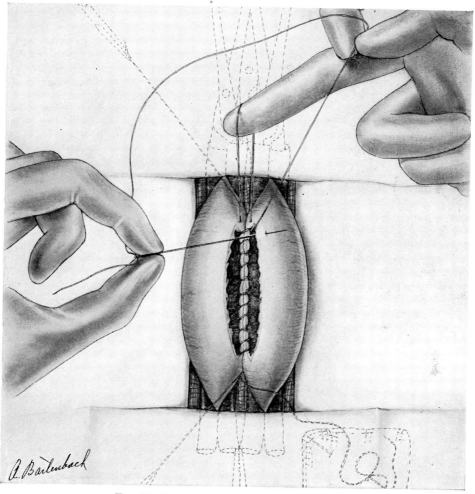

FIG. 90. LATERAL INTESTINAL ANASTOMOSIS.
The intestinal loop is pierced from within outward by the left hand.

intestine below the point where the bowel is opened, a knife should be used].

In order not to cut too deeply, a tissure-forceps should be introduced into the lumen of the bowel and only the anterior wall cut (Fig. 87). Both loops should be opened to the same length.

Step 5. An over-and-over suture is started at the end of the bowel closest to the surgeon, the needle piercing both inner walls as close to the angles of the bowel as possible. Then the inner lip of the left loop is pierced from within outward. This is done with the left hand. The inner lip of the right loop is then pierced from without inward. This is done with the right hand (Fig. 88, A). The two

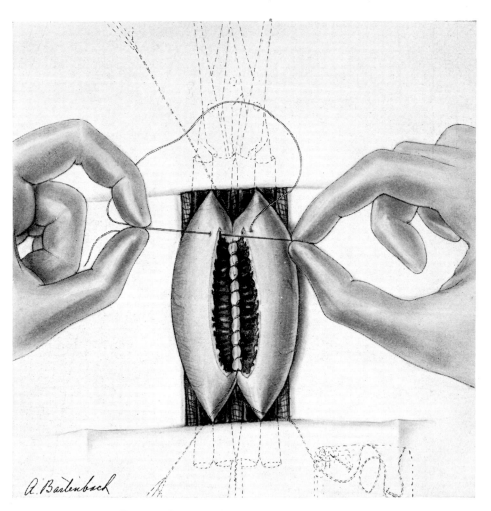

FIG. 91. LATERAL INTESTINAL ANASTOMOSIS.
The loop on the left side is pierced from without inward by the left hand and the needle is grasped by the right hand.

ends of the thread are then tied, and **the knot will be within the lumen of the bowel.** The free end of the thread is clamped and covered by the towel (Fig. 88, B). **[No instruments should lie uncovered by a towel].** The over-and-over suture is then carried through the entire thickness of the intestinal wall, locking each third stitch (Fig. 88, B). As soon as the upper angle is reached, the inner lip is pierced from within outward (Fig. 89, main picture). Then the needle pierces the lip of the opposite side from without inward (Fig. 89, insert). The suturing is then continued in the form of a continuous Connell suture or as an over-and-over suture.

The Connell suture has been described elsewhere as an inter-

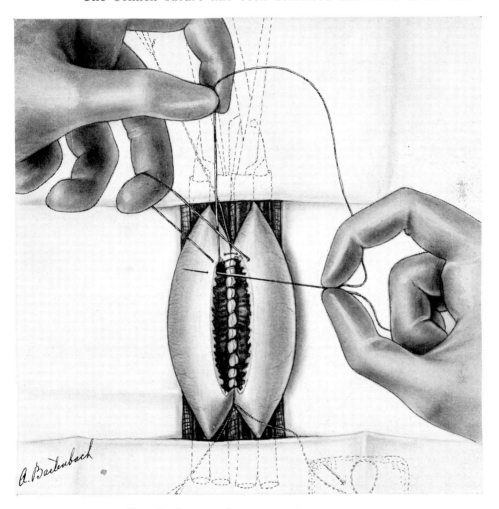

FIG. 92. LATERAL INTESTINAL ANASTOMOSIS.
The thread is used as a tissue forceps. The loop of the left side is pierced from within outward by the right hand.

rupted stitch. It will now be described in detail, as a continuous suture. When the needle and thread are within the bowel, the needle pierces the lip from within outward (Fig. 90). It then crosses the wound and pierces the lip of the opposite side from without inward (Fig. 91), and then the same lip from within outward (Fig. 92), so that loops are formed which are resting on the mucosa. In order not to use tissue-forceps for holding the edges of the wound, which would unnecessarily traumatize them, the thread is used as a tissue-forceps (Figs. 90, 92). One hand should not be used continually for this suturing, since that would require a constant change of the position of the surgeon's body.

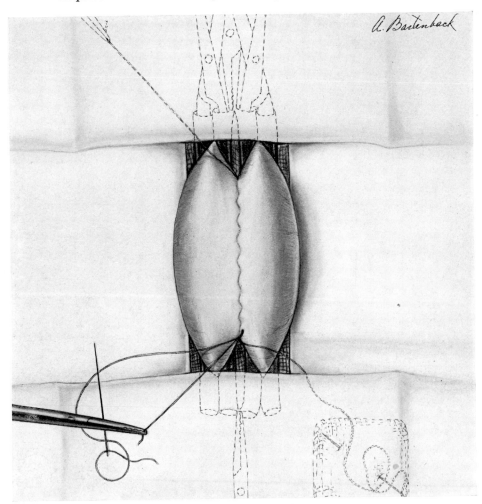

FIG. 93. LATERAL INTESTINAL ANASTOMOSIS.
The suturing of the anterior wall is completed and the ends of the thread are tied to each other.

The hands should be changed; passing from without inward **the left hand should be used for the left loop (Fig 91) and the right hand for the right** (Fig. 89, insert); passing from within outward the reverse is true, namely, **the right hand for the left loop (Fig. 92) and the left hand for the right loop (Fig. 90)**. In order not to lose time by taking the needle from one lip with one hand and inserting it with the other hand, **it should be caught by the hand which will make the next movement.** Thus, in piercing the left lip from without inward the **left hand should be used and the needle grasped by the right hand** (Fig. 91).

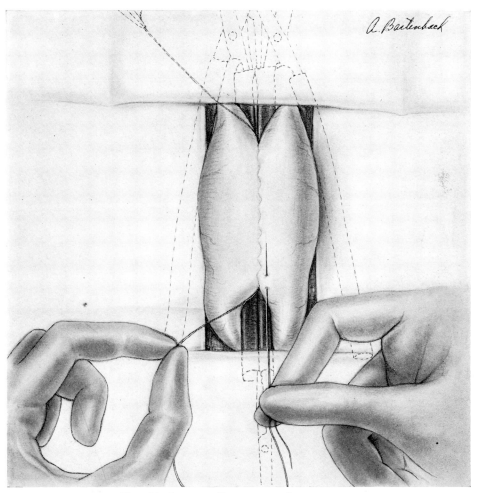

FIG. 94. LATERAL INTESTINAL ANASTOMOSIS.
The clamps are released; the seromuscular suturing is made by the right hand on the right side.

Let us recapitulate. In piercing the **right loop** from without inward, the right hand is used. But the needle is drawn out by the left hand, and then pierces the lip from within outward by this hand. The needle is grasped by the left hand and penetrates the wall of the left loop **(with the left hand)** from without inward. The needle is caught by the right hand and penetrates the wall of the left loop from within outward **(by the same hand),** and so on. This can be given **mnemonically** in the following way:

On passing the needle from without inward the hands should be changed; on passing from within outward, they should not be changed.

When the anterior lips are sutured, the thread is tied to the end

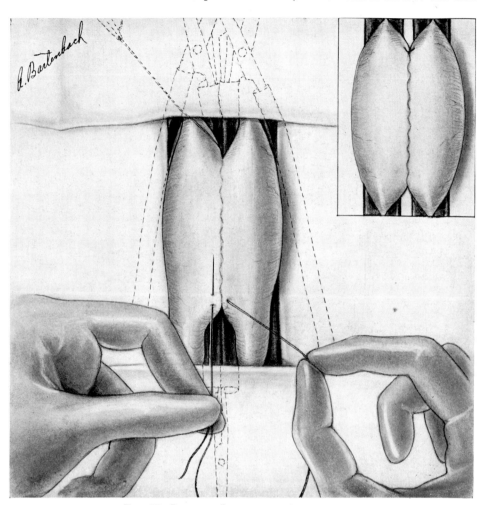

FIG. 95. LATERAL INTESTINAL ANASTOMOSIS.
The clamps are released; the seromuscular suturing is made by the left hand on the left side.

which was left long when the over-and-over suture began (Fig. 93). The ends are then cut short. In this way, the thread and the knot will cut through the edge of the lip. However, this is of no importance, since this will take place only in from four to five days by which time the seromuscular layer, which is a reinforcing layer, will be strong enough.

Step 6. The clamps are unlocked and left in place with wide-opened blades so that the anastomosed loops rest on the central blades (Fig. 94). The sponge which was placed behind the clamps is removed, and the ends of the blades are covered by a towel in order that the thread shall not be caught in them. The needle with the thread left after completion of the first row of the seromuscular suture then

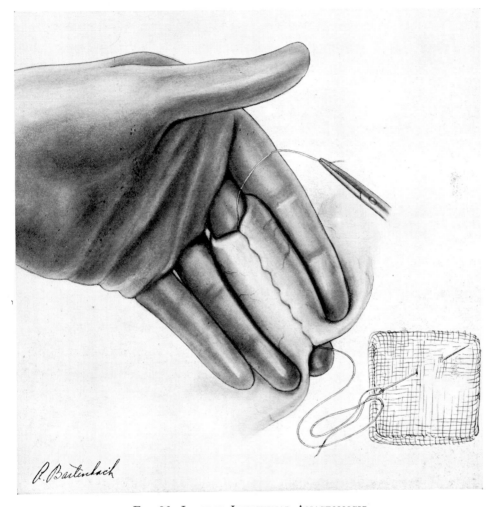

FIG. 96. LATERAL INTESTINAL ANASTOMOSIS.
Alternate method of suturing the anterior wall (See text).

continues the Cushing seromuscular suture, moving **away** from the surgeon to the assistant. **The right hand** is used for sewing the right loop (Fig. 94) and the **left hand** for the left loop (Fig. 95), and the needle is grasped with the hand with which the surgeon is going to make the next move. This suturing is continued in the described manner until the end of the incision on the assistant's side is reached. The thread on the needle is tied with the clamped thread on the assistant's side, and the ends are cut short (Fig. 95, ins.).

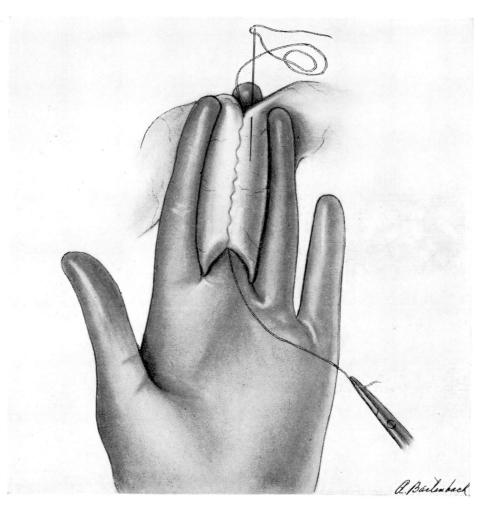

FIG. 97. LATERAL INTESTINAL ANASTOMOSIS.
Alternate method of suturing the anterior wall (See text).

ALTERNATE METHOD OF SUTURING THE SEROMUSCULAR LAYER.

Step 6. The clamps are loosened from the bowel. The sponge behind the clamps is removed, and the anastomosed loops are placed on the palmar surface of the middle finger of the left hand. With the index- and fourth fingers of this hand the anastomosed loops are immobilized (Fig. 96). The hand is then turned in the opposite direction (Fig. 97), and with the needle left after completion of the first row of the seromuscular suture the suturing of the seromuscular layer **is continued toward the surgeon.** When this line is completed, the thread is tied to the end of the thread left at the beginning of the operation.

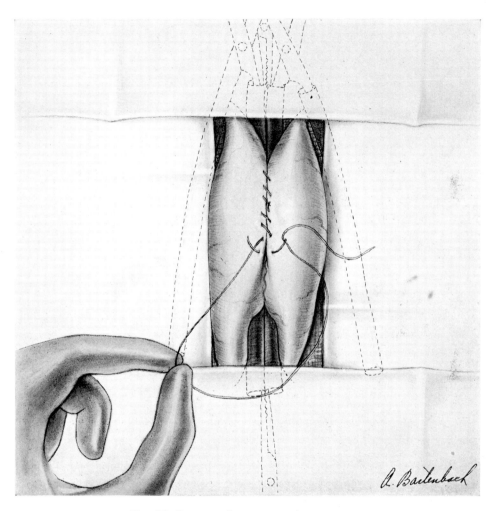

FIG. 98. LATERAL INTESTINAL ANASTOMOSIS.
Seromuscular suturing by the Wysler (Dupuytren) suture.

As may be seen from this description the walls of the bowel are stitched in two layers. The outer is seromuscular and, therefore, is **aseptic.** The inner is an over-and-over suture, which is **contaminated.** However, this contaminated inner layer is surrounded on all sides by the **aseptic seromuscular layer.**

In the case of lateral **intestinal** anastomosis, the Connell suture may be used advantageously. In the case of lateral anastomosis between the **stomach** and a loop of small bowel, however, it is better to use an over-and-over (glover) suture instead of the Connell suture. The reason for this is that in the Connell suture the edges of the wound are **inverted, and if the wound bleeds, it will bleed inside and the surgeon will not know about it.** In the case of an over-and-over suture the **edges are everted,** and if bleeding occurs it would be outside and, being detected, can easily be checked.

Instead of using a Cushing right-angle suture for a seromuscular-seromuscular suture, we may use a continuous **seromuscular-seromuscular suture (continuous Wysler suture).** The operation is essentially the same as previously described in lateral intestinal anastomosis, with variations in some steps:

LATERAL INTESTINAL ANASTOMOSIS WITH CONTINUOUS (WYSLER'S) SEROMUSCULAR SUTURE.

This is performed in a manner similar to that described in the previous operation, with this difference only that a continuous seromuscular suture of the Wysler type is used instead of the Cushing suture at the beginning and at the end of the operation (Fig. 98).

II. LATERAL INTESTINAL ANASTOMOSIS WITH THE AID OF A MURPHY'S BUTTON.

As has already been mentioned, mechanical devices, such as the Murphy button, the Jaboulay button, or Harrington's segmented ring are seldom used. However, the Murphy button is occasionally used today, and for this reason we include here the description of the technic.

Step 1. A fold of bowel-wall, three inches in length, is grasped axially by an intestinal clamp in such a way that at least one and one-half inches of the bowel-wall lie free above the blade. The same is done with another loop of bowel.

Step 2. A seromuscular incision one inch long is made on each bowel (Fig. 99, insert).

Step 3. A purse-string suture is made around each seromuscular incision (Fig. 99, insert). The exposed mucosa of each loop of the bowel is cut through, and the male half of a Murphy button is introduced into one loop and the female half into the other loop (Figs. 99 and 100). The ends of the thread are tightly tied in the furrow of each half of the button and cut short. [When introducing the halves of the button into the lumen of the bowel they should be held by an artery-forceps which catches the tubular projection of each. Otherwise, they will slip, and it will be difficult to hold them while tying the purse-string]. As soon as the halves of the button are fastened, they are brought together and the male half is inserted into the female. In this manner the serous coverings will come into close approximation (Fig. 101). When the part of the wall caught between the halves of the button sloughs away the button will become loose and will be expelled per rectum.

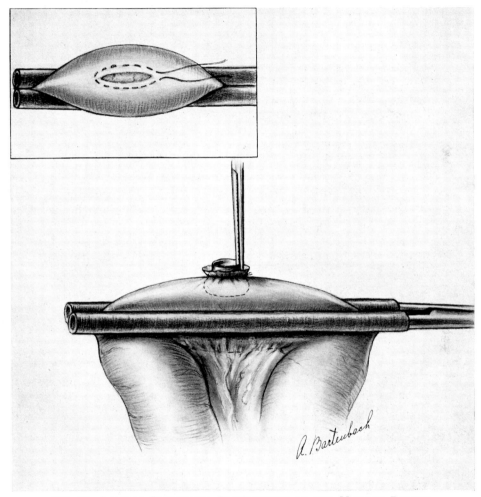

FIG. 99. LATERAL INTESTINAL ANASTOMOSIS BY THE MURPHY BUTTON.

There are some complications which may arise when performing intestinal anastomosis with the Murphy button:

1. The efficiency of the anastomosis, that is, the "water tightness" of it, is just as much in the hands of the instrument-maker as in those of the surgeon.

2. Occasionally, the parts of the wall caught in the button do not slough away, and the button may remain permanently fixed in the loop, producing great narrowing of its lumen, and finally even an intestinal obstruction.

B.   RESECTION OF A BOWEL WITH END-TO-END INTESTINAL ANASTOMOSIS.

End-to-end intestinal anastomosis is used as one of the methods of

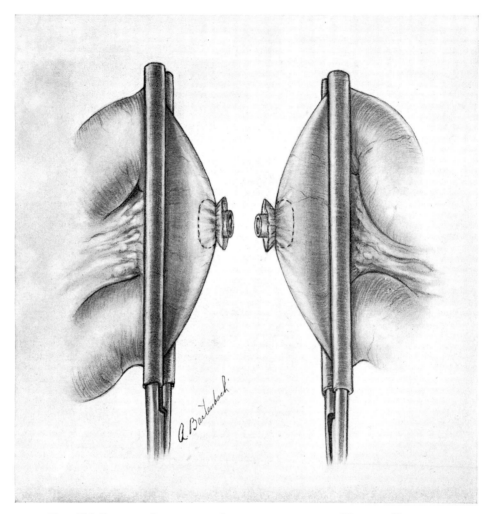

FIG. 100 LATERAL INTESTINAL ANASTOMOSIS BY THE MURPHY BUTTON.
Each half of the button is inserted.

restoring the continuity of the intestinal tract after removal of a portion of a bowel. It was first suggested by Littré, in 1711, and was first performed by Ramdohr, court surgeon of the Duke of Braunschweig. He invaginated the proximal into the distal loop. The dangerous feature of invagination lay in the fact, that at that time the differentiation between the proximal and distal ends of the bowel was not known. This knowledge is absolutely essential in performing the invagination method of anastomosis, since **the distal loop must always be the recipient loop.** Duverger, in 1739, was the first who made an end-to-end anastomosis by suturing the

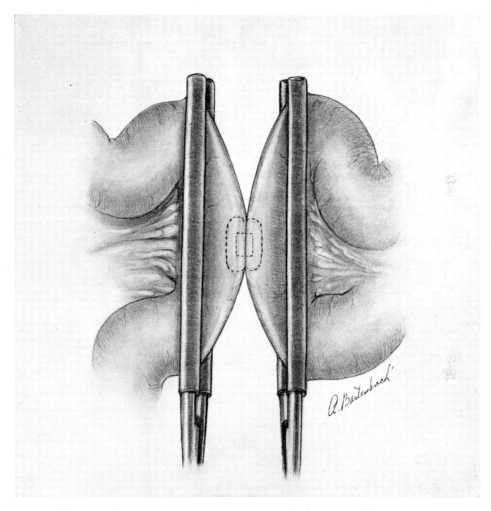

FIG. 101. LATERAL INTESTINAL ANASTOMOSIS BY THE MURPHY BUTTON.
The halves of the button are clamped together.

edges of all the layers of each loop. He did this over the trachea of a lamb in the form of the "four masters suture."

Indications—Chief among these are:

1. Gangrene of the bowel due to strangulation in a hernial sac.
2. Multiple stab-wounds or gunshot wounds of a bowel, when con-

templated repair in several places will produce constriction of the bowel to such an extent that the passage of the intestinal contents will become difficult.

3. Stricture of a bowel due to previous ulcerations which are healed.

4. Malignant changes in the bowel.

5. Irreducible intussusception of a bowel.

6. Tumor or injuries of the mesentery involving the blood-supply of the bowel.

Schede proved that enterectomy and end-to-end anastomosis should not necessarily be immediately consecutive steps of the operation. It might happen that before the operation the loop of the bowel, situated proximally to the place of obstruction, becomes greatly distended and inflamed. Should an end-to-end anastomosis then be performed immediately after resection of the constricted portion, the distended portion contracts and there may result marked tension on the suture-line with yielding of some of the stitches, resulting in leakage and peritonitis.

How Much of the Intestines can be Removed?

As the length of the bowel varies in different individuals, it is clear that the quantity which can be removed will vary with the case. This can be stated relatively to the whole length of the bowel only. Beneke, after comparing the height of an individual and the length of his small bowel in a series of cases, stated that for every 100 cm. of body-length there are about 387.5 cm. of small bowel. Experiments on dogs and observations of patients have shown that about half of the length of the small bowel can be removed safely. It is immaterial whether this will be the upper half or the lower half, though from the physiological point of view, we should expect that the removal of the upper half will lead to more serious consequences than the removal of the lower half.

The **age** is a very important factor in determining this question. Relatively more can be removed from a young person than from an old one, since in the former the vicarious ability of the remaining part is greater than in an adult. Thus, in Ruggi's case, 330 cm. (10 ft. 10 in) were removed successfully from a boy eight years old. The largest piece of bowel removed from a human being successfully was on a patient, reported by Brenner, when 540 cm. (17 ft. 10 in.) of small bowel were removed.

End-to-end anastomosis may be performed:

I.   By suture methods.

II. By mechanical devices.

I.   END-TO-END ANASTOMOSIS BY THE SUTURE METHOD.

Step 1. The loop of the bowel which is to be resected is drawn out and crushing-clamps are placed on each end of this loop (Fig. 102);

the clamps should be placed obliquely so that more of the bowel-wall on the mesenteric border will be left. The reason for this is twofold: 1. It widens the lumen, so that a stricture will not follow after completion of the anastomosis. 2. The blood-supply to the free border of the bowel is better assured in this way.

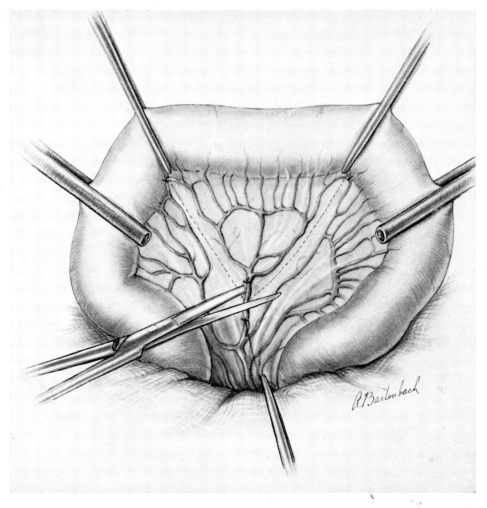

FIG. 102. END-TO-END ANASTOMOSIS BY THE SUTURE METHOD.
The mesenteric artery and the arcuate vessels are tied; scissors ready to cut the mesentery between the two ligatures.

Step 2. From the point where each crushing-clamp is placed the intestinal contents are "milked out" for two inches. On each side of the clamp at a distance of two inches from each crushing-clamp an intestinal clamp covered with rubber tubing is placed (Fig. 102). The operative field is walled off from the peritoneal cavity by towels soaked in normal salt-solution.

Step 3. The mesenteric vessels which furnish the blood-supply to the bowel to be resected are ligated by two ligatures and cut between (Fig. 102). The arcuate artery on the side of each crushing-clamp is ligated between this clamp and the intestinal clamp close to each crushing-clamp. This should be done with a round curved intestinal

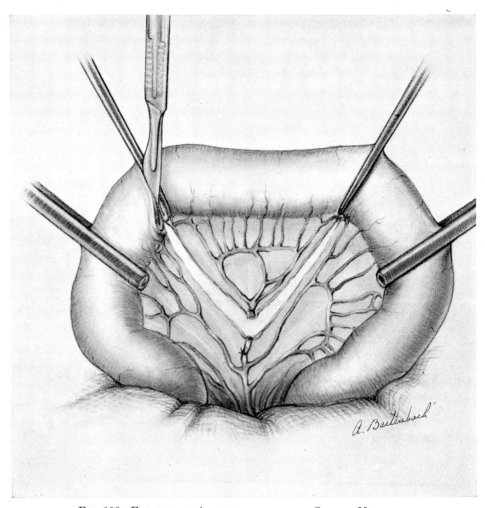

FIG. 103. END-TO-END ANASTOMOSIS BY THE SUTURE METHOD.
The mesentery is cut in a V-shape; the knife begins to cut the bowel.

needle, care being taken to catch also the seromuscular layer of the adjoining intestinal wall (Fig. 102).

Step 4. The mesentery is cut in a V-shape, the apex of which is the stump left after ligation of the mesenteric vessels. Then only should the bowel be cut by the knife just lateral to each crushing-forceps (Fig. 103).

Step 5. Suturing of the ends of the bowel is begun, using for this purpose **Maunsell's mesenteric stitch** (Fig. 104, A), the ends of the thread being left long and grasped by an artery forceps, so that they may be used as a traction-suture. Another traction-suture is placed on the free (antimesenteric) border of the bowel. This

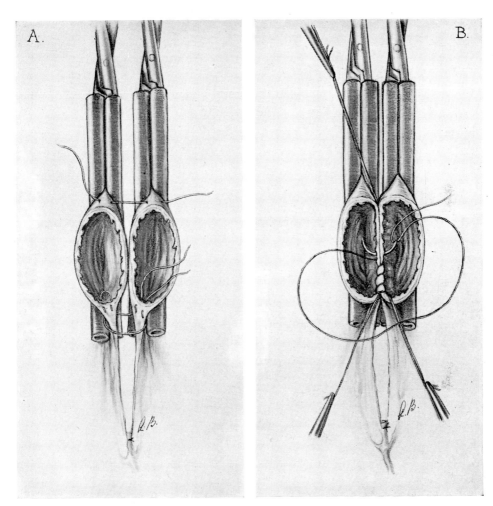

FIG. 104. END-TO-END ANASTOMOSIS BY THE SUTURE METHOD.
A. Maunsell mesenteric stitch inserted; guy stitch is inserted on the free border of the bowel;
B. Suturing the posterior wall by an over-and-over suture.

suture penetrates the seromuscular layer only (Fig. 104, A), and is placed close to the edge of the open end of the bowel. This is tied with one knot, so that later, when this thread is cut, the minute hole in the bowel-wall will be sealed. A through-and-through suture is started on the posterior wall at the mesenteric border (Fig. 104, B) each bite of which should be at a distance of one-eighth of an inch from the other and also from the edges of the lips. Each third stitch is either locked or a back-stitch is made. When the second traction-suture is reached, it should be left intact and the suture is continued either in the form of a Connell suture

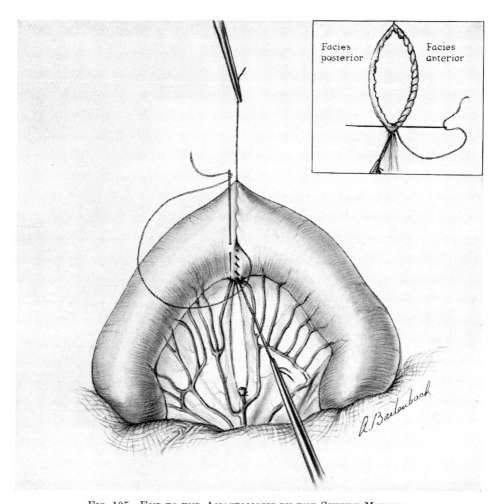

FIG. 105. END-TO-END ANASTOMOSIS BY THE SUTURE METHOD.
MAIN PICTURE. Reinforcing the over-and-over suture by a seromuscular suture.
INSERT. Showing the needle at the mesenteric border passing from the anterior to the posterior surface of the bowel.

or as an over-and-over suture until the mesenteric border again is reached. The thread attached to the needle is tied with the thread left long at the beginning of the suture, and the ends are cut short.

Step 6. The over-and-over suture is now reinforced by a seromuscular suture which starts from the antimesenteric border. The ends of the thread which were on the antimesenteric border and which have been used as a traction-suture are now cut short. The seromuscular suture continues in the form of a Cushing right-angle continuous suture (Fig. 105), so as not to produce a diaphragm. When the mesenteric border is reached, the needle is passed to the

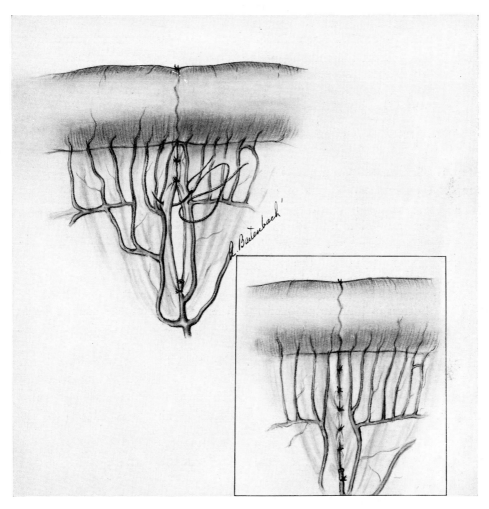

FIG. 106. END-TO-END ANASTOMOSIS BY THE SUTURE METHOD.
Closure of the opening in the mesentery.

other side of the bowel by penetrating the mesentery very close to the wall of the bowel (Fig. 105, insert), which is then turned so as to make the posterior wall face anteriorly [this can be accomplished by drawing the traction-suture applied to the mesenteric border through the hole in the mesentery, and by drawing the end of the thread of the seromuscular suture on the free border in the opposite direction]. A continuous right-angle Cushing suture, or a continuous Wysler suture, is continued. making a back-stitch after each third stitch, until the free border of the bowel is reached. Then the beginning and the end of this seromuscular suture are tied together and cut short. The ends of the thread of the Maunsell mesenteric stitch are also now cut short. The bowel is replaced in its proper position so that the anterior wall faces anteriorly and the posterior wall posteriorly.

Step 7. The slit in the mesentery is closed by a continuous suture or by interrupted sutures (Fig. 106), **care being taken not to injure any blood-vessel lying close to the edge of the mesenteric wound.**

II. END-TO-END ANASTOMOSIS BY A MECHANICAL DEVICE (MURPHY BUTTON).

Step 1. The same as Step 1 of the previous operation.

Step 2. The same as Step 2 of the previous operation.

Step 3. A purse-string suture is made one-half inch away from each crushing-clamp.

Step 4. The same as Steps 3 and 4 of the previous operation.

Step 5. The male half of the button is introduced into one open end of the bowel, its tubal projection being held by an artery-forceps while tying the ends of the purse-string. The female half of the button is then introduced into the open end of the other loop in the same manner. The male tube is inserted into the female (Fig. 107).

Step 6. The line of anastomosis is reinforced by a few seromuscular stitches.

Step 7. An additional stitch is placed on the mesentery close to the button.

Step 8. The slit in the mesentery is closed as shown in Step 7 of the previous operation (Fig. 107, insert).

C. END-TO-SIDE INTESTINAL ANASTOMOSIS.

Definition.

This is an implantation of an open end of a bowel into the lateral wall of another bowel.

Indications.

1. Most frequently it is used in cases of resection of the cecum or colon, as in an ileo-sigmoidostomy.

2. In colo-colostomy.

3. In the Roux "Y" method of gastro-enterostomy.

4. In Maydl's method of jejunostomy.

This operation can be performed either by the suture method or with the aid of some mechanical device such as the Murphy button.

We will now describe an end-to-side anastomosis between two loops of small bowel, leaving implantation of an end of a small bowel into the lateral wall of a large bowel to be described in the Chapter on "The Surgery of the Large Bowel".

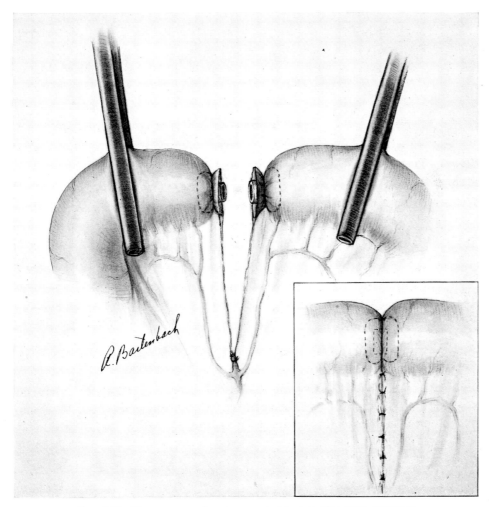

FIG. 107. END-TO-END ANASTOMOSIS BY THE MURPHY BUTTON.

I.   END-TO-SIDE ANASTOMOSIS BY THE SUTURE METHOD.

1. Gould Method.

Step 1. A loop of small bowel is grasped and the intestinal contents are "milked out" for a length of six inches. Three intestinal clamps, the blades of each covered with rubber tubing, are placed, one at one end of the "milked out" gut, another at the other end, and the third between the other two, in such a manner that it will be two inches away from the clamp on the proximal end and four inches away from the clamp on the distal end of the gut. The middle clamp is placed obliquely.

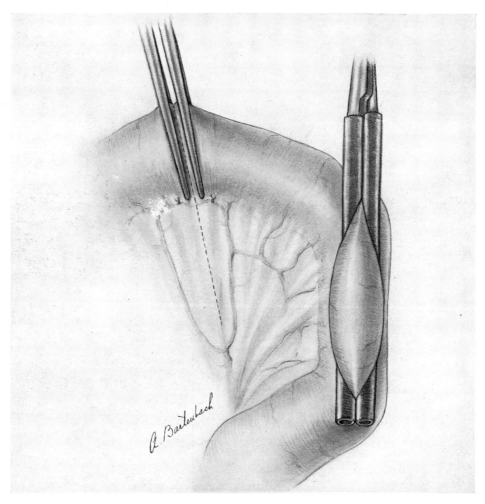

FIG. 108. END-TO-SIDE ANASTOMOSIS BY THE SUTURE METHOD.
The bowel is clamped between two forceps; a fold of bowel is clamped axially.
(See text: Alternate Method of End-to-side Anastomosis).

Step 2. The arcuate vessels are ligated at two points close to the middle clamp and between it and the proximal clamp, and the jejunum is divided, the incision passing between the two ligated arcuate vessels. Then the proximal part will be left open with one clamp at a distance of two inches from its open end, and the distal loop will be held by two intestinal clamps.

Step 3. The free border of the proximal segment is cut longitudinally for one-half to one inch and the sharp edges so produced are trimmed. In this way, the lumen of the bowel will be increased.

Step 4. The receiving bowel is opened for one and one-half inches on its free border.

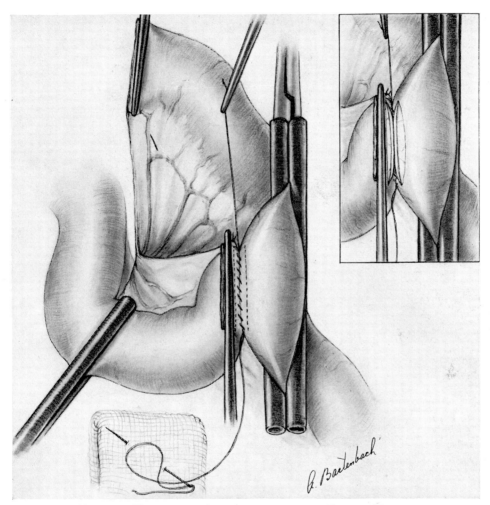

FIG. 109. END-TO-SIDE ANASTOMOSIS BY THE SUTURE METHOD.
(See text: Alternate Method of End-to-side Anastomosis).

Step 5. The proximal loop of the divided bowel is brought to the lateral wall of the distal loop so that the mesenteric border lies at the lower angle (which means that the mesentery will face upward). The lower end of the incision is attached to the mesenteric border of the entering bowel by a mattress-suture. A guy-stitch is placed on each side of this mattress-suture with the free ends lying inside the lumen of each bowel. Each of these threads penetrates the middle of the lip of the entering and receiving bowel. The edges will thereby be everted and the suturing facilitated. The over-and-over suturing is done in the usual way, this layer being reinforced by a second layer of Lembert sutures (interrupted).

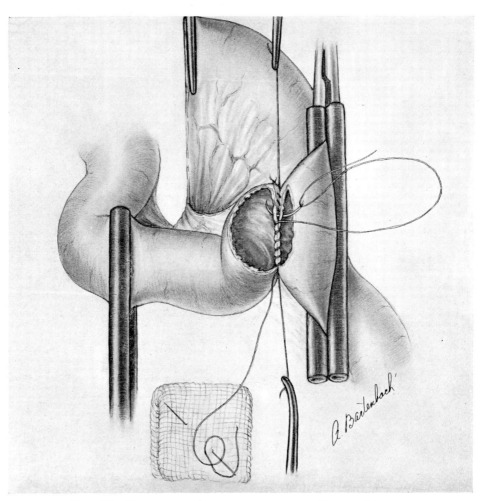

FIG. 110. END-TO-SIDE ANASTOMOSIS BY THE SUTURE METHOD.
Suturing of the posterior wall.
(See text: Alternate Method of End-to-side Anastomosis).

Step 6. The lip of the mesentery is sutured either to the wall of the jejunum, to the mesojejunum, or to the posterior abdominal wall (if this be possible). This is done to prevent the occurrence of internal strangulation.

Step 7. The open end of the distal loop of the bowel may be closed blindly, brought outside, or implanted into another hollow viscus, this depending on the reason for which the operation has been done.

2. Alternate Method of End-to-side Anastomosis.

Step 1. Two crushing-clamps are placed closely together and obliquely

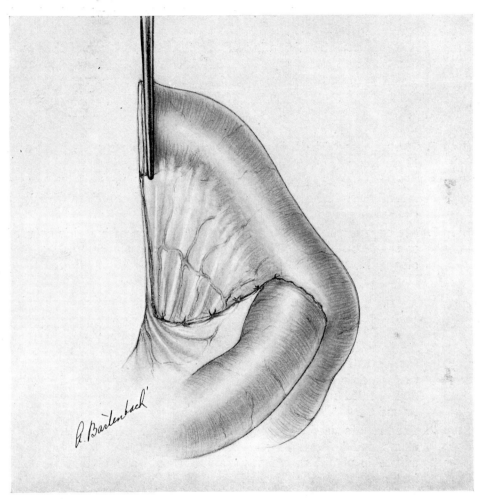

Fig. 111. End-to-Side Anastomosis by the Suture Method.
The mesentery of the entering bowel is sutured to the mesentery of the receiving bowel.

upon a loop of bowel, and this loop and its mesentery are cut between the clamps, remembering however, **to cut first the mesentery and then the bowel** (Fig. 108).

Step 2. A longitudinal fold of the recipient bowel is grasped by an intestinal clamp. The entering loop of bowel is then brought to this fold in such a way that its mesentery faces upward (Fig. 109).

A seromuscular suture is made between these two loops (Fig. 109), and after this is completed the last stitch is locked, and the threaded needle is placed on a piece of gauze beneath the towel.

Step 3. The contents of the entering loop are "milked out" for a distance of three inches, and an intestinal clamp is applied transversely to its long axis, and locked tightly enough to prevent escape of the intestinal contents but not enough to interfere with the blood-supply (Fig. 109).

Step 4. A seromuscular incision is made on the recipient loop of the bowel and also on the entering loop of the bowel just below the clamp. The seromuscular layer will begin to curl and cover the seromuscular line of suture, so that when the lumen of the bowel is opened this suture will not be contaminated (Fig. 109, right upper insert).

Step 5. The mucosa of both loops is incised, thus opening the lumina of these loops (Fig. 110).

Step 6. The operation is now completed as described in the technic of a lateral intestinal anastomosis, starting with that step in which the over-and-over sutures are to be placed (Fig. 110).

Step 7. The edge of the mesentery of the divided loop of bowel is sutured to the mesentery of the recipient loop, thus preventing a possible strangulation of the bowel (Fig. 111).

II. END-TO-SIDE ANASTOMOSIS BY MECHANICAL DEVICES (MURPHY BUTTON).

Step 1. An intestinal loop is "milked out" for a distance of six inches. One intestinal forceps clamps the proximal end perpendicularly to its axis, another grasps the distal portion of the gut axially, and a third midway between grasps the gut perpendicularly to its axis.

Step 2. The arcuate vessels are ligated in two places close to the middle clamp and between it and the proximal clamp. A purse-string suture is placed proximally around the intestinal loop one-half inch away from the middle intestinal clamp.

Step 3. A seromuscular incision one inch long is made on the fold held axially by the distal intestinal clamp. A purse-string suture is made around this incision.

Step 4. The bowel is cut obliquely between the middle and proximal intestinal clamps in such a manner that the plane of the incision passes between the ligated arcuate vessels.

Step 5. The male half of the Murphy button is introduced into the open end of the proximal loop and fixed in the same manner as already described (Fig. 112).

Step 6. The mucosa of the antimesenteric border of the distal loop is incised and the female half of the button introduced and fixed exactly as described in the side-to-side anastomosis by the Murphy button. The male half of the button is then inserted into the female half (Figs. 112, 113). The site of union is reinforced by a seromuscular suture.

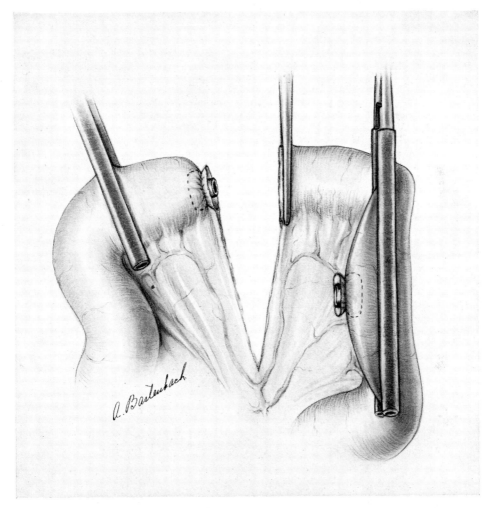

FIG. 112. END-TO-SIDE ANASTOMOSIS BY THE MURPHY BUTTON.

Step 7. The edges of the mesentery are sutured either to the wall of the recipient bowel or to its mesentery or to the peritoneum of the posterior wall (Fig. 113).

Step 8. The open end of the distal bowel may be treated according to the aim of the operation.

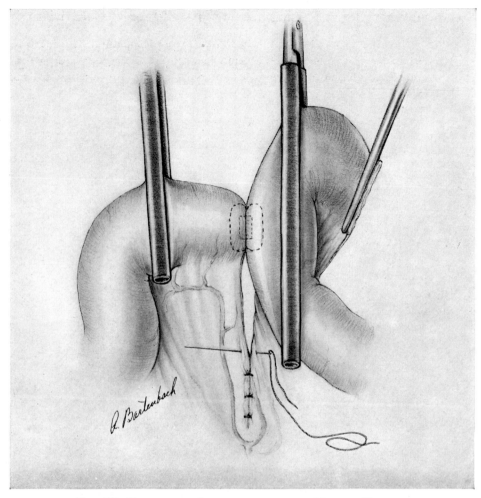

FIG. 113. END-TO-SIDE ANASTOMOSIS BY THE MURPHY BUTTON.
The end of the divided piece of bowel is inserted into the side of the other loop of bowel.
Suturing of the mesenteric edges to each other.

BLIND CLOSURE OF AN OPEN END OF A BOWEL.

This procedure is an essential step in several operations. Thus, it is a routine step in gastrectomies of the type of Billroth II and its modifications. It is also used as one of the steps in what is known as the "Haberer-Finney Modification of Billroth I". It might be used in cases of enterectomies when, after resection of a loop of bowel, the continuity is reëstablished by a lateral intestinal anastomosis between the remaining parts of the bowel after blind closure of the end of each loop. There are different methods of performing this:

a. Over-and-over Suture Method

b. Purse-string Method

a. BLIND CLOSURE BY THE OVER-AND-OVER SUTURE METHOD.

Step 1. After the bowel is cut between two crushing-clamps, the closure
of either or both of these ends is accomplished in the following
manner: A seromuscular suture starts from the antimesenteric

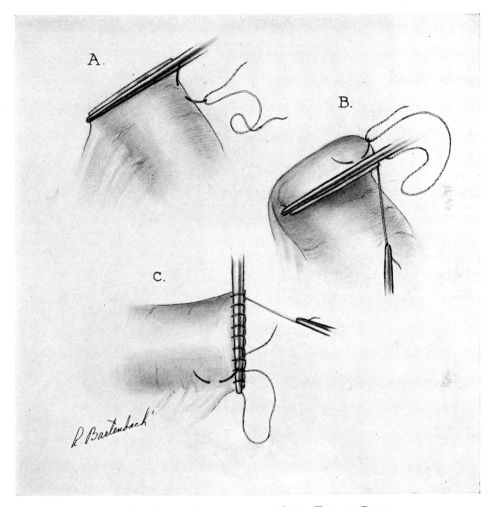

FIG. 114. BLIND CLOSURE OF AN OPEN END OF BOWEL.
A. Starting the suturing at the antimesenteric border;
B. Turning the clamp in order to expose the side on which the suture is to be inserted;
C. Inserting the last stitch.

border of the bowel, the first bite being placed at the distance of
one-half inch from the lower border of the blade of the clamp and
directed **toward it** (Fig. 114, A). The thread is carried over the
clamp with each successive stitch until the mesenteric border is
reached. [In order to make the side of the bowel on which the

surgeon is going to take a bite visible to him, the assistant should turn the clamp each time thereby exposing the sides of the bowel alternately (Fig. 114, B)]. Each bite is taken close to the clamp and parallel to it, the last bite being one-half inch **from the clamp** on the mesenteric border and directed **away from it** (Fig. 114, C).

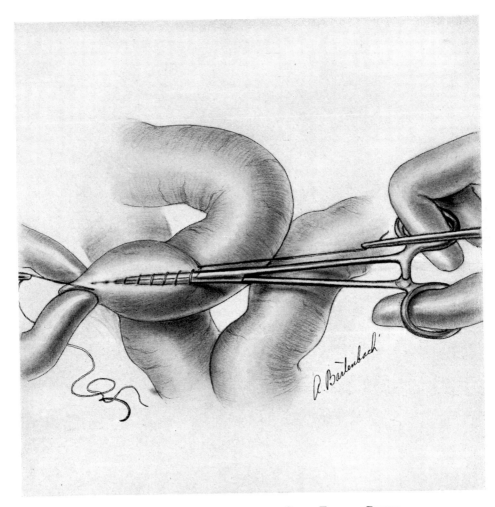

FIG. 115. BLIND CLOSURE OF AN OPEN END OF BOWEL.
Invaginating the end of the bowel.

Step 2. The assistant holds both ends of the thread. The surgeon holds the bowel between the index-finger and the thumb of his left hand one and one-half inches away from the clamp (Fig. 115). With the right hand he takes the handles of the crushing-clamp and gently opens it so that the opened blades shall not tear the thread. The blades are then closed again, and pressing with the tips of the clamp on the crushed end of the bowel, he slowly draws out the clamp while the assistant is pulling the ends of the thread apart (Fig. 115). By this maneuvre the end of the bowel will become invaginated.

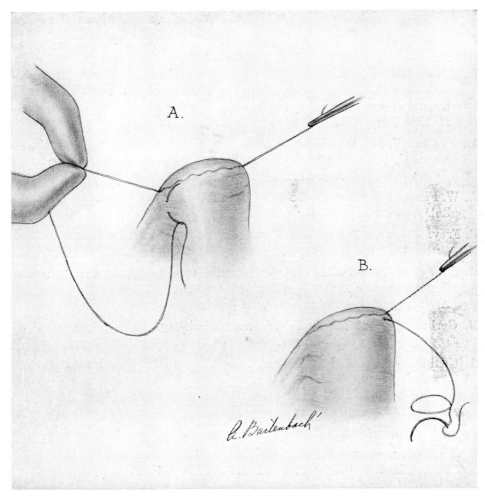

FIG. 116. BLIND CLOSURE OF AN OPEN END OF BOWEL.
A. Starting the second row of sutures;
B. The second row completed.

Step 3. With the needle left on the thread, the seromuscular suture is continued in a direction opposite to the direction of the first layer (Fig. 116, A) until the beginning of this suture is reached (Fig. 116, B), when the ends of the thread are tied.

b.   BLIND CLOSURE BY THE PURSE-STRING METHOD.

Step 1. A crushing-clamp is applied to the bowel which is then cut through flush with the blade.

Step 2. A purse-string seromuscular suture is inserted about one-half inch away from the clamp. The bowel is held in the left hand and the clamp removed by the right hand. The end of the bowel is invaginated as described above, and the assistant ties the ends.

BIBLIOGRAPHY.

M. E. Connell. An experimental contribution looking to an improved technique in enterorrhaphy, whereby the number of knots is reduced to two, or even one.
Medical Record, 42:335-337; y. 1892.

M. E. Connell. Intestinal anastomosis—by a new method, without plates and with but two knots, either silk or catgut sutures may be used.
Journ. Am. Med. Ass. 21:150-154; y. 1893.

A. W. Fischer. Studien zur Seit-zu-Seitanastomose am Darm.
Zbl. f. Chir., 58:930-934; y. 1931.

R. Frey. Ueber die Technik der Darmnaht.
Bruns Beiträge zur klin. Chir. 14:1-136; y. 1895.

R. Galli & G. Bendandi. Studio sperimentale sul trapianto dello sfintere ileo-cecale nelle anastomosi fra tenue e colon.
Arch. ital. di chir. 38:527-574; y. 1934.

H. Gerber. Über einseitige Dickdarmausschaltung.
Bruns Beiträg. z. klin. Chir. 160:399-416; y. 1934.

A. Gould. An improved method of end to lateral intestinal anastomosis. A new matress stitch.
Boston Med. & Surg. Journ. 151:707-708; y. 1904.

A. Gridnev. Circulus vitiosus coli.
Zbl. f. Chir. 61:2362-2363; y. 1934.

F. Harrington. Segmented ring for intestinal anastomosis.
Boston Med. and Surg. Journ. 147:521-522; y. 1902.

C. E. Holm. The fate of the sidetracked loop of ileum following lateral anastomosis for complete, benign obstruction.
Surg. Gynec. Obst. 56:746-751; y. 1933

H. Jansen. Ein neues Verfahren zur totalen Ausschaltung ohne aussere Fistelbildung.
Arch. f. klin. Chir. 163:614-625; y. 1931.

G. Luquet. Technique de quelques procédés: d'abouchement de l'intestin grêle dans le gros intestin après résection.
Paris chirurgical, 23:197-209; y. 1931.

G. L. McWhorter. An original method of closure of a partially aperitoneal or short intestinal end.
Surg. Gyn. & Obst. 50:1037-1038; y. 1930.

J. B. Murphy. Cholecysto-intestinal, gastro-intestinal, entero-intestinal, anastomosis and approximation without sutures—original research.
Chicago Med. Recorder. 3:803-840; y. 1892.

A. Plenk. Über die Mesenterialdurchtrennung bei der Resektion des Dünndarmes.
Zbl. f. Chir. 59:1382-1385; y. 1932.

J. Quénu. L'ileo-coloplastie.
Journ. de Chir. 42:15-48; y. 1933.

N. Senn. Enterorrhaphy, its history, technique and present status.
Journ. Am. Med. Assn. 21:215-235; y. 1893.

H. L. Skinner. Extensive resection of small intestine.
Ann. Surg. 93:788-790; y. 1931.

D. V. Trueblood. Intestinal anastomosis. Using simplified basting stitch method.
West. J. Surg. 40:654-658; y. 1932.

J. Wulsten. Heilung einer Thrombose der Vena mesenterica superior durch Resektion des gesamten Dünndarmes.
Zbl. f. Chir. 56:3155-3159; y. 1929.

CHAPTER VI.

ENTEROTOMY. ENTEROSTOMY.

ENTEROTOMY

Definition.

The word enterotomy consists of two Greek words: ἔντερον, bowel and τομή, a cut. It means to make an opening in the bowel which is closed at the same sitting of the operation.

Indications.

    a. Removal of foreign bodies.

    b. As a step in operations for obstructed bowel.

Technic.

The technic varies somewhat, depending on whether the operation is done for the removal of a foreign body or as a step in an operation for intestinal obstruction.

ENTEROTOMY FOR REMOVAL OF A FOREIGN BODY.

Step. 1. The loop of bowel on which it is intended to make the incision is grasped, and two intestinal clamps, the blades of which are covered with tubing, are placed at a right angle to the long axis of the bowel, one proximally to and the other distally from the intended line of incision. The gut is walled off from the peritoneal cavity by gauze-packs, moistened in warm, normal salt-solution.

Step 2. A longitudinal incision is made along the free border of the bowel, the length of which depends upon the size of the foreign body.

Step 3. The foreign body is dislodged and removed.

Step 4. The incision is closed in the following manner: Three over-and-over sutures are inserted. One passing through the upper and lower angles of the incision, the second, passing through adjoining points of the middle of the left lip, and the third passing through adjoining points of the middle of the right lip. The ends of the threads are tied and left long so that they can be used as traction-sutures. The lips of the wound between the traction-sutures are united by over-and-over sutures. When this is done, the ends of the traction-sutures and the ends of the over-and-over sutures are cut short. This layer is reinforced by a second layer of seromuscular sutures in the usual way. **Thus, the bowel, cut longitudinally, is sutured transversely, thereby preventing a narrowing of its lumen.**

ENTEROTOMY AS A STEP IN INTESTINAL OBSTRUCTION.

Enterotomy should be looked upon as an essential step in the treatment of acute intestinal obstruction. It should be performed above the site of constriction, so as to evacuate the toxic intestinal contents.

Step 1. The abdomen is opened.

Step 2. The bowel which is ensnared is located and freed. It is then brought out of the abdominal cavity and "walled off" from the peritoneal cavity by moist packings. The assistant compresses the wall of the bowel in two places: one about ten inches above the site of the former constriction, and the other immediately below this point. He should do this, not

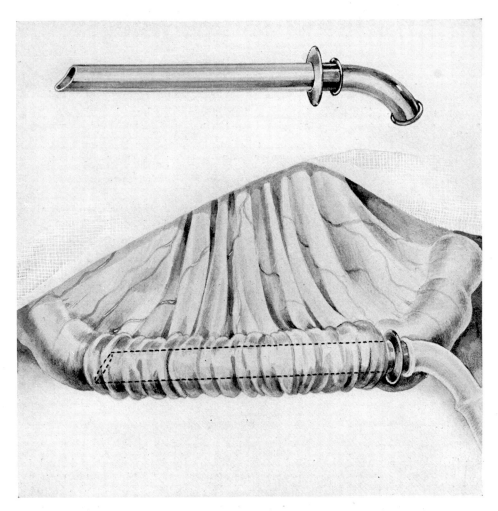

Fig. 117. Enterotomy.
Plaiting the bowel over a glass tube (After Moynihan).

with gloved fingers, because the bowel **is extremely difficult to hold and will slip away, but with a piece of moistened gauze, which will give stability to the gut.**

Step 3. The wall of the bowel is caught on each side of the antimesenteric border by two French vulsellæ about five inches above the seat of the former obstruction. Care must be taken that it is caught **in the healthy portion of the gut.**

Step 4. The free border of the bowel is opened between the two vulsellæ.

Step 5. A glass tube, the length of which is from six to eight inches, to the other end of which a large rubber drainage tube is attached, is introduced into the lumen of the bowel and pushed in the proximal direction for three or four inches. The vulsellæ are then removed from the lips. The bowel, held by a piece of gauze moistened with warm normal salt-solution, is drawn upon the glass tube until it nearly reaches the outer end of the tube. **This should be done with wet warm gauze, which will prevent the fingers from slipping. Thereby there will be no leakage of intestinal contents between the glass tube and the lips of the bowel.** The surgeon draws more and more of the bowel on this glass tube (Fig. 117). [Monks showed that on a tube of six inches in length, **eight or ten feet of bowel can be drawn**]. While pleating the bowel on the tube the intestinal contents will empty through the glass and rubber tubes. **This manipulation should be done very slowly.**

[N. B. The reason for this pleating is that by making a mere opening in the bowel the contents of only one or two of the immediate proximal loops will escape. The rest will remain in the more remote proximal loops. By pleating the intestinal wall on the glass rod, **the contents of many loops will escape**].

Step 6. The bowel is then unpleated from the tube. **This is done very slowly.** As soon as the bowel is all drawn back into the abdomen, the glass tube is slowly withdrawn from the lumen of the bowel. **The assistant tightly holds the opening into the bowel.**

Step 7. The incision into the bowel is closed as described in Step 4 of the previous operation, or in the form of a linear suture which corresponds to the long axis of the bowel.

ENTEROSTOMY.

Definition.

Enterostomy consists of two Greek words: ἔντερον, bowel and στόμα, mouth. It is a surgical procedure by which the lumen of the bowel is opened and remains in communication with the outside world. If it is performed in such a manner that it closes later spontaneously, it is called **temporary enterostomy.** If it does not close spontaneously but requires a special operation for its closure, then it will be a **permanent enterostomy.** Depending on the portion of the bowel which is opened, enterostomy is subdivided into duodenostomy, jejunostomy, ileostomy, appendicostomy, cecostomy and colostomy, the name itself implying where the opening is made. Depending on the portion of the bowel which is opened, enterostomy may serve either as an artificial mouth for feeding the patient **(upper jejunostomy)** or as an artificial anus **(lower ileostomy or colostomy).** In this chapter will be described only the different types of jejunostomy or ileostomy. The colostomy operations will be given in Chapter VIII, "Surgery of the Large Bowel".

Indications.

A. **As an Artificial Anus.** This is done.

1. In some cases of malignant or benign stricture of the cecum, when for some reason, the cecum cannot be removed at the time of operation.

2. In case of obstruction in the lower ileum or cecum, when the strangulation or incarceration cannot be removed at the time of operation, and the surgeon is compelled to be satisfied with releasing "back pressure" by making a "temporary artificial anus".

B. **As an Artificial Mouth (for feeding purposes).** This is done:

1. In case of carcinoma of the pylorus when pylorectomy or gastro-enterostomy for some reason cannot be performed.

2. In case of ulcer of the stomach when the surgeon wants to cure the ulcers by the "Rest Method" (Von Eiselsberg, Lameris, etc.).

3. As a preliminary step in certain operations on the stomach or esophagus.

A. ENTEROSTOMY (ILEOSTOMY) FOR AN ARTIFICIAL ANUS.

TEMPORARY ENTEROSTOMY IN TWO STAGES.

1st Stage.

Step 1. The site of the opening of the abdomen depends upon the location of the loop in which enterostomy is to be made. Thus, for a **high jejunostomy,** the incision should be made in the left upper quadrant [in case a transverse incision is desired it should be made at the level of the umbilicus and directed transversely through the left rectus muscle]. In case of a **low ileostomy,** the incision should be made in the right lower quadrant. [In case the transverse incision is preferred, it should be made transversely through the right rectus muscle at a level midway between the umbilicus and the symphysis pubis].

Step 2. The selected loop is brought out of the abdominal cavity and is anchored at the upper and lower ends of the incision by one suture at each angle. These sutures penetrate the peritoneum and transversalis fascia about one inch from their margin, then pass through the sero-muscular layer of the bowel-wall, and then again pass through the transversalis fascia and peritoneum of the other lip, also at a distance of one inch from its margin (Fig. 118, a).

Step 3. The peritoneum is sutured to the seromuscular layer of the bowel-wall by a series of interrupted sutures. Each stitch should catch the peritoneum about one inch away from its margin (Fig. 118, b).

Step 4. The edges of the skin are sutured to the edges of the peritoneum (Fig. 119).

In this way several things are accomplished:

1st. The bowel is sutured to the peritoneum, so that the peritoneal cavity is shut off from the site of the contemplated opening into the bowel.

2nd. The skin is sutured to the peritoneum, which will prevent the intestinal contents from entering and contaminating the layers of the abdominal wall.

3rd. There will be no bowel spur-formation, which means that spon-

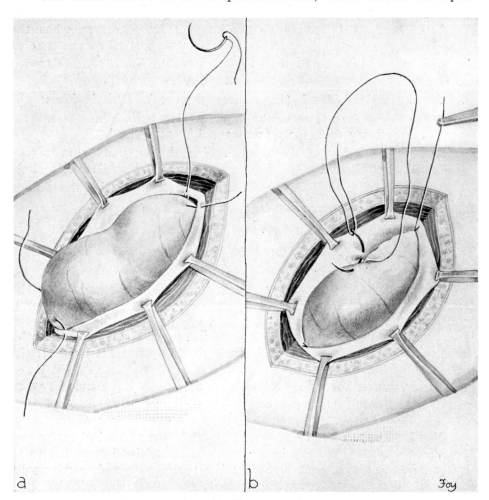

FIG. 118. ENTEROSTOMY.
a. Anchoring the bowel at each end of the abdominal incision.
b. Suturing the seromuscular layer of the bowel to the peritoneum.

taneous closure will be greatly facilitated when the need for enterostomy is over.

Second Stage.

Step 5. One or two days later the bowel is opened by a longitudinal or transverse incision (Fig. 119, insert).

If, however, it is necessary to open the bowel immediately, then the procedure will be as follows: A purse-string suture is placed in the bowel, and the sero-muscular layer of the loop is incised within the purse-string until the mucosa bulges. The protruding mucosa is caught by an Allis forceps and the cone of mucosa thus produced is cut with scissors. A glass

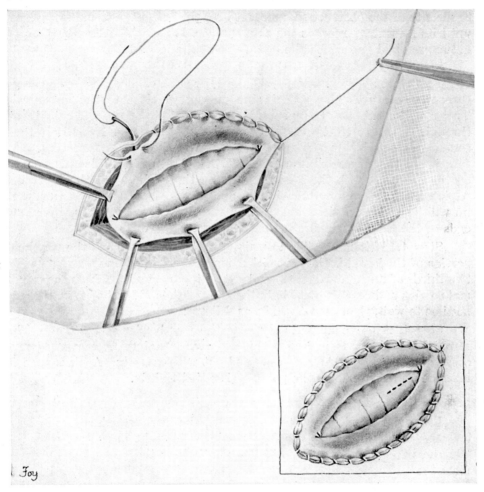

FIG. 119. ENTEROSTOMY.
Suturing the edges of the skin and peritoneum to each other.
INSERT. Opening of the bowel.

tube is immediately inserted into the opening and the ends of the thread are tied snugly around it.

We have described this technic rather in detail, since it is quite frequently used by surgeons both for ileostomy and colostomy. However, we always prefer to attach the loop of bowel (ileum, sigmoid) to the skin in such a manner, **that no sutures pass through the wall of the bowel,** as is described below:

Step 1. The abdomen is opened in the right lower quadrant or by a lower midline incision. The length of the incision should be three to four inches.

Step 2. Any distended loop of ileum is selected, preferably one closest to the site of the obstruction, and it is brought out of the abdominal cavity until its mesentery reaches the skin-surface. It must be determined which is the proximal and which the distal end of the loop.

Step 3. A bite is taken through the entire thickness of the inner lip of the anterior abdominal wall, including the skin. Then, the needle passes through some **avascular** spot in the mesentery close to the mesenteric border of the gut, and then penetrates the outer lip of the abdominal wall through its entire thickness from within outward (Fig. 146, b). It then returns through the mesentery very close to the spot where the first perforation of the mesentery was made (Fig. 146, c). Thus, a loop is formed on the outer lip with the free ends of the thread lying on the inner lip. A piece of rubber tubing is placed on each lip so that the one on the outer lip will lie inside the loop and that on the inner lip will lie between the ends of the thread, which are then tied (Fig. 146, d).

Step 4. If it is possible to wait for two or three days, the proximal portion of the bowel is then cut either transversely (cutting approximately two-thirds of its circumference) or longitudinally, starting from the proximal portion and reaching nearly to the apex of the gut. If however, there is no time to wait, then Step 4 will be as follows:

Step 4. A purse-string is made on the free border of the bowel. The seromuscular layer is incised within this purse-string. The exposed mucosa is caught by an Allis forceps and cut with scissors. A glass tube is inserted and the ends of the purse-string tied tightly.

B.   ENTEROSTOMY (JEJUNOSTOMY) FOR AN ARTIFICIAL MOUTH.

From the physiological point of view, the best procedure would be a duodenostomy, since then the food would be brought in contact with the bile and pancreatic juice close to the point where these secretions pour in from the ampulla of Vater. However, the duodenum should never be used for this purpose, since the unavoidable escape of the duodenal contents onto the skin, with the resulting eczema of the skin, outweigh the advantages of introducing the food close to the stomach.

Jejunostomy (of the proximal jejunal loop) should always be given preference to duodenostomy. The first who performed jejunostomy was Surmay, in 1878. A few methods of performing jejunostomy are given here:

I.   SPIVACK'S METHOD OF TUBO-VALVULAR JEJUNOSTOMY

In this method, a tube and a valve at its base are formed from that portion of the jejunal wall which constitutes and adjoins the antimesen-teric border. The tube is lined with mucosa and for this reason its lumen will not obliterate; the valve will enter the lumen of the tube and stay at its base; it will prevent escape of the intestinal contents outside. Thus, the two difficulties which usually confront the surgeon in this type of opera-tion, namely leakage and obliteration of the channel, are eliminated. The steps of this operation are the same as in the Spivack's tubo-valvular gastrostomy (See pages 306-316 and fig. 172-181).

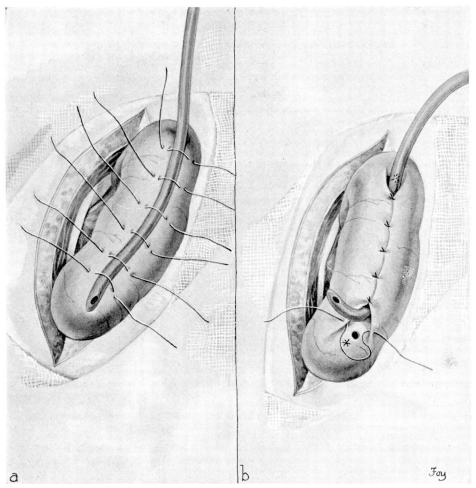

FIG. 120. WITZEL-KAREWSKI METHOD OF JEJUNOSTOMY.

II. WITZEL-KAREWSKI METHOD OF JEJUNOSTOMY

This operation, in which the technic which Witzel used for gastros-tomy was applied to the jejunum, was first performed by Karewski in 1896.

Step 1. The abdomen is opened in the left half of the epigastric region. Whether this incision is longitudinal or transverse depends on the choice of the operator. In case the incision is longitudinal, it should be a left paramedian. In case it is transverse, it should be a left transverse rectus incision at a level one inch above the umbilicus. Its length in either case is three inches.

Step 2. The duodeno-jejunal junction is located by the method of Wölfler-Socin, and the first loop of the jejunum is brought out. Beginning at a distance of eight inches from the duodeno-jejunal junction, the contents of the jejunum are "milked out" for a distance of some inches, and an intestinal clamp is placed at each end of the "milked out" area perpendicularly to the long axis of the bowel.

Step 3. A catheter, size number 12 French, is laid on the wall of the jejunum. A series of interrupted seromuscular sutures are inserted in the bowel-wall over the catheter for a length of three inches (Fig. 120, a). All the threads, with the exception of that one lying close to the eye of the catheter, are tied, thus forming a channel which surrounds the catheter (Fig. 120, b). The wall of the bowel is now incised and the eye-end of the catheter is inserted into the lumen of the bowel, after which the last untied suture is tied, thus closing the opening in the bowel.

Step 4. The bowel is anchored to the peritoneum in two places, one immediately distal to the distal end of the channel and the other immediately proximal to the proximal end of the channel (Fig. 120, b, asterisks); these sutures penetrate the seromuscular layer of the bowel and the peritoneum with the transversalis fascia of the abdomen.

Step 5. The abdomen is closed.

III. MAYDL METHOD OF JEJUNOSTOMY (Fig. 121, a, b).

Step 1. An abdominal incision is made as in the previous operation.

Step 2. A loop of jejunum six inches from the duodeno-jejunal junction is drawn out, and one intestinal clamp, the blades of which are covered with rubber tubing, is placed across it about six inches distally from the duodeno-jejunal junction, and another clamp in the same manner about twelve inches from this junction. The clamps are placed perpendicularly to the long axis of the gut, which they compress just enough to prevent the escape of intestinal contents but not enough to interfere with the blood-supply. The arcuate vessels are ligated at two points, the distance between these points being about one-eighth of an inch. The place of ligation of the arcuate vessels is about three inches distal from the proximal clamps. The bowel is cut obliquely, so that the line of incision runs between the ligated arcuate vessels.

Step 3. The proximal end of the bowel is implanted into the antimesenteric border of the distal loop in such a manner that there will still be left about three inches of the distal end of the jejunum, which should be anchored to the anterior abdominal wall (Fig. 121, a, b). The technic of implantation is exactly as described in **end-to-side anastomosis.**

Step 4. The jejunal tube is anchored separately to each layer of the anterior abdominal wall, that is to the peritoneum and transversalis fascia, to the muscles, to the anterior sheath of the rectus muscle, and to the skin.

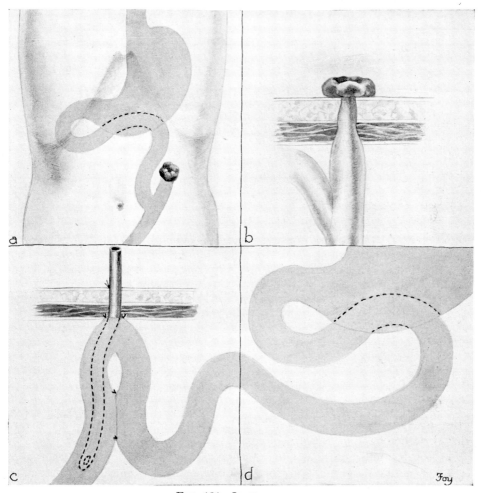

FIG. 121. JEJUNOSTOMY.
a-b. Maydl method;   c-d. Mayo Robson method.

[For a detailed description of anchoring a tube to the anterior abdominal wall see Spivack's tubo-valvular gastrostomy].

IV. MAYO ROBSON METHOD OF JEJUNOSTOMY (Fig. 121, c, d).

Step 1. The abdomen is opened in the left upper quadrant and a loop of jejunum is drawn out as close to the duodeno-jejunal junction as possible, **but without any tension.** A lateral intestinal anastomosis is made between the two limbs placed in an antiperistaltic direction (Fig. 121, c). The technic of the lateral intestinal anastomosis is exactly the same as described in "Lateral Intestinal Anastomosis".

Step 2. A seromuscular incision is made on the knuckle of the loop and a purse-string is made around it. The mucosa is incised, and a catheter is introduced and fastened to the bowel. Care must be taken that the catheter placed into the lumen reaches into the efferent loop beyond the point of anastomosis of the two loops (Fig. 121, c).

Step 3. The bowel is anchored to the peritoneum at two places close to the catheter. The abdomen is closed by tier-suturing.

BIBLIOGRAPHY.

E. Albert. Eine neue Methode der Jejunostomie.
    Wien. Med. Wochenschr. 44:57-59; y. 1894.

U. Bani. La fistolizzazione verso l'intestino, metodo di scelta nelle fistole biliari recidive.
    Policlinico (sez. prat.) 37:659-661; y. 1930.

W. H. Barber. Jejunostomy. A clinical and experimental study of the technic of the operation.
    Ann. Surg. 97:553-576; y. 1933.

M. Cackovic. Ueber totale Verkleinerung (Schrumpfung) des Magens und über Jejunostomie.
    Arch. f. klin. Chir. 65:409-489; y. 1902.

M. Cackovic. Ueber Fisteln des Duodenum.
    Arch. f. klin. Chir. 69:843-856; y. 1903.

V. Carabba. Jejunostomy; an experimental study in a permanent non-leaking yet closable type.
    Ann. Surg. 95:958; y. 1932.

A. Chifflet. Estudio anatomoquirúrgico del ángulo duodenoyeyunal.
    Anales de la Facultad de medicina de Montevideo. 17:382-452; y. 1932.

L. R. Dragstedt, H. E. Haymond & J. C. Ellis. Cannula gastrostomy and enterostomy.
    Surg. Gyn. & Obst. 56:799-801; y. 1933.

R. L. Evans. Value of enterostomy in intestinal surgery.
    Am. J. Surg. 24:53-62; y. 1934.

G. A. Hendon. Simple enterostomy technic.
    Ann. Surg. 94:156; y. 1931.

Jeannel. Chirurgie de l'intestin. y. 1901.

Kelling. Ein sicheres Verfahren der Jejunostomie.
    Zbl. f. Chir. 31:121-124; y. 1904.

M. Kirschner. Die prophylaktische Jejunostomie bei Magenoperationen.
    Arch. f. klin. Chir. 157:561-600; y. 1929.

J. Campos Kunhardt. La yeyunostomia en el tratamiento de la peritonitis aguda generalizada.
Gaceta médica de México. 61:247-269; y. 1930.

K. Maydl. Ueber eine neue Methode zur Ausführung der Jejunostomie und Gastroenterostomie.
Wien. Med. Wchnschr. 42:697-700 and 785-789; y. 1892.

K. Maydl. Weitere Beiträge zur Indicationsstellung der Jejunostomie.
Wien. Klin. Rundschau. 17:3-7 and 24-27; y. 1903.

Nösske. Zur Wertschätzung der Jejunostomie nebst Bemerkungen ueber die Gastroenterostomie.
Deutsche Zeitschr. f. Chir. 72:1-40; y. 1904.

C. A. Perrett. Technique of a new and strictly aseptic method of entero-anastomosis.
Surg. Gyn. & Obst. 44:378-389; y. 1927.

H. J. Shelley. Enterostomy. A consideration of the literature.
Arch. Surg. 25:943-957; y. 1932.

A. Schmechel. Ueber Indikationsbereich und Erfolg der Ileostomie nach dem Prinzip von Witzel.
Deutsche Zeitschr. f. Chir. 241:391-409; y. 1933.

Villard. Jéjunostomie pour ulcère hémorragique.
Lyon chir. 29:251-252; y. 1932.

CHAPTER VII.

ASEPTIC METHODS IN GASTRO-INTESTINAL SURGERY.

The great number of methods employed in gastro-intestinal surgery and known as "aseptic methods" are not aseptic in the true meaning of this word. In order to be aseptic, the lumen of the hollow viscus should not be entered. It is true that there are methods in which the lumen of a hollow viscus is not entered, but these methods are highly impractical and are not employed today. **The methods which are in use are those in which the lumen is entered, but the contamination is negligible, and for such methods the name "aseptic methods" is retained.**

Historical.

One of the earliest methods of "aseptic anastomosis" is the "elastic ligature" method. It was introduced by Silvestri, in 1862, but was soon forgotten. Bardenheuer, in 1888, revived interest in this method, and Mc-Graw, who, more than anybody else popularized and improved the method, described it only in 1891. His technic was as follows:

A seromuscular suture two and a-half inches long is made connecting the walls of the two hollow viscera. A seromuscular incision is made on each of the two viscera at a distance of one-quarter of an inch from the seromuscular suture-line. An elastic ligature, threaded on a special needle, penetrates the mucosa of one hollow viscus close to one end of the seromuscular incision, enters into the lumen of the same viscus and reappears outside of the lumen at the other end of the incision of the same viscus. It then enters into the lumen of the other viscus at a point close to its exit from the first viscus, traverses the lumen of the second viscus and makes its exit at a point close to the point of entrance of the ligature into the first viscus. The two ends are drawn very tight and tied. The original seromuscular suture is continued over the elastic ligature uniting the anterior lips of the seromuscular incision, and this completes the operation.

Usually, due to pressure-necrosis the mucous membrane will slough away, and thus the anastomosis will be established. The elastic ligature will pass *per viam naturales.* As may be seen, the weak points of this operation are:

1. It is not truly aseptic, because the ligature enters into the lumen of the intestine (or stomach).
2. Necrosis of the mucosa will not always take place, and thus the anastomosis **may not be established.**

The **Postnikow method** was as follows: A seromuscular suture was made connecting the two hollow viscera and a seromuscular incision was made on both viscera at a distance of one-quarter of an inch from the suture-line. The mucosa of each viscus was caught with a forceps and drawn out in the form of a cone and tied tightly at its base. The original seromuscular suture was continued to cover the mucosa. As may be seen, this method is truly aseptic, since the **lumina of the viscera were not entered.** However, the results of the anastomosis were uncertain.

The **Boari method** was similar to that of Postnikow with the difference only that, instead of tying the mucosa, caustic material was placed on it, which produced necrosis of the mucosa and thereby established the anastomosis. The same objections which were raised in the case of the Postnikow method hold true in this method.

An important step forward in the development of a "relatively aseptic method" was the discovery by Halsted that the true strength of the union is given by the **submucous layer.** This means that a really strong union can be secured not only by taking a bite through the entire thickness of the wall of the viscus, but also **when the bite includes the entire wall with the exception of the mucosa.** The knowledge of this fact enabled the surgeons to place sutures not entering the lumen and before the viscus was opened, and then to tie the opening as soon as it was made, thus greatly diminishing the possibility of contamination. In this manner, Winiwarter and Halsted performed lateral intestinal anastomosis, Bircher, gastro-enterostomy, and Finney, gastro-duodenostomy. Acting upon the same principle, Parlavecchio did his resection of the bowel with the reëstablishment of its continuity by an end-to-end anastomosis, and Axel Werelius his lateral intestinal anastomosis.

THE PARLAVECCHIO END-TO-END ANASTOMOSIS.

The portion of the bowel to be resected was tied at each end by two ligatures and the bowel cut at each end between the ligatures. The ends of the remaining portions of the bowel were sutured to each other by a series of interrupted seromuscular stitches placed laterally from each ligature, until nearly the entire circumference was sutured. Through the small opening which was still left the ligature which closed each end of the bowel was cut, and the small rent left in the circumference was closed by one or two additional interrupted seromuscular sutures.

This method had, however, several objectionable features:

1. The possibility of contamination was not excluded.
2. A large diaphragn was left which could produce an obstruction, or at least a marked narrowing of the lumen.
3. There was a possibility of hemorrhage.

THE WERELIUS METHOD OF LATERAL INTESTINAL ANASTOMOSIS.

Step 1. A seromuscular suture connected the walls of the two hollow viscera.

Step 2. A silk thread or silver wire, penetrating the entire thickness of the wall, was placed exactly as in the case of the McGraw elastic ligature, entering the lumina of both viscera.

Step 3. The original seromuscular suture was continued anteriorly to cover the silk or silver ligature, leaving only a very small opening through which these ligatures emerged.

Step 4. By sawing movements the walls of the two hollow viscera were broken and the thread released.

Step 5. The small opening was closed by a seromuscular suture.

The objections to this method were:

1. The possibility of hemorrhage.
2. Breaking of the thread.
3. The possibility of sawing off the posterior seromuscular suture-line.
4. The method still made contamination possible.

Bonomo modified the Werelius method. His technic was that of Werelius with the difference only that after making the first seromuscular suture-line he made a seromuscular incision on the wall of each viscus and then introduced a silk thread or silver wire through the mucosa only, completing the operation as Werelius did. In this way, it was easier to saw off the mucosa only instead of the entire thickness of the anterior stomach or bowel-wall. The large blood-vessels exposed by the seromuscular incision could also be ligated before the introduction of the silk or silver suture, thereby preventing the probability of hemorrhage.

The next important step in the development of aseptic intestinal anastomosis was the method suggested by Doyen. He introduced a powerful enterotribe which crushed the wall of the bowel to the thinness of tissue paper. Of the entire thickness of the intestinal wall only the serosa and submucosa were left in the form of thin lamellæ. The blood-vessels were crushed so that there was no danger of hemorrhage.

His technic for the resection of the bowel was as follows: The bowel was crushed at two places by an enterotribe, which was then removed. The groove produced by the enterotribe was tied between two ligatures on each side and the bowel was cut between each of these ligatures. In this way the bowel was resected. The ends of the bowel were brought together by an end-to-end approximation, and a seromuscular row of sutures was introduced in almost the entire circumference, leaving a very small opening through which scissors were introduced to cut the lamella on each side including the ligature. The rent in the seromuscular union was closed by introducing two additional seromuscular sutures. In this way, the anastomosis was reëstablished; there was no hemorrhage and very little contamination.

Parlavecchio made a further technical improvement (Fig. 122). Two crushing-clamps were placed at each end of the bowel, and the latter cut **by the cautery** between the clamps. The ends of the bowel to be anastomosed were brought together so that the clamps lay side by side. A series of interrupted seromuscular sutures were placed over the clamps first on the posterior surface and then on the anterior surface. The clamps were removed and the sutures tied. Thus, we can see, that the crushed wall would not bleed, and the agglutinated ends would prevent the escape of the intestinal contents while the ends of the ligatures were tied. As may be seen, in this operation both Halsted's and Doyen's principles were utilized. A similar procedure was done about the same time by M. O'Hara.

Another prominent feature in the Parlavecchio method was that the **ends were divided by the cautery,** which actually sterilized the intestinal contents which might lie on the surface of the blades.

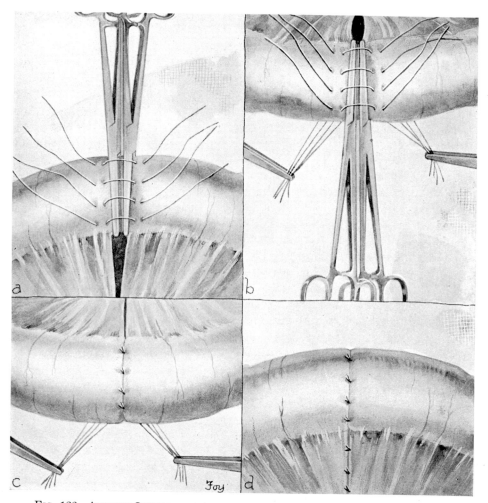

FIG. 122. ASEPTIC INTESTINAL ANASTOMOSIS BY THE PARLAVECCHIO METHOD.

Rostowzew, of Petrograd, greatly popularized the "aseptic intestinal suture". In its essence, his method was practically as was outlined by Parlavecchio, with a few slight technical modifications.

A very popular method in Germany and Austria was that of Moszkowisz, which was a still further technical improvement of the Parlavecchio and Rostowzew methods.

Thus, we may say, that the main factors on which are based the possibility of aseptic intestinal suturing are:

1. The submucous layer is the main holding layer in gastro-intestinal union (Halsted). From the practical point, it means that a strong union between two viscera can be established **without entering into the lumen of a hollow viscus.**

2. Crushing-clamps by crushing the wall, also crush the blood-vessels, thus obviating the danger of hemorrhage (Doyen).

3. Cutting by a cautery renders the field "relatively aseptic".

On these three principles is based the entire structure of all modern "aseptic methods" in intestinal suturing.

As is clear from the above description, **the mucosa is never sutured to the mucosa.** This is of no importance in the suture of bowel to bowel and is by far outweighed by the aseptic features of the operation. However, in surgery of the stomach the reverse is true. The danger, due to contamination is not great, but the complications which may arise from not suturing the mucous layer of the stomach to the mucosa of the other viscus (particularly peptic gastro-jejunal ulcer) are very grave, and for this reason we believe that the **closed aseptic method should never be employed when one of the viscera is the stomach, and that aseptic methods should be reserved only for intestinal work, and especially for the surgery of the large bowel.**

We now describe a few accepted methods of end-to-end, end-to-side and lateral intestinal anastomosis as now employed. Some of these methods are convenient when special enterotribes are not available. However, if the operation is pre-arranged, we consider the work with the Doyen enterotribe or the Rankin or Partipilo clamp much preferable.

END-TO-END ANASTOMOSIS WITH PRELIMINARY BLIND CLOSURE OF THE ENDS OF THE BOWEL (PARKER-KERR METHOD).

Step 1. A crushing-clamp is placed on each end of the bowel to be resected. These clamps are placed obliquely (approximately at 30°), in such a manner that the mesenteric border becomes most prominent. This will secure a better blood-supply and will make the lumen larger. Another clamp is placed to the inner side of each of the previously placed clamps. The arcuate vessels are ligated, and the bowel is cut on each side between each pair of clamps.

Step 2. Each end of the bowel is closed by a basting-suture, the ends of which are left untied. The technic of making a basting-suture was described in Chapter V. [N.B. It must be clearly understood that the word "basting", taken from the seamstress's language, presupposes a loosely placed temporary suture which can easily be removed.]

Step 3. The closed ends of the bowel are brought together, the assistant holding with one hand the beginning sutures and with the other the terminating sutures of each bowel (Fig, 123, a). A continuous seromuscular suture is made on the anterior wall of each end of the bowel (Fig. 123, b) and then another seromuscular suture is made on the posterior surface (Fig. 123, c). The two basting sutures are then withdrawn and the ends of the permanent threads are tied to each other (Fig. 123, d). A second seromuscular suture reinforces the first one.

Step 4. With a finger placed on the wall of either bowel the partially

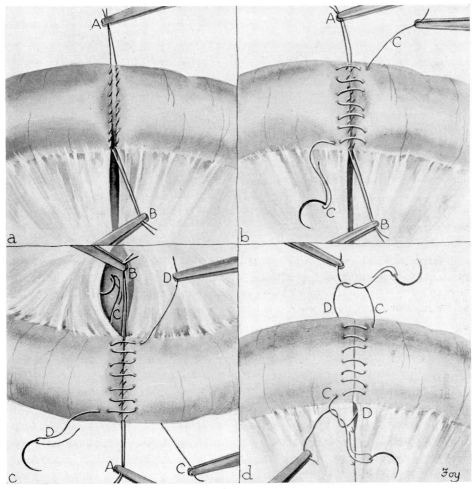

FIG. 123. END-TO-END ANASTOMOSIS BY THE PARKER-KERR METHOD.
a. Each end of the bowel is closed temporarily by a basting-suture and the ends are brought together;   b. Seromuscular suturing of the anterior surfaces of the bowel; c. Seromuscular suturing of the posterior surfaces of the bowel;   d. Basting-sutures withdrawn; tying the ends of the permanent sutures to each other.

agglutinated ends are broken through, so as to restore the continuity at the place of anastomosis.

Step 5. The rent in the mesentery is closed.

A side-to-side and an end-to-side anastomosis may be done by this method, as follows:

LATERAL INTESTINAL ANASTOMOSIS (PARKER-KERR METHOD).

Step 1. A fold of one bowel is grasped by a crushing-forceps, and this fold is cauterized flush with the surface of the blades. Closure of the bowel is made over the blades of the clamp by a basting-suture.

Step 2. Step 1 is repeated on another loop of bowel.

Step 3. The two loops of bowel are placed side-by-side, and the assistant holds with one hand the beginning sutures and with the other hand the terminating sutures of each bowel. A seromuscular continuous suture connecting the posterior surfaces of the two bowels is made, and then is continued on the anterior wall until the entire circumference is sutured. Each third stitch is locked, or a back-stitch is made so as to prevent a purse-string action. The basting-sutures are pulled out and the ends of the thread are tied to each other. A second seromuscular suture reinforces the first.

END-TO-SIDE ANASTOMOSIS (ILEO-SIGMOIDOSTOMY) (PARKER-KERR METHOD).

Step 1. The arcuate vessels of the terminal part of the ileum are ligated, and crushing-clamps are placed obliquely at the site of the intended division. The bowel is cut by the cautery.

Step 2. Each end of the bowel is closed. The distal end is closed permanently, and therefore should be reinforced by another seromuscular suture. The proximal end is closed temporarily by a basting-suture.

Step 3. A fold of the sigmoid is grasped in a crushing-clamp. The size of the fold should be equal to the diameter of the proximal end of the ileum to be implanted into the sigmoid. The protruding part of the sigmoid is "shaved off" by the cautery and sutured with a basting-suture.

Step 4. The proximal end of the ileum and that portion of the sigmoid where the basting-suture lies are brought end-to-side. A seromuscular suture is made, connecting the posterior walls of each, and this is continued anteriorly until the entire circumference is sutured. Each third stitch is locked or a back stitch is made in order to prevent purse-string action. The basting-sutures are pulled out and the ends of the seromuscular thread are tied to each other. A finger is introduced into the newly made anastomosis by invaginating the wall of the bowel.

Step 5. The rent in the mesentery is closed in the usual manner.

The method of Parker-Kerr accomplishes the anastomosis without any special intestinal clamps. An ordinary Kocher or Ochsner clamp, round needles and thread are all that is necessary. However, if special enterotribes are at our disposal the work is much facilitated.

We shall present now an end-to-end, an end-to-side, and a lateral anastomosis with the aid of the Partipilo or the Rankin clamp. All these procedures can be performed by either of the clamps. However, we shall demonstrate some of the operations with one and some with the other clamp so that the surgeon may familiarize himself with each of them.

LATERAL INTESTINAL ANASTOMOSIS WITH THE
RANKIN CLAMP (FIG. 124).

Step 1. The two loops of the bowel to be united are grasped by the

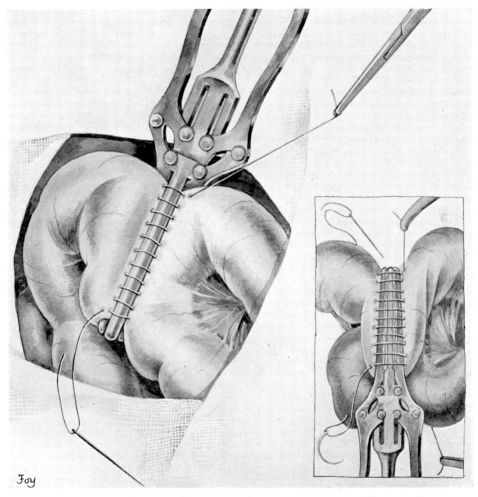

Fig. 124. Aseptic Lateral Intestinal Anastomosis by the Rankin Clamp.

blades of the Rankin clamp which are closed tightly. The clamp is then turned so that its posterior surface faces anteriorly. A seromuscular suture is then started on this surface from the handles of the blades toward the tip (Fig. 124). After completing the suture of the posterior surface, the clamp is turned back so that the anterior surface faces anteriorly.

Step 2. The folds of the bowel projecting above the blades are "shaved off" by the cautery.

Step 3. Another seromuscular suture is carried over the blades, beginning at their tip, until the other end of the "shaved off" portion is reached (Fig. 124, insert). The assistant takes with one hand the two ends of the thread on one side and with the other hand the two ends on the other side. The surgeon slightly separates the lateral blades from the middle one and then gently pulls out the forceps, depressing the tip, while the assistant pulls the ends in one hand away from those in the other hand. This will bury the crushed part of the walls. The ends of the thread on each side of the bowel are tied to each other with moderate firmness in order to prevent purse-string action and are cut short.

Step 4. This seromuscular layer is reinforced by another layer of seromuscular sutures. The agglutinated site of the anastomosis is broken by a finger, thus rendering the lumen patent.

END-TO-END ANASTOMOSIS BY THE PARTIPILO CLAMP (FIGS. 125, 126, 127).

The contents of the bowel are "milked out", the mesenteric and the arcuate blood-vessels ligated and the mesentery cut in a "V"-shape as in the ordinary method of enterectomy described in Chapter V. Then:

Step 1. A Partipilo clamp grasps each end of the bowel in a direction perpendicular to its long axis, immediately lateral to the site of the contemplated line of incision. [Care should be taken to see that the bowel at each end is grasped by the symmetrical portions of each clamp] (Fig. 125). A strong Ochsner or a Payr clamp is placed medially and close to each Partipilo clamp, and the bowel is divided by the cautery between each Partipilo and Ochsner clamps. Thus a portion of the bowel is resected.

Step 2. Two Partipilo clamps are brought together and set so that the prongs of one clamp fit into the indentations of the other clamp and fastened by a screw. Thus the two clamps of the Partipilo instrument become immobile as if they were parts of one instrument (Fig. 126).

Step 3. The clamp is turned in such a manner that the posterior surface of the bowel faces anteriorly (Fig. 126, a). A seromuscular suture starts at the point most remote from the tip of the blades and to the right of the surgeon and runs over the clamp until the point on the bowel closest to the tip of the blade is reached. The last bite is made on the bowel lying to the left of the surgeon. The clamp is then turned to its original position so that the anterior surface of the bowel faces anteriorly. Another seromuscular suture is made over the blade, starting at the point closest to the tip of the blade and to the right of the surgeon. The last bite of this continuous suture is made at the point of the bowel farthest from the tip of the blades and to the left from the surgeon. Thus, on each end of the bowel are present a thread on a needle and a thread clamped by an artery-forceps (Fig. 126, b).

Step 4. The surgeon grasps the two threads lying on his side of the bowel with his left hand. The assistant grasps the threads lying on his side. The surgeon now releases the lock of each part of the Partipilo clamp, **however not changing the mutual relationship of the parts of the clamp** (Fig. 127). The clamps are now **slowly** withdrawn. While removing the clamp the assistant pulls his two threads away from the bowel. As soon

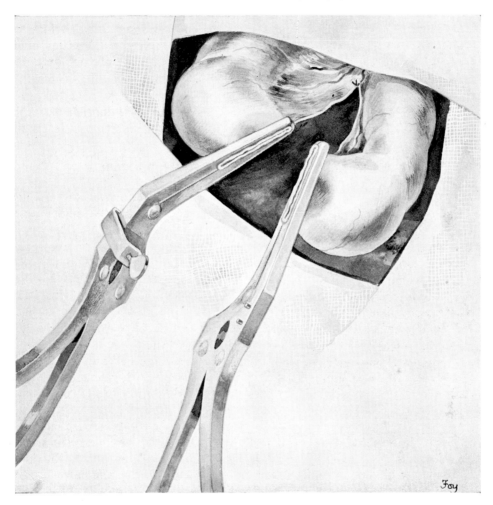

FIG. 125. ASEPTIC END-TO-END INTESTINAL ANASTOMOSIS BY THE PARTIPILO CLAMP.
Each half of the Partipilo clamp holds a divided end of the bowel.

as the clamp is removed, the surgeon pulls his two threads away from the bowel. The surgeon and the assistant tie the ends of the threads to each other with moderate firmness, so as to prevent the purse-string action of these threads. The ends are then cut short.

Step 5. The suture-line is reinforced by another seromuscular suture.

Step 6. The diaphragm thus produced is then broken by invaginating with the finger the wall of the bowel.

Step 7. The rent in the mesentery is closed in the usual manner.

END-TO-SIDE ANASTOMOSIS BY THE PARTIPILO CLAMP (ILEO-SIGMOIDOSTOMY).

Step 1. The Partipilo clamp is placed obliquely on the terminal por-

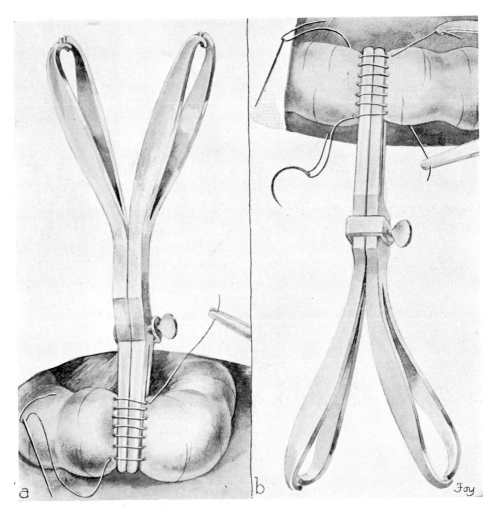

FIG. 126. ASEPTIC END-TO-END ANASTOMOSIS BY THE PARTIPILO CLAMP.
a. Seromuscular suturing of the posterior surfaces of the bowel;
b. Seromuscular suturing of the anterior surfaces of the bowel.

tion of the ileum (at least six inches away from the ileo-cecal junction) in order to secure a larger lumen and a better blood-supply. Any crushing-clamp (Kocher or Ochsner) is placed distally but very close to the Partipilo clamp. The bowel is cut by the cautery between the Kocher and the Partipilo clamps. The end of the ileum connected with the cecum is closed by the over-and-over suture method.

Step 2. A fold of the free border of the sigmoid is grasped by the other half of the Partipilo clamp and is cut by the cautery. The clamps are set as one unit by inserting the prongs into the indentations and are fastened by the screw. The compound Partipilo clamp is then turned so

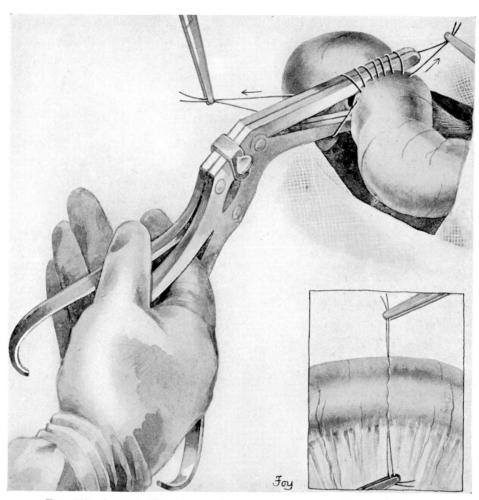

Fig. 127. Aseptic End-to-end Anastomosis by the Partipilo Clamp.
The clamp is unlocked and ready to be removed.

that the posterior surface faces anteriorly, and a seromuscular suture is inserted until the posterior half is united. The clamp is then returned to its normal position and another seromuscular suture is made until the anterior half of the circumference is united.

Step 3. The assistant takes with one hand the short end of one thread and the needle-end of the other thread and in the other hand the short end of the other thread and the needle end of the first thread. **The surgeon opens each half of the Partipilo clamp, not touching the screw so that the mutual relationship of the individual clamps of the compound Partipilo instrument is not altered.** The clamp is gently removed, depressing the tip of the blades, so that the crushed part is buried, while the assistant pulls the threads in the opposite direction. The short end is then tied to the threaded end on each end of the bowel with moderate force so as to prevent purse-string action, and the ends are cut short.

Step 4. This seromuscular layer is reinforced by another layer of seromuscular suturing.

Step 5. The rent in the mesentery is closed.

BIBLIOGRAPHY.

Bardenheuer. Experimentelle Beiträge zur Abdominal—Chirurgie.
Inaugural Dissertation, y. 1888; p. 68.

M. Behrend, W. Belk, and C. Herrman. Clinical versus experimental anastomosis of the hollow viscera.
Journ. Am. Med. Ass. 83:1807-1812; y. 1924.

L. A. Bidwell. A handbook of intestinal surgery. New York, 1911.

J. R. B. Branch Aseptic intestinal anastomosis in resections of the large bowel.
Surg. Gyn. & Obst. 47:678-679; y. 1928.

J. E. Briggs & L. R. Whitaker. An electrosurgical method for aseptic anastomosis of the intestine.
New Engl. J. Med. 206:662-666; y. 1932.

W. C. Burket & W. B. McClure. An aseptic method of intestinal anastomosis.
Surg. Gyn. & Obst. 35:816-819; y. 1922.

J. Gillette Burns. Aseptic end-to-end anastomosis of the intestine.
Annals of Surgery, 81:670-673; y. 1925.

F. K. Collins. Aseptic resection of intestine.
Annals of Surg. 76:738-744; y. 1922.

F. K. Collins. Aseptic intestinal resection and anastomosis without sutures.
West. J. Surg. 43:260-264; y. 1935.

Doyen. Nouveau procédé d'entérorrhaphie. XI Congr. français.
Paris, 1897.

J. Fraser and N. Dott. Aseptic intestinal anastomosis.
Brit. J. Surg. 11:439-454; y. 1924.

J. Fraser. Value of the closed methods in resection of the colon.
Lancet 1:1198; y. 1926.

W. D. Gatch. Aseptic intestinal anastomosis.
Journ. Am. Med. Ass. 59:185-189; y. 1912.

W. D. Gatch. Remarks on intestinal anastomosis with a description of a simple aseptic technic.
Am. J. Surg. 20:341-354; y. 1933.

W. S. Halsted. Blind-end circular suture of the intestine, closed ends abutted and the double diaphragm punctured with a knife introduced per rectum.
Ann. Surg. 75:356-364; y. 1922.

W. Hartert. Ein neuer Weg zur Wahrung vollkommener Asepsis bei Magendarmoperationen.
Bruns Beitr. zur klin. Chir. 99:475-558; y. 1916.

C. F. Horine. Aseptic technik for the resection of intestine.
Annals of Surg. 76:745-754; y. 1922.

H. H. Kerr. Intestinal anastomosis; with a report on the aseptic basting stitch method.
Surg. Gyn. & Ob. 17:496-500; y. 1913.

H. H. Kerr. The development of intestinal surgery.
Journ. Am. Med. Ass. 81:641-647; y. 1923.

K. H. Martzloff & G. E. Burget. Aseptic end-to-end anastomosis and method for making closed intestinal loop suitable for physiologic studies.
Arch. Surg. 23:26-37; y. 1931; correction 23:542; y. 1931.

L. Moszkowicz. Aseptische Darmoperationen.
Arch. f. klin. Chir. 86:887-906; y. 1908.

L. Moszkowicz. Ueber aseptische Magen-und Darmoperationen.
Arch. f. klin. Chir. 91:888-920; y. 1910.

T. McGraw Upon the use of the elastic ligature in the surgery of the intestine.
Journ. Am. Med. Ass. 16:685-694; y. 1891.

M. O'Hara, Jr. A method of performing anastomosis of hollow viscera by means of a new instrument.
Am. Journ. of Obst. and Diseases of Women and Children. 42:81-90; y. 1900.

E. M. Parker and H. Kerr. Intestinal anastomosis without open incisions by means of basting stitches.
Johns Hopkins Hospit. Bull. 19:132-137; y. 1908.

A. V. Partipilo. End-end to side anastomosis.
Am. J. Surg. 5:378-380; y. 1928.

A. V. Partipilo. A closed aseptic and quick method of gastro-intestinal anastomosis.
Am. J. Surg. 6:362-363; y. 1929.

V. Pleth. A simple and practical method of performing anastomosis by means of two knitting needles.
Am. Journ. of Surg. 20:170-172; y. 1906.

V. Pleth and Vera W. Pleth. A contribution to intestinal surgery. Aseptic intestinal anastomosis (entero-enterostomy and gastro-enterostomy).
Am. Journ. of Surg. 23 (old series): 221-223; y. 1909.

P. Postnikow. Die zweizeitige Gastroenterostomie.
Zbl. f. Chir. 19:1018-1021; y. 1892.

S. Pringle. Aseptic resection of the intestine.
Brit. J. Surg. 12:238-243; y. 1924.

F. W. Rankin. An aseptic method of intestinal anastomosis.
Surg. Gyn. Obst. 47:78-88; y. 1928.

F. W. Rankin & A. S. Graham. Aseptic end-to-side ileocolostomy; clamp method. Technic and statistical data.
Ann. Surg. 99:676-681; y. 1934.

M. Iw. Rostowzew. Aseptische Darmnaht.
Arch. f. klin. Chir. 82:462-485; y. 1907.

M. Iw. Rostowzew. Eine neue Modification der aseptischen Darmnaht.
Arch. f. klin. Chir. 95:31-47; y. 1911.

John E. Scarff. Aseptic end-to-end suture of intestine.
Annals of Surg. 83:490-495; y. 1926.

J. E. Sweet. The technique of the surgery of the gastro-intestinal tract.
Surg. Gyn. Obst. 44:811-823; y. 1927.

R. P. Wadhams & V. Carabba. Electro-surgical aseptic intestinal anastomosis.
Surg. Gyn. Obst. 60:1082-1092; y. 1935.

Jerome P. Webster. Aseptic end-to-end intestinal anastomosis.
Annals of Surg. 81:646-669; y. 1925.

A. Werelius. A new method of lateral anastomosis.
Surg. Gyn. Obst. 2:308-309; y. 1906.

Wullstein. Ueber aseptische Darmoperationen.
Arch. f. klin. Chir. 87:886-892; y. 1908.

CHAPTER VIII.

SURGERY OF THE LARGE BOWEL.

I. APPENDECTOMY.

Definition.

This word is composed of the Latin word **appendix,** which means "appendage", and the Greek suffix ἐκτομῆ, excision. It signifies, "excision of the appendix". The term "appendicitis" was coined by Reginald Fitz in 1886.

Indications.

Any disease of the appendix requires its removal, since the diseased appendix may rupture and lead to fatal peritonitis, or it may act as a focus from which the disease may be carried to other abdominal or pelvic organs either by hematogenous or lymphogenous extension or by continuity of tissue.

Anatomy.

The appendix takes its origin from the posterior and medial surface of the cecum, three-fourths of an inch below the ileo-cecal junction, at the place where the three longitudinal tænia coli meet. This point is quite constant. From it the appendix may extend in different directions (Fig. 128). The length of the appendix varies from one-fourth of an inch to twelve inches, its average length being three inches. However, cases of hypoplasia of the appendix are described in which its length was only one-twelfth of an inch. In such cases, it becomes extremely difficult to recognize whether or not we are dealing with the appendix. The most common position of the appendix is given below in the order of decreased frequency:

1. Partially behind the cecum.
2. To the medial side of the cecum in the direction toward the spleen, but not reaching the brim of the pelvis. In some cases it hangs over the brim of the pelvis.
3. Retrocolic and totally retrocecal.
4. Pre-ileal.
5. Post-ileal.

Congenital absence of the appendix vermiformis is an exceptionally rare occurrence. In a most excellent article published in 1925, Dorland collected thirty-eight cases (including his own) in which he covered the subject to that date. Spivack, in 1932, added an additional nine cases (including two of his own). Green in 1934, reported another case, thus making a total of forty-eight cases up to date. This number represents a group of cases in which the appendix was not found on the operating-table, and another group in which it was not found on the dissecting-table. Whereas the second group is absolutely reliable, the first group leaves some doubt, and, therefore, we may consider that the **actual number of cases of absence of the appendix is smaller than has been reported.** But even if we accept this number as correct, we must admit that congenital absence of the appendix is a very rare occurrence, and **one should not be satisfied, in case the appendix is not found, in believing that it is a case of congenital absence.**

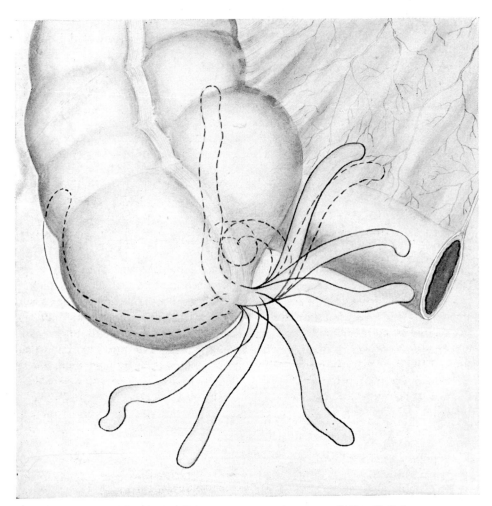

FIG. 128. DIFFERENT POSITIONS OF THE APPENDIX (After Kelly).

The blood-supply of the appendix is derived chiefly from the appendicular artery. This artery is very often seen as a branch of the ileo-colic artery. In other instances, it springs from the superior mesenteric artery below the origin of the ileo-colic artery, and then it is just one of the five terminal branches of this artery. It runs in the meso-appendix from its root to its tip giving off on its way several small branches. **This artery has very poor anastomotic connections with the cecal branches of the ileo-cecal artery, and, therefore, it has many characteristics of a terminal artery. Thus, when the artery is plugged, gangrene of the appendix ensues easily.**

The appendicular artery passes on its way to the appendix behind the terminal portion of the ileum before it enters the meso-appendix. There-fore, in case the terminal portion of the ileum is filled with fecal material, **it may compress the appendicular artery and predispose the appendix to vascular disturbances.**

Occasionally, the appendix receives some blood-supply from the cecal branches. They pass over the base of the appendix in the direction toward its tip, but usually they do not reach the tip. **It is very important to keep in mind this occasional distribution of the blood-vessels in connection with some methods of treating the stump.**

METHODS OF LOCATING THE APPENDIX.

In many instances there is no difficulty in locating the appendix. How-ever, in some cases this is a very difficult procedure, and it requires an exact knowledge of the anatomy to find it. Occasionally, it is not easy even to find the cecum, especially when the "gridiron" incision is employed. Under such circumstances it is well to use Monks method to locate the cecum. This is as follows:

Monks Rule:

The index-finger of the right hand is introduced into the abdomen and placed on the brim of the pelvis. This finger is moved over the brim of the pelvis until the pulsation of the external iliac artery is felt. The finger then follows the pulsation of this artery upward to the upper edge of the brim, and continues beyond upward and laterally until it reaches the blind end of a pouch. This pouch actually is the lower end of the root of the mesentery. In front of the index-finger will lie the terminal part of the ileum (Fig. 76). With the right thumb and the index-finger this part of the ileum is caught and delivered outside the abdominal cavity. A few inches away from this point the cecum will be located.

Monks method of locating the terminal portion of the ileum is excel-lent, providing that the lowermost portion of the root of the mesentery reaches the right sacro-iliac joint, which is normal. However, in some cases the root of the mesentery takes an entirely different direction, as was shown by Stopnitzki and others (Fig. 74). Under such circumstances, Monks rule will not be applicable.

As soon as the cecum is located it is turned upward, so that the pos-terior surface becomes anterior. About three-fourths of an inch below the ileo-cecal junction (and in the reversed position of the cecum, **this is above and not below the junction**) will be seen the point of convergence of the three tænia coli, where the appendix takes its origin.

In about nine per cent. of all cases the appendix lies entirely **retrocecal or retrocolic** and it may be difficult to find it, unless the cecum or colon is mobilized and the posterior surface turned anteriorly. However, the surgeon hesitates to mobilize the cecum or colon (which means opening the retroperitoneal space) until he is reasonably sure that the appendix is

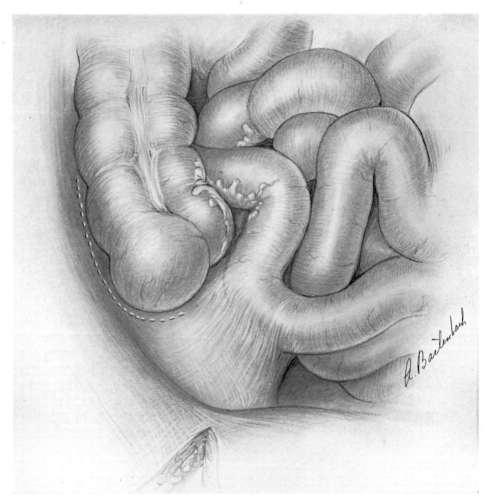

FIG. 129. THE SPIVACK RULE.
The terminal portion of the ileum is attached to the brim of the pelvis. No appendix is seen. The dotted line shows where the cecum should be mobilized in order to find the retrocecal appendix.

actually located there. In order to ascertain this, Spivack, in 1931, described a very simple method as follows:
Spivack's Rule (Figs. 129 and 130).

If the terminal part of the ileum is attached to the brim of the pelvis, then, in ninety per cent. of all cases, the appendix is retrocecal or retrocolic.

This, of course, will justify mobilization of the cecum or colon, after which its posterior surface is turned anteriorly, when the appendix will be clearly exposed (Fig. 130). **The reverse also holds true, namely: If there is a retrocecal appendix, in ninety per cent. of such cases the terminal portion of the ileum will be attached to the brim of the pelvis.**

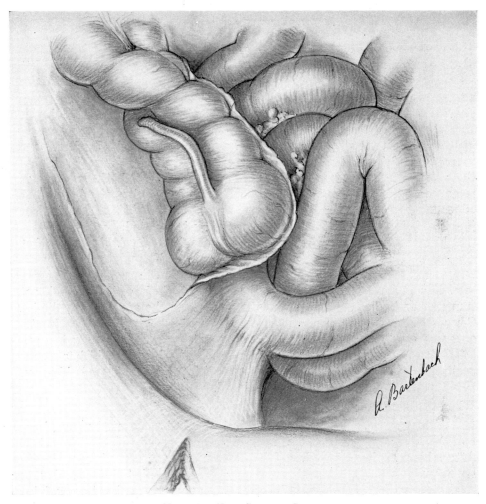

FIG. 130. THE SPIVACK RULE.
The terminal portion of the ileum is attached to the brim of the pelvis; the posterior surface of the cecum is turned anteriorly; the appendix lies on the posterior wall of the cecum.

The surgical significance of this fact is as follows: In removal of a retrocolic or retrocecal appendix in the acute stage of inflammation, nothing else should be done. But if a **retrocolic or retrocecal** appendix is removed in the quiescent stage, then the operation should be supplemented by mobilization of the terminal ileum, and bringing it to its normal anatomical position, since this kink (known as **Lane's kink**) predisposes to intestinal obstruction. However, occasionally in the case of a retrocecal or retrocolic appendix, the organ cannot be seen even after the cecum and colon are mobilized and the posterior wall turned anteriorly, since it may be covered with the visceral peritoneum of the cecum or colon to such an extent that it will not be exposed until the serosa is incised. In several of our cases, the appendix was found after the wall of the cecum was carefully palpated and its serosa incised.

Another important point to bear in mind is that occasionally a portion of the appendix is embedded in the wall of the cecum, with the rest of the viscus projecting from the wall of the cecum in the usual manner. In such a case, the uninitiated may remove only this projecting part of the appendix, so that he actually performs an **amputation of the appendix instead of an appendectomy,** and the patient may have subsequent attacks of appendicitis after an "appendectomy" has been performed. In these cases, the appendix should be dissected from the wall of the cecum by incising the serosa of the cecum on each side of it, after which the appendix is removed in the usual manner as described below. When the base of the appendix (in the reversed position of the cecum) lies **above** the ileocecal junction it is a sign that the **entire** appendix is isolated.

In exceptional cases the appendix may be found in the left side of the abdomen. This may be due either to the fact that a complete situs inversus is present, so that the location of the appendix on the left side is only a part of a general picture, or that some pathological condition, such as a tumor or an abscess has displaced the cecum and the appendix to the left. Complete situs inversus is a rare occurrence. It is met with approximately once in four thousand autopsies, and then as a rule the appendix is on the left side. The presence of the appendix on the left side with a normal position of the other abdominal and thoracic structures, is probably never noted unless it is pathologically displaced.

When to Operate.

All surgeons agree that the patient should be operated upon if seen within thirty-six to forty-eight hours after the onset of the initial attack. After this time has elapsed, and if the symptoms of spreading peritonitis appear, many surgeons prefer not to operate at all, but to employ the "Ochsner method of treatment", resorting to operation only at some future time when all the acute symptoms have disappeared. Still, there are just as many surgeons who believe that the patient should be operated upon whenever the diagnosis is made, irrespective of how many hours have elapsed since the beginning of the attack, unless general peritonitis is already present. It is our practice within the first 60 hours after the initial attack, always to operate.

Operative Technic.

Various incisions are used for appendectomy. They belong to all types of abdominal incision, namely, longitudinal, transverse or oblique. For their description, see Chapter II. Personally, we prefer to employ the "gridiron" incision in acute cases and the transverse incision for the "interval" type.

Step 1. The abdomen is opened.

Step 2. The cecum is located. If this is difficult to find, then the terminal portion of the ileum is located by Monks method (Fig. 76), after which it becomes a simple procedure to find the cecum. The latter is brought outside the abdominal wound and the appendix is located as described above.

Step 3. The part of the meso-appendix which lies close to the distal end of the appendix is caught by an artery-forceps. **[The appendix itself should never be grasped by an artery-forceps or by any other instrument]** (Fig. 131, insert). The appendix and exposed part of the cecum are surrounded by moist laparotomy sponges.

Step 4. Ligation of the Appendicular Artery. There are several ways of doing this:

The meso-appendix is pierced by a curved arterial forceps very close to the base of the appendix (Fig. 131, insert). The jaws of the clamp are opened and grasp one end of a thread, which is drawn through the opening, the other end passing around the meso-appendix, after which both ends are tied (Fig. 131, main picture). The thread should not be tied very close to the body of the appendix. In case it is difficult to do this, it can be facilitated by lifting the body of the appendix by an Allis forceps (which should not grasp the wall of the appendix itself, but the meso-appendix), the blades embracing the body of the appendix with their concave surfaces. The mesentery is then divided between the ligature and the body of the appendix. The ends of the ligature are cut short.

[An alternate method of tying the appendicular artery is as follows: A clamp is placed on the meso-appendix, which is divided between the clamp and the body of the appendix. If the entire meso-appendix is not caught by the first clamp, another is used to clamp the rest of the meso-appendix, which again is divided between the second clamp and the body of the appendix. The meso-appendicular stump is then ligated].

Step 5. The appendix is put on the stretch by the artery-forceps which was applied to the tip of the meso-appendix, and is crushed at its base (Fig. 132). **[The utmost care should be taken to see that the appendix is crushed at its base, since occasionally, as already mentioned, a portion of the appendix is embedded in the wall of the cecum for a distance of from one-fourth to one-half inch. It is then necessary to separate this embedded portion from the wall of the cecum before the crushing-clamp is applied].** The crushing-clamp is now removed and re-applied just a little distally to the crushed base of the appendix. The appendix is then tied in the groove formed by this clamp (Fig. 132), and the ends of the ligature are cut short.

Step 6. A purse-string is placed around the appendix at a distance of one-third of an inch from its base. Each seromuscular bite of this purse-string is made at a distance of one-third of an inch from each other. The first bite is taken at the mesenteric border by piercing the two leaflets of the meso-appendix. The purse-string suture is continued until half of the circumference is covered. Then one loop is left long (Fig. 132), and the

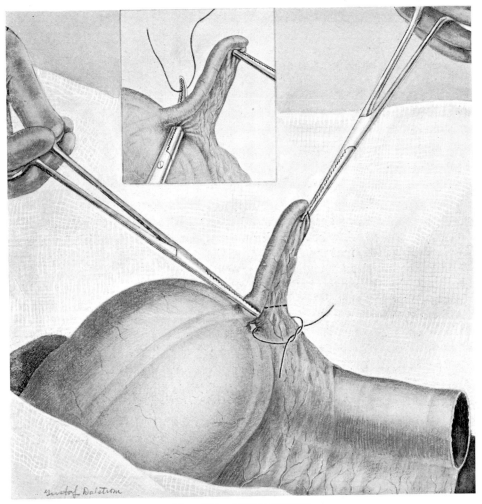

FIG. 131. APPENDECTOMY.
INSERT. An artery forceps penetrates the meso-appendix and grasps the ligature.
MAIN PICTURE. The meso-appendix is tied; the base of the appendix is clamped.

purse-string suture is continued until the entire circumference is covered (Fig. 132). The needle is then placed aside on a piece of gauze. The surgeon grasps with the left hand the forceps holding that portion of the meso-appendix which is still attached to the appendix and puts the organ on the stretch. With his right hand the appendix is "shaved off" at its base by cutting it just below the clamp between this and the tied knot. [The knife is soaked in phenol. The stump is well cleansed with the side of the knife, while the appendix is partially connected with the cecum. After the appendix is cut off entirely, the stump is cleansed with alcohol. The removed appendix with the two attached forceps and also the knife are put aside in a special basin.] The surgeon then grasps the purse-string

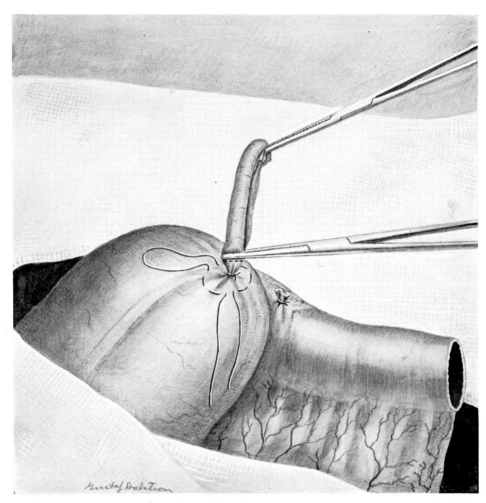

FIG. 132. APPENDECTOMY.
A purse-string suture with a large loop is inserted. (For other details see the text).

in the following way: The two ends of the purse-string are caught between the thumb and index-finger of his left hand, and the long loop of the purse-string by the middle finger of the same hand (Fig. 133). With the right hand, armed with anatomical tissue-forceps, the surgeon grasps the appendicular stump and presses it downward into the wall of the cecum, pulling in the meantime with the left hand the purse-string suture away from the wall of the cecum and releasing first the loop which rested on the middle finger, **while the assistant supports the cecum with his right hand.** [The bowel should always be grasped with a pledget of moist gauze and not by the gloved fingers.] In this way, the stump will be buried and the ends of the purse-string suture tied and cut short. This suture is reinforced by several interrupted seromuscular sutures.

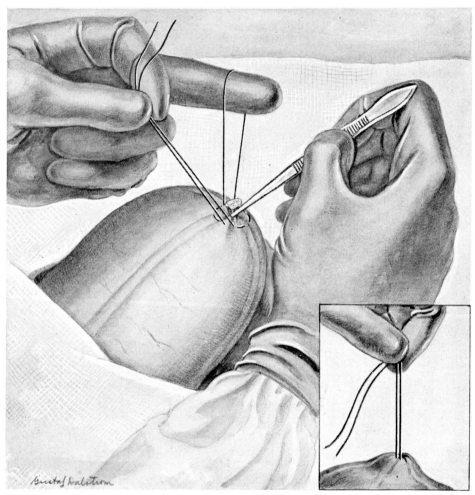

FIG. 133. APPENDECTOMY.
Invagination of the appendicular stump without the aid of the assistant.

By employing this particular maneuvre, the surgeon does not depend on his assistant either for tying the purse-string or for invagination of the stump. The fear of closing the ileo-cecal opening by a careless invagination of the stump seems to us to be unfounded. [N. B. Instead of cutting the appendix by a knife, the cautery may be used.]

Step 7. The abdomen is closed.

With reference to the management of the stump, we wish to state that the burying of the stump in the wall of the cecum is the method most commonly used by the majority of surgeons. However, there are some surgeons who do not bury the stump. They consider, and quite justly, that it is not a scientific procedure to bury diseased tissue in the wall of another viscus. For this reason, other procedures have been suggested as follows:

1. **Ligation and cauterization of the stump which is allowed to drop free into the peritoneal cavity;**

2. **Inversion of the stump into the lumen of the cecum (Dawbarn method).**

This method was suggested by Robert H. M. Dawbarn, in 1891. Edebohls, in 1894, suggested the same inversion method, and not knowing of the work of Dawbarn thought that it was original with him. Many surgeons erroneously call this the "Edebohls method"; however, the latter himself recognized the priority of Dawbarn. Recently, the same method has been suggested again as a "new method" of dealing with the appendicular stump, the author evidently being unaware of the old Dawbarn method.

In this method the stump is not ligated. A purse-string is made as previously described. A crushing-clamp is applied to the base of the appendix, and another clamp is placed just distally to the first. The appendix is cut between the two clamps. The purse-string is caught in the manner described above. The forceps occluding the base of the appendix is removed, and an anatomical tissue-forceps grasps the agglutinated end of the stump and inverts it from without inward into the lumen of the cecum. The ends of the purse-string are then tied to each other. The rest of the operation is as already described.

Some find as an objection to this method that bleeding may occur, particularly in those cases in which some of the branches of the ileo-cecal artery pass from the cecal wall to the appendicular wall. However, we think that this objection is not valid, since at the time that the crushing-forceps was applied to the base of the appendix it also crushed the blood-vessels which are therein contained. **We believe this method to be a very good one and without any serious objections.**

3. **Deaver Method** (cutting the appendix flush with the cecum).

In this method the entire appendix is removed without leaving a stump. The edges of the opened cecum are closed in two layers; the first by an over-and-over suture and the second by a seromuscular suture. Deaver recommended this method, but advised limiting its use to the experienced surgeon.

In some cases it is more convenient to remove the appendix starting at its base. This is known as the **retrograde appendectomy.** It is particularly applicable when there is a long appendix which is bound down so that its tip cannot be seen or cannot be easily delivered through the wound, or in the case of an acute gangrenous appendicitis, in which the tip is

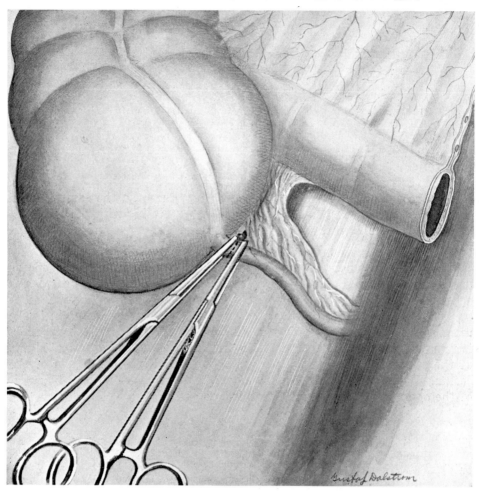

FIG. 134. RETROGRADE APPENDECTOMY.
The base of the appendix is clamped by two artery-forceps.

gangrenous and the surgeon would prefer to deal with the gangrenous part as the last step of the operation.

Technic of Retrograde Appendectomy (Figs. 134, 135).

Step 1. The same as Step 1 in the previous operation.

Step 2. The same as Step 2 in the previous operation.

Step 3. Two crushing-forceps are placed at the base of the appendix perpendicularly to its long axis (Fig. 134); the forceps proximal to the cecum is then removed and the crushed base of the appendix is tied. The appendix is cut between the thread and the crushing-forceps. The stump

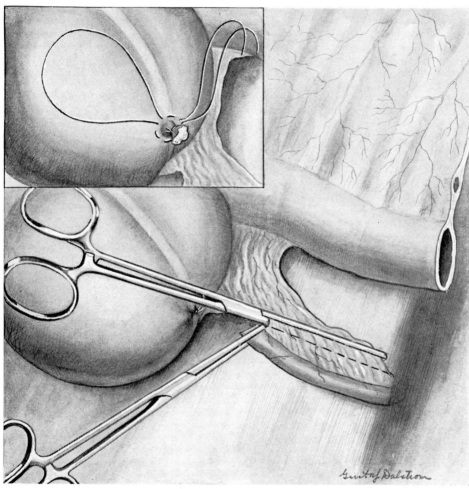

FIG. 135. RETROGRADE APPENDECTOMY.
INSERT. A purse-string suture is inserted for invagination of the stump.
MAIN PICTURE. The meso-appendix is clamped and ready to be incised.

is cleansed with phenol and alcohol. A purse-string suture is made, and the stump is buried as previously described (Fig. 135, insert).

Step 4. The appendix is put on the stretch by the artery-forceps which holds its severed end. A straight arterial clamp is applied to its mesentery. If the latter is too long, or if the entire appendix cannot be delivered at once, another artery-forceps is applied to the remainder of the meso-appendix, which is then cut between the arterial clamp and the body of the appendix (Fig. 135). The clamped mesenteric stump should be ligated.

Step 5. The abdomen is closed in the usual way.

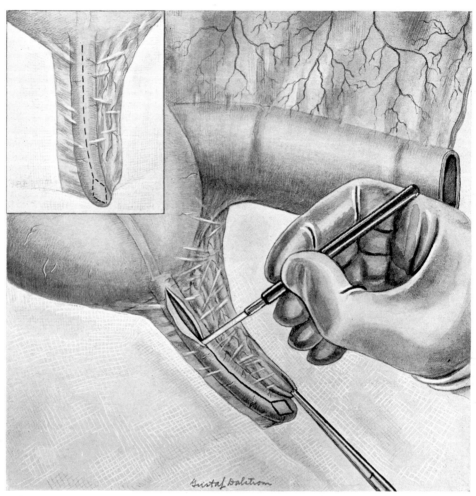

FIG. 136. SUBSEROUS APPENDECTOMY.
Incision of the serosa and shelling out the mucous tube of the appendix.

SUBSEROUS APPENDECTOMY.

This operation was first performed by Poncet, in 1899, and reported in the same year by Vignard. Poncet coined the expression "subserous appendectomy". Poncin, in 1901, and Delore, in 1902, reported several cases of subserous appendectomy performed in different French clinics. In 1905, Isaacs, of New York, reported several cases of subserous appendectomy, which he called "**decapsulation of the appendix**". He, evidently, was not aware of the fact that this technic had been already described, and thought the procedure to be a new method of appendectomy.

This method was originally employed only for those cases in which so many adhesions were present between the appendix and the surrounding structures that it was deemed inadvisable or even dangerous to separate

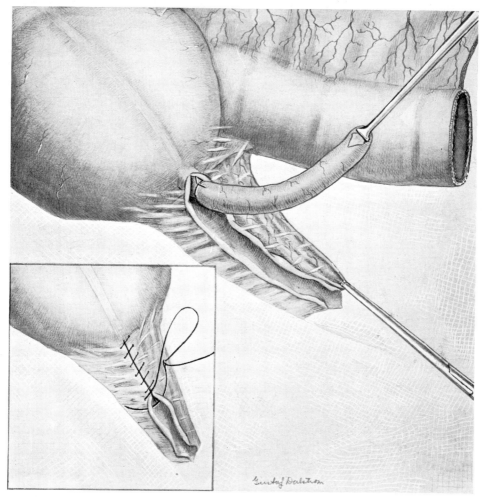

FIG. 137. SUBSEROUS APPENDECTOMY.
MAIN PICTURE. The mucous tube is shelled out and ligated at its base.
INSERT. The tube is removed; suturing of the serous layer of the appendix.

them. Recently some surgeons are employing it as a routine procedure for all appendices whether they be adherent or free. **However, we believe that this method should be employed only in those cases in which dense adhesions are present and not in cases in which the appendix can be readily separated from the surrounding structures.**

Technic.

Step 1. The abdomen is opened, the cecum and appendix located, and the latter walled off from the rest of the peritoneal cavity.

Step 2. The meso-appendix of the tip of the organ is grasped by an artery-forceps and the appendix is put on the stretch. A seromuscular incision is made beginning at the tip of the appendix in the form of a

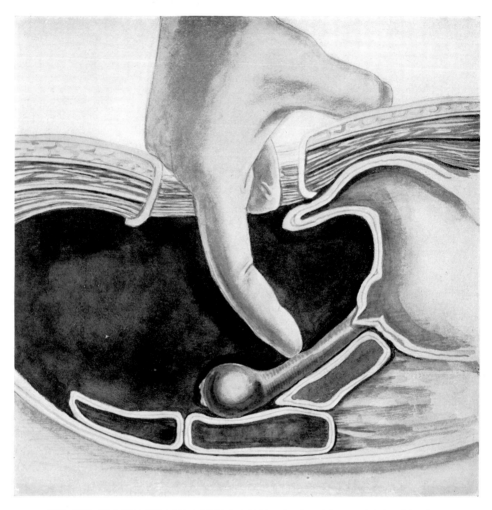

Fig. 138. Correct Method of Exploration of an Appendicular Abscess.
(After Bosch-Arana).

racquet, and this is continued as a linear incision along the entire length of the antimesenteric border until its base(*i.e.* its junction with the cecum) is reached (Fig. 136). Both seromuscular lips are reflected so as to isolate the mucous tube in its entire circumference at least in one place (close to the tip, since this is the safest point in case the mucosa is accidentally torn). A hook is placed around this completely isolated mucous tube, and the isolation is continued until the base of the appendix is reached (Fig. 137), which is then crushed and cut between two clamps. The proximal crushed end is tied and the stump sterilized, after which it is buried by a purse-string suture. The seromuscular lips are then sutured to each other (Fig. 137, insert).

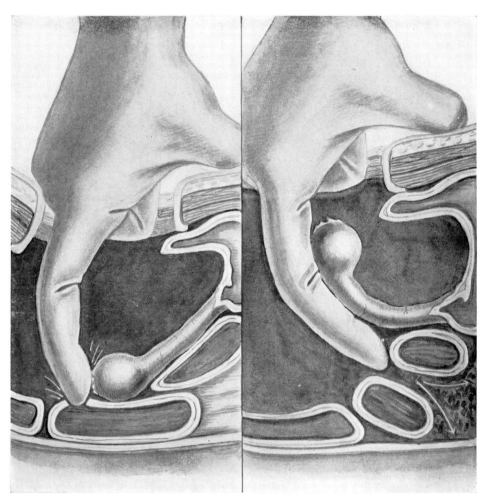

FIG 139. INCORRECT METHOD OF EXPLORATION OF AN APPENDICULAR ABSCESS.

THE TREATMENT OF AN APPENDICULAR ABSCESS.

The position of an appendicular abscess is just as variable as the position of the appendix. Thus, it may be situated in the iliac, lumbar, subhepatic, or subphrenic regions or in the pelvic cavity. In treating such abscesses, the same rules should be applied as in the treatment of abscesses in any other region, namely:

1. To make the opening at the most prominent point of the abscess.

2. To make it at the lowest point in order to facilitate drainage.

When the abscess is exposed and it is ascertained that its periphery is adherent to the anterior abdominal wall, the latter should then be well protected by laparotomy sponges in order to prevent its infection by the

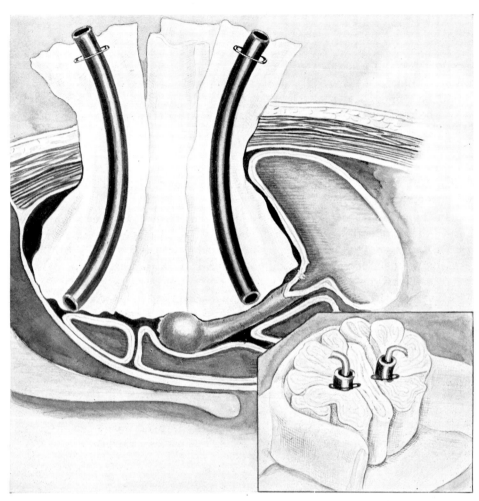

FIG. 140. DRAINAGE OF AN APPENDICULAR ABSCESS (After Bosch-Arana).

contents of the abscess. If the abscess is not adherent to the wall (and, therefore, the general peritoneal cavity is opened), then it (*i.e.* the peritoneal cavity) should be walled off from the abscess by many laparotomy sponges, and then only the abscess should be opened, its contents evacuated, and the cavity carefully examined. **No rough handling is permissible,** since the examining finger may break through the wall of the abscess-cavity and start a general peritonitis (Fig. 139). The reason for examining the cavity (Fig. 138) is chiefly to ascertain its extent in order to know, whether the abdominal incision is sufficient for draining purposes, or whether an additional incision will be required. For drainage, a split rubber tube is very good. It is introduced in several places to afford the best drainage (Fig. 140). The drain should never be removed too soon, since this may lead to early closure of the skin-wound before the deeper structures have had time to granulate and to become obliterated.

It has been a debatable question, whether the appendix should be searched for and removed while opening the abscess. It is now generally accepted that if the appendix lies free and presents itself in the cavity it should be removed. Otherwise, no search for it should be made, and it should be removed a few months later as a type of "interval" appendix.

CLOSURE OF THE APPENDECTOMY INCISION.

In the case of appendectomy performed for catarrhal appendicitis the abdomen is closed without drainage.

In the case of gangrenous appendicitis, or if free pus or fluid has been found in the abdominal cavity, opinions differ: The majority of surgeons drain the abdomen; however, some close the peritoneal cavity entirely by suturing the peritoneum only, and then either **drain the rest of the anterior abdominal wall,** or close it completely, depending on the gravity of the infection. In the case of extremely grave infection they suture the peritoneum only, and pack the more superficial structures of the wound with hot moist gauze, not suturing them at all. The reason for doing this is that they believe that it is impossible to drain the numerous pockets of the abdominal cavity, that the peritoneum will take care of the infection (and if it cannot take care of itself, no drains will save the patient), while the fascia and muscles have to be helped against the infection. This opinion (that the peritoneum is less vulnerable to infection and will take care of itself, thus eliminating the necessity of drainage after appendecomy) has been emphasized for the last twenty years by Karl A. Meyer.

II. RESECTION OF THE LARGE BOWEL.

The amount of bowel resected depends on several factors:

1. **The character of the pathology present in the wall of the bowel.**

   If it is a case of tuberculosis, the amount of bowel to be removed will be slightly larger than the size of the affected area. If it is a case of carcinoma of the bowel, the amount to be removed is much larger than the actual size of the pathology present in the wall, since other considerations, such as the invasion of lymphatic glands and the vascular distribution in the bowel, necessitate far more extensive resection.

2. **The manner of the distribution of the blood-vessels in the bowel.**

This is actually the main factor which requires vast resection of the bowel in case of carcinoma with lymphatic involvement. Removal of the lymphatic vessels and primary glands makes imperative the ligation of the accompanying blood-vessels, and this certainly requires the resection of a large amount of bowel.

3. **The lymphatic drainage of the wall of the bowel.**

In the case of carcinoma of the bowel the disease is disseminated by the lymphatic vessels. The primary seat of the disease may be small, but the lymphatic vessels running from this small area may reach lymphatic glands which are situated far remote from this primary seat, and this will necessitate the removal of all this lymphatic area. The removal of such a vast area of lymphatic vessels and glands will require the ligation of a large number of blood-vessels and this means the removal of a large portion of bowel. **The importance of an exact knowledge of the lymphatic drainage for intelligent surgical treatment of carcinoma of the bowel becomes paramount.**

4. **Mechanical considerations in restoring the continuity of the intestinal tract.**

In some cases, mechanical considerations will warrant the removal of more bowel than the pathology would indicate, since otherwise anastomosis of the remaining parts may become impossible. Thus, in the case of a benign tumor of the ascending colon it may become impossible to bring the cecum to the hepatic flexure, and in such a case it may become imperative to remove the entire cecum and to bring the ileum to the hepatic flexure, which is not a difficult procedure.

In the case of resection of the bowel for any cause except malignancy, the technic is exactly the same as outlined in Chapter V. The continuity of the tract may be restored either by an end-to-end, an end-to-side or a side-to-side anastomosis. This can be done either by open methods or by the "closed aseptic methods". It is well to emphasize again that in surgery of the large bowel the "closed aseptic methods" offer the greatest advantage, greatly reducing the mortality.

We would emphasize again that removal of the carcinomatous bowel alone and not the carcinomatous glands also makes the operation incomplete and makes certain a recurrence.

The most important contributions to our knowledge of the lymphatic drainage of the walls of the small and large intestines have been made by Clado, Cunéo, Polya and von Navratil, and Jamieson and Dobson. These investigators used in their work the method of Gerota of injecting the lymphatic vessels. The outline, given below, is taken from Jamieson and Dobson. It is, however, in accordance with the results obtained by the other above mentioned investigators.

In order to do a radical operation, the following facts should be remembered:

1. **In the case of carcinoma of the appendix or cecum** we must remove the last six inches of the ileum, the appendix, the cecum, the ascending colon and about one-third of the right side of the transverse colon with their lymphatic areas (Fig. 141, a, b).

2. **In the case of carcinoma of the hepatic flexure** we must remove the

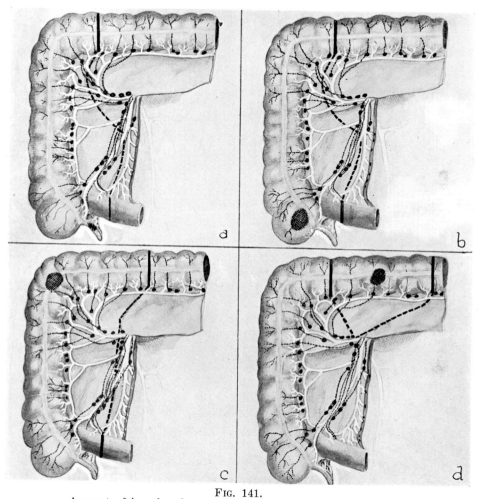

FIG. 141.
Amount of bowel to be removed depends on the seat of cancer
(After Jamieson and Dobson).
a. Carcinoma of the appendix;   b. Carcinoma of the cecum;   c. Carcinoma of the hepatic flexure;   d. Carcinoma of the transverse colon.

terminal six inches of the ileum, the appendix, the cecum, the ascending colon, the hepatic flexure and about half of the transverse colon with their lymphatic areas (Fig. 141, c).

3. **In the case of carcinoma of the middle portion of the transverse colon** we must remove that part of the transverse colon which includes the

diseased portion of the gut and three inches of healthy gut on each side of it with the corresponding portion of the transverse mesocolon (Fig. 141, d).

4. **In the case of carcinoma of the splenic flexure** we must remove the left third of the transverse colon, the splenic flexure and the descend-

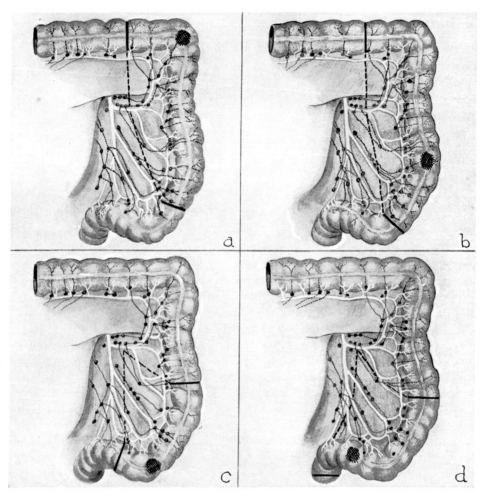

FIG. 142. AMOUNT OF BOWEL TO BE REMOVED DEPENDS ON THE SEAT OF CANCER.
a. Carcinoma of the splenic flexure;   b. Carcinoma of the upper portion of the sigmoid;
c. Carcinoma of the lower portion of the sigmoid;   d. Carcinoma of the recto-sigmoid junction.

ing colon down to the sigmoid flexure with their lymphatic areas (Fig. 142, a).

5. **In the case of carcinoma of the descending colon** we must remove the left third of the transverse colon, the splenic flexure, the entire descending colon and the upper part of the sigmoid flexure with their lymphatic areas (Fig. 142, b).

6. **In the case of carcinoma of the lower portion of the sigmoid flexure
    and the upper portion of the rectum** we must remove the entire sig-
    moid flexure and the upper half of the rectum with their lymphatic
    areas (Fig. 142, c, d).

A. RESECTION OF THE CECUM (CECECTOMY).

This operation is done usually in combination with the removal of the
terminal portion (six to eight inches) of the ileum and a part of the ascending colon.

Indications.

It is done for extensive tuberculosis of the cecum.

Technic.

Step 1. The abdomen is opened by one or other of the usual incisions:

  a.   Transverse incision;

  b.   Incision through the right semilunar line.

In the case of a longitudinal incision through the right semilunar line,
Step 2 will be as follows:

Step 2. Two large retractors reflect the lateral lip of the wound. The
cecum and ascending colon are mobilized by incising the parietal peritoneum covering the posterior abdominal wall just lateral to them. (Fig.
129). The inner lip of peritoneum thus produced is grasped by an artery-
forceps and separated from the posterior wall of the abdomen by the
index-finger of the left hand placed behind it. This separation is continued
by moving the finger progressively closer to the median line. Thus, the
cecum and ascending colon will be lifted and will hang as on a mesentery,
becoming as movable as the loops of the small bowel, so that finally it will
be possible to deliver them outside the abdominal cavity. [In mobilizing
the cecum and colon **care must be taken not to injure the right ureter and
the right internal spermatic or ovarian artery.**] After the mobilization
of the cecum and colon is accomplished, the forceps holding the inner lip
of the parietal peritoneum of the posterior abdominal wall, and the retractors, should be removed.

Step 3. At a point of the ileum about six inches away from the ileo-
cecal junction the arcuate vessels are ligated exactly as is shown in
Chapter V "Resection of the Small Bowel". In the same manner, the
arcuate vessels of the ascending colon are ligated just above the place
where the colon should be divided.

Step 4. The mesentery on which hangs the terminal part of the ileum,
the cecum and the ascending colon is put on the stretch, and the ileo-colic
artery and as many branches of the right colic artery which give blood
supply to that part of the ascending colon which must be removed are tied.
The ligation of the vessels can be done either by clamping the mesentery

with artery-forceps and cutting it between them, or by piercing the mesentery by a forceps and introducing a thread through this perforation.

Step 5. Two crushing-clamps are placed very close to each other on the terminal portion of the ileum and between the ligatures which tied the arcuate vessels in such a way that they lie perpendicular to the long axis of the ileum. An intestinal clamp, the blades of which are covered

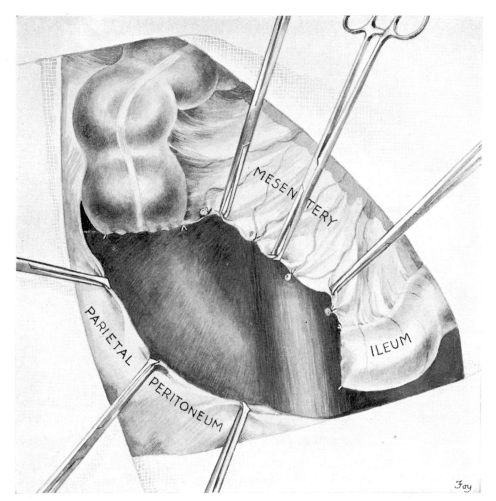

FIG. 143. PERITONIZATION OF THE POSTERIOR WALL OF THE ABDOMEN.

with rubber tubing, is placed across the bowel perpendicularly to its long axis and two inches proximal to the proximal clamp. The bowel is cut ("shaved off") between the two crushing-clamps so that nothing is left on the proximal crushing-clamp. Both stumps are sterilized over the blade with phenol and alcohol (unless the bowel was cut by the cautery). The stump of the distal part of the ileum is covered with gauze which is tied to the clamp to prevent its slipping; the end of the proximal loop of the ileum is closed by the "suture over the clamp" method. The intestinal clamp which held the ileum is now removed.

Step 6. Two crushing-clamps are placed very close to each other on the large bowel between the ligatures which tied the arcuate vessels. An intestinal clamp is placed across the bowel perpendicularly to its long axis, and two inches distal from the distal crushing-clamp. The bowel is cut, preferably by the cautery, transversely between the two crushing-clamps. This cut should be very close to the distal crushing-clamp so that nothing is left on the clamp [if it is cut by a knife, the cut end of the bowel should be sterilized by phenol, followed by alcohol]. As soon as the large bowel is cut, the diseased portion loses its entire attachment to the body and is removed. The open end of the large bowel is then closed by the "suture over the clamp" method.

Step 7. A lateral intestinal anastomosis is now made between the terminal portion of the ileum and the ascending colon, the transverse colon, or the sigmoid flexure. [If this anastomosis is made between the ileum and the ascending colon, care should be taken to see **that no large blind pouch is left either on the ileum or on the colon.**]

Step 8. By stitching the lateral lip of the parietal peritoneum to the remnant of the mesentery the bed of the cecum and ascending colon will be peritonized (Fig. 143).

As has already been noted, if the cecum, or even the appendix, is removed because of a malignant growth, then the **mere removal of the terminal six inches of ileum and of the appendix and the cecum is not sufficient.** In such cases it is necessary to remove **the terminal six inches of the ileum, the cecum, the ascending colon and the right third of the transverse colon.** This is what is known as:

B. THE FRIEDRICH OPERATION.

This operation is performed for malignancy of the appendix alone, or of the appendix and cecum, or of the appendix, cecum and ascending colon.

Step 1. Abdominal section is made.

Step 2. The same as Step 2 of the previous operation, with the exception only that the incision of the parietal peritoneum lateral to the ascending colon should be made upward to the level of the hepatic flexure, and that when stripping the inner lip of the parietal peritoneum the finger should reach upward and medially to the second part of the duodenum as well as to that portion of the third part of the duodenum where the superior mesenteric artery crosses the bowel.

Step 3. The same as Step 3 in the previous operation.

Step 4. The same as Step 4 of the previous operation, with the understanding, of course, that not only the branches of the right colic artery, but **the artery itself should be ligated very close to its origin either from the ileo-colic artery or from the superior mesenteric artery,** and that the attachment of the lateral few inches of the transverse colon should be separated from the duodenum.

Step 5. The same as Step 5 in the previous operation.

Step 6. The same as Step 6 in the previous operation.

Step 7. A lateral intestinal anastomosis is made between the terminal portion of the ileum and the transverse colon or the sigmoid flexure.

Step 8. The bed of the cecum, ascending colon and of the removed portion of the transverse colon is peritonized by suturing in the manner described above.

C.   RESECTION OF THE COLON FOR CARCINOMA OF THE HEPATIC FLEXURE.

Due to the course of the lymphatic drainage from the hepatic flexure, it is necessary to remove the last six to eight inches of the terminal ileum, the cecum, the ascending colon, the hepatic flexure, and two to three inches of the transverse colon together with the glands into which the lymphatic vessels of these regions drain (Fig. 141, c). **Since, in order to remove all the lymphatic glands from this region, it will be necessary to ligate the middle colic artery close to its origin, therefore, it will be necessary to resect about half of the transverse colon, otherwise there might result gangrene of the right half of the colon.** The technic is exactly the same as in the previous operation, with the difference only that the middle colic artery and vein must be ligated.

D.   RESECTION OF THE TRANSVERSE COLON.

In the case of malignancy of the central portion of the transverse colon, since the lymphatics do not spread beyond the limits of the part of the bowel affected, it is sufficient in order to effect a radical cure to resect only the affected part of the bowel with two to three inches of healthy tissue on each side of the growth (Fig. 141, d).

Technic.

Step 1. The abdomen is opened by a midline or a transverse incision.

Step 2. Ligation is made of the gastrocolic ligament for a length corresponding to the length of the portion of the transverse colon to be removed. This is done in the following manner:

The gastrocolic ligament is grasped between two tissue-forceps between which it is cut (Fig. 144). [Care should be taken not to cut through the transverse mesocolon which lies so close to the gastrocolic ligament that they appear as a single layer.] A curved artery-forceps is introduced into the opening in the gastrocolic ligament, and this opening is enlarged by spreading the blades. The index-finger of the left hand is then introduced and gently separates the gastrocolic ligament, which lies in front of the finger, from the transverse mesocolon, which lies behind the finger (Fig. 231). Two artery-forceps are then placed on the gastrocolic ligament, one on each side of the intended line of incision, and the ligament is cut sectionally between the forceps. The finger acts as a protector for the transverse mesocolon (Fig. 231).

Step 3. Those branches of the middle colic artery which give the

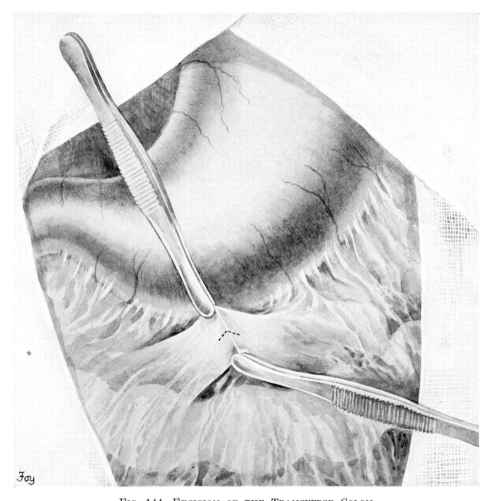

FIG. 144. EXCISION OF THE TRANSVERSE COLON.
The gastrocolic ligament is cut between two tissue-forceps.

blood-supply to the portion of the bowel to be resected, must be ligated, and also the arcuate vessels at the ends of the section of the bowel to be removed.

Step 4. The part of the omentum attached to the resected portion of the colon is cut away from the rest of the omentum. The cutting should be done between two artery-forceps.   [Large bites of the omentum should not be taken.]

Step 5. An artery-forceps is placed at each end of the bowel to be resected and a Partipilo clamp just lateral to each of these clamps.   The bowel is cut between each artery-forceps and the Partipilo clamp by a knife, or still better by the cautery.

Step 6. The continuity of the colon is restored by making an end-to-end anastomosis as described in Chapter VII.

Step 7. The lips of the transverse mesocolon are sutured together.

Step 8. The abdomen is closed.

E. RESECTION OF THE SPLENIC FLEXURE.

If it is necessary to remove the splenic flexure on account of malignancy, the radical operation then is very extensive because of the necessity of removing the spleen, since the lymphatics of the splenic flexure drain also into those of the spleen.   However, surgeons usually confine their work to removal of the left half of the transverse colon, the splenic flexure, and the descending colon, and then restore the continuity of the intestinal tract by making an end-to-end, an end-to-side or a side-to-side anastomosis between the remaining parts of the transverse colon and the sigmoid flexure.   All three procedures do not offer mechanical difficulties, since both the transverse colon and the sigmoid are movable.

Step 1. Abdominal incision is made (left semilunar or transverse).

Step 2. The descending colon is mobilized precisely in the same manner as was described in "Mobilization of the Ascending Colon".

Step 3. The costocolic ligament is divided between two clamps [this loosens the fixed portion of the splenic flexure].   The left half of the transverse colon is separated from the stomach by severing the gastro-colic ligament in the manner described in the previous operation.

Step 4. The left branch of the middle colic artery and the ascending branch of the left colic artery are ligated, and the mesentery is divided longitudinally between the artery-forceps in the same way as described in the previous operation. The mesocolon is divided along the line shown in Fig. 142, a.

Step 5. Arterial clamps and Partipilo crushing-clamps are placed on the bowel precisely in the same manner as described in the previous operation, and the bowel is divided between each arterial and Partipilo clamp by a knife, or preferably by the cautery.

Step 6. An end-to-end anastomosis is made between the remaining portions of the bowel.

Step 7. The denuded bed of the descending colon is peritonized by suturing the lateral lip of the parietal peritoneum to the remnants of the mesocolon. If it is impossible to bring these together, the parietal peritoneum must be mobilized.

Step 8. The abdomen is closed.

If it is decided to reëstablish the lumen of the intestinal tract by making a lateral intestinal anastomosis, the procedure then is somewhat different, thus:

Steps 1 to 4 the same as in the previous operation.

Step 5. Two arterial clamps are placed on each end of the bowel to be removed. The bowel is resected between each pair of clamps, and each end of the bowel is closed blindly.

Step 6. A lateral intestinal anastomosis is made in the usual way.

Step 7. The denuded bed of the descending colon is peritonized precisely in the same way as described in Step 7 of the previous operation.

Step 8. The abdomen is closed.

F. REMOVAL OF THE DESCENDING COLON.

Due to the lymphatic arrangement, in the case of malignancy of the descending colon this portion of the colon should be removed together with the splenic flexure and the left half of the transverse colon. The difference in the amount of bowel removed in cases of malignancy of the splenic flexure and of malignancy of the descending colon is that in the latter the lower end of the resected bowel should be at the upper part of the sigmoid flexure. The technic of resection is precisely the same as described in "Removal of the Splenic Flexure".

G. REMOVAL OF THE SIGMOID FLEXURE.

In the case of malignancy of the sigmoid flexure, it is necessary to remove the lower half of the descending colon and the entire sigmoid flexure down to the sigmoido-rectal junction. The technic is essentially the same as that in the case of resection of the splenic flexure with some additional steps which are described below.

Step 1. Abdominal section is made through the left semilunar line.

Step 2. The descending colon is mobilized in its lower half precisely as described in "Mobilization of the Ascending Colon". However, if it is seen that after the resection of the lower half of the descending colon there will be difficulty in making an end-to-end anastomosis between the upper portion of the descending colon and the rectum, then it will be necessary to mobilize the entire length of the descending colon and the splenic flexure. The sigmoid portion of the bowel should be mobilized in the following way:

An incision is made in the parietal peritoneum just lateral to the sigmoid. This incision is carried downward to the brim of the pelvis, and then still further downward to the place where the peritoneum of the urinary bladder (in the male) or the uterus (in the female) is reflected onto the anterior wall of the rectum [this is usually at the level of the second or third sacral vertebra]. This part of the bowel is mobilized precisely as in mobilization of the ascending colon [while doing this care should be taken not to injure the left spermatic artery and left ureter]. The reflection of the peritoneum from the bladder (in the male) or the uterus (in the female) onto the rectum is cut across in front of the rectum. Then the parietal peritoneum is incised one inch away from the right side of the rectum and sigmoid. When the promontory is reached, if the middle sacral artery is in the way, it should be ligated and cut between two ligatures. The leaflets of the parietal peritoneum from which the descending colon and sigmoid are suspended, are treated precisely in the same manner as described for resection of any other portion of the large bowel. The rest of the operation differs, depending on whether it is desired to reëstablish the continuity of the gastro-intestinal tract or to resort to the formation of an artificial anus. In the latter case the next step will be:

Step 3. Two crushing-clamps are placed on the rectum which is cut between them. The distal end is closed blindly.

Step 4. A crushing-clamp is placed at the proximal end of the gut to be removed, and two inches proximal to it an intestinal clamp, the blades of which are covered with rubber, is placed across the bowel which is cut off just proximal to the distal clamp, and the gut removed. The proximal end of the bowel is then attached to the anterior abdominal wall.

If, however, it is decided to reëstablish the continuity of the gastro-intestinal tract, then:

Step 3. A crushing-clamp is placed on the distal end of the gut to be removed, and another on the proximal end. Two inches proximal to the proximal clamp an intestinal clamp is placed across the gut, which is cut distal to the distal clamp and proximal to the proximal crushing-clamp. The continuity of the intestinal tract is then reëstablished either by a plain end-to-end anastomosis or with the aid of a rubber tube.

Step 4. The assistant everts the lower segment of the rectum. A rubber tube is introduced into the proximal end of the sigmoid and secured there by a chromic catgut stitch. The other end of the rubber tube is inserted into the everted portion of the rectum until its end protrudes through the anus. The assistant then pulls this tube downward so that a portion of the upper segment of the rectum is telescoped through the entire length of the lower segment. These ends are then sutured to each other by a series of over-and-over interrupted sutures, after which the bowel is pulled upward so as to replace in its normal position the everted portion of the rectum and anus.

Step 5. The abdomen is closed.

Step 6. The coccyx is removed, thus exposing the line of anastomosis, which is reinforced by another layer of interrupted seromuscular sutures.

H. RESECTION OF A BOWEL IN SEVERAL STAGES.

This type of operation belongs to the earliest group of operations in which, because of high mortality of the one-stage operation, the surgeons preferred to perform it in several stages. With the improvement in surgical technic this type is now reserved only for those cases in which intestinal obstruction is already present and the patient cannot stand more than a mere colostomy. A very widely used method for this class of cases is:

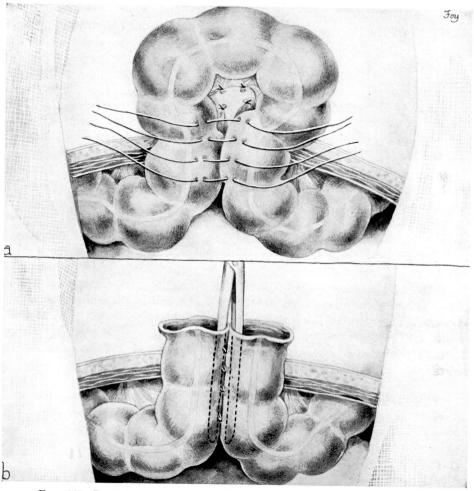

FIG. 145. RESECTION OF THE LARGE BOWEL BY THE MIKULICZ METHOD.
a. Suturing two loops by interrupted seromuscular sutures;
b. Crushing the wall by an enterotribe.

Mikulicz Method.

This is done in four stages.

Technic.

1st. Stage.

Step 1. The abdomen is opened by a left gridiron or by a left para-rectus incision.

Step 2. The sigmoid is located. The mesentery of the sigmoid is ligated and cut in a "V" shape. [It should be kept in mind, that not only the blood-vessels distribution, but also the area of lymphatic drainage, should be considered before deciding the amount of bowel to be removed].

Step 3. The portions of the bowel lying in close proximity to the portion to be removed are laid side by side. A seromuscular suture connects them either on one or on both sides (Fig. 145, a).

Step 4. A suture fixes each loop of the "double-barrel" to the peritoneum in its vicinity.

Several days (4 to 7) later the second stage is performed.

2nd. Stage.

Step 1. The bowel lying on the skin is resected, leaving only about one and one-half inches of bowel above the surface of the skin.

Several days later (5 to 7 after the 2nd. Stage) the 3rd, stage is done:

3rd. Stage.

Step 1. An enterotribe with blades four inches long is introduced into the lumen of each bowel-opening (Fig. 145, b) ; the lock is closed slightly. Each day the enterotribe is locked a little firmer than on the previous day. In a few days (on the average, five to seven) the intestinal wall between the two loops is crushed, so that a spur is no longer present.

Two or three days after this the next stage is done:

4th. Stage.

Step 1. The edges of the intestinal wound are freshened and mobilized. [Care should be taken not to mobilize the loops behind the peritoneum]. The intestinal lips are sutured to each other by an over-and-over suture and then reinforced by a sero-serous suture.

The skin is closed either immediately or a few days later.

III. COLOSTOMY.

The word colostomy is composed of two Greek words: κόλον, colon and στόμα, mouth; it is an artificial communication between the lumen of a bowel and the outside world.

The site of the colostomy depends on the location of the pathology. As it is done more frequently for malignancy of the rectum than for any other portion of the bowel, it is usually done in the sigmoid flexure. However, the opening is infrequently made in the cecum, the ascending colon, the transverse colon or in the descending colon. The opening may be temporary only, and then the operation is called "temporary colostomy", or it may be made as a permanent affair and then it carries the name of a "permanent colostomy".

If the communication has been established intentionally it it called an **"artificial anus"**, and if the communication came spontaneously as the result of pathological changes in the bowel-wall it is then called a **"fecal fistula"**. If the opening is made in the appendix, it is called **appendicostomy**, if in the cecum, **cecostomy**, if in the sigmoid flexure, **sigmoidostomy**.

The site of the abdominal incision depends on the part of the bowel to be opened. Thus, in the case of cecostomy it will be in the right iliac region; in the case of making an opening in the transverse colon, it will be a longitudinal or a transverse incision in the epigastric region; and in the case of a sigmoidostomy, in the left inguinal region.

Historical.

An excellent article on "The Origins and Evolution of Colostomy" was written by Tilson Dinnick, of London, and published in the British Journal of Surgery, in July, 1934. We quote freely from this article for the historical review of colostomy.

Accidental colostomies, due to injury of the bowel were known from remote antiquity. The earliest suggestion of this occurrence is probably that which is mentioned in the Bible, in the "Book of Judges", where we read that Ehud stabbed Eglon, the King of Moab "and his dirt ran out and he died". Coelius Aurelianus states that Praxagorus (who lived four hundred years before Christ), among the different methods used to cure ileus suggested making an opening in the abdomen, incising the bowel, evacuating its contents, and then closing the bowel and the abdominal wall.

However, the credit for deliberately advocating the use of colostomy to relieve obstruction is given to the French surgeon Littré, who, in 1710, advocated this procedure in the case of an imperforate anus in an infant. The first who actually performed it, in the form of a right inguinal colostomy (cecostomy), was Pillore, a surgeon of Rouen, who did it in 1776 on a patient suffering from carcinoma of the rectum. Duret, in 1793, was the first who performed a left lumbar colostomy on an infant for imperforate anus. Thus, he preceded Callisen, to whom erroneously is given the credit for being the first who introduced lumbar colostomy.

The first colostomy made in the transverse colon was done by Fine, of Geneva, in 1797. It was done as an error, since he thought, at the time of operation, that he was doing an ileostomy, and only the subsequent autopsy on the patient showed that instead of the ileum the transverse colon had been opened. Callisen, of Copenhagen, published in 1800 his "Systema Chirurgiæ Hodiernæ" in which he advised performing a lumbar colostomy. Although he does not claim originality for this method, and mentions the names of several men who did it before him, nevertheless many erroneously consider him as the originator of this operation. Freer, of Birmingham, was the first to perform a colostomy in England, in 1815.

However, this operation has been used only occasionally by a few daring surgeons. Only since Amussat, of Paris, described in detail its technic, in 1839, has lumbar colostomy become the operation of choice. It held this position until Allingham, Jr. showed, in 1887, the advantage of the inguinal approach, which, together with other types of anterior abdominal approach, replaced entirely the lumbar route.

F. T. Paul, in 1890, described his glass-tube, which enabled the surgeon to open the bowel immediately, whenever it was deemed necessary. Schitzinger was the first who, in 1881, divided the exteriorized bowel completely, thus making two openings which were entirely separated from each other.

By using the "two-stage" method, in which the bowel is delivered and attached to the skin as the first stage, and opened a few days later as the second stage, this operation becomes a safe procedure. The only difficulty that confronts the surgeon now is making the opening "watertight" and "gastight". Many ingenuous devices have been offered to make the opening "water-and gas-tight", but the last word has not yet been said.

Indications.

1. In the case of an obstruction of the large bowel.
2. As a preliminary step to removal of the rectum.
3. As a preliminary step in surgery of the rectum, when it is not necessary to remove the latter.
4. To give rest to the bowel in certain pathological conditions, such as ulcerative colitis, etc.
5. Appendicostomy or cecostomy has been used lately by some surgeons as a routine procedure in the treatment of perforation of the appendix with peritonitis.

The technic of colostomy varies, depending on whether a permanent or a temporary colostomy is to be established.

A. PERMANENT COLOSTOMY OR ARTIFICIAL ANUS.

In making a permanent colostomy several factors must be taken into consideration:

1. All the fecal material should escape through the colostomy opening. **No fecal material should pass into the distal loop.** This can be accomplished by making a spur between the designated proximal and distal loops, and then by making the opening in the proximal loop.
2. The opening should be "watertight". This means that no fecal material should escape through the opening involuntarily. Many ingenuous methods have been devised to accomplish this requirement, but the great majority of them are unsatisfactory. This is the reason why surgeons rely more on different mechanical appliances (such as cups), on diet or on a constipation-habit of the patient, than on mechanico-physiological apparatus made of the human structures.
3. No loop of small bowel should be caught between the large bowel and the abdominal wall to which it is attached, in order not to produce an intestinal obstruction.

4. There should be no retraction of the proximal loop into the abdominal cavity or into the abdominal wall.

5. There should be no prolapse of the proximal loop.

a. Left Inguinal Colostomy.

Step 1. The abdomen is opened by a "gridiron" incision precisely as for appendectomy, with this difference only that the incision is made on the left side. The length of the incision is three inches (Fig. 146, a).

Step 2. The index-finger of the right hand is introduced behind the lateral lip of the abdominal incision and is directed laterally until it reaches the lateral border of the abdominal cavity. It then moves downward until the posterior abdominal wall is reached, and then medially until the mesosigmoid is reached. Then the finger follows the mesosigmoid until the mesenteric border of the sigmoid flexure is reached, which is then grasped by the finger and brought outside the abdominal cavity.

Step 3. The proximal portion of the sigmoid is drawn outside the abdominal cavity until it is placed on a moderate stretch. The drawn-out portion of the bowel is placed in the form of a horse-shoe. The mesenteric border of the arch thus produced at its summit should lie about one and one-half inches above the level of the skin.

Step 4. With the Pagenstecher linen thread, or a silk thread, the middle of the inner lip of the abdominal wall is pierced through its entire thickness (skin, fascia, external oblique muscle, internal oblique muscle, transversus abdominis muscle, transversalis fascia and the peritoneum). Then the needle passes through a bloodless spot on the mesentery about one inch away from the mesenteric border of the bowel (Fig. 146, b), then through the entire thickness of the lateral lip of the abdominal wall from within outward, then again through the mesentery very close to the point where the thread previously passed through, and the thread is brought over the inner lip. Thus, a loop of thread will lie on the skin of the outer lip with its two ends resting on the inner lip (Fig. 146, c). A rubber tube is then placed in the loop and another between the free ends of the thread, which are tied snugly (Fig. 146, d). The reason for placing the rubber tubes is to prevent the thread from cutting through the skin, while the ends are snugly tied. The wound is then covered with gauze abundantly impregnated with vaseline. The opening of the bowel is postponed for four or five days, after which the "second stage" is performed.
Second Stage.

Step 5. The proximal loop of the bowel is opened by a transverse incision the length of which is about two-thirds of its circumference. This incision should not lie very close to the skin, so that in case of a future retraction of the loop it will not slip behind the level of the skin. [The technic, as described above is highly recommended by Moynihan for use in the permanent as well as in the temporary type of colostomy.]

If, however, after completing the "First Stage" of the operation, the patient begins to complain of severe gas-pain and Step **5** cannot be postponed at least for 24 hours, or if it is an acute case of obstruction of the colon in which the opening in the bowel must be made immediately, then as there is no time for the formation of protective adhesions, it is necessary to introduce a rubber, or still better, a glass tube. Then Step **5** will be as follows:

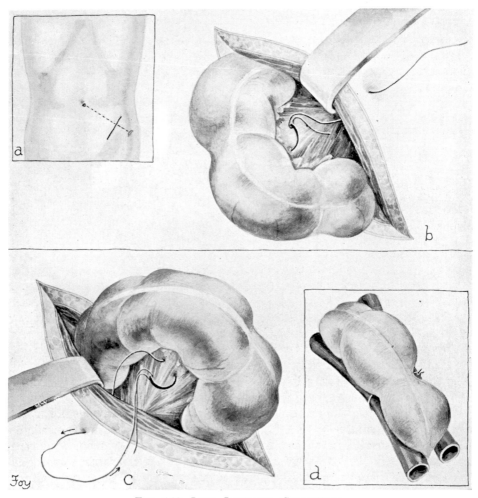

FIG. 146. LEFT INGUINAL COLOSTOMY.
a. Skin incision;
b. Suturing the mesocolon to one of the abdominal lips;
c. Suturing the mesocolon to the other abdominal lip;
d. Final view.
(Pictures b, c and d are seen from the left side of the patient).

Step 5. A purse-string seromuscular suture is made on the free (antimesenteric) border of the proximal limb. The diameter of the circle should be about half an inch. The wall of the bowel is caught inside of the purse-string by an Allis forceps and is opened by one snip of the scissors.

Then the Allis forceps is drawn upward, which will prevent the escape of the intestinal contents. A glass tube is immediately introduced and the ends of the purse-string are tied snugly around the tube.

This operation, performed as described above, is very simple; its execution requires only about ten minutes. The single suture will keep the spur above the skin until adhesions are formed. As can be seen, the bowel is sutured at no point to any layer of the abdominal wall.

In order to give support to the protruding bowel Audry and later Mixter made a bridge consisting of the entire thickness of the anterior abdominal wall, which acted as a good support for the protruded bowel. Their technic is as follows:

b. Audry-Mixter Method.

Step 1. A ⌐ -shape incision is made through the skin, superficial and deep fascia until the anterior sheath of the left rectus muscle is reached. This incision starts at the level of the umbilicus at the lateral border of the left rectus muscle, and runs first vertically downward (AB) for a length of two inches. Then another limb of the incision is made (BC) perpendicular to the first one and runs medially until the midline is reached. It is then turned downward along the median line (CD) for another two inches, and then laterally perpendicular to the linea alba until it reaches the lateral border of the left rectus muscle. The incision is then turned downward parallel to the linea alba (EF) for another two inches (Fig. 147, insert). The quadrangular flap BCDE is then reflected laterally (Fig. 147). The rectus muscle is then split from the point A downward to the point F (that is for the length of six inches), and the posterior sheath and the peritoneum are opened longitudinally along the same line AF.

Step 2. The sigmoid is located and brought outside. The loop for the colostomy is selected precisely in the same manner as described in the previous operation.

Step 3. A longitudinal incision two inches in length, is made in the mesosigmoid perpendicular to the long axis of the bowel. The middle of each lip of the split rectus muscle is sutured to the other through the rent in the mesosigmoid. Then the quadrangular skin-flap is protruded through the rent in the mesocolon and replaced in its original position and sutured to the adjoining skin (Fig. 148, a). The bowel is covered with vaseline and the opening into it is deferred for a few (four or five) days.

The Second Stage of the Audry-Mixter Colostomy.

Step 4. The protruding part of the bowel is cut away at a distance of one inch above the skin. In this manner two openings will be produced, separated from each other by a bridge of skin two inches in length, and the contents of the proximal loop cannot escape into the distal loop (Fig. 148, b). The opening of the distal loop may serve for the purpose of medication.

This method was first described by Audry, and Mixter described it later, being unaware of the work of the former.

Although this method prevents the escape of the contents from the proximal into the distal loop, and also the retraction of the bowel, nevertheless **it is not watertight, a most distressing condition to the patient.**

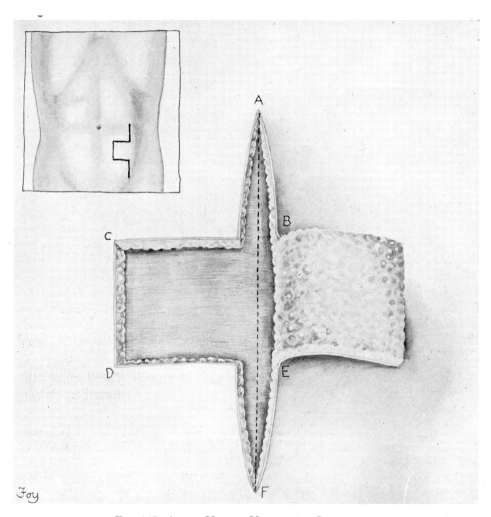

FIG. 147. AUDRY-MIXTER METHOD OF COLOSTOMY.
INSERT. Skin incision.
MAIN PICTURE. The cutaneous flap is reflected.

The same type of flap incision " ⌐ " made only lateral from the outer border of the rectus muscle, is used by some surgeons, and is known as the **Jeannel incision.**

In order to make the colostomy opening watertight Kurtzahn, in 1920, suggested two methods. One consisted in making two tubes from two skin-

flaps and then carrying each tube through a subcutaneous channel around
the portion of the bowel on which the colostomy opening was contemplated;
these two tubes met below the gut so that they encircled it in the form of
a sphincter. However, in a later work in the same year he suggested another
method, which is as follows: A skin-tube is made out of a skin-flap. This

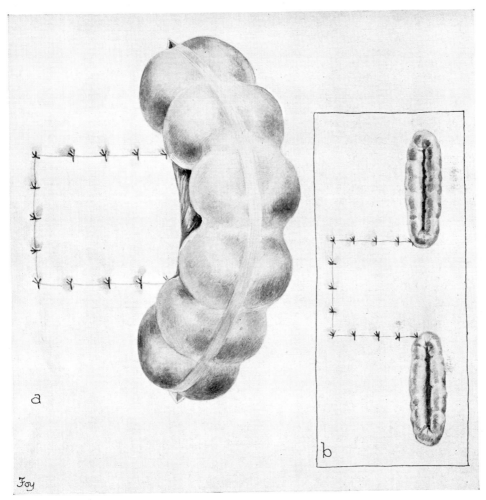

Fig. 148. Audry-Mixter Method of Colostomy.
a. The skin-flap is sutured in its original position.
b. Two openings in the bowel separated by a bridge of skin.

tube is carried through a hole in the mesosigmoid, which is brought outside the abdominal cavity, and then the tube is fastened to the other lip
of the skin. Thus, the sigmoid rests on a skin-tube. A metalic rod is placed
in the lumen of the tube. A pellet is placed outside on the bowel, so that
the latter is compressed between these two foreign bodies. This method

was further improved by R. Haecker, in 1923, and since that time has been used by many surgeons, many of whom have been well pleased with the method.

c. Kurtzahn-Haecker Method.

Step 1. A quadrangular skin-incision is made in front of the left rectus muscle at the level of the umbilicus (Fig. 149, a). The width of this

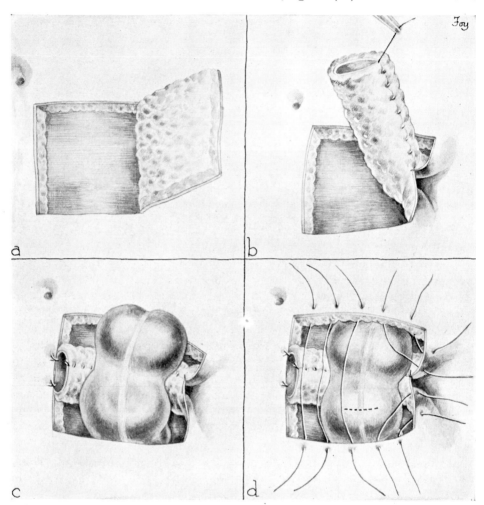

FIG. 149. KURTZAHN-HAECKER METHOD OF COLOSTOMY.
a. The cutaneous flap is made; b. Formation of a tube from the flap; c. The tube is carried through an opening in the mesosigmoid and sutured to the opposite side; d. Closure of the skin over the bowel.

incision is 6cm. and the length about 5cm. The base of this incision lies on the left semilunar line. This flap is reflected from the underlying tissues and transformed into a tube (Fig. 149, b).

Step 2. The abdomen is opened by a longitudinal incision, running along the lateral border of the rectus muscle. The sigmoid is delivered outside. A hole is made in the mesosigmoid through which the skin-tube is carried to the inner lip of the opened abdomen. Here it is fixed at two points to the skin of the inner lip (Fig. 149, c).

Step 3. The upper lip is sutured to the lower one over the bowel, leaving a small opening in the skin in the lower angle through which the bowel is seen (Fig. 149, d).

Step 4. The bowel is opened at the lower angle, a few days after Steps 1 to 3 have been performed.

A clamp with rubber tubing on its blades is applied in the following manner: One blade of the clamp passes through the cutaneous canal, lying behind the gut. Another blade lies on the skin in front of the gut. The clamp is locked. Thus, not only feces but even gas will not pass through the clamped bowel.

However, the objection to this method lies in the fact that mechanical appliances are required to make the opening watertight. In order to eliminate any mechanical appliances, **Spivack devised a method in which a tubo-valvular apparatus is made out of the bowel, which makes the opening watertight without employing any mechanical appliances.**

d. **Spivack Tubo-valvular Colostomy** (Fig. 150).

1st Stage.

Step 1. The abdomen is opened by a left "gridiron" or left pararectus incision. The sigmoid is delivered outside the abdomen. A slit is made in the mesosigmoid, and the lips of the anterior abdominal wall are sutured to each other in layers. Thus the bowel rests on the bridge of the anterior abdominal wall.

Step 2. Several seromuscular-seromuscular sutures are inserted in the proximal loop of the sigmoid (Fig. 150, a, b). The distance between the insertions of each thread is about three-fourths of an inch. The distance between the successive threads is half an inch. These threads are placed so as to be inserted into the entire circumference of the bowel. The ends of each thread are tied and cut short.

2nd Stage.

The bowel is cut transversely a few days after the first stage. **Thus, we have a valve at the proximal portion of the bowel not far from its mouth. This will prevent the escape of feces.**

In those cases in which a permanent ileostomy is contemplated for extensive pathology of the large bowel but in which the cecum is not pathologically altered, Spivack devised the following operation:

e. **Spivack Method of Construction of an Artificial Rectum and Anus.**

This operation consists in dividing the terminal portion of the ileum, implanting the proximal end of the divided bowel into the cecum, bringing outside the abdominal cavity the distal end of the divided ileum and fastening it to the anterior abdominal wall, dividing the cecum completely from the ascending colon and closing blindly both ends of the divided bowel. Thus, a receptacle is formed (from the cecum) for the storage of feces. An artificial rectum is formed (from the terminal portion of the ileum). An artificial sphincter ani is formed (from the ileo-cecal valve).

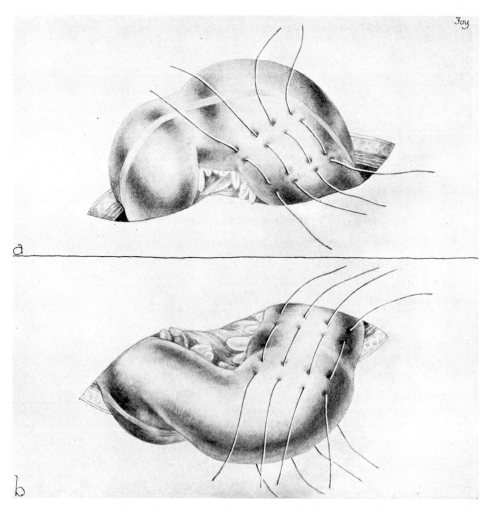

FIG. 150. SPIVACK TUBO-VALVULAR COLOSTOMY.
a. Inserting sero-serous sutures on one side of the bowel;
b. Inserting sero-serous sutures on the other side of the bowel.

Technic.

The operation is performed as a two-stage method.

1st Stage.

Step 1. The abdomen is opened on the right side by a "gridiron" incision.

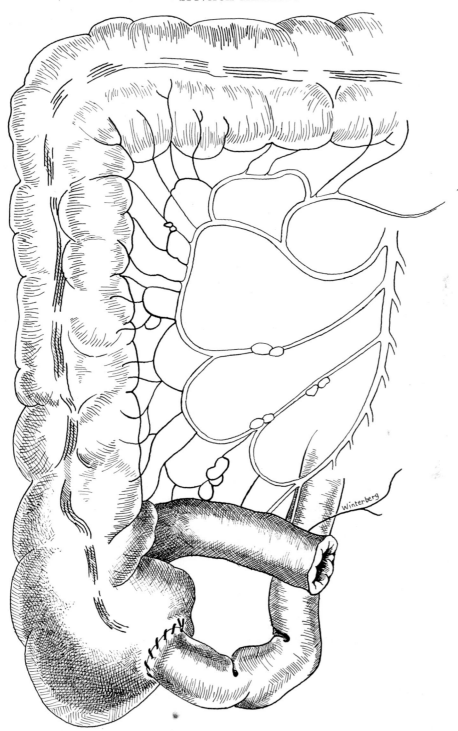

FIG. 151. SPIVACK METHOD OF THE FORMATION OF AN ARTIFICIAL ANUS.
The terminal ileum is divided and the proximal portion implanted into the cecum.

Step 2. The terminal portion of the ileum is cut transversely between two crushing-clamps at a distance of three inches from the ileo-cecal junction.

Step 3. The appendix is removed. The end of the proximal portion of the divided ileum is implanted into the anterior wall of the cecum (Fig. 151). The distal end of the divided ileum is brought outside the abdominal cavity and fastened to the layers of the anterior abdominal wall (Fig. 152).

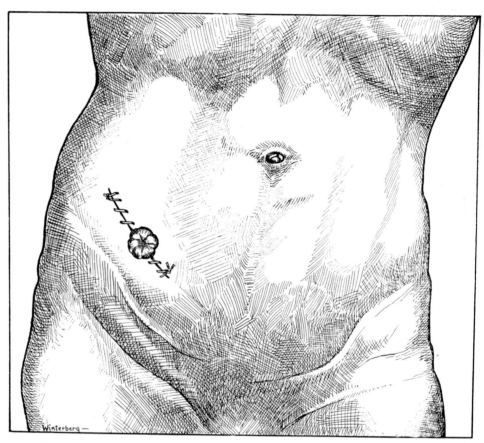

FIG. 152. SPIVACK METHOD OF THE FORMATION OF AN ARTIFICIAL ANUS.
The distal end of the divided ileum serves as an abdominal anus.

A few days later, the second stage is performed:

2nd Stage.

Step 1. The abdomen is opened by a transverse incision which runs on the right side from the anterior axillary line to the lateral border of the right rectus muscle. This incision is made at the level of the umbilicus (Fig. 154). After the skin is incised, its lips are retracted, and the abdominal cavity is entered through a muscle-splitting incision.

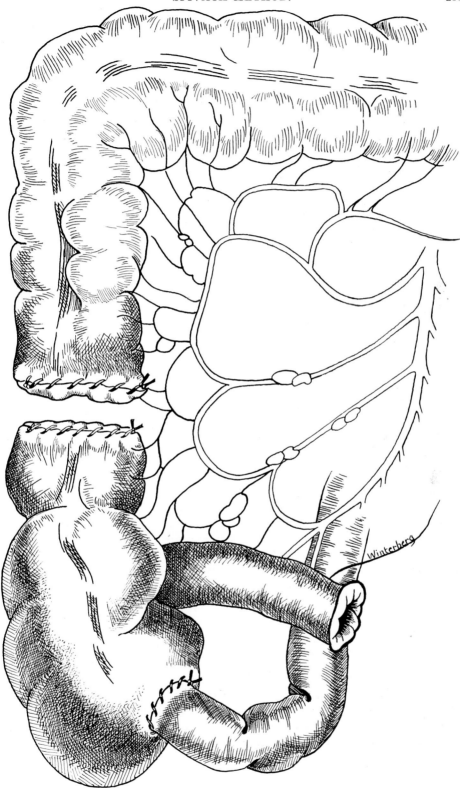

Fig. 153. Spivack Method of the Formation of an Artificial Anus.
The cecum is divided transversely and each end is closed blindly.

Step 2. The cecum and the adjoining portion of the ascending colon are mobilized and brought outside the abdominal cavity. Two crushing-clamps (Payr or Doyen) are placed across the colon very close to each other; the bowel is cut between the clamps by the cautery. Each end of the divided bowel is then closed blindly (Fig. 153).

Step 3. The abdomen is closed in layers.

The final view is seen in Fig. 154.

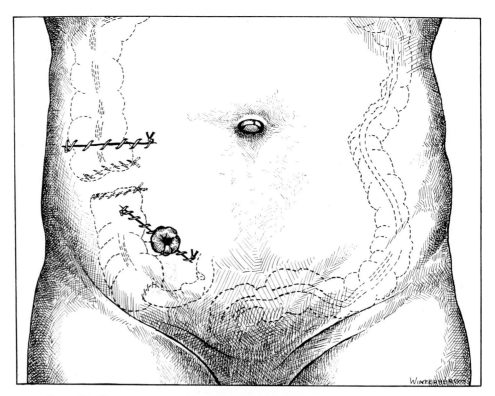

FIG. 154. SPIVACK METHOD OF THE FORMATION OF AN ARTIFICIAL ANUS.
Final View.

B. TEMPORARY COLOSTOMY.

The prerequisites for temporary colostomy are the same as for permanent colostomy, and they have already been enumerated in the subchapter on permanent colostomy. In addition to them, temporary colostomy offers some other difficulties, since, in the latter, two of the prerequisites are antagonistic to each other:

a. In order that the fecal material should not pass into the distal loop it is necessary **to make a marked spur. The larger the spur, the more assured we are that the contents will not escape into the distal loop.**

b. It is easier to close the opening (when the necessity for it no longer exists) when the bowel does not form a spur. **If a spur is present, the smaller the spur, the easier it is to close the opening.** This is the reason why it is such a difficult task to make a truly satisfactory temporary colostomy, and this explains also why so many different methods have been suggested.

Technic.

Step 1. The same as Step 1 in Left Inguinal Colostomy.

Step 2. The same as Step 2 in Left Inguinal Colostomy.

Step 3. The proximal part of the sigmoid flexure is drawn outside the abdominal cavity until it is placed on a moderate stretch. Care should be taken to see that **only part of the intestinal wall protrudes outside of the wound and that no spur is formed.**

Step 4. The abdominal wall is sutured to the circumference of the sigmoid flexure. The needle and the thread pass through the peritoneum and the transversalis fascia only and through the seromuscular layer of the bowel. It is best to suture with interrupted stitches, placing them at a distance of three-fourths of an inch from each other, **and penetrating the peritoneum and the transversalis fascia at a distance of one inch from their edges** (Fig. 118, b). The bowel should be attached to the ends of the abdominal incision in such a manner that the thread penetrates the peritoneum and the transversalis fascia of one lip, then through the seromuscular layer of the bowel, penetrating the tænia longitudinalis coli, and then through the peritoneum and the transversalis fascia of the other lip. In this manner, there is no danger of the slipping of a loop of the small bowel between the large bowel and the skin, thereby eliminating the danger of possible incarceration or strangulation of a loop of small bowel.

Step. 5. The edges of the peritoneum and of the transversalis fascia are sutured to the edges of the skin of the same lip. **Thus, the thickness of the abdominal wall will be sealed and the chance of its contamination by intestinal contents will be greatly minimized** (Fig. 119).

Second Stage.

The second stage is done four or five days after the first stage.

Step 6. A longitudinal incision, about one and a half inches in length, is made along the free (antimesenteric) border of the proximal portion of the bowel.

If, however, the patient has severe "gas-pains", immediately after the operation, or if it is necessary to open the bowel within twenty-four hours after performing the first stage, then a glass tube should be inserted in the manner already described.

However, we prefer, if possible, not to suture the bowel to the peritoneum.

The appendix and cecum are used quite frequently as the seat of the colostomy opening. The performance of cecostomy in the case of intestinal obstruction dates back to the year 1776, when Pillore, of Rouen, performed it on a patient suffering from cancer of the rectum.

Appendicostomy as a type of colostomy was first suggested in 1884, by C. B. Keetley, at a meeting of the London Medical Society, when he "suggested that when it was necessary to empty the cæcum at once, the vermiform appendix might be made use of as a spout". The first who actually utilized this idea of Keetley was R. F. Weir, who reported, in 1902, that he performed appendicostomy. He, evidently, was not aware of the suggestion of Keetley. In 1909, Groves performed an appendicostomy **as one of the important steps in the treatment of peritonitis accompanying a ruptured appendix.** This operation (appendicostomy) for the treatment of peritonitis due to a ruptured appendix has since been largely replaced by cecostomy, so that now **many surgeons use as a routine procedure an appendicostomy or a cecostomy in all cases of ruptured appendix.**

C. APPENDICOSTOMY.

Technic.

Step 1. The abdomen is opened by a McBurney incision.

Step 2. The cecum is located. The appendix is found and delivered outside the abdominal cavity. The meso-appendix is clamped close to the tip of the appendix, which enables the surgeon to secure a firm hold on the appendix. The meso-appendix is ligated. A purse-string suture is placed on the cecum half an inch away from the base of the appendix. The appendix is clamped close to its base by two clamps, and is removed by an incision made between these two clamps. The forceps, clamping the base of the appendix is now replaced by two or three Allis forceps each of which grasps the edge of the appendicular stump. A catheter No. 14F. is introduced into the cecum through the patent appendicular stump. A bite is inserted now through the wall of the appendicular stump and the wall of the catheter, thus fastening the catheter. The latter is now invaginated, thereby inverting also the appendicular stump. The ends of the purse-string are tied and cut short.

Step 3. The catheter is brought outside the abdominal cavity either through the original abdominal incision or through a stab-wound. In the latter case the original incision is closed.

D. CECOSTOMY.

The first cecostomy, as already mentioned, was performed by a Frenchman, Pillore, of Rouen, in 1776, to relieve a patient from intestinal obstruction due to carcinoma of the rectum. It is employed now for all cases of obstruction of the ascending colon, and by some surgeons also for obstruction of the transverse and even the descending colon. Many surgeons are also using it is a routine procedure in the treatment of ruptured appendix with ensuing general peritonitis. The technic employed may be either as in the Stamm, Witzel, or Spivack methods of gastrostomy.

E. CLOSURE OF AN ARTIFICIAL ANUS.

The technic of closure of an artificial anus differs according to whether we are dealing with a temporary or a permanent colostomy. In the first case, it is simpler because, while performing the colostomy, every effort was made to facilitate its closure at some future time. Whereas, in the case of a permanent colostomy, its closure was not contemplated at all at the time when the operation was done, and, as a matter of fact, every effort was made at that time to prevent ultimate closure of the opening.

I. **Closure of a Temporary Colostomy.**

Step 1. The edges of the opened end of the bowel must be refreshed.

Step 2. The opening is closed by over-and-over sutures either by penetrating symmetrical points of the opposite lips, or by uniting the upper angle of the opening with the lower, and then suturing the symmetrical points of the newly formed lips. The over-and-over layer is reinforced by a seromuscular layer of sutures.

Step 3. The adhesions formed between the bowel and the abdominal wall are separated, and the lips of the abdominal wound, except the skin, are sutured to each other.

Step 4. The skin-lips are sutured together.

II. **Closure of a Permanent Colostomy.**

The main difficulty in repairing an artificial anus is to destroy the spur. This was described as the 3rd Stage of the Mikulicz operation. As soon as this is done, the remainder of the operation is merely a simple closure of a temporary colostomy.

An over-cautious surgeon who fears to crush the spur on account of the possibility of crushing some intestinal loop, may adopt the following technic:

Step 1. An elliptical incision is made around the artificial anus penetrating the skin and superficial fascia only. This incision should lie at a distance of one or one and one-half inches away from the edges of the opening (Fig. 155, upper half). The inner flap is reflected up to the colostomy opening and the edges of this flap are sutured together so that they entirely cover the colostomy opening (Czymanoffsky technic. Fig. 155, lower half).

Step 2. The limbs of the bowel which form the artificial anus are detached from the anterior abdominal wall.

Step 3. The portion of the sigmoid which forms the artificial anus is resected in the same manner as described in "Resection of the Sigmoid Colon", and the continuity of the intestinal tract is restored either by an end-to-end, an end-to-side, or a lateral intestinal anastomosis.

Step 4. The abdomen is closed.

F. CLOSURE OF A FECAL FISTULA.

When a fecal fistula is the result of some pathological change in the bowel or of a surgical accident its closure becomes a complicated procedure. In many cases dense adhesions are formed before the surgical interference

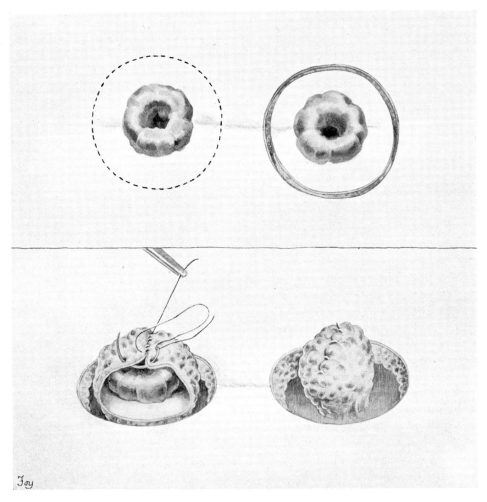

FIG. 155. CZYMANOFFSKY METHOD OF THE REMOVAL OF A FECAL FISTULA.
Upper left. Skin incision around the fistula; Upper right. The skin and superficial fascia are incised; Lower left. Suturing of the edges of the skin over the fistula-opening; Lower right. The external opening of the fistula is covered by skin. The surgeon is ready to proceed with the removal of the fistula.

takes place. The skin is the seat of a severe dermatitis or eczema, and this makes the intervention still more complicated. These are the reasons why many surgeons advocate always attempting the closure by injecting different kinds of paste into the fistulous tract with the aim of ultimate spontaneous closure. However, if the mechanical means fail, one must resort to surgery.

As there are many forms of fistulæ, depending on their location and etiology, there can hardly be outlined a single operative procedure which will satisfactorily take care of all the cases. However, a few general facts should be remembered: Care should be taken to diminish the irritation of the skin. (The care of the skin is a very important feature in the pre-operative management). **Attempts should never be made to close the fistula by operating upon the skin-opening.** It is advisable to open the abdomen some distance from the fistula in order to reach the bowel-end of the fistula. This end of the fistula is cut, and the opening in the bowel is closed in two layers—the first, over-and-over, and the second, sero-muscular. Then an attempt is made to follow the fistula and dissect it out. If, however, this is difficult on account of dense adhesions, it may be left alone, since being disconnected from the bowel it will eventually close spontaneously.

BIBLIOGRAPHY.

K. Abel. Über 1363 nach der Rehnschen Methode operierte Wurmfor-satzentzündungen.
Deutsche Zeitschr. f. Chir. 241:293-296; y. 1933.

F. V. Abramovitch. Operative treatment of acute appendicitis in all stages.
Vestnik Khirurgii (No. 58-60) 20:201-207; y. 1930.

F. M. Al Akl. Modification of the Dawbarn technique for dealing with the appendicial stump.
Am. J. Surg. 25:26-27; y. 1934.

J. Alfredo. Ano ilíaco continente.
Revista di cirugía de Buenos Aires. 12:881-890; y. 1933.

H. W. Allingham, Jr. Inguinal colotomy; its advantages over the lumbar operation, with special reference to a method for preventing fæces passing below the artificial anus.
Brit. Med. Journ. II:874-878; y. 1887.

H. W. Allingham, Jr. Fifty cases of left inguinal colotomy, with remarks on their points of special interest.
Brit. Med. Journ. 1:1013-1016; y. 1892.

J. Z. Amussat. Mémoire sur la possibilité d'établir un anus artificiel dans la region lombaire sans pénétrer dans le péritoine.
Paris, Germer-Baillière, 1839-1841.

V. Aubert. Technique d'anus lateral à éperon epiploíque.
Journ. de Chir. 40:649-658; y. 1932.

Ch. Audry. Un nouveau procédé de Colostomie iliaque. Colostomie trans-pariétale.
Arch. prov. de Chir. 1:347-351; y. 1892.

W. W. Babcock. The operative treatment of carcinoma of the rectosigmoid with methods for the elimination of colostomy.
Surgery, Gynecology & Obst. 55:627-632; y. 1932.

R. Badolle. De la douleur à gauche dans l'appendicite aiguë ou subaiguë.
Lyon Chir. 29:235-239; y. 1932.

H. L. Baker. The repair of intestinal fistulæ.
Annals of Surgery. 95:687-699; y. 1932.

J. F. Baldwin. The prevention of fecal fistula after appendectomy.
Annals of Surg. 95:704-714; y. 1932.

Willard Bartlett. A self-inverting suture for the appendix stump.
Surg. Gyn. & Obst. 16:98-99; y. 1913.

Battle. Modified incision for removal of the vermiform appendix.
Brit. Med. Journ. II:1360; y. 1895.

M. Behrend. Fecal fistula after appendectomy.
Annals of Surgery, 96:158-159; y. 1932.

R. J. A. Berry. The anatomy of the vermiform appendix.
Rep. Laborat. of the Royal College of Phys. Edinb. 6:65-71; y. 1897.

R. R. Best. Abdominal incision in lesions of the rectum and recto-sigmoid as related to the colostomy.
Surg. Gynec. & Obst. 59:194-197; y. 1934.

W. Billington. Appendicostomy in diffuse septic peritonitis.
Brit. Med. Journ. 1:77-78; y. 1909.

J. A. Blake. Malposition of the appendix as a cause of functional disturbances of the intestine.
Annals of Surg. 42:394-398; y. 1905.

J. C. Bloodgood. Intestinal obstruction due to volvulus or adhesions of the sigmoid colon, with a report of five cases, and a study of the etiological factors.
Annals of Surgery 49:161-182; y. 1909.

G. Bosch Arana. Sincronización técnica de la apendicectomía retrograda.
La Semana Médica 39:1361-1380; y. 1932.

G. Bosch Arana. Técnica sincronizada de la apendicectomía apicobasal.
La Semana méd. 39:1841-1851; y. 1932.

G. Bosch Arana. Sincronización quirúrgica del absceso y peritonitis localizadas apendiculares.
La Semana Médica. 40:2089-2108; y. 1933.

G. Bosch Arana. Sincronización standard. Síntesis abdominal en la apendicitis.
La Semana Médica. II:1149-1163; y. 1933.

E. Braatz. Kann ein doppelter Wurmforsatz praktische Bedeutung bekommen?
Zbl. f. Chir. 56:1346-1348; y. 1929.

J. I. Bradley. Congenital absence of the vermiform appendix.
Arch. of Surg. 18:1904-1908; y. 1929.

M. M. Brea. Técnica de la invaginación del muñón apendicular.
La Semana méd. 1:2005-2017; y. 1934.

H. Burkard. Einfache Naht zur Versenkung des Appendixstumpfes.
Zbl. f. Chir. 61:2550-2551; y. 1934.

H. Bűrkle-de la Camp. Zur Versorgung des Appendixstumpfes.
Zbl. f. Chir. 59:2082-2086; y. 1932.

F. Caesar. Behelfsmässiger Verschluss des Bauchafters.
Zbl. f. Chir. 61:2967; y. 1934.

C. P. Caplesco. Remarques sur l'appendicite rétro-cæcale.
Bul. Acad. de Med. Paris. 104:173-178; y. 1930.

A. Ceballos & H. Taubenschlag. Tratamiento del ano contra natura y de las fístulas estercorales por el método intra-peritoneal a distancia.
La Semana Médica. 39:370-379; y. 1932.

P. Clairmont. Casuistischer Beitrag zur Radicaloperation der Kothfistel und des Anus præternaturalis.
Arch. f. klin. Chir. 63:670-714; y. 1901.

H. S. Clogg. Cancer of the colon: a study of 72 cases.
Lancet II:1007-1012; y. 1908.

R. C. Coffey. Colonic polyposis with engrafted malignancy.
Ann. Surg. 83:364-380; y. 1926.

Harrison Cripps. Nine cases of inguinal colotomy for malignant disease of the rectum: recovery.
Brit. Med. Journ. II:760-762; y. 1888.

Harrison Cripps. Complications arising in inguinal colotomy.
Brit. Med. Journ. II:966-967; y. 1895.

C. B. Davis. Pauchet closure.
Surgical Clinic of North America. 10:259-264; y. 1930.

R. H. M. Dawbarn. A study in technique of operation upon the appendix.
Internat. Journ. of Surg. 8:139-141; y. 1895.

J. B. Deaver. Appendicitis; its history, anatomy, clinical aetiology, pathology, symptomatology, diagnosis, prognosis, treatment, technic of operation, complications and sequels.
4th Ed. y. 1913.

Y. Delagenière. Traitement des appendicites aiguës par l'incision et le drainage de Henry Delagenière: technique et résultats d'après 2352 observations.
Arch. franco-belges de chir. 34:126-131; y. 1934.

P. Descomps. Les zones accolées du péritoine. Leur décollement opératoire.
Revue de Chirurgie. 60:451-498; y. 1922.

T. Dinnick. The origins and evolution of colostomy.
Brit. Journ. Surg. 22:142-154; y. 1934.

Mario Donati e Federico Alzona. Le stenosi ileo-coliche di posizione.
Archivio Italiano di Chirurgia. 3:1-104; y. 1921.

W. A. Newman Dorland. Congenital absence of the vermiform appendix.
Internat. Clinics. 4:44-54; y. 1925.

C. Dukes. Simple tumors of the large intestine and their relation to cancer.
Brit. Journ. Surg. 13:720-733; y. 1926.

P. Duval & H. Welti. La fermeture intraperitoneale de fistules et anus coliques chirurgicaux. Technique operatoire. Resultats.
Arch. franco-belges de Chir. 32:101-106; y. 1930.

E. R. Easton & W. J. Watson. Analysis of 100 complicated cases of acute appendicitis; primary cecostomy or enterostomy as a life-saving procedure.
Surg. Gyn. Obst. 58:762-767; y. 1934.

A. Ebner. Neuerungen aus dem Gebiet der chirurgischen Appendicitis-behandlung.
Deutsche Zeitschr. f. Chir. 103:594-607; y. 1910.

J. F. Erdmann & J. H. Morris. Polyposis of the colon.
Surg. Gyn. & Obst. 40:460-468; y. 1925.

J. M. T. Finney, Jr. An analysis of complications and deaths occurring in appendicitis.
Am. J. Surg. 20:772-799; y. 1933.

H. Finsterer. Die Chirurgie des Dickdarms.
Arch. f. klin. Chir. 164:349-397; y. 1931.

E. H. Fiske & H. E. Rhame. New incisional approach to the appendix.
Am. Journ. Surg. 25:19-25; y. 1934.

W. B. Gabriel. Appendicostomy.
Post-grad. Med. Journ. 9:136-142; y. 1933.

S. G. Gant. Diseases of the rectum, anus and colon.
W. B. Saunders & Co. y. 1923.

E. Gehrels. Der Operative Verschluss des künstlichen Afters ohne Sporn-quetschung.
Arch. f. klin. Chir. 117:705-715; y. 1921.

W. Gemmill. Acute appendicitis: treatment by immediate or delayed operation.
Birmingham Med. Rev. 8:226-230; y. 1933.

J. H. Gibbon. The Kerr technic in resection of the colon.
Ann. Surg. 96:102-106; y. 1932.

D. Giordano. Peculiarità di sintomi e modalità di interventi in appen-diciti.
La Riforma Medica. 46:123-128; and 239-243; y. 1930.

R. J. Gladstone. Congenital absence of the appendix of the caecum.
Journ. Anat. & Physiol. 49:414-417; y. 1914.

R. J. Gladstone & C. P. G. Wakeley. The relative frequency of the various
positions of the vermiform appendix; as ascertained by an analysis
of 3,000 cases, with an account of its development.
Brit. Journ. of Surg. 11:503-520; y. 1924.

W. Goldschmidt. Sphinkterersatz bei Anus præternaturalis.
Zbl. f. Chir. 48:961-962; y. 1921.

W. Goldschmidt. Zum Sphinkterersatz beim Anus præternaturalis.
Zbl. fur Chir. 51:2800-2803; y. 1924.

Sir Henry M. W. Gray. Some problems of drainage.
Surg. Gynec. & Obst. 39:221-228; y. 1924.

James T. Greeley. A new method of treating the stump in appendectomies.
Surg. Gyn. Obst. 12:593; y. 1911.

E. W. H. Groves. Appendicostomy in conditions of acute peritonitis.
Annals of Surg. 50:1334-1341; y. 1909.

E. B. Gurd. A specific technique for the treatment of acute perforated
appendicitis.
Am. J. Surg. 17:52-58; y. 1931.

Alberto Gutiérrez. Cierre intraperitoneal de los anos y fístulas colónicas
(técnica de Avelino Gutiérrez).
Revista de cirugía de Buenos Aires. 13:349-356; y. 1934.

V. Hacker. Colostomie mit Sphincterbildung aus dem linken musc. rectus
abdominis.
Bruns Beitr. z. klin. Chir. 23:628-642; y. 1899.

V. Von Hacker. Zum Verschluss des Anus præternaturalis im allgemeinen
und über ein dabei verwendetes Verfahren der einzeitigen, blutigen
Sporndurchtrennung im besonderen.
Zbl. f. Chir. 47:1066-1072; y. 1920.

R. Haecker. Zur Frage des Sphinkterersatzes bei Anus præternaturalis.
Zbl. f. Chir. 50:827-829; y. 1923.

W. Sampson Handley. The surgery of the lymphatic system.
Brit. Med. Journ. 1:922-928 and 1378-1379; y. 1910.

H. Hans. Sauerbruch'sche Untertunnelung als Sphinkterersatz beim Anus
præternaturalis.
Zbl. f. Chir. 48:1348-1349; y. 1921.

S. C. Harvey. The one-stage operation for resection of the cecum and
proximal colon.
New England Journ. of Med. 211:1039-1044; y. 1934.

F. Hesse. Über den Wert der Anus praeter.-Verschlussplastik nach
Haecker-Kurtzahn.
Chirurg. 4:921-926; y. 1932.

H. Hilarowicz. Zur Frage der Versenkung des Appendixstumpfes nach Appendektomie.
Zbl. f. Chir. 59:2407-2408; y. 1932.

L. J. Hirschmann. Median colostomy.
Surg. Gyn. Obst. 50:903-906; y. 1930.

N. Hortolomei. Soll man den Appendixstumpf nach Appendectomie versenken oder nicht?
Zbl. f. Chir. 58:2379-2381; y. 1931.

E. H. Hutchins. Sigmoidostomy after radical operations for rectal cancer.
Surg. Gyn. & Obst. 44:225-229; y. 1927.

I. Iriarte & C. Olivera. Técnica de la apendicectomía subserosa.
La Semana Médica. 40:2101-2106; y. 1933.

A. E. Isaacs. Decapsulation of the appendix.
Medical Record. 67:574-576; y. 1905.

Jabez N. Jackson. Membranous pericolitis.
Surg. Gyn. & Obst. 9:278-287; y. 1909.

Jabez N. Jackson. Membranous pericolitis and allied conditions of the ileocæcal region.
Annals of Surgery. 57:374-401; y. 1913.

Jalaguier. Appendicite à rechute. Excision de l'appendice pendant une periode de calme. Guérison.
Bullet. et. mém. Soc. de Chir. de Par. n. s., 18:349-350; y. 1892.

J. Kay Jamieson & J. F. Dobson. Lectures on the lymphatic system of the cæcum and appendix.
Lancet 1:1137-1143; y. 1907.

J. Kay Jamieson & J. F. Dobson. The lymphatics of the colon.
Annals of Surg. 50:1077-1090; y. 1909.

Jeannel. De la colostomie iliaque d'après le procédé d'Audry.
Arch. prov. de Chir. Paris. 3:96-100; y. 1894.

A. F. Jonas. Undescended cecum and vermiform appendix. Report of cases.
Journ. Am. Med. Ass. 76:1821-1823; y. 1921.

E. S. Jones. Appendicostomy in cases of ruptured appendix associated with diffuse general peritonitis.
Ann. Surg. 99:640-649; y. 1934.

E. S. Judd & L. W. Polloch. Diverticulitis of the colon.
Ann. Surg. 80:425-438; y. 1924.

M. B. Jukelson. Soll man nach überstandenem Appendikularabscess im Interval appendektomieren?
Arch. f. klin. Chir. 169:59-68; y. 1932.

M. Kappis. Die Hautkanalplastik zum Verschluss des Anus iliacus.
Zbl. f. Chir. 51:1728-1732; y. 1924.

C. B. Keetley. Discussion of the Medic. Soc. of London.
Brit. Med. Journ. II:1112; y. 1894.

C. B. Keetley. Appendicostomy.
Brit. Med Journ. II:863; y. 1905.

H. Kelly & E. Hurdone. The vermiform appendix and its diseases.
W. B. Saunders & Co. y. 1905.

J. Kinscherf. Der Verschluss des Anus præternaturalis.
Zbl. f. Chir. 47:151-152; y. 1920.

O. Kleinschmidt. Über die Bildung eines verschliessbaren Anus præternaturalis nach Kurtzahn-Haecker.
Zbl. f. Chir. 52:626-631; y. 1925.

H. Köhler. Eine seltene Lageanomalie des Wurmforsatzes.
Zbl. f. Chir. 53:1115-1116; y. 1926.

H. Körbl. Die Continenzverhältnisse nach den radicalen Operationen des
Mastdarmkrebses.
Arch. f. klin. Chir. 101:449-481; y. 1913.

W. Körte. Die chirurgische Behandlung der malignen Dickdarmge-
schwülste.
Arch. f. klin. Chir. 102:563-650; y. 1913.

Kurtzahn. Eine neue Möglichkeit der Bildung eines künstlichen Sphink-
ters.
Deutsche Med. Woch. 46:461-463; y. 1920.

Kurtzahn. Zur Erzielung der Kontinenz bei Anus præternaturalis.
Deutsche Med. Wchnschr. 46:546-547; y. 1920.

Kurtzahn. Verfahren zur Erzielung der Kontinenz bei Anus præternaturalis.
Deutsche Zeitschr. f. Chir. 167:129-138; y. 1921.

Sir W. Arbuthnot Lane. The operative treatment of chronic intestinal
stasis.
4th Ed. H. Frowde, Hodder & Stoughton. y. 1918.

R. Lascaux. L'appendicectomie dans les appendicites rétro-cæcales.
Presse méd. 42:685-687; y. 1934.

O. A. Levin. So-called chronic appendicitis and cecum mobile.
Vestnik Khirurgii (No. 58-60) 20:208-216; y. 1930.

H. Lilienthal. Permanent colostomy.
Annals of Surg. 52:384-387; y. 1910.

P. E. Lineback. Studies on the musculature of the human colon, with
special reference to the tæniæ.
Am. Journ. of Anat. 36:357-383; y. 1925-1926.

G. M. Linthicum. Plastic abdominal incision for colostomy.
Surg. Gyn. & Obst. 31:197-198; y. 1920.

P. Lockhart-Mummery. Methods of closing fæcal fistulæ.
  Surgery, Gyn. & Obst. 29:312-314; y. 1919.

K. Logothetopulos. Erleichterung der Appendektomie bei Längs—und
Querschnitt und Vereinfachung der Eröffnung des Peritoneums.
Zbl. f. Gynäk. 57:878-879; y. 1933.

Lusk. Discussion on "Cancer of the rectum" in the New York Surgical
Society.
Annals of Surg. 72:383-384; y. 1920.

B. Masci. Trecento appendicectomie senza affondamento del moncone.
Policlinico (sez. prat.) 37:1021-1022; y. 1930.

C. Walter Mattingly. Cecostomy in the treatment of the ruptured appendix
and peritonitis.
New Orleans Medical and Surgical Journal. 87:31-32; y. 1934.

K. Maydl. Zur Technik der Kolotomie.
Zbl. f. Chir. 15:433-439; y. 1888.

W. Mayo. Surgery of the large intestine.
Annals of Surg. 50:200-228; y. 1909.

C. H. Mayo & W. A. Hendricks. Carcinoma of the right segment of the
colon.
Ann. Surg. 83:357-363; y. 1926.

C. H. Mayo & C. F. Dixon. A new type of permanent colostomy.
Ann. Surg. 87:711-717; y. 1928.

E. Melchior. Zur Technik der Verschlusses eines Anus præternaturalis.
Zbl. fűr Chir. 46:179-180; y. 1919.

E. Melchior. Die Therapie der akuten Appendizitis.
Fortschr. d. Therap. 6:23-27; y. 1930.

K. Mermingas. Der Lumbalschnitt bei der Appendektomie.
Zbl. f. Chir. 58:706-708; y. 1931.

K. Mermingas. Zur Schnittführung bei der Appendektomie.
Zbl. f. Chir. 59:1747; y. 1932.

K. Mermingas. Die Appendektomie ohne folgende Muskelnaht.
Zbl. f. Chir. 60:553; y. 1933.

K. Meyer & J. Spivack. On the relationship between retrocecal appendix
and Lane's kink and its surgical significance.
The Amer. Journ. of Surg. 25:12-13; y. 1934.

L. P. Minkh. Undeferred operations in acute appendicitis in all stages
of its development.
Vestnik Khir. (No. 52) 18:119-128; y. 1929.

E. Moen. Zur Behandlung der perforierten Appendicitis, besonders der
Bauchwandbehandlung.
Zbl. f. Chir. 59: 1980-1981; y. 1932.

G. H. Monks & J. B. Blake. The normal appendix; its length, its mesentery, and its position or direction, as observed in 656 autopsies.
Boston Med. & Surg. Journ. 147:581-583; y. 1902.

A. Monteiro. Fermeture aseptique de l'anus artificiel. (Méthode trans-péritoneale).
Rev. sud.-amer. de méd. et de chir. 2:705-710; y. 1931.

A. Monteiro. Nouvelle incision angulaire voie d'acces simultanée à la vésicule biliaire et à l'appendice.
Rev. sud.-amer. de méd. et de chir. 3:573-578; y. 1932.

R. T. Morris. Length and position of the appendix.
Med. Rec. 48:862-863; y. 1895.

L. Moszkowicz. Die Dickdarmresektion nach der Vorlagerungsmethode.
Arch. f. klin. Chir. 116:260-275; y. 1921.

B. Moynihan. Abdominal operations.
II:1-97 and 184-212; y. 1926.

A. Mülleder. Appendicitis und primärer Bauchdeckenschluss.
Wien. klin. Wchnschr. 43:1501-1505; y. 1930.

J. Murard. De la fermeture intrapéritoneale des anus contre nature du gros intestin.
Bull. et mém. Soc. nat. de chir. 56:1032-1037; y. 1930.

F. Neuman. Cure aseptique de l'anus caecal temporaire. Technique opéra-toire.
Bull. Acad. roy. de méd. de Belgique. 14:141-150; y. 1934.

E. D. Newell. Peritoneal drainage; with especial reference to drainage or non-drainage following appendectomy when the appendix is ruptured.
Transactions of the South. Surg. Ass. (1929) 42:322-328; y. 1930.

O. Nordmann. Die Entwicklung der Dickdarmchirurgie in den letzten 25 Jahren.
Arch. f. klin. Chir. 142:312-367; y. 1926.

W. H. Ogilvie. The preservation of the ileocecal sphincter in resection of the right half of the colon.
Brit. J. Surg. 19:8-24; y. 1931.

V. Pauchet et P. Le Gac. Cure d'un anus transverse gauche par iléo-colo-rectostomie.
Bull. et mém. Soc. chir. de Paris. 26:120-122; y. 1934.

F. T. Paul. A method of performing inguinal colotomy, with cases.
Brit. Med. Journ. II:118-123; y. 1891.

C. H. Peck. Diverticulitis of the colon. Clinical types and treatment.
Ann. Surg. 81:322-325; y. 1925.

G. Piotet. Indications opératoires et technique opératoire des appendicites. Fausses appendicites. Colites et péritonites d'origine extra-appendiculaire.
Schweiz. med. Wchnschr. 65:154-156; y. 1935.

E. Polya & D. von Navratil. Untersuchung über die Lymphbahnen des Wurmfortsatzes und des Magens.
Deutsche Zeitschr. f. Chir. 69:421-456; y. 1903.

Poncin. De l'appendicectomie sous-séreuse; procédé de M. le Professeur Poncet.
Thésis de Lyon. 1900-1901.

V. M. Popovici. Les muscles de la paroi anterieure de l'abdomen et recherches topographiques sur appendice.
Rev. de Chir. 67:679-722; y. 1929.

E. E. Pribram. Die Therapie der Rectumcarcinome nach den Erfahrungen der Leipziger Klinik.
Arch. f. klin. Chir. 120:1-34; y. 1922.

F. W. Rankin & J. A. Bargen. Vaccination against peritonitis in surgery of the colon.
Arch. Surg. 22:98-105; y. 1931.

F. W. Rankin. Total colectomy; its indication and technic.
Ann. Surg. 94:677-704; y. 1931.

Reclus et Verneuil. Valeur comparative de l'anus iliague et de l'anus lombaire dans le cancer du rectum.
Rev. de Chir. V:394-395; y. 1885.

J. Rotter. Zur chirurgischen Behandlung der Coloncarcinome.
Arch. f. klin. Chir. 102:651-683; y. 1913.

D. Sarafoff. Zur Technic der künstlichen Darmfistel mit Hinblick auf ihren späteren Spontanverschluss.
Zbl. f. Chir. 60:198-212; y. 1933.

E. Schmidt. Ein Appendektomiezeichen.
Zbl. f. Chir. 61:1090; y. 1934.

J. Schnitzler. Die häufigsten Indikationen für die Anlegung einer Darmfistel und die Art ihrer Nachbehandlung.
Ärztlich. Praxis, 6:121-122; y. 1932.

H. Schridde. Über den angeborenen Mangel des Processus Vermiformis.
Virchow Arch. 177:150-166; y. 1904.

G. Schubert. Dauererfolge der Schubertschen Scheidenplastik.
Chirurg. 3:796-801; y. 1931.

E. Schwarz. Zur Chirurgie des Dickdarmes.
Zbl. f. Chir. 59:86-101; y. 1932.

A. M. Shipley. Appendicitis with peritonitis; treatment without drainage.
South. Surg. 3:308-315; y. 1934.

W. E. Sistrunk. Practical considerations with regard to permanent colostomies.
Surg. Gyn. Obst. 28:436-439; y. 1919.

D. Smith. Two-stage procedures in abdominoperineal resection of the sigmoid and rectum for cancer.
Tr. Am. Proct. Soc. 33:103-113; y. 1932.

A. L. Soresi. Latero-posterior incision for appendectomy.
Am. Journ. Surg. 11:552-556; y. 1931.

R. Soupault & R. Leibovici. Technique opératoire de l'amputation du rectum cancéreux par voie abdomino-périneale avec abaissement du colon du périnée.
Journ. de chir. 38:816-838; y. 1931.

C. B. Spalding. Some interesting appendices.
Kentucky Med. Journ. 12:639-645; y. 1914.

J. L. Spivack. Congenital absence of the appendix vermiformis.
The American Journal of Surgery. 13:297-300; y. 1931.

J. L. Spivack. Eine neue Methode zur Anlage eines künstlichen Afters.
Bruns Beiträge zur klinischen Chirurgie. 156:51-62; y. 1932.

Abraham Strauss. Clinical aspect of disease of the extraperitoneal appendix vermiformis.
Surg. Gyn. Obst. 21:318-321; y. 1915.

J. E. Struthers. Multiple polyposis of the intestinal tract.
Ann. Surg. 72:649-664; y. 1920.

P. Sudeck. Ueber die Gefässversorgung des Mastdarmes in Hinsicht auf die operative Gangrän.
Münch. med. Wchnschr. 2:1314-1317; y. 1907.

B. R. Sworn & G. M. Fitzgibbon. An analysis of 2126 cases of acute appendicitis.
Brit. Journ. Surg. 19:410-414; y. 1932.

L. T h e v e n o t. L'appendicectomie sous-séreuse. (Appendicectomie de Poncet).
Revue de Chirurgie. 35:222-233; y. 1907.

Franz Torek. Zur Frage der Versenkung des Appendixstumpfes.
Zbl. für Chir. 59:204; y. 1932.

F. Treves. Hunterian lectures on the anatomy of the intestinal canal and peritoneum in man.
Brit. Med. Journ. 1:415-419; y. 1885.

M. G. Tschernjachowski. An intra-abdominal receptacle of feces.
Letopis Russkoi Chirurgii. y. 1898.

G. Tschmarke. Bemerkungen zur Indikation und Technik des operativen Dünndarmfistelverschlusses.
Arch. f. klin. Chir. 169:754-773; y. 1932.

D. del Valle, A. Yódice & R. A. Ciarlo. Ano contranatura.
La Seman. méd. 39:1428-1433; y. 1932.

R. C. Webb. Drainage in appendicitis.
Journal-Lancet. 53:23-27; y. 1933.

R. F. Weir. A new use for the useless appendix, in the surgical treatment of obstinate colitis.
Med. Record, 62:201-202; y. 1902.

P. W. Willis. When to and when not to operate.
West. Journ. Surg. 40:195-200; y. 1932.

O. Witzel. Zur Indikation und Technik der Kolostomie und Enterostomie.
Zbl. f. Chir. 21:937-941; y. 1894.

W. L. Wolfson. Right hemicolectomy with ileocolic tube drainage.
Am. Journ. Surg. 16:478-484; y. 1932.

John A. Wyeth. Colostomy for permanent fecal fistula.
Journ. Am. Med. Ass. 35:1458-1459 y. 1900.

J. Yovtchitch. Appendicectomie sans ligature du moignon appendiculaire.
Presse méd. 42:1039; y. 1934.

I. D. Zhitnyuk. Treatment of the stump of the appendix after appendectomy.
Novy khir. Arkhiv, 28:250-255; y. 1933.

PART II.

CHAPTER IX.

ANATOMY OF THE STOMACH. ITS STRUCTURE, NERVE- AND BLOOD-SUPPLY. ITS LYMPHATIC DRAINAGE.

The stomach is the most dilated portion of the gastro-intestinal tract. Its form and position present great variations not only in different individuals but even in the same individual, depending to the degree to which it is filled, the size and the position of the adjacent organs, etc. Much light on the size, the position and the form of the stomach has been thrown by X-Ray examination, which altered many previous conceptions concerning them in the living individual.

Shape: Generally it is piriform.

Size: This varies according to the degree of distention. In a fully distended stomach, the length is ten to eleven inches, the width four to four and one-half inches, its antero-posterior diameter three to four inches, the average capacity about two and one-half pints, and its weight about four and one-half ounces.

The stomach has two surfaces:

a. The anterior. **b.** The posterior.
Two borders:

a. The greater curvature, and **b.** The lesser curvature.
The stomach is divided into four portions:

a. The cardia. b. The fundus. c. The body proper. d. The pylorus (Fig. 156).

Position of the Stomach.

It lies in the epigastric and left hypochondriac regions.

The cardia lies about four inches behind the sternal end of the seventh left costal cartilage, about one-half to one inch to the left from its junction with the sternum. From the posterior aspect of the body, the cardia lies at the level of the **tenth** thoracic vertebra.

a. **The cardia** is the esophageal opening into the stomach. To the left side of the cardia is the **incisura cardiaca** which separates it from the fundus.

b. **The fundus** is the uppermost portion of the body. It is usually filled with gas. It lies in the left hypochondrium, and its dome reaches the level of the sternal end of the left fifth costal cartilage.

c. The body of the stomach extends to the angular notch on the small curvature and to the notch on the greater curvature at which the pylorus starts.

d. The pylorus begins at the angular notch of the lesser curvature and at the notch on the greater curvature and extends to the beginning of the duodenum.

The pylorus itself is subdivided into a larger portion, **the antrum,** and a smaller tubular portion adjoining the duodenum, **the pyloric canal.**

The **pylorus** lies near or on the median line of the body and at the level of the first lumbar vertebra. In the distended stomach, it lies one to one and one-half inches to the right of the middle line. Its position on the surface of the anterior abdominal wall corresponds to a point one-half inch to the right from the midline at the level of a line drawn around the body midway between the jugular notch of the sternum and the symphysis pubis **(Addison line).**

Structure.

The wall of the stomach consists of four layers:

a. The tunica serosa. **b.** The tunica muscularis. **c.** The tunica sub-mucosa. **d.** The tunica mucosa.

a. The tunica serosa. This is peritoneum corresponding to the visceral peritoneum of the bowel, and consists externally of endothelium which rests on a fibro-elastic layer, which is attached to the next layer, the tunica muscularis.

b. The tunica muscularis. This consists of three layers, an external layer of longitudinal fibers, a middle layer of circular fibers, and an inner layer of oblique fibers.

c. The tunica submucosa. This consists of a layer of connective tissue. It contains the blood-vessels, lymphatics and nerves (the **plexus of Meissner).** These pass into and subdivide in the mucosa.

d. The tunica mucosa. This is a dense layer which is thickest near the pylorus. Its surface is much larger than that of any other layer of the stomach, and, therefore, it is plicated and forms numerous folds or ridges which, during distention of the stomach, are completely effaced. These folds run mostly in a longitudinal direction, especially near the pyloric end of the stomach.

The glands of the stomach are situated in the mucosa and are of two varieties: **the fundus glands** and the **pyloric glands.**

The **fundus glands** lie in the fundus and the body, including the region of the lesser and the greater curvatures.

The **pyloric glands** lie in the pyloric region.

The fundus glands secrete hydrochloric acid; the pyloric glands secrete mucus **(Bensley).**

THE BLOOD-SUPPLY OF THE STOMACH (Figs. 156 and 157).

This is derived from the three terminal branches of the celiac artery:

a. The left gastric artery.

b. The hepatic artery.

c. The splenic artery.

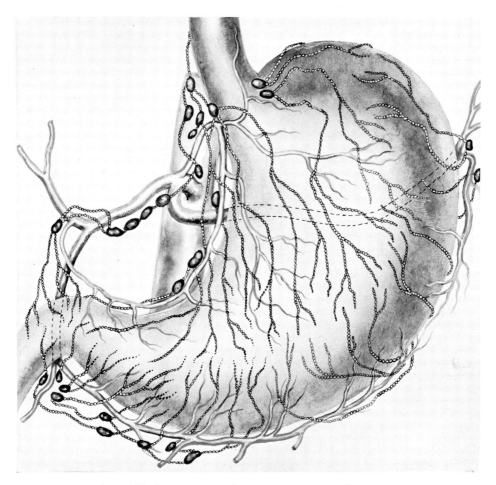

FIG. 156. ARTERIES AND LYMPHATICS OF THE STOMACH.
ANTERIOR VIEW (after Polya and von Navratil).

a. **The left gastric artery** takes its origin from the celiac artery and runs upward and to the left. Then it makes a curve, pierces the left gastro-pancreatic ligament, and runs along the lesser curvature between the two layers of the lesser omentum. Before piercing the left gastro-pancreatic ligament, it gives off an esophageal branch which inosculates with the lowest of the esophageal branches of the thoracic part of the aorta.

The left gastric artery in its course along the lesser curvature inosculates with the right gastric artery, which is a branch of the hepatic artery, so that these two arteries form, as it were, a single artery which runs along the lesser curvature. From this single trunk six to eight

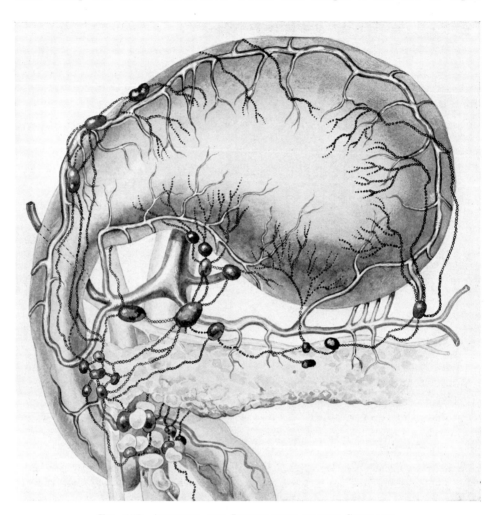

FIG. 157. ARTERIES AND LYMPHATICS OF THE STOMACH.
POSTERIOR VIEW (Polya and von Navratil).

branches take their origin, and some of these run across the anterior, and others across the posterior wall of the stomach.

b. **The hepatic artery** takes its origin from the celiac artery and runs transversely to the right. On its way it pierces the right gastropancreatic ligament, and then changes its course to an upward direction and finally breaks into a right and left hepatic artery. Before thus dividing, it gives off two branches:

1. **The gastro-duodenal artery,** which runs behind the first portion of the duodenum to its lower border where it breaks into two terminal branches, the **right gastro-epiploic artery** and the **superior pancreatico-duodenal artery.**

2. **The right gastric artery,** which runs along the right side of the lesser curvature to the left, where it inosculates with the left gastric artery as described above.

The right gastro-epiploic artery runs along the greater curvature from right to left and inosculates with the **left gastro-epiploic artery,** which is a branch of the **splenic artery.** These two gastro-epiploic arteries form, as it were, a single artery which runs along the greater curvature of the stomach and which gives off four or five branches to each wall of the stomach. These **vasa brevia** anastomose with each other and with the short arteries **(vasa brevia)** derived from the right and the left gastric arteries.

c. **The splenic artery** is the largest branch of the celiac artery. It runs at first behind the stomach, then behind the gastro-splenic ligament until it reaches the spleen. On its way it gives off branches to the fundus and to the upper part of the body of the stomach, and finally the left gastro-epiploic artery which, as already mentioned, inosculates with the right gastro-epiploic artery (Figs. 156 and 157).

THE LYMPHATICS OF THE STOMACH.

An accurate knowledge of the lymphatic drainage of the stomach is essential if the operative treatment of malignant disease occuring therein is to be attended with any degree of success.

The lymph-vascular and lymph-glandular arrangements in and around the stomach have been studied by many observers, the most distinguished of whom are Cunéo, Most, Borrmann, Lengemann, Polya and von Navratil, and Jamieson and Dobson.

To Mikulicz is due the credit of being the first who demonstrated the principles and the methods upon which the rational operative treatment of cancer of the stomach must be based. The investigations of Most, Borrmann, and Lengemann were made in his clinic.

The lymphatic system of the stomach consists of lymph-vessels and lymph-glands. According to Cunéo, the stomach may be divided into three parts, according to the direction of the lymph-flow. A line drawn from the apex of the fundus to the middle of the pyloric canal divides the stomach into the upper and the lower portions.

The direction of the lymph-vessels of the upper portion is parallel to the lesser curvature. The portion of the stomach below this line may be subdivided by a perpendicular line drawn from the left side of the cardiac opening to the greater curvature.

The course of the lymph-vessels of the left portion of this divided lower portion of the stomach is toward the left gastro-epiploic artery, and of the right portion is toward the right gastro-epiploic artery.

The lymphatic vessels all drain into the lymphatic glands, which are arranged in certain groups. As the glands follow closely the course and the distribution of the blood-vessels, they bear the same names as the blood-vessels.

Therefore, the glands in this region are associated with:

<blockquote>
A.   The left gastric artery.
B.   The hepatic artery.
C.   The splenic artery.
D.   The celiac artery.
</blockquote>

A.   THE GLANDS ASSOCIATED WITH THE LEFT GASTRIC ARTERY ARE:

<blockquote>
a.   The lower coronary (Jamieson and Dobson), or the anterior left gastric glands.
b.   The upper coronary (Jamieson and Dobson), or the posterior left gastric glands.
c.   The paracardial glands.
</blockquote>

a.   **The lower coronary or the anterior left gastric glands.** These glands lie along the left half of the lesser curvature in close proximity to the left gastric artery and between the leaflets of the gastro-hepatic omentum. They extend to the right paracardial gland, and receive their **afferent** vessels from the entire length of the lesser curvature. The number of these glands is variable. Polya and von Navratil found on an average only two or three. Their **efferent** vessels discharge into the posterior left gastric glands.

b.   **The upper coronary or the posterior left gastric glands.** This group lies along the main trunk of the left gastric artery at the point where the artery pierces the left gastro-pancreatic ligament. **They are the most constant and the most important glands of this region.** Their **afferent** lymph-vessels run from the **anterior left gastric gland group and from the right, left and posterior paracardial glands.**
In addition, they receive, as Polya and von Navratil pointed out, the afferent vessels from the lesser curvature of the stomach. [This observation is one of great significance from the surgical point of view.] Their **efferent** vessels drain into the celiac glands.

c.   **Paracardial Glands.**
Some authors subdivide these into two groups, the **right** and the **left,** while others subdivide them into three groups, **the right, the left,** and the **posterior paracardial glands.** The paracardial glands, together

with their lymphatics, form a "girdle", an expression coined by Most. **The right paracardial glands** are constant. They receive their **afferent** vessels directly from the lesser curvature of the stomach and from the retro-paracardial and left paracardial glands (Polya and von Navratil). Their **efferent** vessels drain into the posterior left gastric glands. **The left paracardial glands,** according to Cunéo, are not as constant at the right paracardial glands. Polya and von Navratil and Jamieson and Dobson consider them as constant glands. Their **afferent** vessels come from the fundus, and their **efferent** vessels drain into the upper coronary (the posterior left gastric) glands. **The posterior paracardial glands** lie on the posterior aspect of the stomach between the layers of the gastro-phrenic ligament. Their **afferent** vessels come from the neighboring portion of the cardia, and their **efferent** vessels drain into the posterior left gastric glands.

B.   THE GLANDS ASSOCIATED WITH THE HEPATIC ARTERY.

These may be subdivided into three groups:

   a.   Those in connection with the gastroduodenal artery.
   b.   Those in connection with the trunk of the hepatic artery.
   c.   Those in connection with the pyloric artery.

a. The glands in connection with the gastro-duodenal artery are subdivided into three groups:
An upper group, lying near the bifurcation of the gastro-duodenal artery.
A lower group, lying along the right gastro-epiploic artery below the greater curvature of the stomach.
A retropyloric group lying along the side of the gastro-duodenal artery behind the pylorus.

The "upper" and "lower" groups are termed "**subpyloric**" by Polya and von Navratil. Jamieson and Dobson term only the "upper" group as "subpyloric".

The "upper group" or the "subpyloric" (J. and D.) consists of four or five glands and occasionally more, lying beyond the pylorus at or near the point of bifurcation of the gastro-duodenal artery. They lie in the angle formed by the first and second portions of the duodenum. Their **afferent** vessels come from the pylorus and duodenum, and they receive also the **efferent** vessels from the "lower group". Their **efferent** vessels run in three directions:

   1.   To the glandular chain along the hepatic artery.
   2.   Across the pancreas to the glands of the celiac artery.
   3.   To the glands lying in the root of the mesentery.

The "lower" group, two to seven in number, lie along the right gastro-epiploic artery between the layers of the great omentum. They lie **below** the artery and are apt to wander downward into the great omentum. Their **afferent** vessels drain the lower third of the stomach along the right half of the greater curvature, and their **efferent** vessels discharge into the glands of the upper group.

The retropyloric glands, inconstant, lie behind the pylorus on the anterior surface of the pancreas beside the gastro-duodenal artery. Their **afferent** vessels come from the "upper" group and also directly from the posterior surface of the pylorus and the duodenum.

b. **The glands in connection with the main trunk of the hepatic artery (the right suprapancreatic glands).**—These glands are few in number and lie along the trunk of the hepatic artery at the upper border of the pancreas. Their **afferent** vessels drain the region of the upper border of the pylorus (occasionally, a **"suprapyloric"** gland lies in the path of one or more of the vessels). They receive also the **efferent** vessels of the "upper gastro-epiploic" group. These glands are, therefore, both **primary** and **secondary.** Their **efferent** vessels drain into the glands around the celiac artery.

C. THE GLANDS ALONG THE SPLENIC ARTERY.

The glands drain the "isolated" area of the stomach. Only one or two small glands of this group lie in the hilum of the spleen and in the gastrosplenic omentum. The main group lies along the trunk of the splenic artery at the upper border of the pancreas, and these are called the **suprapancreatic glands.** They receive their **afferent** vessels from the left half of the greater curvature and from the fundus, and their **efferent** vessels run into the glands of the celiac artery.

D. THE GLANDS IN CONNECTION WITH THE CELIAC ARTERY.

These glands are few in number but large in size. They lie beside the celiac artery between the origin of the left gastric and splenic arteries. They are recipients of all the groups of glands previously mentioned. Their **efferent** vessels discharge partly into the receptaculum chyli and partly run behind the pancreas to the glands lying in the root of the mesentery.

As may be seen from the above description, there are two different groups of glands: One group receives its vessels directly from the stomach and constitutes the **"primary"** group of glands. Another group receives its **afferent** lymphatics from the glands of the first group and they constitute the "secondary" group. There are certain groups which are both "primary" and "secondary".

From the surgical point of view, it is extremely important to differentiate the "primary" from the "secondary" glands. Thus, in case of cancer of the stomach the "primary" glands are, or may be, very early involved. In partial gastrectomy, this first cordon of glands should be removed. These glands are:

1. The lower coronary (O. T.) or the anterior left gastric group (B. N.).
2. The upper coronary (O. T.) or the posterior left gastric group (B. N.).
3. The right paracardial group.
4. The suprapyloric group.
5. The right suprapancreatic group.
6. The gastro-epiploic (the upper and the lower) group.
7. The retropyloric group.

Glandular invasion occurs early in cancer of the stomach. According to Cunéo, this was found to be correct in all cases in which an autopsy was performed, and in 87.5 per cent. of the specimens removed by gastrectomy. An invasion of the glands of the lesser curvature is most frequently found. According to Cunéo, this is present in 91.4 per cent. of all the cases, and the glands on the greater curvature are affected in 62.5 per cent.

THE NERVE-SUPPLY OF THE STOMACH.

The nerve-supply of the stomach is derived both from the central and the sympathetic nervous systems. The right and the left vagus nerves represent the central system, and branches coming from the sympathetic celiac represent the sympathetic system. Both vagi nerves pass through the esophageal opening of the diaphragm, the left vagus nerve ramifying on the anterior wall and the right on the posterior wall of the stomach.

BIBLIOGRAPHY.

B. M. Bernheim. Partial and total devascularization of stomach.
Ann. Surg. 96:179-183; y. 1932.

R. Borrmann. Das Wachstum und die Verbreitungswege des Magencarcinoms vom anatomischen und klinischen Standpunkt.
Jena, 1901.

W. Budde. Über die Motorik des Magens.
I Mitteilung: Der Pylorusreflex.
Arch. f. klin. Chir. 171:136-148; y. 1932.

L. H. Clerf & W. F. Manges. Congenital anomalies of esophagus, with special reference to congenitally short esophagus with portion of stomach above diaphragm.
Ann. Otol. Rhin. & Laryng. 42:1058-1068; y. 1933.

Cunéo. De l'envahissement du Systeme lymphatique dans le Cancer de l'estomac.
Thèsis, Paris, 1900.

E. D'Arcy MacCrea. The nerves of the stomach and their relation to surgery.
Brit. Journ. of Surg. 13:621-648; y. 1926.

C. Dienst. Zu den problemen der Magensekretion; zur Physiologie; zur Pathologie.
Zeitschr. f. d. Ges. Exp. Med. 83:718-734; y. 1932.

L. Findlay & A. B. Kelly. Congenital shortening of oesophagus and thoracic stomach resulting therefrom.
Proc. Roy. Soc. Med. (Sec. Laryng.) 24:85-102; y. 1931.

P. Giraud & Astier. Ectopie thoracique droite de l'estomac chez un enfant de 22 mois.
Bull. Soc. de pédiat. de Paris, 30:352-357; y. 1932.

E. Gjőrup. Un cas d'oesophage double et estomac double.
Acta paediat. 15:90-98; y. 1933.

B. T. Horton. Pyloric block, with special reference to musculature, myenteric plexus and lymphatic vessels.
Arch. Surg. 22:438-462; y. 1931.

J. Kay Jamieson & J. F. Dobson. Lectures on the lymphatic system of the stomach.
Lancet, I:1061-1066; y. 1907.

Lengemann. Die Erkrankungen der regionären Lymphdrüsen beim Krebs des Pars pylorica des Magens.
Verhandl. d. Deutsch. Ges. f. Chir. 31:483-519; y. 1902.

R. K. S. Lim. The gastric mucosa.
Quarterly Journ. of Microscop. Science, 66:187-212; y. 1922.

M. Lucien & A. Beau. La cravate de Suisse; considérations anatomiques et historiques.
Presse méd. 42:59-61; y. 1934.

J. P. Madigan. Case of megalogastria and megaduodenum.
South. Med. Journ. 27:939-943; y. 1934.

A. Most. Ueber die Lymphgefässe und die regionären Lymphdrüsen des Magens in Rücksicht auf die Verbreitung des Magencarcinoms.
Arch. f. klin. Chir. 59:175-180; y. 1899.

E. Polya & D. von Navratil. Untersuchung über die Lymphbahnen des Wurmforsatzes und des Magens.
Deutsch. Zeitsch. f. Chir. 69:421-456; y. 1903.

A. Rosselet & O. Mengis. Sur une anomalie congénitale de l'estomac.
Acta radiolog. 15:438-442; y. 1934.

H. Shay, A. B. Katz & E. M. Shloss. Experimental studies in gastric physiology; evaluation of rôle of duodenal regurgitation in control of acidity in man. (Boldyreff Theory).
Arch. Int. Med. 50:605-620; y. 1932.

H. Shukry. Shape, position and movements of stomach of normal children.
Journ. Egypt. Med. Ass. 14:361-380; y. 1931.

J. R. Varela de Seijas y Aguilar. Dextrogastria y megacolon.
Progresos de la clin. 42:22-27; y. 1934.

CHAPTER X.

GASTROTOMY.

The word "gastrotomy" consists of two Greek words: γαστήρ, stomach and τέμνειν, to cut. It means "to cut the stomach". This term is applied to cases in which the opening and the closure of the stomach is done in one sitting.

This is the earliest of all gastric operations, and was first performed by Dr. Daniel Schwaben, in 1635, on a farmer who accidently swallowed a knife. The patient survived the operation. However, the closed stomach opened and formed a fistula, so that instead of an intended "gastrotomy" it became accidentally a gastrostomy.

Indications.

1. Removal of foreign bodies from the stomach.
2. Removal of foreign bodies from the lower end of the esophagus.
3. Dilatation of the lower end of the esophagus.
4. Exploration of the interior of the stomach in case of bleeding gastric ulcer.
5. Removal of a polypus projecting into the lumen of the stomach.
6. Checking of a hemorrhage from the suture line of a previously performed gastro-enterostomy or partial gastrectomy.

Technic.

Step 1. The abdomen is opened through a longitudinal or a transverse incision.

Step 2. The omentum is grasped and gently drawn down. Thus, the anterior wall of the stomach is brought into view. The assistant catches the anterior wall of the stomach in two places close to the greater curvature. [The stomach should never be held with gloved fingers, because it will slide and make it a very difficult task for the assistant to hold it. **The stomach should always be held with a piece of gauze in each hand.** This gauze should always be moistened in warm normal salt-solution.] The anterior wall of the stomach is walled off by four laparotomy sponges, placed one to the left, another to the right, the third above and the fourth below the intended line of the incision of the anterior stomach-wall. A laparotomy sponge with a hole in its center is placed on the anterior wall of the stomach in such a manner that the hole corresponds to the intended line of incision. (Fig. 158, insert). This sponge is held attached to the stomach by two Allis forceps. The assistant now holds the stomach by holding these two Allis forceps.

Step 3. An incision is made through the seromuscular layer of the anterior wall of the stomach. The mucosa, which will then protrude, is

caught by an Allis forceps and put on the stretch. It will then acquire
the form of a cone. This is cut by scissors just below the point where the
Allis forceps holds the mucosa (Fig. 158). The tube of a suction-apparatus
is introduced into the lumen of the stomach and its contents sucked out.
The incision of the stomach is then enlarged so that the proper examination of its lumen becomes possible (Fig. 159).

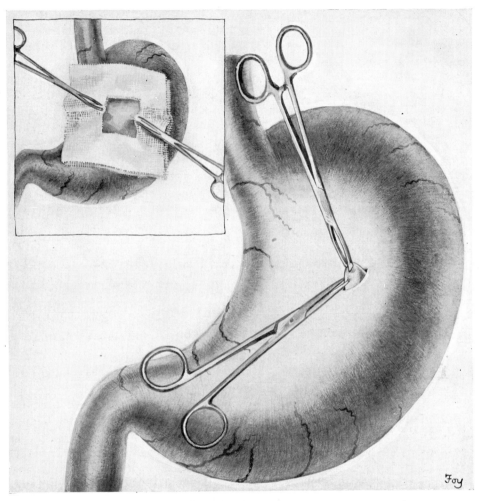

FIG. 158. GASTROTOMY.
INSERT. A portion of the stomach is isolated.
MAIN PICTURE. Scissors ready to cut the anterior stomach-wall.

Step 4. The operation within the lumen of the stomach is performed
according to the conditions for which the gastrotomy was indicated.

Step 5. The stomach-opening is closed by over-and-over sutures reinforced by a layer of seromuscular sutures, continued or interrupted.

Step 6. The abdomen is closed.

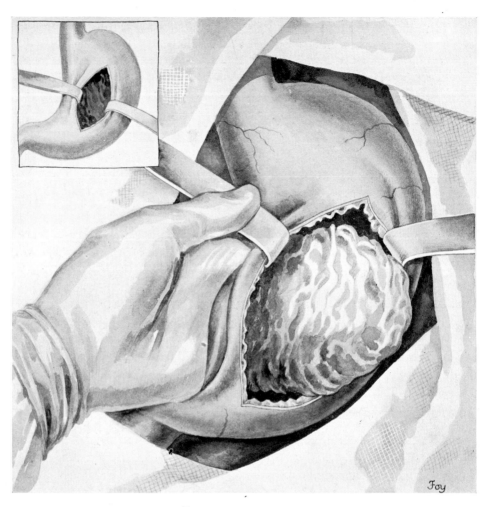

FIG. 159. GASTROTOMY.
INSERT. The lips of the incised anterior gastric wall are retracted.
MAIN PICTURE. The posterior wall is delivered through the incision in the anterior wall.

BIBLIOGRAPHY.

F. G. Moehlau. Gastrotomy in the 17th Century.
    Buffalo Med. Journ. 35:395-397; y. 1895-1896.

H. Taubenschlag. Cuerpos extraños del estómago y del ciego, extraidos
    por gastrotomía y cecotomía.
    Bol. y trab. de la Soc. de cir. de Buenos Aires. 13:708-715; y. 1929.

K. Urban. Bericht über eine verschluckte, die durch Gastrotomie entfernt
    wurde.
    Wien. Klin. Wchnschr. 43:780-781; y. 1930.

CHAPTER XI.

GASTROSTOMY.

Definition.—The word "**gastrostomy**" is derived from two Greek words: γαστήρ, **stomach** and στόμα, **mouth.** It signifies a "gastric fistula", which connects the lumen of the stomach with the outside world.

Indications.—Gastrostomy is performed:

A. For the purpose of feeding the patient through the stomach-opening when for some reasons the esophagus cannot be used for this purpose.

B. For some therapeutic purposes.

A. The usual cases which prevent feeding through the esophagus are:

1. Constriction of the esophagus due to benign or malignant tumors.

2. Constriction of the esophagus due to the healing of ulcers produced by swallowing corrosive material.

3. Constriction of the esophagus which occurs from time to time after deep X-Ray therapy of the neck. This therapy is employed in case of malignancy of some of the structures of the neck, such as the larynx or the thyroid.

4. Diverticuli of the esophagus, when part of the food passes into the diverticulum, stagnates there and produces esophagitis. In order to control the inflammation, it is best not to feed the patient through the mouth.

5. Aneurysm of the aorta which compresses the esophagus.

6. Tumors of the posterior mediastinum.

B. For therapeutic purposes, the gastrostomy is performed in those cases in which it is desired to dilate the cardiac end of the stomach, and also occasionally for gastroscopy and duodenoscopy.

Historical.

Gastrostomy was one of the earliest operations performed by surgeons in the abdominal cavity. As mentioned already in the chapter on "gastrotomy", the first case of gastrostomy was performed rather accidentally, in 1635, when Daniel Schwaben performed a gastrotomy on a patient who swallowed a knife. However, the opening in the stomach did not close, and thus a fistula was formed. But as a deliberately planned operation it was not until Egelberg, a Norwegian military surgeon, advised its performance in cases of esophageal stricture, at a meeting of the Christiania Medical Society, in 1837. However, he did not perform the operation. Bassow, a professor of surgery at Moscow University, in 1842, and Blondlot, in 1843, performed it on dogs. Sédillot, a French surgeon of Strassbourg, was the first to perform the operation on a human being. He did his first operation in 1849 and the second in 1853. Both patients died from peritonitis, a usual sequel of the abdominal operations in pre-antiseptic days. Since then there were many unsuccessful attempts to do this operation on a human being. The first successful operation was performed by Sidney Jones, in 1875. This was the thirty-third attempt to do it on a human being. Verneuil, modifying Sédillot's method, was the first who did it successfully in France.

The operation performed by Verneuil was such a rarity that his patient made a source of livelihood of it, going from city to city demonstrating his fistula. This method was used by many surgeons until 1886, when Von Hacker proposed his technic. At that time one serious difficulty usually confronted the surgeon, namely, the opening of the stomach was not watertight and the acid gastric contents, escaping from the lumen of the stomach, either contaminated the peritoneal cavity, thus producing fatal peritonitis, or irritated the skin, producing painful eczemas. To obviate this danger of leakage of the gastric contents into the peritoneal cavity, the early operators preferred to perform a "two-stage" operation. They sutured the anterior wall of the stomach to the anterior abdominal wall, deferring the opening of the stomach for four or five days until strong adhesions were formed between these two structures. But these methods were also not entirely satisfactory, since they did not prevent the leakage of the gastric contents through the new opening. Various ingenuous devices were offered to make the stomach water-tight:

1. The formation of a cone from a part of the stomach, the cone being placed in such a way that it was compressed by different devices. To this class belong:
    a. The Hahn method and its modifications (Heussner).
    b. The Ssabanejew-Frank method and its modifications (Helferich, Jaboulay, Lucy).
2. An attempt to make a sphincter out of the abdominal wall:
    a. The Von Hacker method.
    b. The Girard method.
3. An attempt to form a sphinchter out of the stomach wall itself:
    a. The Ullmann method.
4. Operations in which a canal is made out of the anterior gastric wall, this canal being lined with serosa:
    a. The Witzel method.
    b. The Kader method.
    c. The Stamm method.
    d. The Fontan method.
5. Operations in which a canal is made in the thickness of the anterior gastric wall and which is not lined with serosa:
    a. The Marwedel method.
    b. The Schnitzler method.
    c. The Fischer method.

6. The formation of a tube out of the anterior wall of the stomach, this tube being lined with mucous membrane:

   a. The Depage method.
   b. The Janeway method.
   c. The Beck-Carrel (Jianu) method.
   d. The Hirsch method.

7. The formation of a tube from the anterior wall of the stomach which is lined with mucosa. The tube has a valve at its base.

   a. The Spivack method.

8. The formation of a tube from a loop of jejunum which is implanted into the anterior wall of the stomach:

   a. The Tavel method.

Until recently the most commonly used methods were those of Stamm and Witzel, and they will be described first. Since Spivack described his method it has become the operation of choice with many surgeons. In his operation a new principle is introduced, namely, **a valve is made from the stomach-wall, situated at the base of the tube which it hermetically closes. This principle has been successfully applied to other hollow viscera to make them watertight.**

In addition to those methods, there are several others that are used quite often in some surgical clinics. Some of these are of interest because the principle of the operation is used in other procedures, although in gastrostomy they are discarded.

THE STAMM METHOD.

This was suggested in 1894.

Step 1. The stomach is walled off with towels from the rest of the peritoneal cavity. A seromuscular incision half an inch in length is made on the anterior wall of the stomach. This incision lies midway between the greater and the lesser curvatures (Fig. 160, insert).

Step 2. A purse-string suture is placed around this incision. This is done with the right hand while working to the left and above the incision (Fig. 160), and with the left hand while working to the right and below the incision (Fig. 161). One link of the purse-string chain is left as a large loop. [It is well to remember the rule: **In order not to obscure the operative field from the assistants, the posture of the surgeon's body should not be changed, but hands and instruments only should be changed.**]

Step 3. The protruding mucosa is caught by an Allis forceps and placed on the stretch so that it will form a cone. Then the mucosa is cut by scissors beneath the Allis forceps (Fig. 161, insert). [It should not be cut by the knife, since even if the knife is very sharp, the blade very frequently, **instead of going through the mucosa, slides along its surface** and separates the mucosa from the seromuscular layer. By scissors the mucosa can be cut with one stroke.]

Step 4. As soon as the stomach is opened, the Allis forceps is lifted upward. This will eliminate leakage of the gastric contents from the opening. The tube of a suction-apparatus is inserted into the lumen of the stomach and the contents are sucked out. A rubber tube, size No. 20 of the French scale, one end of which is held by a Kocher forceps, is introduced

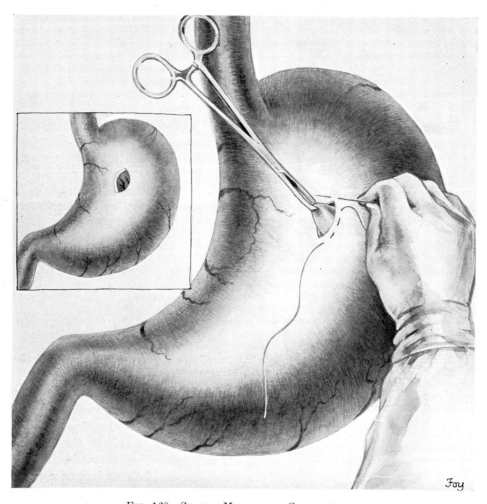

FIG. 160. STAMM METHOD OF GASTROSTOMY.
INSERT. Seromuscular incision on the anterior wall of the stomach.
MAIN PICTURE. Inserting the purse-string suture with the right hand on the left side of the seromuscular incision.

into the lumen of the stomach for a distance of one inch (Fig. 162). **The Allis forceps and Kocher hemostat are held together** (Fig. 163). By this maneuver the rubber tube becomes immobilized and will not slip downward or upward, which is important in performing the next step. The open end of the rubber tube is clamped by an artery-forceps.

Step 5. The rubber tube is fastened to the stomach-wall by a thread attached to a round curved needle (Fig. 163). The Kocher clamp which holds the rubber tube is now withdrawn from the lumen of the stomach.

Step 6. The loop which was left in the purse-string is caught by the index-finger of the left hand and its two free ends are held between the thumb and the middle finger of the same hand. The rubber tube is caught

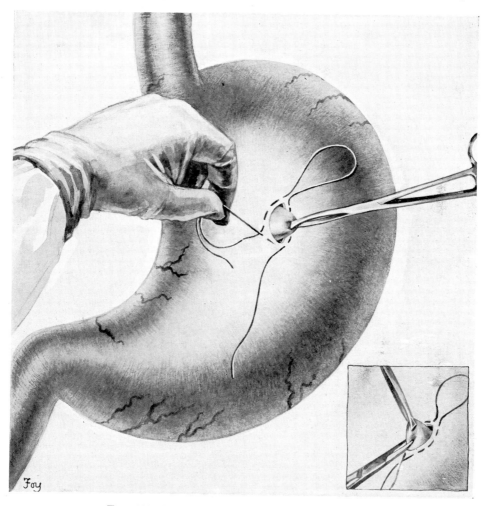

FIG. 161. STAMM METHOD OF GASTROSTOMY.
Inserting the purse-string suture with the left hand on the right side of the seromuscular incision.

by the right hand. The assistant removes the Allis forceps which was attached to the mucosa within the purse-string. By lifting the thread with his left hand and by pressing down the rubber tube with his right hand, the surgeon thereby invaginates the tube into the stomach-wall (Fig. 164). By letting the loop drop from his index-finger and by continuing to pull the thread upward with his left hand, the rubber tube becomes tightly attached to the stomach. The ends are then tied to each other. A clamp is then placed on the thread, and this serves as a good "guy-suture" while another purse-string suture is made around the tube (Fig. 165).

Step 7. A second purse-string suture is made precisely as is described

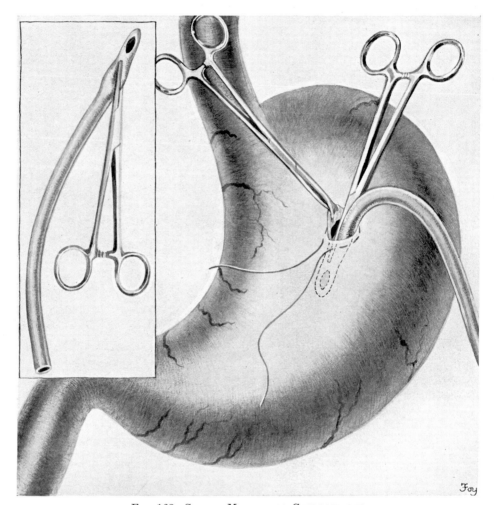

FIG. 162. STAMM METHOD OF GASTROSTOMY.
Inserting the catheter into the lumen of the stomach.

in Step 2. This suture should be at a distance of three-fourths of an inch away from the tube. The bites should be half an inch apart (Fig. 165).

Step 8. The tube is invaginated in the same manner as described in Step 6. The "guy-suture" should be cut short before this invagination is made.

Step 9. The anterior wall of the stomach is fastened to the anterior abdominal wall at two places in the following manner: A round curved needle takes a bite through the posterior sheath of the rectus muscle and the peritoneum of one lip of the anterior abdominal wall. Then it pierces the seromuscular layer of the stomach just above the tube. Then the needle passes through the posterior sheath of the rectus muscle and the

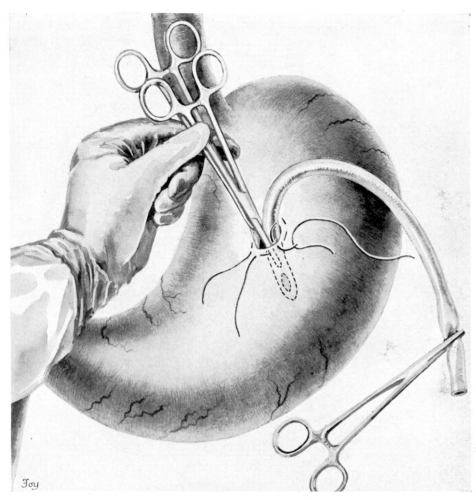

FIG. 163. STAMM METHOD OF GASTROSTOMY.
Immobilizing the catheter by holding the Allis and the Kocher forceps together while the transfixing suture is inserted through the tube and the stomach-wall.

peritoneum of the other lip of the abdominal wall, and the ends are tied and cut short.

Step 10. The stomach is fastened to the anterior abdominal wall below the tube precisely in the same manner as described in Step 9.

Step 11. The peritoneum is closed in the usual manner above and below the rubber tube. The muscles, fascia and skin are sutured in tiers above and below the rubber tube. Care should be taken to leave just enough space so as not to constrict the rubber tube.

As may be seen from this description, a canal has been formed out of the anterior wall of the stomach lying in a direction perpendicular to its anterior surface. This canal is lined with serous membrane. It can be

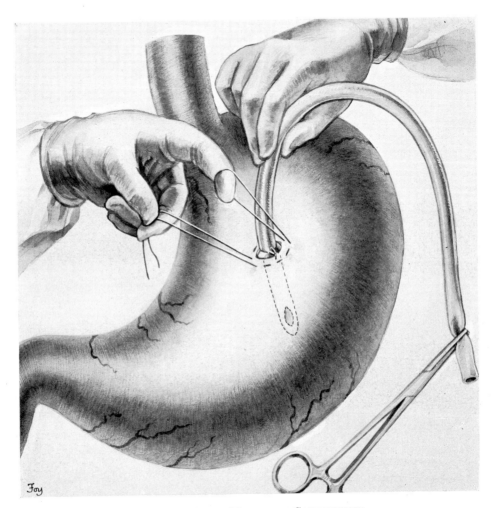

FIG. 164. STAMM METHOD OF GASTROSTOMY.
Invagination of the catheter.

made on a small and contracted stomach, which is the great advantage of the method, since it is well known that in cases of stricture of the esophagus the stomach is usually small and contracted. The operation is very simple in its technic, which is also a very important factor, because, as a rule, patients object to such an operation as gastrostomy and they submit to it only when they are extremely emaciated and dehydrated.

On the other hand, the disadvantage of this method is that the canal is lined with serosa. As is well known, two serous surfaces brought together and constantly irritated by the periodic introduction of a rubber tube have a tendency to become adherent to each other, *i.e.*, there is a tendency for the canal to become obliterated, with the result that after

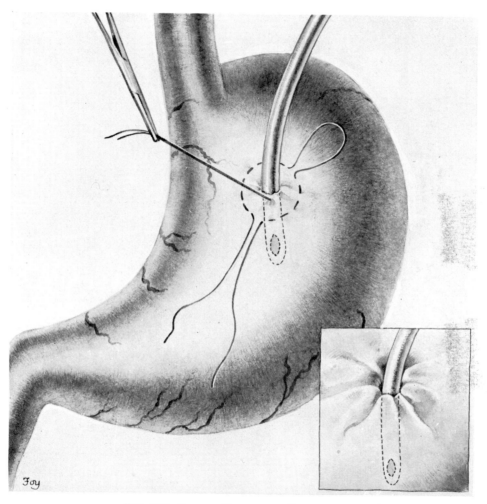

FIG. 165. STAMM METHOD OF GASTROSTOMY.
Inserting another purse-string suture around the catheter.

a few weeks or months it becomes progressively more difficult to introduce a rubber tube to feed the patient.

Notwithstanding this disadvantage, the method is that most commonly used in the United States. It has been erroneously attributed to Emanuel Senn, and is often called "Senn's method". However, this method was described by Stamm, Professor of Surgery in Wooster University, Cleveland, Ohio, and was published in 1894. Senn described a different method, which was published later in 1896.

THE WITZEL METHOD.

This method was suggested in 1891, and is characterized by the

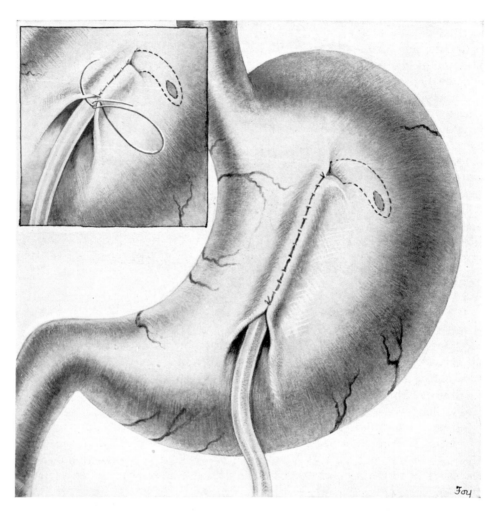

FIG. 166. WITZEL METHOD OF GASTROSTOMY.

formation of a channel from the anterior stomach-wall which is lined with serosa. In Witzel's original article a few of the steps differ from those given below. However, we can still call it the Witzel method, **because the principle and the final results are precisely the same as described by Witzel.**

Step 1. The same as Step 1 in the Stamm method with the difference only that the incision is made on the fundus.

Steps 2 to 6 are precisely the same as in the Stamm operation.

Step 7. The rubber tube is laid on the anterior wall of the stomach in a direction **away from the cardia.** A series of seromuscular interrupted or continuous sutures is made on each side of the tube. The distance of each bite from the tube should be about half an inch. The length of the channel thus formed will be three inches (Fig. 166).

Step 8. The stomach is fastened to the anterior abdominal wall at two points, one proximal to the proximal end and the other distal to the distal end of the tube. The method of fixation of the stomach is precisely the same as described in the method of Stamm under Step 9.

Until Stamm published his method in 1894, Witzel's method was used in nearly all the clinics of Continental Europe. His method has a decided advantage over all the older methods, because here a canal is formed, a sort of a very short esophagus. This canal, three inches long, runs parallel to the curvatures of the stomach and is lined with serosa. Although this method has definite merits, it has also some objectionable features, **which are common to all the methods in which the canal is lined with serosa, namely that the canal has a tendency to become obliterated, making it increasingly difficult to introduce the rubber tube and feed the patient.**

In order to overcome this difficulty, G. Marwedel offered his method:

THE MARWEDEL METHOD (FIG. 167, c).

This method was suggested in 1896.

Technic.

Step 1. A seromuscular incision is made on the anterior stomach-wall three inches in length and situated midway between the greater and lesser curvatures.

Step 2. The mucosa is caught at the upper angle of the incision by an Allis forceps and pulled tightly so that it forms a cone.

Step 3. The mucosa is cut by scissors just below the Allis forceps.

Step 4. A rubber tube is inserted into the lumen of the stomach for a distance of one and one-half inches and is fastened at the opening of the mucosa. The adjoining portion of the rubber tube lies on the outer surface of the mucosa (Fig. 167, c).

Step 5. The seromuscular lips of the stomach are sutured to each other over the rubber tube (Fig. 167, c).

Step 6. The stomach is fastened to the anterior abdominal wall at two places. This should be done precisely as described in Steps 9 and 10 of the Stamm method.

Although the Marwedel method has some advantages as compared with the Witzel method, inasmuch as it can be performed on a smaller stomach, nevertheless, in order to place a rubber tube in the canal it is necessary to separate the seromuscular layer from the mucosa for a considerable width. Another disadvantage is that the rubber tube being introduced into the channel from time to time is liable to tear the posterior wall of the channel which consists only of mucosa. **In all, we may say that this method has no advantages over the Witzel method and very few surgeons use it.**

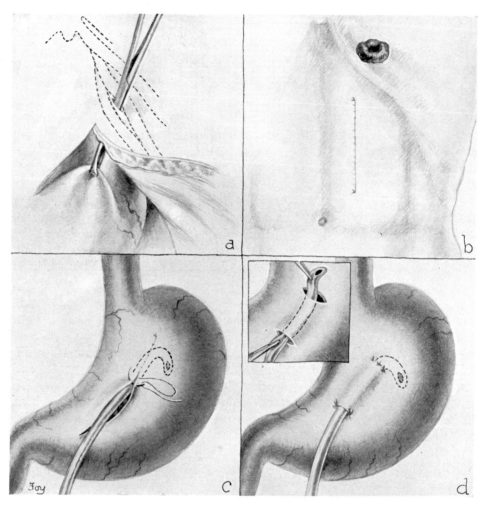

FIG. 167. TYPES OF GASTROSTOMY.
a and b. Hahn method;   c. Marwedel method;   d. Schnitzler method.

THE SCHNITZLER METHOD.

Another modification of the Witzel method was described by Schnitzler in 1896. This operation is of interest in that in addition to its use in gastrostomy, the principle is utilized by other surgeons in certain other operations, such as gastropexy and the transplantation of ureters.

Technic.

Step 1. The same as Step 1 in the Stamm method.

Step 2. A second longitudinal incision, half an inch long, is made through the seromuscular layer of the anterior wall of the stomach two inches closer to the cardia than the first incision. The wall of the stomach between these two incisions is undermined by a curved artery-forceps introduced behind the seromuscular layer of the stomach-wall (Fig. 167, d). One end of a rubber tube is caught by the jaws of the artery-forceps protruding from the lower opening of the canal and is drawn through the canal.

Step 3. The lips of the lower incision are sutured to each other at the side of the rubber tube.

Step 4. An opening into the stomach is made by incising the mucosa, which was exposed after the upper seromuscular incision was made, and the protruded end of the tube is inserted into the lumen of the stomach.

Step 5. The seromuscular lips of the upper incision are sutured to each other.

Step 6. The stomach is fastened to the anterior abdominal wall at two points precisely in the same manner as described in the Witzel method.

The final results are the same as in the Marwedel method.

THE KADER METHOD.

This method was suggested in 1896. In it the canal is also formed from the anterior stomach-wall, but instead of lying parallel to that wall, as in the Witzel method, it lies perpendicular to it. The canal in this method is also lined by the serosa. The description given below has some technical deviations from the method described by Kader. The final result, however, is precisely the same as in Kader's original description.

Step 1. The stomach is walled off from the rest of the peritoneal cavity by towels. A seromuscular incision, the length of which is half-an inch, is made through the anterior wall of the stomach. This incision lies midway between the greater and lesser curvatures.

Step 2. The protruding mucosa is caught by an Allis forceps and pulled upward so that a cone is formed. The mucosa is cut by scissors beneath the forceps.

Step 3. The Allis forceps holding the mucosa is drawn upward. This eliminates the leakage of gastric contents from the opening. The tube of the suction-apparatus is inserted into the lumen of the stomach and the gastric contents, if there are any, are sucked out. A rubber tube, No. 20 of the French scale, with its end held by a Kocher forceps, is inserted into the lumen of the stomach for a distance of one inch. The Allis forceps and the Kocher hemostat are held together by the same hand. By this maneuver the rubber tube becomes immobilized and will neither slip downward nor move upward, which is important for the next step.

Step 4. A round curved intestinal needle penetrates the edge of the mucosa and the adjoining wall of the rubber tube. The ends of the thread are tied, and the Kocher clamp which holds the end of the rubber tube is removed from the lumen of the stomach.

Step 5. Two seromuscular-seromuscular sutures are placed on each side of the rubber tube. The distance between the rubber tube and each

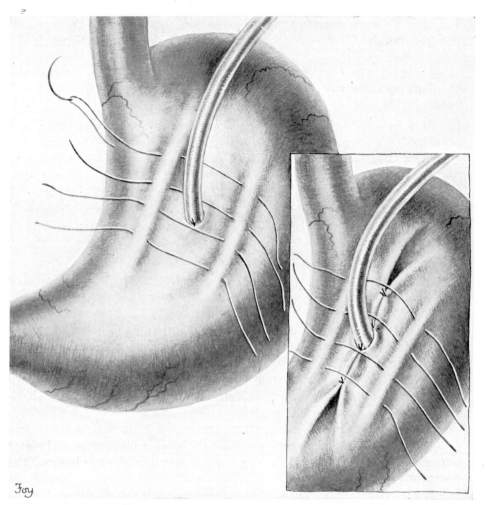

FIG. 168. KADER METHOD OF GASTROSTOMY.

adjoining stitch, as well as the distance between the first and second seromuscular-seromuscular sutures, is about three-fourths of an inch. The distance between two bites of the same suture is a little more than one inch (Fig. 168, main picture). The ends of each suture are tied and cut short.

Step 6. Step 5 is repeated, using the same distances (Fig. 168, insert).

As already mentioned, in most of the methods of gastrostomy the surgeon encounters several difficulties. One of them is that the canal is lined with serosa and therefore has a tendency to become obliterated. Another difficulty is that the canal is not watertight.

In order to overcome these difficulties, many surgeons tried to make a canal out of the stomach-wall, and lined it with mucosa, and in order to make it watertight they placed it in a subcutaneous canal and compressed it from the outside by means of a bandage. To this type belong the method of Ssabanejew and its modifications **(Helferich, Jaboulay and Lucy).**

THE SSABANEJEW METHOD.

This operation was first performed by a Russian surgeon, Ssabanejew, in May, 1890, and was pubished in "Vratch" in the same year.

Step 1. The abdomen is opened by a left midrectal incision (Fig. 169, insert).

Step 2. A small incision, which is half an inch long and penetrates the skin and the superficial fascia only, is made in the fifth left intercostal space immediately to the left of the sternum (Fig. 169, insert). Then, with a curved forceps, the skin and the superficial fascia are undermined in the direction toward the opening in the abdomen, so that a channel is formed leading into the abdominal cavity (Fig. 169).

Step 3. The anterior wall of the stomach is grasped by an Allis forceps close to the fundus and brought to the tips of the blades of the artery-forceps which protrude from the subcutaneous canal. The stomach is then grasped and drawn through the subcutaneous canal (Fig. 170, a) by the artery-forceps (or by an Allis forceps).

Step 4. The base of the small cone protruding from the upper end of the subcutaneous canal is sutured to the lips of the skin (Fig. 170, a).

Step 5. The abdominal wound is closed (Fig. 170, b).

Step 6. The small cone is opened and its edges are sutured to the skin (Fig. 170, b).

As may be seen a canal is formed which is lined with mucous membrane and therefore has no tendency to become obliterated. However, it is not watertight, and it is necessary to keep continuously a bandage over the subcutaneous canal for its compression, thus rendering the stomach watertight. **Another disadvantage of this method is that it requires a large stomach. In case of stricture of the esophagus the stomach is usually small and contracted.**

The same operation was described a few years later, namely, in 1893, by Rudolf Frank, of Vienna, and it is called by many the "Ssabanejew-Frank operation".

Although this operation is not very much used today, we have described it in detail not only because it is used even now by some surgeons, but also because in it for the first time was suggested the idea of forming a subcutaneous tunnel for making hollow viscera watertight. This idea has been utilized by some surgeons for certain colostomy operations.

In order to increase the watertightness of the stomach, Helferich modified Ssabanejew method. All the steps of his operation are the same as in the original Ssabanejew method with the difference only that after Step 3 of the original method is completed, he twists the small cone of

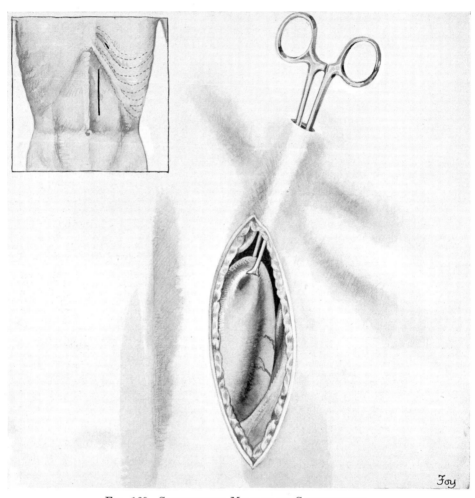

FIG. 169. SSABANEJEW METHOD OF GASTROSTOMY.
INSERT. Skin-incision on the abdomen and the chest-wall.
MAIN PICTURE. Grasping the stomach by an Allis forceps.

the upper wound 180 degrees and then sutures the incised mucosa to the lips of the upper skin-wound.

Jaboulay, in 1894, modified the Ssabanejew method by making the smaller skin-incision just a little to the left of the umbilicus instead of in the fifth intercostal space and connecting the two skin-incisions by a sub-

cutaneous canal (Fig. 171, a). Then the cone of the stomach is more angu-
lated than in the Ssabanejew method and also for this reason more watertight. Moreover, this operation can be performed on a small and contracted
stomach.

Lucy, in 1899, instead of making the smaller incision close to the
median line, made it close to the lateral border of the rectus muscle. His

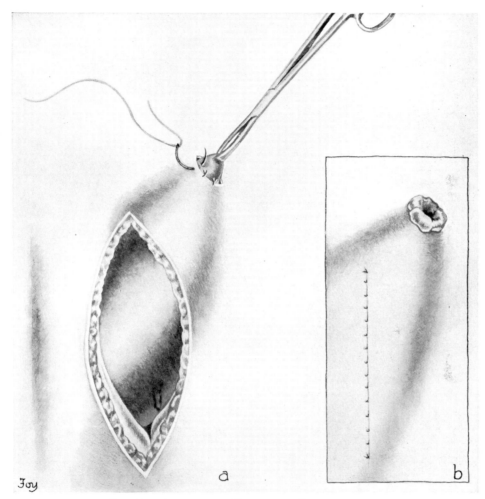

FIG. 170. SSABANEJEW METHOD OF GASTROSTOMY.
a. The stomach-cone is drawn through a subcutaneous canal;
b. The cone is opened. Final view.

method has the same features as the Jaboulay method (Fig. 171, b).

The method of Ssabanejew and its modifications eliminate one complication, namely, the possibility of obliteration of the canal. However, the
disadvantages of this method are that the operation cannot always be
performed, since it requires a large stomach, and also that the stomach

is not watertight. Even when the bandage is in place compressing the canal, the stomach may leak, and without the bandage it leaks freely.

Depage, of Brussels, in 1901, suggested forming a tube of the anterior wall of the stomach. He made a reversed "**U**"-shape flap of the anterior stomach-wall (Fig. 172, d) and formed of it a tube, which he sutured to the anterior abdominal wall in such a manner that on the cutaneous sur-

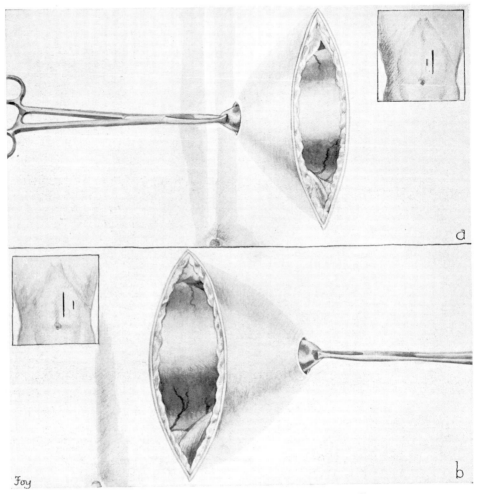

FIG. 171. MODIFICATIONS OF SSABANEJEW'S METHOD OF GASTROSTOMY.
a. Jaboulay modification;
b. Lucy modification.

face only a small pinkish opening was seen leading into the tube. It is easy to feed the patient through such an opening, and it does not become obliterated. **However, the great drawback to this method is that the stomach is not watertight; indeed, it leaks more than in many of the previously described methods.**

Carl Beck, and Alexis Carrel of Chicago, in 1905, suggested a method of esophagoplasty in which they formed a flap on the greater curvature of the stomach by making incisions on both the anterior and posterior walls, the base of the flap being placed toward the cardia. This method, as mentioned already, was designed as a form of esophagoplasty and not as a new method of gastrostomy. In 1912, Amza Jianu, of Bucharest, de-

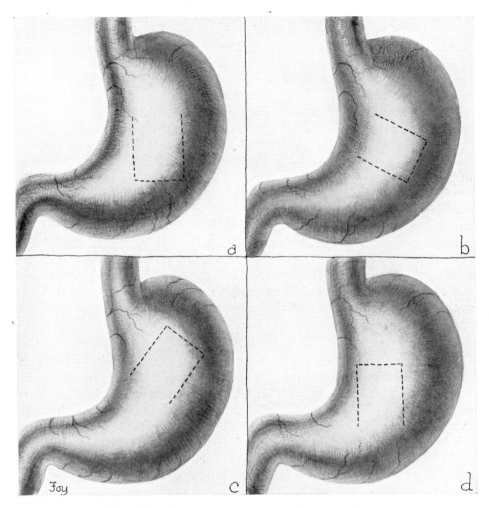

FIG. 172. FLAPS OF THE ANTERIOR STOMACH-WALL.
a and b. Janeway flap;   c. Hirsch flap;   d. Depage flap.

scribed the same method, and this is erroneously called by many surgeons the "Jianu method."

Janeway, in 1913, described a method which actually is identical with the Depage method with the difference only that he made a flap which is reversed to that employed by Depage (Fig. 172, a, b).

Hirsch, in 1911, suggested forming a flap from the anterior gastric wall, the base lying near the cardia and the free end close to the pylorus (Fig. 172, c).

The great drawback to all these flap-methods is that the stomach is not watertight and the gastric contents leak just as much as in the older methods.

THE TAVEL METHOD.

In this method, described in 1906, Professor Tavel, of Bern, formed a short esophagus out of a loop of the jejunum. He resected a small portion of the jejunum, three inches long, leaving it hanging on its vascular pedicle, and implanted its anal end into the anterior wall of the stomach. Its oral end he brought outside and attached it to the skin (this short segment of the jejunum he brought to the anterior wall of the stomach by cutting the transverse mesocolon and the gastro-colic ligament). Thus, he believed, the escape of gastric contents through the tube would be more difficult because the food would have to go in an antiperistaltic direction. However, in this method, **only one aim was actually accomplished,** namely, that the canal did not become obliterated, since it was lined with mucosa. **But the gastric contents still escaped whenever intragastric pressure was increased,** as for example when the patient coughed or strained. Another great disadvantage of this operation is that the technic is very complicated and not commensurable to the results obtained. Therefore, the method is not used at all. We mention it not merely because of its historical interest but also to show **how dissatisfied the surgeons were with the numerous methods suggested and how persistent they were in the search for better methods.**

THE SPIVACK METHOD.

In order to eliminate the possibility of leakage, Spivack, in 1929, described a method, the characteristic feature of which is **the formation of a valve at the base of the tube.** This valve allows the food to be introduced into the lumen of the stomach, and hermetically closes the stomach whenever the intragastric pressure is increased, thus preventing an escape of the food through the tube. **Therefore, it makes the stomach watertight.**

In this operation the tube and the valve are formed from a flap of the anterior wall of the stomach (Fig. 172, a, b, c, d).

Technic.

Step 1. A quadrangular area is outlined on the anterior wall of the stomach three inches long and two inches wide [if, however, the stomach is not large enough for this, it may be made two and one-half inches long and two inches wide]. An Allis forceps is placed at each angle of this quadrangular area (Fig. 173). **[It should be emphasized here, that although Spivack made his flap as a reversed U ("∩") nevertheless, this is not an essential feature of his method. The flap may be made in any direction]** (Fig. 172).

Step 2. A seromuscular suture is made between the points A and B and C and D. The distance between A and B or C and D is from one to one and one-third inches. An artery-forceps is placed behind the threads connecting A with B and C with D. The ends of the thread which connects A with B are tied and clamped. The ends of the thread which connects

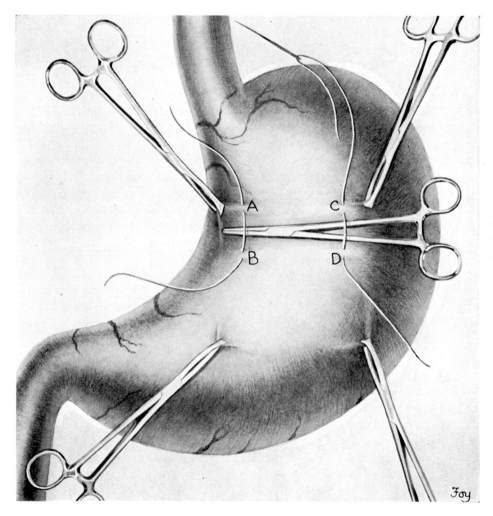

FIG. 173. SPIVACK TUBO-VALVULAR GASTROSTOMY.
Doubling the anterior gastric wall.

C with D are also tied, and an artery-forceps is placed on one end of the thread and with the other end of the thread on the needle the next step is performed (Fig. 174). Before starting the next step, the two Allis forceps which have been placed previously at points close to A and C are withdrawn.

Step 3. The two ridges thus formed are sutured together by a continuous seromuscular suture (Fig. 174, insert). Thus, the upper half of the flap is doubled. The artery-forceps or probe, lying behind the bridge, is now withdrawn.

Step 4. Two seromuscular vertical incisions connecting the points

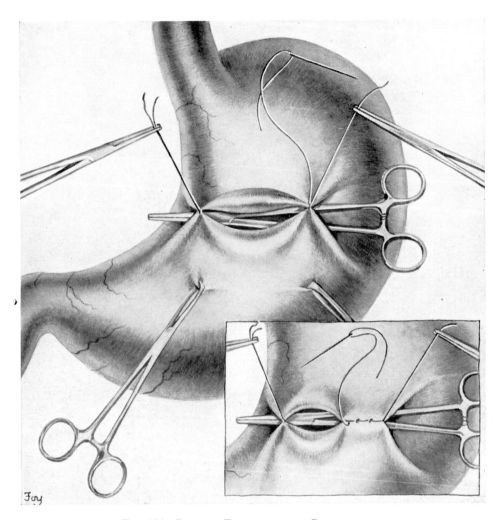

FIG. 174. SPIVACK TUBO-VALVULAR GASTROSTOMY.
Doubling the anterior gastric wall (continuation).

AB and CD with the lower angles of the guadrangular area are made, and also a transverse incision connecting these lower angles with each other (Fig. 175). [In order to prevent the contraction of the seromuscular layer while making the transverse incision, each lower angle of the flap is caught by an Allis forceps before the transverse incision is made. If large blood-vessels are seen on the mucous membrane they may be ligated before the mucosa is opened. We prefer to ligate only the blood-vessels which lie close to the stomach-wall and not those which are close to the flap. Still, if desired they all may be ligated before the mucosa is incised (Fig. 175)].

Step 5. The exposed mucosa is cut and the flap reflected. A valve at the base of the flap is then clearly seen (Fig. 176). Two buttonhole

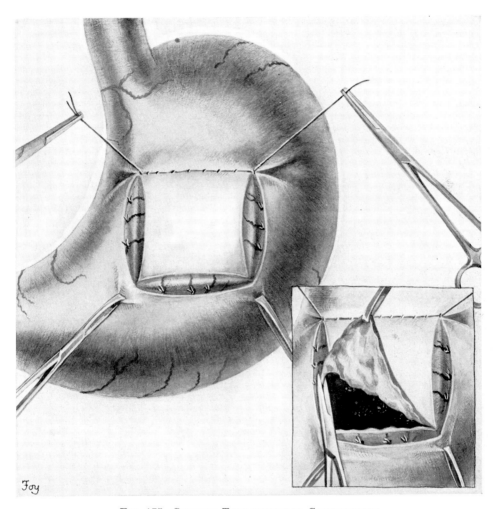

FIG. 175. SPIVACK TUBO-VALVULAR GASTROSTOMY.
MAIN PICTURE. A seromuscular incision is made.
INSERT. The stomach is opened.

sutures are then made, one penetrating the upper two corners of the flap and the other passing through two points at the base of the flap (Fig. 176). The ends of both are tied and clamped. The lower angle of the stomach-incision is grasped by an Allis forceps (Fig. 176). The ends of the two previously made sutures, which are the beginning and the end of the seromuscular suture which connected the ridges to each other, are now cut short.

Step 6. An artery-forceps is inserted into the stomach through the tube thus formed. The opening into the stomach is closed by an over-and-over suture, as also are the lips of the tube. When the first layer is completed it is reinforced by a second seromuscular layer (Figs. 177 and 178).

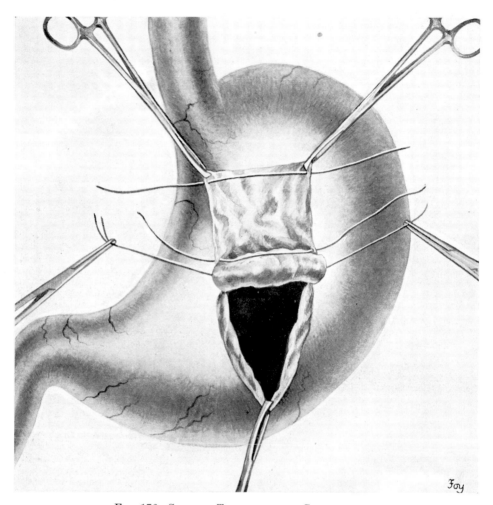

FIG. 176. SPIVACK TUBO-VALVULAR GASTROSTOMY.
The valve is exposed. Beginning the construction of a tube.

Step 7. The weak spot at the junction of the suture-line of the tube with that of the stomach is now reinforced by three interrupted seromuscular sutures (Fig. 179, insert).

Step 8. The anterior wall of the stomach is sutured to the parietal peritoneum. A bite is taken on the parietal peritoneum and the posterior sheath of the rectus muscle of one lip, then through the seromuscular layer of the stomach at a point just below and proximal to the base of the tube, and then through the peritoneum and the posterior sheath of the rectus muscle of the other lip, and the ends are tied. The same is done to connect the peritoneum and the transversalis fascia of one lip with the stomach at a point lying below and distal to the base of the tube, and then with the

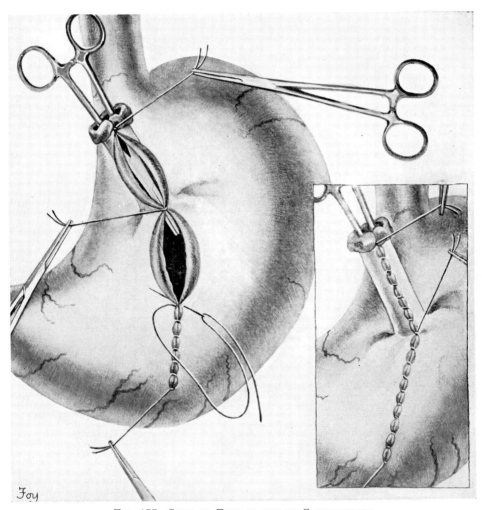

FIG. 177. SPIVACK TUBO-VALVULAR GASTROSTOMY.
Suturing the tube and closure of the opening in the stomach.

peritoneum and the transversalis fascia of the second lip. **Before tying the thread care should be taken to see that the tube is not constricted** (Fig. 179). The rest of the peritoneal cavity is then closed in the usual manner.

Step 9. The wall of the tube is then sutured to the muscles and to the anterior sheath in the same manner as described in Step 8 (Fig. 180, a).

Step 10. The skin is attached to the tube in four places (Fig. 180, b). The sutures penetrate the subcuticular layer of one lip of the skin and then the seromuscular layer of the wall of the tube at a distance about **half an inch** from its open end, so that a portion of the tube will protrude above the surface of the skin, thus eliminating the danger of retraction of the mouth of the tube below the skin surface. The mucosa covers the portion

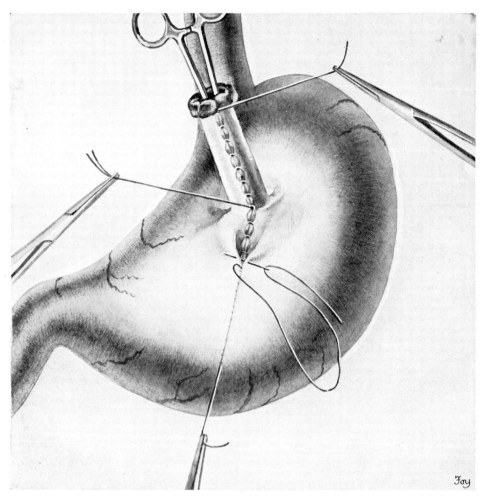

FIG. 178. SPIVACK TUBO-VALVULAR GASTROSTOMY.
Inserting the seromuscular suture layer on the wall of the stomach and on the tube.

of the tube which protrudes above the skin in the form of a rosette (Fig. 180, c), thus preventing the harmful action of the air upon the serous layer of the protruding portion of the tube.

A tube is thus formed, which is lined with mucosa and, therefore, the canal will not become obliterated. The valve at the base of the tube assures the watertightness of the stomach.

Before attaching the tube and the stomach to the anterior abdominal wall, McNealy carries the tube through an opening in the omentum (Fig. 181, main picture). Thus, not only is the junction of the tube and of the stomach reinforced but also the suture-line of the anterior stomach-wall is protected.

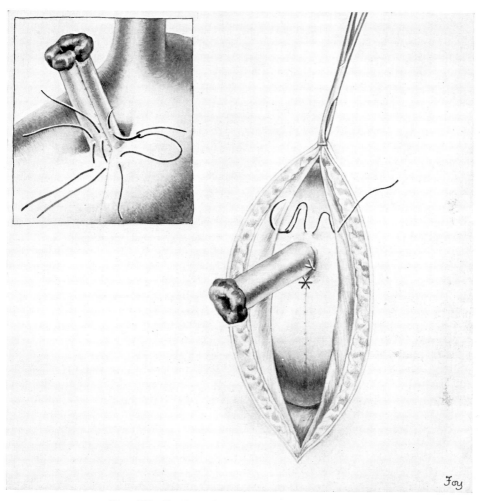

FIG. 179. SPIVACK TUBO-VALVULAR GASTROSTOMY.
INSERT. Making a cuff around the base of the tube.
MAIN PICTURE. Suturing the stomach to the parietal peritoneum.

Spivack's method can be used also on a small and contracted stomach.
However, being confronted with a case of a very small and contracted stomach Spivack modified his usual technic in the following manner:

Step 1. The same as Step 1 in the previous operation (Fig. 173).

Step 2. The same as Step 2 in the previous operation (Fig. 174).

Step 3. The crests of the two ridges are united by a continuous seromuscular suture. The gastro-colic ligament is cut between the points E and F, and part of the posterior wall of the stomach is drawn out (Fig. 182, ins.). The gastro-epiploic artery (or arteries) is ligated between two ligatures at E and F (Fig. 182, ins.).

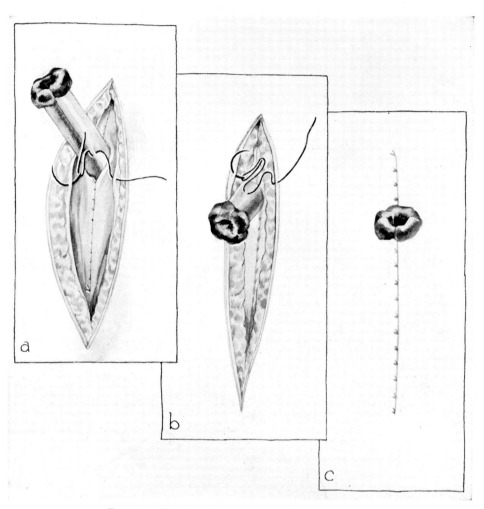

FIG. 180. SPIVACK TUBO-VALVULAR GASTROSTOMY.
a. Suturing the anterior sheath to the tube;
b. Suturing the subcuticular layer to the tube;
c. Final view.

Step 4. The same as Step 4 in the previous operation (Figs. 175 and 182).

Step 5. The same as Step 5 in the previous operation (Figs. 175, 176).

Step 6. The same as Step 6 in the previous operation (Figs. 177, 178)

Step 7. The same as Step 6 in the previous operation (Fig. 179, ins.).

Step 8. The gastro-colic ligament is sutured to the stomach at the places where it was cut in Step 3 (Fig. 182).

Step 9. The same as Step 8 in the previous operation (Fig. 179, main picture).

Step 10. The same as Steps 9 and 10 in the previous operation (Fig. 180).

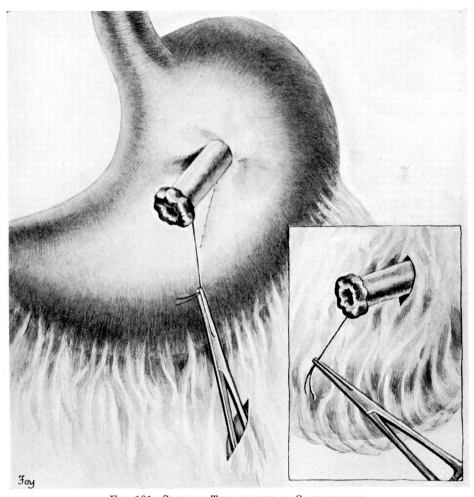

FIG. 181. SPIVACK TUBO-VALVULAR GASTROSTOMY.
Covering the line of the incision on the stomach by omentum (McNealy).

In this variation, the posterior wall is also utilized for making the tubo-valvular gastrostomy.

The Spivack method eliminates the two difficulties which confront the surgeon. In his method, the channel does not become obliterated and the stomach remains watertight. We consider **this tubo-valvular gastrostomy as the operation of choice.**

Of all the methods described we recommend:

The **Stamm** method in case of a **temporary** gastrostomy for a short duration.

The **Spivack** method in case of a **temporary** gastrostomy for a long duration.

The **Spivack** method in case of a **permanent** gastrostomy.

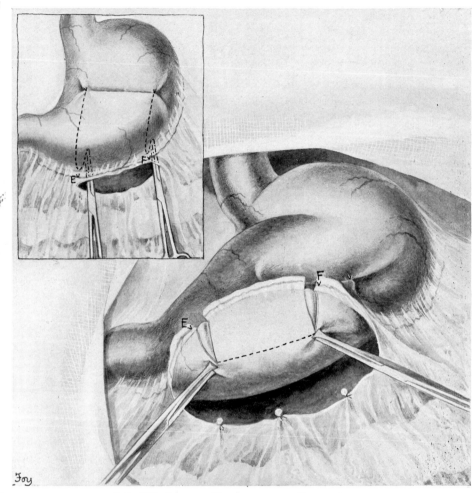

FIG. 182. SPIVACK TUBO-VALVULAR GASTROSTOMY.
Utilization of a part of the posterior stomach-wall in case the stomach is small and contracted.

In the case of a temporary gastrostomy for a long duration, the Spivack method may be used, and when the necessity for it has passed, the tube can be removed under local anesthesia. As is evident from the method of fixing the tube, it will **not be necessary to open the peritoneal cavity, because the tube lies extra-peritoneally.**

BIBLIOGRAPHY.

Albrecht. Über die Torsion des vorgezogenen Magenstückes.
Inaug. Diss. Greifswald, 1895.

C. Beck & A. Carrell. Demonstration of specimens illustrating a method of formation of a prethoracic esophagus.
Ill. Med. Journ. May. 1905, pp. 463-464.

Bérard & Colson. Gastrostomie de Fontan pour néoplasme de l'oesophage datant d'un an, avec maintien d'un état général parfait et possibilité d'alimentation par les voies naturelles depuis dix mois.
Lyon Chir. 32:64-65; y. 1935.

C. H. Golding Bird. Note on the after-treatment of gastrostomy cases.
Brit. Med. Journ. 1:16-17; y. 1896.

M. R. Bookman. An improved gastrostomy.
Surg. Gyn. & Obst. 21:132; y. 1915.

Maurice Bremond. A propos de la Gastrostomie.
Les Annales d'oto-laryngologie, y. 1932, pp. 675-677.

V. Carabba. Gastrostomy; clamp method.
Am. Journ. Surg. 27:484-486; y. 1935.

A. Carless. Gastrostomy.
Edinb. Med. Journ. 12 (New series) : 25-35; y. 1902.

F. S. Castillón. Gastrostomias.
Ars Medica, 9:10-36; y. 1933.

C. Cornioley. Un nouveau Procédé de Gastrostomie définitive.
Lyon Chir. 21:529-535; y. 1924.

E. Crone-Munzebrock. Zur Technik der Gastrostomie.
Zbl. f. Chir. 53:2075-2076; y. 1926.

D'Agostino. Nuovo processo di "gastrostomia sfinterica".
Arch. Ital. di chirurg. 3:285-292; y. 1921.

L. Defontaine. Un procédé de gastrostomie.
Bull. et Mém. Soc. de Chir. 43:1982-1983; y. 1917.

A. Depage. Nouveau procédé pour la gastrostomie.
Journ. de chir. et annales de la société belge de chirurgie. 1:715-718; y. 1901.

H. Donovan. Gastrostomy for carcinoma of the oesophagus.
Lancet, II:1434; y. 1932.

L. R. Dragstedt, H. E. Haymond & J. C. Ellis. Cannula gastrostomy and enterostomy.
Surg. Gyn. & Obst. 56:799-801; y. 1933.

Dreesmann. Gastrostomie bei Ulcus ventriculi.
Allg. ärtzl. Ver. Köln. 11, Feb. 1918.
Münch. med. Wochenschr. 65:802; y. 1918.

E. Fenger. Ueber Anlegung einer kűnstlichen Magenöffnung am Menschen durch Gastrotomie.
    Virchow Arch. 6:350-384; y. 1854.

F. Fischer. Mittheilung űber Magenfistelbildung.
    Verhandl. der Deutsch. Gesellschaft fűr Chirurgie, 24:229-239; y. 1895.

Fontan. Sur une nouvelle opération de gastrostomie.
    La Semaine Med. 16:423; y. 1896.

Fontan. Une nouvelle opération de gastrostomie (Procédé valvulaire).
    Assoc. franç. de chir. Proc.—verb. (etc.).
    Paris, 1896, X, 411-415.

Fracassini. La gastrostomia.
    La clinica chirurgica; y. 1901.

Rudolf Frank. Eine neue Methode der Gastrostomie bei Carcinoma oesophagi.
    Wien. klin. Wchnschr, 6:231-234; y. 1893.

M. L. Gernez. Sur la gastrostomie permanente.
    Bull. et mémoir. de la Société Nationale de Chirurgie, 55:1107-1110; y. 1929.

Gernez & Ho-Dac-Di. Nouvelle technique de gastrostomie.
    Presse méd. 38:191-192; y. 1930.

M. M. Ginsberg. Zur Technik der Gastrostomie.
    Zbl. f. Chir. 57:1718-1721; y. 1930.

Girard. Neue Methode der Gastrostomie mit Sphinkterbildung.
    Korr. -Bl. f. Schweiz. Ärzte, y. 1888, p. 345.

Guillot. De la gastrostomie par torsion de la muqueuse.
    Gazette des hôpitaux. 75:1405-1407; y. 1902.
    (Description of the method of Souligoux).

V. Hacker. Über die Verwendung des Musculus rectus abdominis zum Verschlusse der kűnstlichen Magenfistel.
    Wien. med. Wchnschr, 36:1073-1077 and 1110-1114; y. 1886.

E. Hahn. Eine neue Methode der Gastrostomie.
    Zbl. f. Chir. 17:193-195; y. 1890.

C. E. Haines. Preventing leakage after gastrostomy.
    Journ. Am. Med. Ass. 84:1495; y. 1925.

G. Hauck. Zur kűnstlichen Epithelisierung der Witzelfistel nach Narath.
    Deutsch. Zeitschr. f. Chir. 171:125-129; y. 1922.

Heussner. Über eine neue Methode zur Anlegung von Magenfisteln.
    Zbl. f. chir. 23:986; y. 1896.

M. Hirsch. Plastischer Ersatz des Oesophagus aus dem Magen.
    Zbl. f. Chir. 38:1561-1564; y. 1911.

C. J. Imperatori. Accidental perforation of the esophagus; Gastrostomy, recovery. A plea for retrograde dilatation in small sized strictures.
Ann. Otol. Rhin. & Laryng. 42:799-801; y. 1933.

Jaboulay. Procédé pour pratiquer la gastrostomie et la cystostomie.
Gazette Hebdomadaire de médicine et de chirurgie, 31:89-90; y. 1894.

H. H. Janeway. The relation of gastrostomy to inoperable carcinoma of the esophagus.
Journ. Am. Med. Ass. 61:93-95; y. 1913.

H. H. Janeway. Eine neue Gastrostomiemethode.
Münch. med. Wchnschr. 60:1705-1707; y. 1913.

A. Jianu. Gastrostomie und Oesophagoplastik.
Deutsche Zeitschr. f. Chir. 118:383-390; y. 1912.

S. Jones. Gastrostomy for stricture (cancerous) of esophagus; death from bronchitis forty days after operation.
Lancet. I:678; y. 1875.

B. Kader. Zur Technik der Gastrostomie.
Zbl. f. Chir. 23:665-670; y. 1896.

H. L. Kearney. The retrograde method of dilating cicatricial stenosis of the esophagus.
New Orleans Med. & Sur. Journ. 83:23-26; y. 1930.

O. Langer. Über Gastrostomie.
Inaug. Diss. Kiel, 1884.

Lemarchaud. Contribution à l'étude de la Gastrostomie; ses résultats fonctionelles; orifice étroit sans suture de la muqueuse.
Thèse de Paris, 1900.

K. G. Lennander. Temporäre Gastrostomie bei Magen-oder Duodenal-geschwüren, besonders bei perforierten Geschwüren mit gleichzeitiger Retention.
Deutsch. Ztschr. f. Chir. 92:297-311; y. 1908.

I. A. Liubishkin. Aluminum tube in gastrostomy.
Vestnik Khirurgii (No. 67), 23:106; y. 1931.

N. H. Lowry & S. Sorenson. Spivack's method of gastrostomy.
The American Journal of Surgery, 18:521-528; y. 1932.

B. Lubarsky. Beitrag zur Technik der Gastrostomie.
Zbl. f. Chir. 55:3151-3154; y. 1928.

R. H. Lucy. The after treatment of cases of gastrostomy.
Edinburgh med. journ. 5:46-50; y. 1899.

H. E. Martin and W. L. Watson. The original Janeway gastrostomy.
Surg. Gyn. Obst. 56:72-78; y. 1933.

G. Marwedel. Zur Technik der Gastrostomie.
Bruns Beitr. zur klin. Chir. 17:56-74; y. 1896.

F. G. Moehlau. Gastrostomy in the 17th Century.
Buffalo Med. Journ. 35:395-397; y. 1895-1896.

G. P. Muller & S. Brill. Gastrostomy in carcinoma of the oesophagus.
Ann. Surg. 88:48-57; y. 1928.

G. T. Pack. The Jianu gastrostomy.
Surg. Gyn. Obst. 57:86-92; y. 1933.

V. Pauchet. Gastrostomie tubulaire continente (Procédé de Depage).
Bull. et mém. Soc. de chir. de Paris. 23:158-162; y. 1931.

L. Pénières. De la gastrostomie par la méthode de la valvule ou du plisse-
ment de la muqueuse stomacale.
Arch. prov. de Chir. 2:284-293; y. 1893.

Poirier. Gastrostomie. Manuel opératoire.
Bull. et mém. de la soc. de chirurg. de Paris, 26:475-484; y. 1900.

A. Poncet. De la gastropexie et de la gastrostomie dans les rétrécissements
cancéreux de l'oesophage.
Mercredi médical, 3:145-147; y. 1892.

E. Prud'homme. La Gastrostomie continente.
Le Journal de L'Hotel-Dieu de Montreal,; pp. 1-49 and 103; y. 1932.

E. P. Quain. Prophylactic gastrostomy.
Ann. Surg. 87:395-400; y. 1928.

E. P. Quain. Prophylactic gastrostomy; indications, technic and results
in 44 cases.
Northwest Med. 29:346-352; y. 1930.

H. Schmidt. Die Technik der Gastrostomie.
Inaug. Diss. Kiel, y. 1897.

J. Schnitzler. Zur Technik der Gastrostomie.
Wien. klin. Rundschau; 10:513-514; y. 1896.

E. Schwartz. Gastrostomie par la procédé de la torsion de Souligoux.
Bull. et mém. de la soc. de chir. de Paris. 28:815-819; y. 1902.

C. Sédillot. De la gastrostomie fistuleuse.
Academie de science, 23:222-227; y. 1846.

C. Sédillot. Quelques considérations sur les tumeurs.
Gazette médicale de Strassbourg, 9:398-407; y. 1849.

C. Sédillot. Observation de gastrostomie.
Gazette de Hôp. 26:160-161 and 164-165; y. 1853.

E. J. Senn. Gastrostomy by a circular valve method.
Journ. Amer. Med. Ass. 27:1142-1145; y. 1896.

Th. A. Shallow. Gastrostomy. An improved technic.
Surgic. Clin. of North Am. 4:114-126; y. 1924.

Ch. Souligoux. Gastrostomie par torsion.
Bull. et mém. de la Soc. de chir. de Paris, 37:818; y. 1911.

Ch. Souligoux & Réné Bloch. La gastrostomie continente: procédé de Ch. Souligoux.
Presse méd. 28:857-858; y. 1920.

J. L. Spivack. Eine neue Methode der Gastrostomie.
Bruns Beitr. z. klin. Chir., 147:308-318; y. 1929.

J. L. Spivack. Utilization of the posterior wall of the stomach in valvulo-tubular gastrostomy in case of small and contracted stomach.
Clin. Med. & Surg. 40:212-213; y. 1933.

J. F. Ssabanejew. On a new method of gastrostomy.
Report in Odessa Medic. Society, Sept. 15th. 1890; Vratch, No. 39, y. 1890. Also in Zbl. f. Chir. 20:862; y. 1893.

M. Stamm. Gastrostomy by a new method.
Med. News, 65:324-326; y. 1894.

E. Tavel. Eine neue Methode der Gastrostomie.
Zbl. f. Chir. 33:634-635; y. 1906.

F. Terrier & A. Gosset. Note sur la gastrostomie.
Revue de Chir. 25:164-175; y. 1902.

M. Thorek. Tubo-valvular gastrostomy.
Ill. Med. Journ. 62:347-349; y. 1932.

G. S. Toprover. A new method of gastrostomy.
Vestnik Khir. 34:23-30; y. 1934.

G. S. Toprover. Eine neue Methode der Gastrostomie.
Zbl. f. Chir. 61:1919-1921; y. 1934.

F. Trendelenburg. Ueber einen Fall von Gastrotomie bei Oesophagus-strictur.
Arch. f. klin. Chir. 22:227-234; y. 1878.

Trofimow. The technic of gastrostomy.
Letopis Russkoi Chirurgii; y. 1898.

Turck. A new operation for gastrostomy and one for curettement of carcinoma of the cardia.
Brit. med. journ. II:1546-1547; y. 1898.

E. Ullmann. Zur Technik der Gastrostomie.
Wien. med. Wchschr. 44:1662-1663; y. 1894.

Verneuil. Observation de gastrostomie pratiquée avec succès pour un rétrécissement cicatriciel infranchissable de l'oesophage.
Bull. de l'acad. de médécine, 2nd series. 5:1023-1038; y. 1876.

Villar. Note à propos du manuel opératoire de la gastrostomie.
Bull. et Mémoires de la Soc. de Chir. de Paris, 20:758-761; y. 1894.

Werckmeister. Demonstration einer Canüle für Schrägfisteln (Witzel) am Hunde.
Verhandl. der Deutsch. Gesell. für Chir. 32:55-58; y. 1903.

P. Wertheimer. La gastrostomie transpylorique dans un cas d'ulcère juxtacardiaque.
Lyon Chir. 29:223-225; y. 1932.

P. Wertheimer. Ablation d'un diverticule de l'oesophage cervical, gastrostomie préalable.
Lyon Chir. 30:231-233; y. 1933.

A. R. Whitlow. Unusual occurrence in a gastrostomy.
Lancet II:1316; y. 1933.

H. J. Wing. A new method in gastrostomy. (Describes Spivack's operation).
Clinical Medicine and Surgery. 39:101-104; y. 1932.

Oskar Witzel. Zur Technik der Magenfistelanlegung.
Zbl. f. Chir. 18:601-604; y. 1891.

G. Zechel. Eine plastische Gastrostomie.
Arch. für klin. Chir. 151:805-810; y. 1928.

CHAPTER XII.

PYLOROPLASTY.

Definition.

The term "Pyloroplasty" consists of two Greek words: πυλωρός, pylorus and πλάσσειν, to form.

This operation consists of an enlarging of the pyloric outlet by means of an incision made in one direction which is closed by suturing in the direction perpendicular to the line of incision.

This operation was first performed by Heineke and described by Friedrich Fronmüller, of the former's clinic in Erlangen, in 1886. The next year, Mikulicz, independently and not knowing of the work of Heineke described it, hence the name "Heineke-Mikulicz operation".

Indications.

The indications for this operation are rather limited. It is used in certain cases in which the pyloric outlet becomes narrowed, which frequently is due to scar-formation in a healed pyloric ulcer. This operation was used more extensively at the time when pylorectomy was followed by a great mortality and surgeons preferred to perform a pyloroplasty than to jeopardize the life of the patient by performing a pylorectomy. Many surgeons preferred this operation to gastro-jejunostomy, since in the latter operation, the normal physiological arrangement of the gastro-intestinal tract is disturbed, that is, the duodenum is transformed into an excretory duct conveying bile and pancreatic juice, whereas in the case of pyloroplasty, the physiological conditions remain unaltered.

Surgeons who have had considerable experience with this operation are dissatisfied with the results obtained. Mayo has found that extensive adhesions commonly follow the operation, and that the pyloric opening becomes fixed at a high level. Under such circumstances it is often difficult for the food to pass through the highly situated pyloric outlet.

This operation is now advocated only for cases of pylorospasm, in which there is not an extensive formation of scar-tissue and in which the acidity of the stomach is high. However, in cases in which there is an organic stricture of the pylorus and only a moderate degree of acidity is present, gastro-enterostomy is preferable.

HEINEKE-MIKULICZ OPERATION (FIG. 183).

Technic.

Step 1. Abdominal incision, either longitudinal or transverse.

Step 2. A transverse incision is made through the pylorus and the adjoining part of the duodenum the length of which should be approximately one inch longer than the length of the stricture, and which should extend beyond the stricture both on the gastric and the duodenal sides (Fig. 183, insert). This incision cuts through the entire thickness of the anterior pyloric wall.

Step 3. The middle points of both the upper and lower lips are caught

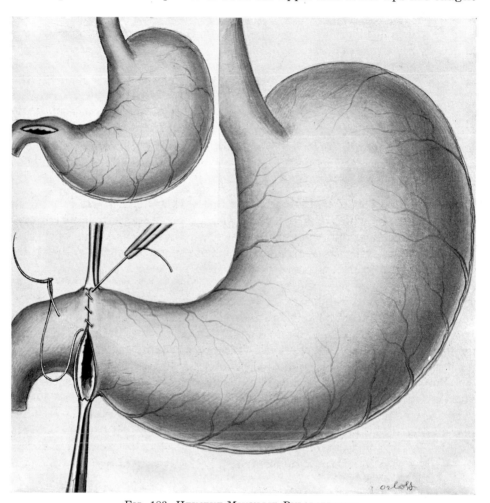

FIG. 183. HEINEKE-MIKULICZ PYLOROPLASTY.
INSERT. A transverse incision is made.
MAIN PICTURE. A transverse slit is transformed into a longitudinal one.

by Allis forceps. The upper lip is drawn upward and the lower lip downward (Fig. 183, main picture).

Step 4. The opening is closed by two layers of sutures. The first includes the entire thickness of the wall and the second, the seromuscular layer, reinforces the first.

C. H. MAYO MODIFICATION OF THE HEINEKE-MIKULICZ PYLOROPLASTY.

The incision in this operation is horse-shoe in shape. It is longer than the incision in the Heineke-Mikulicz operation and not as long as in the Finney gastro-duodenostomy. The line of the "flap incision" is not so close to the greater curvature or to the pyloric angle as in the case of the Finney gastro-duodenostomy, and this makes it possible to remove a pyloric or duodenal ulcer if present. The closure is the same as in the Heineke-Mikulicz operation.

HORSLEY MODIFICATION OF THE HEINEKE-MIKULICZ OPERATION (FIG. 184, LOWER HALF).

This method of pyloroplasty, according to its originator, is suitable only in cases in which there is a small ulcer in the first part of the duodenum, or a small prepyloric ulcer, and also when it is desired to give rest to the stomach after excision of a small ulcer in other regions of that organ. The ulcer is removed as a routine procedure. If the ulcer is of a large size, or if it is farther away than one inch on the duodenal side or two inches on the stomach side of the gastro-duodenal junction, then pyloroplasty is not a suitable procedure and the surgeon should resort either to a gastro-enterostomy or to a pylorectomy.

Technic.

Step 1. An incision one inch long is made on the duodenum and two inches long on the pylorus. [N. B. As a rule, the gastric side of the incision should be twice the size of the duodenal.]

Step 2. A suture connecting the gastric end of the incision with the duodenal end is made, which penetrates, in the stomach, the seromuscular layer only, and, in the duodenum, the entire thickness of its wall (Fig. 184, lower half). The ends of this thread are tied to each other. This transforms the transverse into a longitudinal incision. Another suture connecting the seromuscular layer of the stomach with the entire thickness of the duodenal wall is made half an inch above the first one and its ends are also tied. The rest of the opening is sutured by grasping only the seromuscular layer of the stomach and the entire thickness of the wall of the duodenum.

Step 3. This suture-line is reinforced by a second row of seromuscular sutures, beginning and ending with a purse-string suture.

Step 4. The suture-line is covered by the great omentum, or by the gastro-hepatic omentum, to which it is attached by a few sutures.

RICHARDSON MODIFICATION OF THE HEINEKE-MIKULICZ PYLOROPLASTY.

Step 1. A transverse incision of the Heineke-Mikulicz type is made. The upper and the lower lips are trimmed off so that the opening acquires the shape of a lozenge (Fig. 184, upper half). Thus, all the cicatricial tissues are cut away.

Step 2. The opening is closed in two layers in the same manner as described in the original Heineke-Mikulicz method.

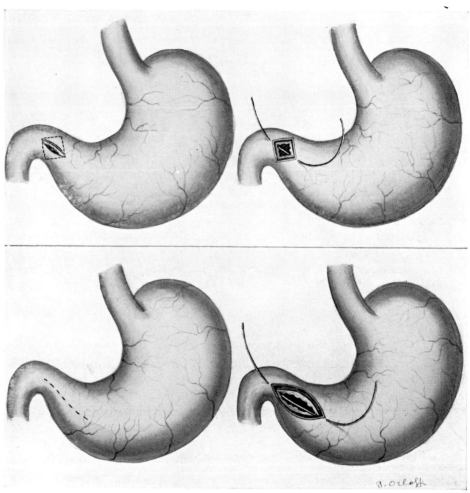

FIG. 184. PYLOROPLASTY.
UPPER HALF. Richardson modification of the Heineke-Mikulicz operation.
LOWER HALF. Horsley modification of the Heineke-Mikulicz operation.

BIBLIOGRAPHY.

J. Chomet. Étude clinique des sténoses pyloriques de l'adulte.
    Gaz. d'hôp. 104:1813-1819; y. 1931.

P. T. Crymble and T. Walmsley "Hypertrophy of the pylorus" in an adult.
    Brit. J. Surg. 20:602-606; y. 1933.

P. Delbet & de Vadder. La gastro-pyloro-duodeno-entérostomie.
    Bull. Acad. de méd. de Paris. 99:274-289; y. 1928.

F. Fronmüller. Operation der Pylorusstenose. Inaug.-Dissert.
Fürth, 1886 (Describes the Heineke method).

J. S. Horsley. Surgery of the stomach and small intestine.
pp. 172, 174. D. Appleton & Co. Publishers. y. 1926.

B. T. Horton. Pyloric block, with special reference to musculature, myenteric plexus and lymphatic vessels.
Arch. Surg. 22:438-462; y. 1931.

E. S. Judd & H. L. Thompson. Hypertrophic stenosis of the pylorus in adults.
Surg. Clin. of North America 13:801-806; y. 1933.

E. S. Judd & J. R. Phillips. Pyloroplasty; its place in treatment of peptic ulcer.
Annals of Surg. 100:196-201; y. 1934.

G. E. Konjetzny. Die Pylorushypertrophie des Erwachsenen als Selbständiges Krankheitsbild.
Med. Welt. 6:728-730; y. 1932.

C. H. Mayo. Gastro-duodenostomy: Its indications.
Surg. Gyn. & Obst. 38:583-587; y. 1924.

C. C. McClure. Hypertrophy of the pyloric muscle in adults.
Surgery, Gyn. & Obst. 52:945-952; y. 1931.

E. P. McNamee. Pyloric stenosis with hypertrophy of pyloric muscle in adult.
Am. Journ. of Roentgenol. 29:24-30; y. 1933.

J. Mikulicz. Zur operativen Behandlung des stenosirenden Magengeschwüres.
Arch. f. klin. Chir. 37:79-90; y. 1888.

C. B. Morton. Stenosis with spasm and hypertrophy in adults; surgical aspects.
Virginia Med. Monthly. 57:46-48; y. 1930.

A. J. Palmén. Zur Pyloroplastik bei pylorospastischen Zuständen Erwachsener.
Zbl. f. Chir. 61:336-338; y. 1934.

E. Payr. Ueber Pylorusmuskeldurchschneidung (extramuköse Pyloromyotomie) zur Behebung spastischer Zustände.
Zbl. f. Chir. 51:2407-2416; y. 1924.

E. Payr. Erfahrungen mit der Pyloromyotomie.
Arch. f. klin. Chir. 138:639-671; y. 1925.

M. H. Richardson. Three cases of pyloroplasty for stricture of the pylorus.
Boston Med. and Surg. Journ. 141:537-542; y. 1899.

E. Spamer. Zur Operation des Pylorospasmus.
Zbl. f. Chir. 61:162-163; y. 1934.

E. Steden. Zur Pyloromyotomie nach Payr.
Bruns Beiträge zur klin. Chir. 138:391-394; y. 1927.

E. W. Twining. Chronic hypertrophic stenosis of pylorus in adults.
Brit. Journ. of Radiol. 6:644-655; y. 1933.

CHAPTER XIII.

OPERATIONS FOR CONGENITAL PYLORIC STENOSIS.

Historical.

The term "Congenital Pyloric Stenosis" was coined rather recently, namely, in 1879, by Landerer. However, the disease has been known probably since 1627. In that year, Fabricius Hildanus (1560-1634) described a condition in an infant which clinically bears a close resemblance to the picture of congenital pyloric stenosis. The infant recovered, and for this reason there is no way of establishing definitely whether or not he actually dealt with a true case of a congenital pyloric stenosis.

The next case was reported by Patrick Blair, in 1717. He recorded the case of a male infant, who "being a month old was seized with a violent vomiting and a stoppage of urine and stool. Some time after both these became more regular, but the vomiting still continued". The infant died when five months old, and the autopsy showed: "The ventriculus was more like to an intestine than a stomach, its length being five inches and its breadth but one inch. The pylorus and almost all of the duodenum were cartilaginous and something inclined to ossification".

Weber, in 1758, recorded the case of a new-born female infant, who "sucked milk without difficulty but soon after she had filled her stomach with this infant nourishment, she returned it by vomiting". She died on the sixth day. The autopsy showed that, "The pylorus was hard to touch like cartilage, and contracted. On incision its substance was seen to be thick, and the tightness of its contraction made the lumen similar."

The next case was reported by George Armstrong, of London, in 1771. It was a description of an autopsy made on an infant who was affected with "watery gripes."

It was found on autopsy that "there was no morbid appearance to be observed anywhere but in the stomach, and this viscus being so full while the intestines were almost empty, looked as if the disease had been chiefly due to a spasm of the pylorus which prevented the contents of the stomach from passing into the duodenum."

Even more clearly, the same disease was described by Hezekiah Beardsley, of New Haven, Connecticut, in 1788. On autopsy it was found that "the pylorus was invested with a hard compact substance or scirrhosity which so completely obstructed the passage into the duodenum as to admit with the greatest difficulty the finest fluid; whether this was the original disorder or only a consequence may perhaps be a question."

The first case recorded in Germany was in 1842 by Siemon-Dawosky. He was the first man to mention the projectile type of vomiting.

The name, **"Congenital Pyloric Stenosis"**, as mentioned already, was coined by Landerer, in 1879.

Indications.

Cases of congenital pyloric stenosis come to the surgeon as a rule only after medical treatment has failed, although it is true that there are many cases presenting clinical symptoms of congenital pyloric stenosis which

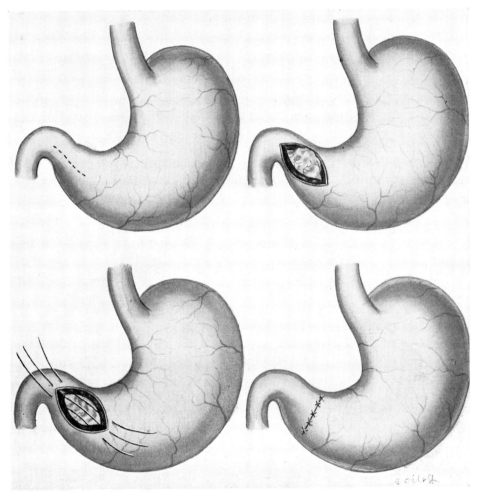

FIG. 185. CONGENITAL PYLORIC STENOSIS.
Fredet-Weber operation.

respond to medical treatment. For this reason the majority of surgeons believe that each child should be first given medical treatment, and if this fails, that is, if the child after being under the physician's care still continues to lose weight, then only should one resort to surgery. However, under prolonged medical treatment a good surgical risk may become a bad one.

The preöperative management in these cases is of the greatest importance. This, combined with the proper postoperative care, has reduced the mortality of from twenty-eight or thirty per cent. of twenty years ago, to from two to three per cent., which is now the mortality-rate in the hands of the competent surgeon. Some surgeons have reported one hundred consecutive cases without a single death.

The preöperative care consists in giving the infant hypodermoclysis of 200 to 300 c.cm. of normal salt-solution, or of three per cent. glucose in normal salt-solution, twice daily, for two days before the operation, and of one blood-transfusion (100-150-200 c.cm.) immediately preceding the operation. It may also be useful to give another blood-transfusion the day following the operation.

Technic.

The old methods of surgical treatment of this condition were jejunostomy, pylorodiosis, gastro-enterostomy and the Heineke-Mikulicz pyloroplasty. The mortality-rate of these operations was so high that it made them prohibitive. In the case of the Heineke-Mikulicz operation technical difficulties also were added, because it is very difficult to suture in a perpendicular direction the incised thick pyloric ring.

Fredet, in 1907, and Weber, in 1910, suggested an **extra-mucous pyloroplasty** of the Heineke-Mikulicz type. They cut the pylorus longitudinally through the serosa and muscularis only, and sutured it again in a direction perpendicular to the line of the incision (Fig. 185).

The **Fredet-Weber** method is very seldom used now. Its interest however, is not only historical. It served as a transient step in the development of the operation which is used now not only as an operation of choice **but actually as a routine procedure for congenital pyloric stenosis, namely, the Ramstedt operation.**

THE RAMSTEDT OPERATION.

This was performed by Ramstedt for the first time on June 18th, 1912.

Step 1. The abdomen is opened by a **right paramedian incision** one or one and one-half inches long. The lower end of this incision is at the level of the umbilicus.

Step 2. A McFadden forceps (Fig. 186, a) grasps the pylorus and delivers it through the abdominal opening. This forceps is then disengaged and the pyloric tumor is held between the index-finger and the thumb of the left hand (Fig. 186, b).

Step 3. An incision parallel to the pyloric canal is made in the "bloodless area", which is usually situated in the upper third of the anterior wall of the pylorus. **The serosa and only the superficial layer of the muscularis are cut** along the entire length of the pyloric ring. The length of such an incision is on the average about one and one-half inches. [Care should be taken not to make the incision shorter than is necessary, since then the constriction is not relieved. Neither should it be made longer than necessary, particularly on the duodenal end, in order to avoid opening the duodenum.] After the superficial layer of the muscle is incised, the separation of the muscle-fibers is continued by the handle of the knife (Fig. 186, c) until the submucosa is reached. This is done with comparative ease, since the muscle is rather friable. Then, the submucous layer is separated and the mucosa is thus exposed, which immediately bulges through the gap in

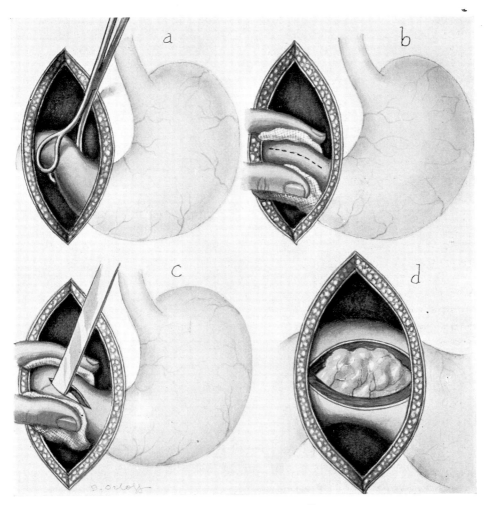

FIG. 186. CONGENITAL PYLORIC STENOSIS.
Ramstedt Operation.

the muscle (Fig. 186, d). The bleeding-points are checked by applying hot sponges. If this fails, they are sutured, using an intestinal curved needle [it is not advisable to apply hemostatic forceps to stop the bleeding, since the tissue is very fragile.] Usually the bleeding will be checked by one of the above mentioned manipulations. However, if it is not, then a small piece of rectus muscle may be incised and sutured over the bleeding area.

Step 4. The abdominal wall is closed in layers.

The sutures for all layers should be of silk, since in emaciated children healing is delayed and if an absorbable suture is used, it may dissolve before healing takes place.

This operation is very simple and requires about 10 to 15 minutes for its performance. It would seem to be a hazardous procedure to leave the mucosa exposed and protruding through the thick seromuscular gap. However, no bad sequelæ have resulted from this. A few weeks after the operation, at the place of the former gap only a small scar can be seen, and a few months after the operation it is difficult to find even the scar at the site of the incision.

The results of the operation are excellent. The infants gain weight and are perfectly normal.

Very few modifications of the Ramstedt operation have been described, a certain sign that the operation in itself is excellent and hardly needs any improvement.

BIBLIOGRAPHY.

R. W. Bolling. Congenital hypertrophic pyloric stenosis.
  Journ. Am. Med. Ass. 85:20-24; y. 1925.

A. Brown. Congenital hypertrophic pyloric stenosis and its operative treatment.
  Ann. Surg. 90:507-516; y. 1929.

D. Browne. Surgical anatomy of Ramstedt's operation.
  Arch. Dis. of Childhood, 6:129-135; y. 1931.

G. Calinich & R. Zenker. Das Schicksal der nach Ramstedt operierten Säuglinge.
  Deutsche Zeitschr. f. Chir. 239:444-452; y. 1933.

A. Castellanos. Sobre los accidentes y complicaciones mas frecuentes de la pilorotomia extramucosa (operación de Fredet-Ramstedt).
  Bol. Soc. cubana de pediat. 6:355-380; y. 1934.

M. B. Clopton & A. F. Hartmann. The Fredet-Ramstedt operation for congenital pyloric stenosis.
  Surg. Gyn. & Obst. 47:527-530; y. 1928.

A. Dietrich. Anatomische Vorbedingungen der kindlichen Pylorusstenose.
  Ztschr. f. Kinderh. 50:705-714; y. 1931.

W. A. Downes. Congenital hypertrophic pyloric stenosis.
  Journ. Am. Med. Ass. 75:228-233; y. 1920.

Fredet. La sténose hypertrophique du pylore chez le nouveau-né.
  Archives des maladies de l'appareil digestif et de la nutrition. 2:393-417; y. 1908.

E. Gohrbandt. Operations des Pylorospasmus der Säuglinge.
Arch. f. klin. Chir. 126:190-193; y. 1923.

L. W. Grove. Ramstedt operation with modified technic for local anaesthesia.
South. Med. Journ. 23:727-728; y. 1930.

H. Haberer. Erfahrungen mit der Ramstedtschen Operation bei der Pylorusstenose der Säuglinge.
Deutsche Zeitschr. f. Chir. 235:91-104; y. 1932.

H. Haberer. Liestungsfähigkeit der Ramstedschen Operation bei der Pylorusstenose der Säuglinge.
Münch. med. Wchnschr. 81:903-908; y. 1934.

B. Heile. Ergänzendes zur Operation des Pylorospasmus der Säuglinge.
Zbl. für Chir. 57:19-24; y. 1930.

B. Hundsdörfer. Weber-Ramstedtsche Operation und Loretasche Dehnung.
Deutsche Zeitschr. für Chir. 212:330-338; y. 1928.

A. Jacobson. Zur operativen Behandlung des Pylorospasmus der Säuglinge.
Arch. f. klin. Chir. 145:189-202; y. 1927.

J. A. Jenkins. Safeguard for danger area in Ramstedt operation for congenital hypertrophy of pylorus.
Australian & New Zealand Journ. of Surg. 4:318; y. 1935.

C. E. Kellett. On the incidence of congenital hypertrophic pyloric stenosis in 17th and 18th centuries.
Arch. of Dis. in Childhood, 8:323-328; y. 1933.

M. Kirschner. Die operative Behandlung der Pylorusstenose des Säuglings.
Zbl. f. Chir. 54:3146-3150; y. 1927.

M. Kirschner. Anmerkungen zur operativen Behandlung des kindlichen Pylorospasmus.
Deutsch. Zeitschr. f. Chir. 227:242-254; y. 1930.

O. F. Lamson. Congenital hypertrophic pyloric stenosis. Treatment of accidental perforation of mucosa during Ramstedt operation.
Surg. Gyn. & Obst. 57:398-399; y. 1933.

T. H. Lanman & P. J. Mahoney. Congenital hypertrophic stenosis of the pylorus.
Surg. Gyn. Obst. 56:205-209; y. 1933.

W. Lehmann. Neuere Anschauungen über die sogen. kongenitale Pylorusstenose.
Ztschr. f. Kinderh. 50:691-704; y. 1931.

G. Luquet & J. Crochet. Pyloroplasties extra-muqueuses.
Rev. de chir. Paris. 51:77-95; y. 1932.

G. D. F. McFadden. Forceps to simplify Ramstedt operation for congenital hypertrophic pyloric stenosis.
Lancet II:1136; y. 1928.

W. Noetzel. Zur Anatomie und Operation des Magenausgangsverengerung der Säuglinge.
Deutsche Zeitschr. f. Chir. 231:614-624; y. 1931.

W. J. Norris. Congenital hypertrophic pyloric stenosis; summary of 100 consecutive cases operated upon at Children's Hospital, Los Angeles, California.
West. Journ. of Surg. 41:377-390; y. 1933.

H. R. Paas. Zur Frage der hypertrophischen Pylorusstenose der Säuglinge, ihrer Behandlung und ihres späteren Schicksals.
Bruns Beitr. zur klin. Chir. 155:383-402; y. 1932.

V. Pauchet. Sténose hypertrophique du pylore chez les nourrissons.
Paris chir. 21:33-44; y. 1929.

C. Ramstedt. Zur Operation der angeborenen Pylorusstenose.
Monatschr. f. Kinderheilkunde, XI:409-411; y. 1912.

C. Ramstedt. Zur Behandlung des Pylorospasmus der Säuglinge.
Deutsche med. Wchnschr. 56:348-350; y. 1930.

C. Ramstedt. Ist die Pyloromyotomie beim kindlichen Pylorospasmus die Methode der Wahl?
Chirurg, 3:449-451; y. 1931.

C. Ramstedt. Die operative Behandlung der hypertrophischen Pylorusstenose der Säuglinge.
Ergebn. d. Chir. u. Orthop., 27:54-105; y. 1934.

L. W. Sauer. Hypertrophic pyloric stenosis.
Arch. of ped. 41:145-170; y. 1924.

A. A. Strauss. Clinical observations of congenital pyloric stenosis.
Journ. Am. Med. As. 71:807-810; y. 1918.

E. Uhr. Die hypertrophische Pylorusstenose des Säuglings.
Deutsch. Zeitschr. für Chir. 235:58-90; y. 1932.

H. L. Wallace & L. B. Wevill. Congenital hypertrophic stenosis of pylorus; analysis of 145 cases treated by operation.
Brit. Med. Journ. I:1153-1157; y. 1934.

W. Weber. Ueber eine technische Neuerung bei der Operation der Pylorusstenose des Säuglings.
Berliner klin. Wchnsch. 47:763-765; y. 1910.

H. Wilke. Grundsätze der Pylorospasmusbehandlung.
Med. Klin. 30:1193-1194; y. 1934.

H. Willi. Gibt es für die Therapie der hypertrophischen Pylorusstenose eine Methode der Wahl?
Jahrb. f. Kinderh. 138:259-279; y. 1933.

W. L. Wolfson. Modified Ramstedt operation for congenital stenosis of pylorus.
Ann. of Surg. 101:965-968; y. 1935.

K. Zoellner. Eine neue chirurgische Behandlungsmethode des Pyloro-spasmus bei Säuglingen.
Deutsche med. Wchnschr. 56:95-96; y. 1930.

CHAPTER XIV.

GASTROPLICATION.

Definition.

This term is derived from the Greek γαστήρ, stomach, and the Latin **plicare,** to fold. It consists in plaiting (or plicating) either the anterior wall of the stomach alone or the posterior stomach-wall as well.

Indications.

The indications for this operation are not very often met with now. It is used **occasionally** in cases of atonic dilatation of the stomach not due to obstruction of the pylorus. It is **occasionally** also used for gastroptosis in connection with some other operation, such as gastro-enterostomy or gastropexy. The first who performed this operation was Heinrich Bircher, of Aarau, Switzerland, in 1890, who published an account of it in 1891.

THE BIRCHER METHOD.

Step 1. The abdomen is opened in the epigastric region.

Step 2. The stomach is drawn out from the abdominal cavity and its anterior wall exposed. A seromuscular suture connects two points close to the pyloric end of the stomach, and another seromuscular suture two points close to the cardiac end of the stomach. The ends of the same thread are tied to each other.

Step 3. A probe is placed behind the two points tied together, so that a furrow with two ridges is formed on the anterior wall of the stomach.

Step 4. The crests of these parallel ridges are sutured to each other by a continuous seromuscular suture. Thus, part of the anterior wall of the stomach is actually doubled.

The disadvantage of this method is that it diminishes only the size of the anterior wall of the stomach, leaving the size of the posterior wall unaltered. Another disadvantage is that by doubling the anterior wall there is formed a very large fold of this wall which protrudes into the lumen of the stomach and forms there a large partition.

In order to eliminate the formation of this large partition in the lumen of the stomach, Weir modified the Bircher method in the following manner:

THE WEIR GASTROPLICATION METHOD.

Step 1. A furrow one inch deep is made on the anterior stomach-wall by pressing a probe upon it. The length of this furrow depends on the length of the stomach in its transverse direction. Eight or ten interrupted seromuscular stitches are taken, thus transforming the furrow into a canal.

Step 2. The probe is then removed and another furrow and canal are made at a distance of one inch below the first one, using the same technic as described in Step 1 (Fig. 187, main picture). This procedure is repeated until the distance between the greater and the lesser curvature is reduced to four or five inches.

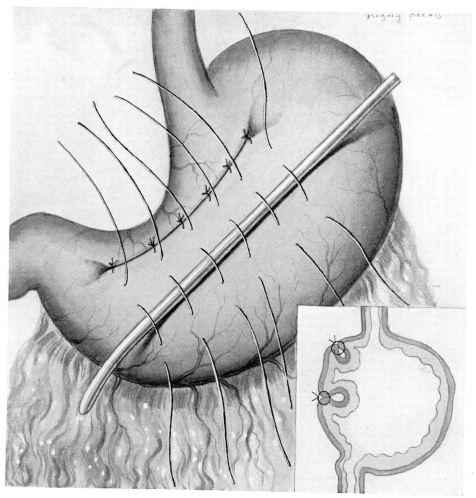

FIG. 187. GASTROPLICATION.
Weir method.

The result is the same as in the case of the Bircher method, with the difference only that the dead spaces on the serous surface are obliterated and the partition in the lumen is eliminated.

In order to overcome the formation of a pouch of the posterior gastric wall, Moynihan supplements the gastroplication with a gastro-enterostomy.

THE MOYNIHAN METHOD OF GASTROPLICATION.

Step 1. A series of interrupted seromuscular stitches are taken in the direction from the lesser to the greater curvature of the stomach. Each thread makes three to four bites and the distance between each successive bite is about one inch (Fig. 188, main picture). Each thread lies at a distance of an inch and a half from the next one. The ends are tied and

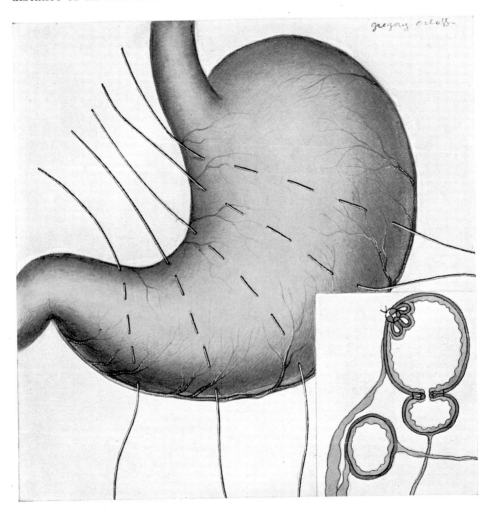

FIG. 188. GASTROPLICATION.
Moynihan method.

cut short.

Step 2. A posterior gastro-enterostomy is performed (For technic of gastro-enterostomy, see Chapter XVI). **This is a very important point of the operation,** since in Step 1 only the anterior wall of the stomach is plaited and the posterior wall of the stomach forms a deep pouch.

THE BRANDT METHOD OF GASTROPLICATION.

To avoid leaving a large pouch formed by the posterior stomach-wall, Brandt in 1894, suggested plicating also the posterior stomach-wall in a manner similar to Bircher's plication of the anterior wall. The main difficulty comes in exposing the posterior wall. Brandt did this by making small holes in the gastro-colic ligament and drawing out parts of the posterior stomach-wall and pleating them. However, this method is complicated and not as effective as the Moynihan method. We will conclude this chapter by stating again that **gastroplication is now very seldom used.**

BIBLIOGRAPHY.

H. Bircher. Eine operative Behandlung der Magenerweiterung.
Korrespondenzblatt für Schweizer Ärzte, 21:713-724; y. 1891.

H. Bircher. Neue Beiträge zur operativen Behandlung der Magenerweiterung.
Korrespondenzblatt für Schweizer Ärzte, 24:553-564; y. 1894.

J. Brandt. Über Gastroplicatio.
Zbl. f. Chir. 21:361-363; y. 1894.

M. Cusani. Ricerche sperimentali sulla "plicatio gastrica".
Clin. chir. 35:1200-1214; y. 1932.

B. G. A. Moynihan. The operation of gastrorrhaphy (gastroplication) with notes of a case.
Lancet, I:1177-1179; y. 1898.

G. Ronfini. Gastroplicatio. Ricerche sperimentali.
Giorn. veneto di sc. med. 9:18-34; y. 1935.

R. F. Weir Gastrorrhaphy for diminishing the size of a dilated stomach.
New York Med. Journ. 56:29-31; y. 1892.

CHAPTER XV.

GASTROPEXY.

Definition.

The word gastropexy consists of two Greek words: γαστήρ, stomach and πηγνύναι, to attach.

It signifies "The fixation of the stomach".

Indications.

The operation is done for gastroptosis, a downward displacement of the stomach. This disease is not a rarity. It is usually met with in women; 95.4 per cent. of all cases of gastroptosis occur in women and only 4.6 per cent. in men (Rovsing).

As gastroptosis is often associated with gastrectasia, some surgeons prefer to resort to gastroplication only for its correction, while others employ gastrofixation, and some both gastroplication and gastrofixation combined. While some are using gastroplication with a posterior gastro-enterostomy, others are using a gastropexy with a posterior gastro-enterostomy, and still others are using a gastropexy with a posterior gastro-enterostomy supplemented by an occlusion of the pylorus. As quite frequently gastroptosis is only a feature of gastrocoloptosis, many believe that not only the stomach but also the colon should be fixed. And finally, there are many not only among the internists but also among the surgeons, **who consider that gastroptosis is a constitutional disease and that it should be treated medically only.**

All the methods of fixation of the stomach can be subdivided into three groups:

A. **Operations in which the stomach, or the ligaments connected with it, are sutured directly to the anterior abdominal wall.**

B. **Operations in which the stomach is fastened in its normal position through some operative procedure on its ligaments without being attached to the anterior abdominal wall.**

C. **Operations in which not only the stomach but also the colon is attached either to the anterior or to the posterior abdominal wall.**

A. OPERATIONS IN WHICH THE STOMACH, OR THE LIGAMENTS CONNECTED WITH IT, ARE SUTURED DIRECTLY TO THE ANTERIOR ABDOMINAL WALL.

1. THE DURET METHOD (FIG. 189).

This is the earliest operative procedure of gastropexy and was performed first by Duret, of Lille, France, in 1896.

Step 1. A midline incision is made from the ensiform process down to the umbilicus, incising all the structures down to but not including the peritoneum.

Step 2. The peritoneum is opened only in the lower half of this incision.

Step 3. The stomach is lifted up. A thread attached to a round

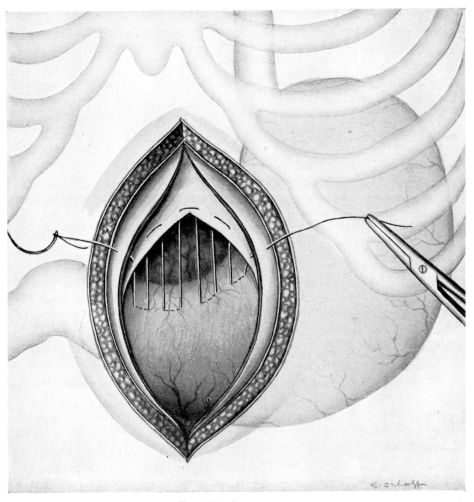

FIG. 189. GASTROPEXY.
Duret method.

curved needle passes through the entire thickness of the left lip of the opened abdomen, except the skin. Then, with the same needle, a bite is taken through the seromuscular layer of the stomach close to the cardiac end of the lesser curvature. This is then carried through the undivided portion of the peritoneum from within outward, and then again penetrates the peritoneum from without inward. Another seromuscular bite is then taken through the anterior stomach-wall a little way from the previous seromuscular bite in the direction toward the pylorus. These movements of catching alternately the peritoneum and the seromuscular layer of the stomach close to the lesser curvature are continued until the antrum is reached. Then the needle pierces the entire thickness of the right lip of the abdomen, with the exception of the skin. The ends of the thread are tied together and cut short only after the anterior sheath is closed. By this maneuvre, the stomach is lifted and fixed to the abdominal wall.

Step 4. The abdomen is closed in layers.

2. THE ROVSING METHOD.

This was first described in 1899.

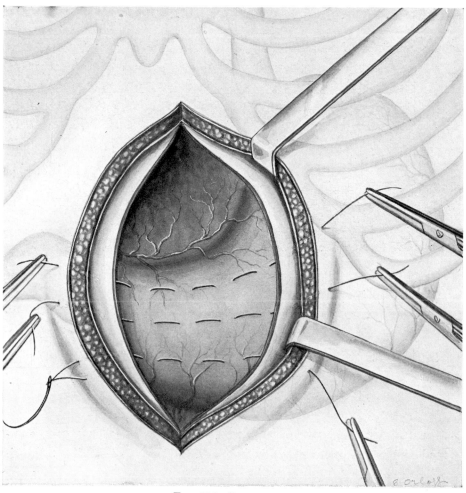

Fig. 190. Gastropexy.
Rovsing method.

Step 1. The abdomen is opened through a midline incision extending from the ensiform process down to the umbilicus.

Step 2. A bite is taken through the entire thickness of the left lip of the abdominal wall from without inward, and then two or three bites are taken through the seromuscular layer of the stomach, and then again through the entire thickness of the right lip of the abdominal wall from

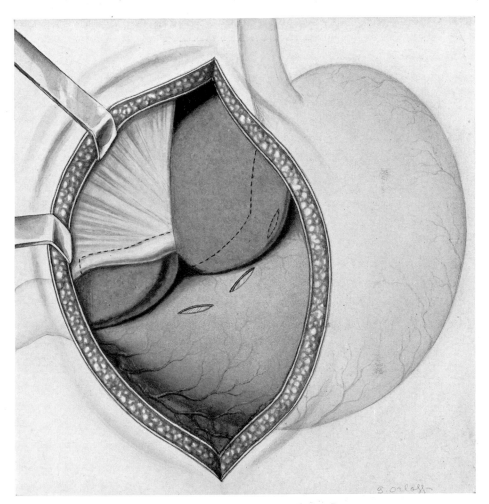

FIG. 191. GASTROPEXY. (Perthes method).
Separating the round ligament from the falciform ligament.

within outward. A second and a third row of sutures are made in a similar manner, each row being one inch below the previous one (Fig. 190). The ends are still not tied.

Step 3. The abdomen is closed in the usual way in layers.

Step 4. A piece of gauze is placed over the sutured abdominal wall, and the three threads which fastened the stomach to the anterior abdominal wall are tied over it and the ends are cut short. The gastrofixation sutures are removed four weeks later.

This method is considered by many as one of the best. However, its disadvantage is the same as in the method of Duret, in that extensive adhesions are formed between the stomach and the anterior abdominal wall, which decrease the mobility of the stomach and in many cases produce distress.

3. THE PERTHES METHOD.

In this method the round ligament of the liver is utilized for the raising and fixation of the stomach.

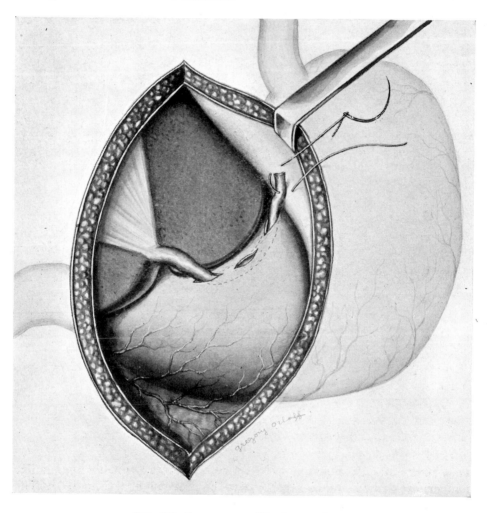

FIG. 192. GASTROPEXY. (Perthes method).
The round ligament is carried through a seromuscular canal in the stomach-wall and sutured to the posterior sheath of the left rectus muscle.

Step 1. The abdomen is opened through a midline incision.

Step 2. The round ligament of the liver is severed very close to its attachment to the umbilicus, and is separated from its attachment to the falciform ligament along its entire length up to the liver (Fig. 191).

Step 3. The upper free end of the round ligament is transfixed by a silk thread, which is inserted into the eye of a grooved director. A seromuscular incision one-quarter of an inch long is made through the anterior stomach-wall just proximal to the pylorus. Another seromuscular incision of the same length is made at a distance of one to one and one-half inches more proximally (Fig. 192). The seromuscular layer between these two incisions is undermined, and with the aid of the grooved director the silk thread with the round ligament are carried through the seromuscular canal thus formed (Fig. 192). A third seromuscular incision is made at a distance of one and a half inches still closer to the cardia, and the seromuscular layer is again undermined between the last two incisions and the round ligament is carried through it. These manipulations are repeated several times until the round ligament lies close to the cardia.

Step 4. The seromuscular lips are sutured over the exposed parts of the round ligament.

Step 5. The free end of the round ligament is fastened either to the posterior sheath of the left rectus muscle, or to the cartilage of the seventh left rib at a point located two inches to the left from the ensiform process (Fig. 192).

Step 6. The abdomen is closed in the usual manner.

As may be seen from this description, Perthes fastens the round ligament of the liver to the anterior wall of the stomach precisely in the same manner as Schnitzler fastens the rubber tube to the anterior stomach-wall in his method of gastrostomy.

4. THE VOGEL METHOD.

Step 1. The abdomen is opened.

Step 2. The round ligament of the liver is cut very close to its attachment to the umbilicus, and is separated from the falciform ligament along its entire length up to the liver.

Step 3. The round ligament is laid upon the anterior wall of the stomach midway between the greater and the lesser curvatures and parallel to them (Fig. 193, insert).

Step 4. A series of seromuscular bites are taken on each side of the round ligament. The distance of each bite from the round ligament is about one-third of an inch, and the distance between each two adjoining sutures is one-half of an inch. Six interrupted seromuscular sutures are made in this manner. Thus, three inches of the round ligament are buried in the anterior stomach-wall (Fig. 193).

Step 5. The free end of the round ligament is brought through the peritoneum, the posterior sheath of the left rectus muscle, the left rectus muscle, and the anterior sheath of this muscle to which it is fastened (Fig. 193).

Step 6. The abdomen is closed in tiers.

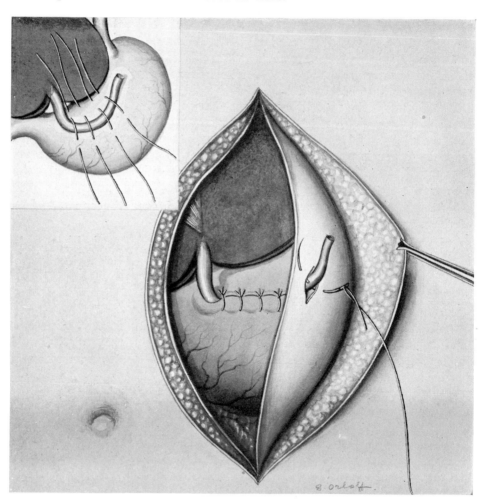

FIG. 193. GASTROPEXY.
Vogel method.

5. THE GÖBBEL METHOD.

This was first described in 1913.

Step 1. The abdomen is opened.

Step 2. A posterior gastro-enterostomy is performed.

Step 3. A strip from the anterior sheath of the left rectus muscle, 12 cm. by 2 cm., is made and detached from the sheath.

Step 4. A seromuscular flap having its base toward the pylorus, is made out of that portion of the anterior stomach-wall which is adjacent to the pylorus (Fig. 194).

Step 5 The pyloric ring is encircled by a portion of the detached aponeurotic strip, and the ends forming the ring around the pylorus are sutured together with silk sutures (Fig. 194).

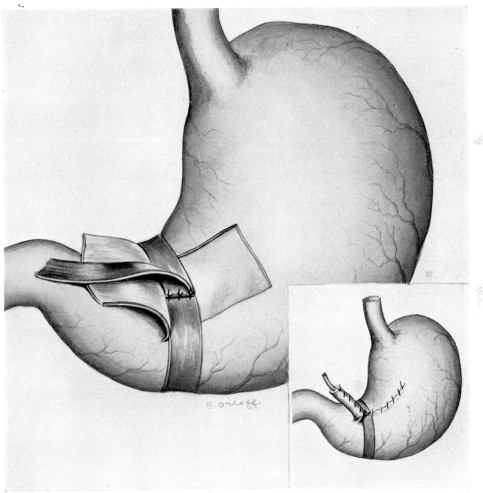

FIG. 194. GASTROPEXY.
Göbbel method.

Step 6. The rest of the aponeurotic strip is laid upon the muscular surface of the seromuscular flap, and the edges of this flap are sutured to each other so as to surround the aponeurotic strip (Fig. 194, insert).

Step 7. The gap in the anterior stomach-wall, produced by making the seromuscular flap, is closed by a series of interrupted or continuous seromuscular sutures (Fig. 194, insert).

Step 8. The newly formed suspensory ligament is brought outside the abdominal cavity by piercing the peritoneum, the posterior sheath of the left rectus muscle, this muscle itself, and its anterior sheath to which it is fastened.

Step 9. The abdomen is closed in tiers.

6.   THE ABRASHANOW METHOD.

This was first described in 1925. The characteristic feature of this method is that three suspensory ligaments are constructed either from the anterior sheath of the rectus muscle or from the fascia lata, two of which are then attached to the **anterior wall of the stomach** [one close to the pyloric and the other to the cardiac end of the lesser curvature], and the third to the **posterior wall of the stomach** close to the mid-point of the lesser curvature.

Step 1. The abdomen is opened by a midline incision.

Step 2. Three strips are cut from the anterior sheath of the rectus muscle or from the fascia lata. The size of the strips is 4 to 5 cm, by 1½ cm.

Step 3. Three small seromuscular incisions are made close to the lesser curvature. One is made two fingers' width to the left from the antrum on the anterior wall of the stomach, another, at the middle point of the lesser curvature, but only on the posterior wall, and the third, below the cardia on the anterior wall of the stomach. A seromuscular canal is undermined in an upward direction for a length of 2 cm., starting from each of the seromuscular openings. Three seromuscular channels are thus formed. Each strip is carried through the seromuscular channel for half of its length, so that a portion of the strip projects from each end of the channel. Each of the small seromuscular incisions is then closed. The two ends of each strip are brought outside the abdominal cavity through the upper angle of the wound, piercing the peritoneum, muscle and the anterior sheath of the rectus muscle, and each end of the strip is sutured to the other end of the same strip and also to the anterior sheath of the rectus muscle.

7.   THE LAMBRET METHOD.

This was described in 1929, by O. Lambret, of Lille, France, who makes an aponeurotic flap of the anterior sheath of the left rectus muscle, the size of which is 12 cm. by 2 cm., and leaves the upper end of it connected with the anterior sheath. The lower end is brought into the abdominal cavity through the seventh intercostal space and is sutured to the greater curvature of the stomach by making a seromuscular-seromuscular canal over it. Finally, the free end of the aponeurotic strip is sutured to the round ligament of the liver. This operation accomplishes the following:

1. It diminishes the size of the stomach. The stomach is **not hanging** on a band as in some other methods, but is **resting on a band.**
2. The pylorus and the first part of the duodenum lie in a straight line.
3. The evacuation of the gastric contents is rapid.

Technic.

Step 1. A midline incision is made through the skin and superficial fascia extending from the ensiform process down to the umbilicus. Two additional oblique incisions, also through the skin and superficial fascia, each of which is about five centimeters long, are made, one at each end of the vertical incision. The flap (which consists of skin, superficial and deep fascia) is then reflected, and the anterior sheath of the rectus muscle is thereby well exposed.

Step 2. An aponeurotic flap, 12 cm. by 2 cm., is made from the anterior sheath of the left rectus muscle, having its base at the upper portion of the muscle. The peritoneal cavity is now opened.

Step 3. A small incision is made in the seventh left intercostal space close to the sternum. The free end of the aponeurotic flap is caught by an artery-forceps brought from within the abdominal cavity through this small opening, and the flap is pulled into the abdominal cavity as far as possible.

Step 4. The aponeurotic strip is placed along the greater curvature of the stomach, the highest point of which lies as high as is required by the position of the stomach. Starting from this point, the greater curvature is then sutured over the aponeurotic strip along the entire length of the greater curvature until the pyloric canal is reached.

Step 5. The free end of the aponeurotic strip is sutured to the round ligament of the liver.

Step 6. The abdomen is closed in tiers.

Manuel Corachan, of Barcelona, made a slight modification in the Lambret technic. Instead of using a strip from the anterior sheath of the rectus muscle he uses a double thread of silk, one end of which he attaches to one costal arch and the other to the opposite costal arch. The rest of the operation is the same as in the Lambret method.

B. **Operations in which the stomach is fastened in its position either by strengthening its normally existing ligaments or by other intra-abdominal fixation.**

1. THE METHOD OF BEYEA-BIER.

This operation consists in pleating the gastro-hepatic ligament. It was first performed by Bier, in November 1897, in Kiehl. However, the report of it was made only in 1900. Beyea performed his first operation in April, 1898, not being aware either of the work done by Duret or by Bier. The technics of Bier and Beyea have a striking resemblance to each other.

Technic.

Step 1. The abdomen is opened.

Step 2. A plaiting of the gastro-hepatic ligament is made in three or four places. Each threaded needle takes three or four bites. The first bite of each thread grasps the seromuscular layer of the stomach very close to the lesser curvature, then two or three bites grasp the gastro-

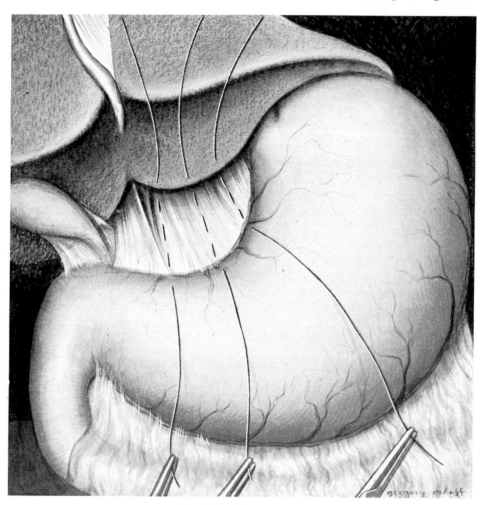

FIG. 195. GASTROPEXY.
Beyea-Bier method.

hepatic ligament, and the upper bite grasps the thickened capsule of the liver close to its transverse fissure (Fig. 195). The ends of the same thread are tied to each other.

Step 3. The abdomen is closed in tiers.

The advantage of this method is that the stomach is not attached to the anterior abdominal wall and, therefore, no extensive adhesions are formed. However, the disadvantages are:

a. The danger of injury to the hepatic, left gastric and pyloric arteries, while doing the pleating.

b. Frequent recurrences of the gastroptosis on account of the thinness and weakness of the gastro-hepatic ligament.

In order to reinforce the pleated gastro-hepatic ligament several methods were suggested:

2. THE ROTHE METHOD.

This was published in 1919. The pleated gastro-hepatic ligament is reinforced by three strips of the fascia lata the size of which is about 5 cm. by 1½ cm. The technic is as follows:

Step 1. A pleating of the gastro-hepatic ligament is made precisely as in the Beyea-Bier method.

Step 2. Three small seromuscular flaps of a reversed U-shape (∩) are made on the anterior wall of the stomach very close to the lesser curvature. These flaps are reflected downward. A strip of fascia lata is sutured into each area of the exposed mucosa. The U-flaps are turned back and sutured in their original position. The other end of each strip is sutured to the lower surface of the liver, which is also scarified in order to make the attachment stronger.

C. OPERATIONS IN WHICH NOT ONLY THE STOMACH BUT ALSO THE COLON IS FIXED.

THE WAUGH-COFFEY OPERATION.

As gastroptosis is frequently associated with ptosis of the cecum and of the ascending colon, Coffey suggested in such cases performing as a routine procedure a colopexy by the Waugh method and a gastropexy by his "hammock" technic.

Technic.

Step 1. The abdomen is opened through a midline incision.

Step 2. A retractor is placed on the right lip of the abdominal wound which is retracted to the right. The cecum is grasped and drawn medially. An incision is made in the parietal peritoneum of the posterior abdominal wall one inch lateral to the cecum and the ascending colon. The lateral lip of the parietal peritoneum is caught by an Allis forceps and detached from the underlying muscles of the posterior abdominal wall.

Step 3. Three seromuscular bites are taken on the cecum, one just medial to the anterior longitudinal tænia coli, another through the tænia coli itself, and the third slightly lateral to it. A fourth bite is taken through the lateral lip of the divided parietal peritoneum of the posterior abdominal wall. This method of suturing starts at the lower angle of the wound by a series of interrupted sutures, and continues in an upward direction, at a distance of one-half of an inch from each other, until the hepatic flexure is reached. The ends of the same thread are then tied to each other. Thus, the Waugh colopexy is completed.

Step 4. The "hammock operation" is now performed in the following manner: A bite is taken on the gastro-colic ligament and another through the parietal peritoneum. of the anterior abdominal wall at a point two and a half inches above the umbilicus. The first stitch should be at the extreme left side of the colon. The next stitch should run medially, and the distance between two bites should be not more than one-half to three-fourths of an inch, so that no loop of bowel can become incarcerated between the two successive stitches. This suturing is carried on until the right side of the gastro-colic omentum is reached.

BIBLIOGRAPHY.

A. Abrashanow. Ein plastisches Verfahren der Gastropexie.
Zbl. f. Chir. 52:1707; y. 1925.

H. Axtell. Gastroenteroptosis and its problems.
Am. Journ. of Surg. 39:132-135; y. 1925.

H. Beyea. The elevation of the stomach in gastroptosis by the surgical plication of the gastrohepatic and gastrophrenic ligaments; an original operation.
Philadelphia Med. Journ. XI:257-262; y. 1903.

H. Beyea. The surgical elevation of the stomach in gastroptosis by suture of the gastro-hepatic omentum.
Journ. Am. Med. Ass. 54:766-770; y. 1910.

E. Bircher. Zur Technik der Gastropexie und Hepatopexie.
Zbl. f. Chir. 45:449-452; y. 1918.

A. Blecher. Beitrag zur chirurgischen Behandlung der Enteroptose.
Deutsche Zeitschr. f. Chir. 56:374-397; y. 1900.
(Describes Bier method).

H. Bőker. Über die chirurgische Behandlung der Gastroptose.
(Dissertation), Kőln, y. 1922.

W. R. Braizew. Eine Methode der chirurgischen Behandlung der Gastroptose.
Zbl. f. Chir. 52:2245-2250; y. 1925.

J. Gonzalez Campo. Concepto clínico de las ptosis gástrica e intestinal.
Progresos de la clín. 39:382-394; y. 1931.

A. P. Cawadias. The modern treatment of gastro-enteroptosis.
Brit. Med. Journ. I:1163-1167; y. 1932.

R. Coffey. Gastroptosis: a method of suspending the stomach in a hammock made of the great omentum.
Philad. Med. Journ. 10:506-513; y. 1902.

M. Corachan. Modification de la technique de Lambret dans la gastropexie.
Bull. et mém. de la Soc. nat. de chir. 59:1192-1194; y. 1933.

B. Davis. A contribution to the surgery of gastroptosis and enteroptosis.
Western Medical Review, I:291-294; y. 1897.

H. Duret. De la gastropexie.
Rev. de Chir. 16:421-433; y. 1896.

E. Eliot, Jr. Hepatoptosis complicated by gastroptosis; a suggestion as to treatment.
The Medical News, 85:913-916; y. 1904.

C. de Ginestet. Technique de la gastro-suspension par le procédé de Lambret.
Bull. et mém. de la Soc. de chir. de Paris, 25:120-128; y. 1933.

R. Gőbell. Die Ergebnisse der chirurgischen Behandlung der Gastroptose.
Arch f. klin. Chir. 144:266-281; y. 1927.

F. A. Hadley. A new operation for cure of gastroptosis.
Journ. of the College of Surg. Australasia, I:236-237; y. 1928.

H. Havlicek. Gastropexie durch Rekonstruktion des Ligamentum hepatogastricum mittels frei transplantierter Fascie.
Zbl. f. Chir. 48:787-789; y. 1921.

A. Jentzer. La ptose gastrique et son traitement chirurgical.
Rev. méd. de la Suisse Rom. 52:335-346; y. 1933.

Klapp & Riess. Die Anheftung des Gastroptotischen Magens an die Rippen.
Arch. f. klin. Chir. 118:125-137; y. 1921.

O. Lambret. Traitement chirurgical de la ptose gastrique par suspension et coulissage de la grande courbure.
La Presse médicale. 37:1613-1616; y. 1929.

O. Lambret & G. Bizard. Traitement chirurgical de la ptose gastrique par la suspension et le coulissage de la grande courbure. (Principes et technique).
Paris chir. 22:33-43; y. 1930.

O. Lambret. Traitement chirurgical de la ptose gastrique par l'operation de suspension-coulissage de la grande courbure.
Arch. de mal. de l'app. digestif; 21:529-545; y. 1931.

E. Liek. Sollen wir den Senkmagen operieren?
Arch. f. klin. Chir. 137:174-182; y. 1925.

L. Losio. Creazione di un diaframma di sostegno allo stomaco ptosico mediante il mesocolon transverso.
Arch. Ital. Chir. 17:61-72; y. 1927.

L. Losio. La correzione dello stomaco ptosico con il processo Losio.
Arch. ital. di chir. 24:213-220; y. 1929.

D. Maluschew. Über die verschiedenen Modificationen der Bier'schen Gastroptoseoperation.
Zbl. f. Chir. 50:55-57; y. 1923.

R. O. Moody. Are diagnoses of enteroptosis, gastroptosis and coloptosis now justifiable?
Am. Journ. of Surg. 7:470-473; y. 1929.

R. Ollenstein. Die operative Behandlung der Gastroptose und deren Erfolge.
Arch. f. klin. Chir. 158:611-626; y. 1930.

E. Pagenstecher. Gastropexie vermittelst des Ligamentum teres.
Münch. med. Wochenschr. 60:24; y. 1913.

E. Paul. Erfahrungen mit der Ptosenoperation nach Perthes.
Arch. f. klin. Chir. 134:698-708; y. 1925.

G. Perthes. Über Operation der Gastroptose unter Verwendung des Ligamentum teres hepatis.
Zbl. f. Chir. 47:818-821; y. 1920.

G. Perthes. Erfahrungen mit der Operation der Gastroptose.
Arch. f. klin. Chir. 120:441-471; y. 1922.

J. Pi-Figueras. Un caso de gastropexia por el procedimiente de Lambret.
Ars. méd. Barcelona, 8:202-208; y. 1932.

B. O. Pribram. Die operative Behandlung der Gastroptose und prinzipielle Bemerkungen zur Ptosenfrage.
Zbl. f. Chir. 60:734-742; y. 1933.

E. Boix Ripollés. Contribución al estudio de la ptosis gástrica.
Rev. méd. de Barcelona, 21:297-344; y. 1934.

A. Rothe. Neue Operationsmethode der Gastro-und Nephroptose.
Zbl. f. Chir. 46:506-509; y. 1919.

A. Rothe. Noch einmal die Gastroptose.
Zbl. f. Chir. 48:1189-1191; y. 1921.

T. Rovsing. Ueber Gastroptose und ihre Operative Behandlung.
Arch. f. klin. Chir. 60:812-834; y. 1900.

T. Rovsing. Die Gastro-coloptosis, ihre pathologische Bedeutung, ihre Krankheitsbilder, Diagnose und Behandlung.
F. C. W. Vogel, publishers. Leipzig, 1914.

A. Rudolf. Erfahrungen über die chirurgische Behandlung der Gastroptose.
Bruns Beiträge zur klin. Chir. 127:223-228; y. 1922.

K. Secher. Über die Beziehungen zwischen Cor pendulum, Gastroptose und Bathygastrie.
Deutsch. Arch. f. klin. Med. 174:341-351; y. 1932.

G. Serra. La ptosi gastrica e la sua cura chirurgica col metodi di Perthes-Vogel e Coffey-Beyea.
Arch. ital. di chir. 39:141-175; y. 1935.

P. Skliaroff. A new method of elevation of the stomach.
Khirurg. 24:45-48; y. 1931.

A. Stengel & H. Beyea. Gastroptosis: Report of a case in which a new operation was undertaken and the patient greatly improved.
Amer. Journ. of the Med. Science, 117:663-675; y. 1899.

A. C. Vietor. Anatomical basis for study of splanchnoptosis; ptosis en masse and its relation to body form; preliminary communication.
New England Journ. of Med. 206:1137-1144; y. 1932.

A. C. Vietor. Anatomic basis for study of splanchnoptosis; paths of visceral descent; preliminary report.
Arch. of Surg. 28:659-683; y. 1934.

Vogel. Ueber Operation der Gastroptose unter Verwendung des Lig. teres hepatis.
Zbl. f. Chir. 47:1101-1102; y. 1920.

Weber. Un cas de libération de l'estomac après accidents consécutifs à une gastropexie.
Bull. et mém. Soc. de chirurgiens de Paris, 25:381-384; y. 1933.

CHAPTER XVI.

EXCISION OF A GASTRIC ULCER. EXCLUSION OF A GASTRIC ULCER. REPAIR OF A PERFORATED GASTRIC ULCER.

I. EXCISION OF A GASTRIC ULCER.

This is usually done when the ulcer is single and not of a large size. If, however, the ulcers are multiple or of a large size, a partial gastrectomy is the operation of choice.

Technic.

This operation is a simple procedure when it is done for removal of an ulcer on the anterior stomach-wall. When the ulcer is situated on the lesser curvature (and this is what actually happens in the great majority of cases), then the procedure is more complicated.

a. REMOVAL OF AN ULCER ON THE ANTERIOR STOMACH WALL.

Step 1. The abdomen is opened by a longitudinal or transverse incision.

Step 2. The stomach is walled off from the rest of the peritoneal cavity. A fold of the anterior wall of the stomach, which includes not only the ulcer but also the surrounding healthy tissues, is grasped by an intestinal clamp.

Step 3. The fold is cut away so that only a portion of the wall, about one-half inch, is left above the blades.

Step 4. The lips of the gastric opening are closed by two layers of sutures. One is an over-and-over, and the other, a seromuscular-seromuscular suture. [Before starting the seromuscular-seromuscular suture, the intestinal clamp releases the fold of the stomach.]

Many surgeons prefer not to use the clamps at all. Then, Step 2 will be as follows:

Step 2. The stomach is walled off form the rest of the peritoneal cavity. Two guy-sutures are placed in the healthy tissues of the stomach so as to facilitate the suturing, which will follow the incision of the diseased area. Two Allis forceps grasp the healthy tissues close to the diseased portion (Fig. 196). The stomach is cut between one of the guy-sutures and the adjoining Allis forceps. The tube of the suction-apparatus is then inserted into the stomach and its contents sucked out. The diseased portion of the stomach-wall, including also the adjoining healthy portions with the two Allis forceps attached to them, is cut away, leaving an opening into the stomach with a guy-suture at each end.

The rest of the operation is the same as Step 4.

b. EXCISION OF AN ULCER ON THE POSTERIOR STOMACH-WALL.

There are three different methods of exposure of an ulcer on the posterior stomach-wall:

1. **Through a slit in the transverse mesocolon.**—The posterior wall of the stomach is pulled through a slit in the transverse mesocolon. This method is applicable only in cases in which the ulcer is small and lies on

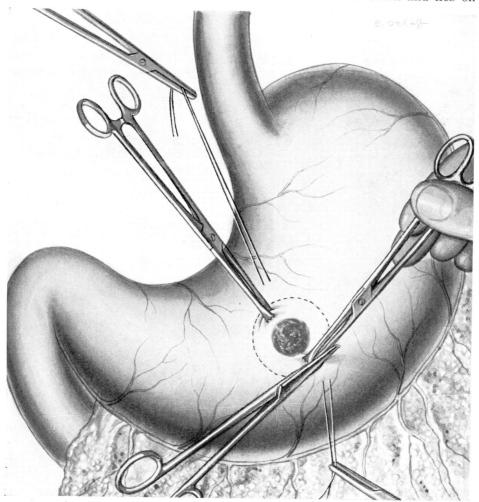

FIG. 196. EXCISION OF AN ULCER IN THE ANTERIOR STOMACH-WALL.

that portion of the posterior stomach-wall which adjoins the "avascular area of Riolan" of the transverse mesocolon. The technic of excision of the ulcer is the same as described in the previous operation.

2. **By cutting the gastrocolic ligament and turning the posterior wall anteriorly** (Fig. 144).—While cutting the gastrocolic ligament **care should be taken not to injure the middle colic artery,** and the technical details of

this are already described elsewhere. The technic of excision of the ulcer is the same as in the previous operation.

3.   **The Transgastric Method.**—This consists in making an incision through the anterior stomach-wall, and then in the removal of a portion of the posterior stomach-wall with the ulcer. However, this method, although still used occasionally, can hardly be recommended, since it is very easy

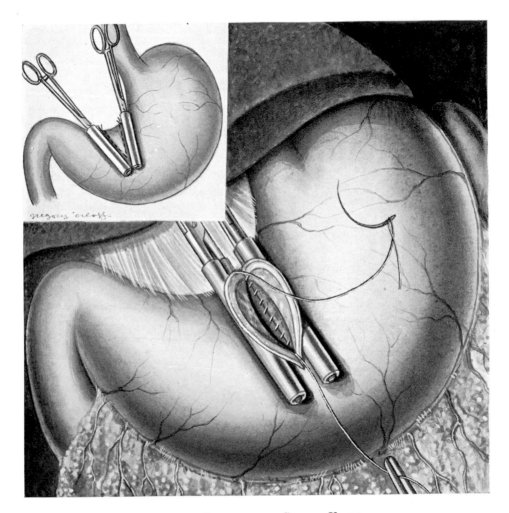

FIG. 197. EXCISION OF A GASTRIC ULCER.
Valla's technic.

to contaminate the lesser peritoneal cavity, and also because in suturing the posterior wall through the transgastric incision it is difficult to place a non-contaminated seromuscular suture.

c. REMOVAL OF AN ULCER ON THE LESSER CURVATURE
(VALLA'S TECHNIC).

Step 1. The artery which runs along the lesser curvature is ligated in two places, one inch distal and one inch proximal from the indurated area.

Step 2. The gastro-hepatic ligament is cut for a length slightly greater than the distance between the ligated points of the artery.

Step 3. Two intestinal clamps, the blades of which are covered with rubber tubing, are placed across the stomach in such a manner that one clamp lies proximal to the proximal point of the ligated artery and the other distal to the distal point of the ligated artery (Fig. 197, insert). The clamps lie in such a manner that the posterior blades meet at an angle on the posterior wall of the stomach and the anterior blades at an angle on the anterior wall (Fig. 197, insert). Thus, the two clamps separate a wedge-shaped portion of the stomach, which contains the gastric ulcer, from the rest of the stomach.

Step 4. The "V" -shape portion of the stomach is cut away, leaving about one-half of an inch of the stomach-wall protruding from each clamp, which are then placed side-by-side (Fig. 197, main picture). The two openings are sutured to each other precisely as described in the Chapter on "Lateral Intestinal Anastomosis."

Step. 5. The opening in the gastric-hepatic ligament is closed.

II. EXCLUSION OF A GASTRIC ULCER.

This procedure is performed in cases in which the ulcer penetrates into one of the surrounding viscera (as the pancreas) and cannot be separated from it. The operation consists in excising the ulcer from the stomach, leaving the ulcer connected with the pancreas, and suturing the opening in the stomach. **Thus, the ulcer becomes "extragastrectomized",** as it were.

These ulcers are usually located on the posterior gastric wall. The approach to them is either through:

      1. The gastro-colic ligament; or

      2. The anterior gastric wall.

The technic of the operation differs somewhat depending on the route of approach.

a. **In case of gastro-colic approach,** the operation is as follows:

Step 1. The gastro-colic ligament is cut.

Step 2. The greater curvature of the stomach is lifted so as to make the posterior wall face anteriorly.

Step 3. A circular incision is made on the healthy portion of the posterior wall of the stomach surrounding the ulcer. This will free the stomach from the surrounding structures when it can be fully reflected. **The ulcer is carefully and thoroughly disinfected.**

Step 4. The opening in the stomach is closed by two layers of sutures, the first being over-and-over and the second seromuscular-seromuscular.

Step 5. The lips of the gastro-colic ligament are sutured to each other.

b.   In case of transgastric approach, the operation is as follows:

Step 1. After the abdomen is opened and the stomach is "walled off" from the rest of the peritoneal cavity, the anterior stomach-wall is opened

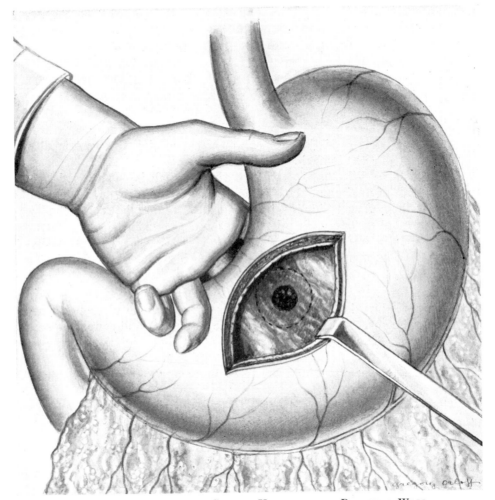

FIG. 198. EXCLUSION OF A GASTRIC ULCER ON THE POSTERIOR WALL.

and its lips are separated from each other, thereby exposing the mucous surface of the posterior wall.

Step 2. A circular incision is made through the posterior wall of the stomach surrounding the ulcer, starting in the healthy mucosa at a distance of one inch from the edges of the ulcer (Fig. 198). In order to facilitate this cutting, the index- and the middle fingers of the left hand of the surgeon are introduced behind the posterior wall of the stomach (through an opening made in the gastro-hepatic ligament) in such a manner that the index-finger lies to one side and the middle finger to the other side of the ulcer. The fingers lying behind the posterior wall of the stomach will prevent the possibility of injuring the pancreas while the cutting takes place. The surface of the ulcer is now thoroughly disinfected.

Step 3. The opening in the stomach is closed by a series of over-and-over mattress-sutures.

The "extragastrectomized" ulcer either absorbs or shrinks. Cases are reported in which patients so treated were clinically cured.

III. REPAIR OF A PERFORATED GASTRIC OR DUODENAL ULCER.

Step 1. After the abdomen is opened the stomach (or the duodenum) is walled off from the rest of the peritoneal cavity.

Step 2. An over-and-over suture is made penetrating the healthy tissues. If the indurated portion is too large it should first be excised. The number of sutures required for closure depends on the size of the opening. In ordinary cases of perforation, when the opening is very small, two sutures suffice. The sutures should be of an **insoluble** material such as linen or silk.

Step 3. The closed opening is covered either by the great omentum or by the gastro-hepatic ligament, depending on the location of the perforation.

BIBLIOGRAPHY.

P. Adreani. Contributo alla conoscenza del trattamento dell'ulcera gastrica col metodo Schiassi (discontinuità nervosa vagosimpatica).
Il Policlinico, 37:873-877; y. 1930.

J. Armour. A lesser curvature gastroplasty. (Flap exteriorization of ulcer. The formation of a gastric pouch).
Canad. Med. Ass. Journ. 23:756-761; y. 1930.

D. C. Balfour. The surgical treatment of hemorrhagic duodenal ulcer.
Ann. of Surg. 96:581-587; y. 1932.

O. Bsteh. Technik der Resektion tiefsitzender Duodenalulcera.
Arch. f. klin. Chir. 175:114-120; y. 1933.

H. Bürckle-de la Camp. Zur Pathologie und Chirurgie der peptischen Schädigungen des Magen-Darmkanals.
Deutsche Zeitschr. f. Chir. 220:31-88; y. 1929.

G. Cavina. Intorno al trattamento dell'ulcera duodenale cronica ed in modo particolare intorno alla operazione di Starr Judd.
Arch. ital. di Chir. 37:165-203; y. 1934.

M. Chaton. Note sur un procédé d'excision des ulcus gastriques (procédé du cone muqueux).
Bull. et mém. Soc. nat. de Chir. 53:857-859; y. 1927.

A. Ciminata. Zur Resektion des tiefsitzenden Duodenalgeschwüren.
  Zbl. f. Chir. 61:334-336; y. 1934.

F. G. Connell. Fundusectomy. A new principle in the treatment of gastric
  or duodenal ulcer.
  Surgery, Gyn. & Obst. 49:696-701; y. 1929.

F. G. Connell. Resection of the fundus of the stomach for peptic ulcer.
  Ann. of Surg. 96:200-203; y. 1932.

J. B. Deaver & V. G. Burden. The pyloric sphincter and duodenal ulcer.
  Ann. of Surg. 94:818-827; y. 1931.

L. Durante. Duodeno-sfinterectomie anteriori.
  Arch. ital. di chir. 36:422-444; y. 1934.

J. M. T. Finney. The surgery of gastric and duodenal ulcer.
  Am. Journ. of Surg. 1:323-343; y. 1926.

H. Finsterer and F. Cunha. The surgical treatment of duodenal ulcer.
  Surg. Gyn. & Obst. 52:1099-1114; y. 1931.

M. Friedemann. Der Streit um den Pfortner. Zugleich ein Beitrag zum
  Thema: "Salzsäure und Magengeschwür".
  Zbl. f. Chir. 61:2658-2670; y. 1934.

Von Haberer. Chirurgische B e h a n d l u n g des Magen-und Duodenalgeschwürs.
  Zbl. f. Chir. 58:958-964; y. 1931.

Von Haberer. Zur operativen Behandlung des nicht resezierbaren Duo-
  denalgeschwüres.
  Zbl. f. Chir. 58:3145-3153; y. 1931.

J. Hohlbaum. Zur chirurgischen Behandlung des Kardianahen Magen-
  geschwürs.
  Arch. f. klin. Chir. 162:574-581; y. 1930.

J. B. Hume. Sympathectomy for chronic gastric ulcer.
  St. Barthol. Hosp. Rep. 66:28-29; y. 1933.

E. S. Judd & G. W. Nagel. Excision of ulcer of the duodenum.
  Surg. Gyn. & Obst. 45:17-23; y. 1927.

M. Kirschner. Meine Technik der Resektion beim chronischen Magen-Duo-
  denalgeschwür. Technik der Treppen-oder Schlauch und der Pallia-
  tivresektion.
  Chirurg. 4:417-421; y. 1932.

W. J. Klug. Sattlers Operationsmethoden am ulcuskranken Magen des
  Menschen im Tierexperiment.
  Deutsche Zeitschr. f. Chir. 208:33-40; y. 1928.

M. Madlener. Die "palliative" Resektion bei der Magengeschwürskrank-
  heit.
  Zbl. f. Chir. 54:450-454; y. 1927.

S. L. Malinovski. A new operative method in the treatment of gastric ulcer.
Novy khir. Arkhiv. 31:317-320; y. 1934.

Mallet-Guy & R. Peycelon. Documents pour l'étude chirurgicale des grandes hemorrhagies gastriques par ulcère.
Journ. de Chir. 40:809-827; y. 1932.

K. A. Meyer and W. A. Brams. Some indications for surgical treatment of peptic ulcer of the stomach and duodenum.
Illin. Med. Journ., September 1926.

K. A. Meyer, W. A. Brams and W. N. Graves. Final results of the operative treatment of gastric ulcer.
Annals of Surgery, June 1925.

F. Mandl. Zur Resektionsbehandlung des Ulcus duodeni.
Wien. klin. Wchnschr. 43:974-978; y. 1930.

L. M. Moriconi. Escisione transgastrica dell'ulcera gastrica.
Riforma med. 43:677-681; y. 1927.

N. N. Nasaroff. Combined operations in gastric ulcer.
Vestnik Khir. (No. 61). 21:53-55; y. 1930.

R. Nissen. Zur Resektion des tiefsitzenden Duodenalgeschwűrs.
Zbl. f. Chir. 60:483-485; y. 1933.

V. Pauchet. Technische Einzelheiten bei Resektionen von riesengrossen Geschwűren am Magen.
Arch. f. klin. Chir. 167:440-442; y. 1931.

V. Pauchet. Ulcus gastrique haut situé traité par la résection en gouttière.
Tech. Chir. 25:137-152; y. 1933.

I. Philipovici. New method of resection of duodenal ulcer.
Rev. de chir. Bucuresti, 36:487-490; y. 1933.

B. Schiassi. The role of the pyloro-duodenal nerve supply in the surgery of duodenal ulcer.
Annals of Sur. 81:939-948; y. 1925.

B. Schiassi. La discontinuita nervosa vago-simpatica nella cura dell'ulcera gastrica.
Arch. ital. di Chirurgia, 17:1-37; y. 1927.

M. E. Steinberg. Exclusion operation for duodenal ulcer; an experimental and clinical study.
Am. Journ. of Surg. 23:137-147; y. 1934.

V. P. Voznessensky. Method of excision in ulcer of small curvature of the stomach.
Vestnik Khir. 14:13-38; y. 1928.

W. Walters. The choice of surgical procedures for duodenal ulcer.
Ann. of Surg. 96:258-268; y. 1932.

A. J. Walton. The surgical treatment of simple ulcers of the body of the stomach.
Lancet, I:1070-1075; y. 1931.

C. A. Wells. High gastric ulcer. A suggested operation.
Brit. Med. Journ. I:778-779; y. 1933.

W. Wynen. Experimenteller Beitrag zur Frage der Absteppung von Ulcus-kranken Magenteilen durch die Naht nach Sattler.
Deutsche Zeitschr. f. Chir. 201:252-255; y. 1927.

PART III.

CHAPTER XVII.

GASTRO-ENTEROSTOMY.

Definition

The term GASTRO-ENTEROSTOMY consists of three Greek words: γαστήρ, stomach, ἔντερον, bowel and στόμα, mouth. It is an artificial communication between the lumen of the stomach and that of a bowel. If the communication is established between the lumen of the stomach and the duodenum, jejunum, ileum or colon, it is called respectively gastro-duodenostomy, gastro-jejunostomy, gastro-ileostomy and gastro-colostomy. When using the word **gastro-enterostomy** we usually presume that gastro-jejunostomy is done. No one intentionally does a gastro-ileostomy or a gastro-colostomy, yet such procedures have been performed in error.

EVOLUTION OF GASTRO-ENTEROSTOMY.

The first gastro-enterostomy was performed on Sept. 28, 1881, by Anton Wölfler, at that time one of the assistants in the surgical clinic of Prof. Billroth, in Vienna, at the suggestion of Prof. Nicoladoni. Some writers believe that the idea originated with Villar and that Wölfler only first executed it. Wölfler made the anastomosis between the lumen of the stomach and one of the loops of the small bowel. He brought this loop in front of the omentum, the transverse colon, and the gastrocolic ligament, and sutured it to the **anterior** wall of the stomach, performing thus a **gastro-enterostomy antecolica anterior,** or the **anterior gastro-enterostomy.** This operation afforded good drainage for the stomach-contents and was considered a successful operation, thus introducing a new surgical procedure.

There is hardly any operation in the entire field of abdominal surgery, which caused so many controversies as this operation, both from the standpoints of indications and of technic.

Indications

Some surgeons could hardly find any indications for its performance, advocating the use of some other operation, such as gastrectomy, jejunostomy or pyloroplasty.

Another group of surgeons suggested quite a wide field of indications for gastro-jejunostomy and advocated its use in case of:

    1.   Pyloric stenosis.

    2.   Gastric ulcer.

3. Duodenal ulcer.

4. Hour-glass stomach.

5. Perigastritis.

6. Functional disturbances of the stomach.

Let us analyze each of the above enumerated group of indications:

1. **Pyloric stenosis of benign origin** in adults may be treated either by pyloroplasty, pylorectomy or gastro-enterostomy. In the United States, the majority of surgeons are performing gastro-enterostomy, although there is quite a large number who prefer one or another type of pyloroplasty or pylorectomy.

Pyloric stenosis due to malignancy should be treated by pylorectomy, if the case is still mechanically operable, and by gastro-enterostomy in the case in which pylorectomy is **mechanically impossible.**

There are many cases which are inoperable from the **pathological** point of view (metastasis to the liver, etc.), but **mechanically** it is still possible to make a resection (no adhesions to surrounding structures), and for such cases we believe **pylorectomy should be given preference to gastro-jejunostomy.**

2. **Gastric Ulcer.**

The conservative group of surgeons are performing gastro-jejunostomy without excision of the ulcer. The more radical group perform gastro-jejunostomy with excision of the ulcer, and the most radical group prefer to perform a gastrectomy. In the United States, the majority of surgeons are performing a gastro-enterostomy with excision of the ulcer. In Continental Europe, and particularly in Germany, gastrectomy is the operation of choice.

3. **Duodenal Ulcer.**

There is no unanimity of opinion in the handling of the duodenal ulcer. The conservative group of surgeons consider that duodenal ulcer should not be treated surgically at all. **Only when complications arise, such as perforation or hemorrhage, or when the ulcer does not yield to medical treatment employed for a considerable length of time, should one resort to surgery.** The less conservative group (and this, probably, is the majority) perform gastro-enterostomy without excision of the ulcer. The more radical group perform gastro-jejunostomy with excision of the ulcer, and the most radical perform either partial gastrectomy alone, or duodenectomy of the first part of the duodenum in combination with a partial gastrectomy. **The majority of surgeons in the United States are performing gastro-jejunostomy without excision of the duodenal ulcer.**

4. **Hour-glass Stomach.**

In the early days of gastro-jejunostomy many surgeons employed this operation to remedy this gastric condition. Nowadays, the majority prefer to employ a "sleeve resection" of the stomach.

However, in those rare cases in which the hour-glass stomach is adherent to its bed, so that gastrectomy is technically difficult or impossible to perform, it may be necessary to resort either to anterior gastro-enterostomy with an entero-anastomosis **(Wölfler-Braun method)**, or to some type of gastro-plastic operation **(Wölfler or Kammerer type)**.

5. Perigastritis.

Some surgeons still use gastro-jejunostomy for this condition but the more radical group prefer a partial gastrectomy. **Von Eiselsberg and his school believe that jejunostomy is the operation of choice for this condition.** There is still another group of surgeons, who believe that for this condition the treatment should be purely medical.

6. Functional disturbances of the stomach.

At the time when the indications for gastro-enterostomy were numerous, some surgeons advocated the use of gastro-enterostomy for these conditions. Now probably hardly any surgeon would perform gastro-jejunostomy for these ailments.

TECHNIC OF GASTRO-ENTEROSTOMY.

Many different methods of gastro-enterostomy have been suggested. These differ from each other depending on whether the jejunum is sutured to the anterior or to the posterior wall of the stomach, whether the incision in the stomach runs longitudinally, obliquely or transversely, whether it is located immediately above the greater curvature or higher up, leaving a pouch, and whether it lies on the antrum, body or fundus of the stomach.

There are methods in which the loop of jejunum is brought in front of the colon and sutured to the **anterior** wall of the stomach, others in which the jejunum is brought in front of the colon and sutured to the **posterior** stomach-wall, others in which the jejunum is brought behind the colon and sutured to the **posterior** stomach-wall, and others in which the jejunum is brought behind the colon and sutured to the **anterior** stomach-wall.

Some methods were suggested in which the loop of the jejunum was taken very close to the duodeno-jejunal junction, and in others far away (16 to 24 inch.) from this junction. There are methods in which the incision in the jejunum runs parallel to its long axis, and others in which the incision runs perpendicularly to its long axis. Also there are methods in which the jejunum is completely severed in a direction perpendicular to its long axis, and then the distal end of the severed loop is implanted into the stomach and the proximal end into the antimesenteric border of the distal loop.

There are methods in which the gastro-jejunostomy is supplemented either by a lateral intestinal anastomosis between the afferent and efferent loops of the bowel or by a gastrostomy. And, in addition, to all the different methods already mentioned, if we consider that each of them was performed either by a suture method or by the use of a mechanical appliance, and if we remember that these mechanical appliances were numerous such as the Murphy button, the Senn decalcified bone-plates, the Ramaugé aluminum ring, the Abbé catgut plates, the Mayo Robson bobbin, the Penrose soft-rubber plates, the Brockow arteries of an ox, the Dawbarn potato plates, the Baracz turnip plates, etc., we can realize how many methods have been actually described.

In addition to all these methods a number of "aseptic anastomosis" methods have been suggested in which attempts were made not to open the lumen of the stomach or of the bowel at all. And finally, the introduction of the so called "relatively aseptic methods" greatly increased the number of the different methods suggested. However, of all this multitude of methods, **only three or four have stood the test of time and are used to-day and these methods we will describe in detail.**

The large number of gastro-enterostomies suggested can be subdivided into two groups:

A.   Anterior gastro-enterostomy.

B.   Posterior gastro-enterostomy.

A.   Anterior Gastro-enterostomy.

This is characterized by suturing the jejunum to the anterior wall of the stomach.

The subdivisions of anterior gastro-enterostomy are:

1. **The anterior antecolic antiperistaltic gastro-enterostomy (Gastro-enterostomia antecolica anterior antiperistaltica—the original Wőlfler method).**

In this variety, the jejunum is brought to the stomach in front of the transverse colon and placed in such a manner that its peristalsis runs in the direction opposite to the peristalsis of the stomach. This variety is now very seldom used.

2. **The anterior antecolic iso-peristaltic gastro-enterostomy (Gastro-enterostomia antecolica anterior isoperistaltica—t h e Wőlfler-Lűcke-Rockwitz method).**

This is characterized by placing the loop of the jejunum in front of the transverse colon on the anterior wall of the stomach in such a manner that the peristalsis of the stomach and of the jejunum move in the same direction. This variety is used now quite extensively in all cases in which anterior gastro-enterostomy is performed in combination with entero-anastomosis (**Wőlfler-Braun method**).

3. **Anterior retrocolic gastro-enterostomy (Gastro-enterostomia retrocolica anterior—the Billroth-Brenner-Brammann method).**

This is characterized by making an opening in the transverse meso-colon and another in the gastrocolic ligament and bringing the loop of the jejunum through both openings and suturing it to the anterior wall of the stomach.

In this manner, the jejunum will not compress the colon anteriorly and produce symptoms of low colonic obstruction. **This method is obsolete now.** However, in the pioneer days of gastro-enterostomy it was used quite frequently.

4. Gastro-enterostomia antecolica anterior by the "Y method" (the second method of Wőlfler; Roux method).

This is characterized by a transverse division of the jejunum, and an implantation of the distal open end of the jejunum into the stomach and of the proximal end of the severed jejunum into the lateral border of the distal loop of the jejunum.

This method eliminates the occurrence of a regurgitant vomitus but introduces a new complication more frequently than any other method, namely, the formation of a gastro-jejunal ulcer.

This method was first suggested by Wőlfler, but commonly it is known as the Roux "Y method". It is seldom used now by any surgeon, but in the pioneer days of gastro-enterostomy it was used quite frequently.

5. Gastro-enterostomia antecolica anterior by the Chaput method.

This method is characterized by a transverse division of a loop of the jejunum each end of which is closed blindly, then by making a lateral anastomosis between the stomach and the distal portion of the divided jejunum, and then by making a lateral intestinal anastomosis between the proximal and the distal loops of the divided jejunum.

The object of this operation was to prevent the possibility of regurgitant vomitus and to obviate the more difficult technic of making an end-to-side anastomosis. **This operation is obsolete.**

6. Anterior antecolic gastro-enterostomy with an entero-anastomosis (Wőlfler-Braun method).

This method consists in making an anterior gastro-jejunostomy and in supplementing this at the same sitting by a lateral intestinal anas-tomosis between the afferent and efferent loops of the bowel.

The object of this method is to obviate the possibility of a regurgitant vomitus, since should the food pass from the stomach into the afferent loop, it will then change its direction and enter the efferent loop as soon as it reaches the stoma between the two loops of the bowel (Fig. 209).

This method, namely, the Wőlfler-Braun method, is the best operative procedure in all cases in which anterior gastro-enterostomy is indicated, and is considered as the standard operation.

B. **Posterior Gastro-enterostomy (Gastro-enterostomia posterior).**

This is characterized by suturing the jejunum to the **posterior wall** of the stomach. The subdivisions of posterior gastro-enterostomy are:

1. **Posterior retrocolic gastro-enterostomy (Gastro-enterostomia retrocolica posterior—Courvoisier method).**

This method is characterized by making one opening in the transverse mesocolon and another in the gastro-colic ligament, and by bringing the loop of the jejunum through both openings and suturing it to the posterior wall of the stomach.

Courvoisier, indeed, is the originator of the posterior gastro-enterostomy.

This method is obsolete.

2. **Posterior retrocolic gastro-enterostomy (Gastro-enterostomia retrocolica posterior—Von Hacker method).**

This method is characterized by making an opening in the transverse mesocolon, then by pushing the posterior wall of the stomach through this opening into the general peritoneal cavity, and then by suturing a loop of the jejunum to this protruded posterior wall of the stomach.

In this method the gastro-colic ligament is left intact.

3. **Gastro-enterostomia retrocolica posterior with a very short jejunal loop (Petersen method) and with the incision on the stomach running either in an oblique direction (Mayo method) or in a vertical direction (Moynihan method).**

Posterior gastro-jejunostomy is done now by nearly all surgeons by this method.

In order to understand the stimuli which moved the surgeons to search for new methods and for improvements of the old ones, let us analyze the complications which arose from time to time after the performance of a gastro-enterostomy. These complications were:

1. Surgical shock.
2. Peritonitis.
3. Hemorrhage.
4. Inanition.
5. Regurgitant vomitus ("Vicious circle").
6. Post-operative gastro-jejunal ulcer.
7. Internal strangulation of the bowel:
     a. Due to the non-closed slit of the transverse mesocolon.
     b. Due to the suturing of the slit of the mesocolon to the jejunum or to the anastomotic line.
8. Retrograde intussusception into the stoma.
9. Formation of a gastro-jejuno-colic fistula.
10. Gastro-enterostomy disease.

1. Shock.

This was the most frequent cause of death in the pioneer days of gastro-enterostomy. Nearly fifty per cent. of all cases of death were due to shock following the operation.

The main reason for this was that the patients were operated upon when they were already in a bad condition. Another reason was that the technic was very crude. The handling of the tissues was not gentle [in order to find a high jejunal loop, nearly the entire length of the small bowel was handled]. The pre-operative management consisted, among other things, in the administration of a great number of cathartics, thus increasing the further dehydration of the patients. With the improvement in the surgical technic and in the pre-operative preparation of the patients this cause of death became practically *nil*.

2. **Peritonitis** was second in frequency as a cause of death. Nearly twenty five per cent. of all deaths were attributed to this cause. Undoubtedly, the percentage of death due to peritonitis was much higher, since in many cases in which the death was attributed to shock peritonitis was also present. It is not to be wondered at that peritonitis was of such frequent occurrence. At that time antiseptic methods were in vogue, the greatest importance being laid on the use of the phenol-spray for the prevention of infection. The importance of using strictly sterile instruments and sponges was not yet appreciated. The stomach- or intestinal-clamps were used infrequently, and the escape of the gastro-intestinal contents was, therefore, quite frequent. The importance of "walling off" the opened stomach and bowel from the peritoneal cavity was not yet appreciated and, therefore, the contamination of the abdominal cavity by the escaped contents was of common occurrence.

But with the advent of the "aseptic period" in surgery, which replaced Listerism, with the introduction of the stomach- and intestinal-clamp, thus minimizing the possibility of escape of the gastro-intestinal contents, the possibility of peritonitis was greatly diminished. **Barker, in 1886, and Lauenstein, in 1888, still further minimized the possibility of contamination of the peritoneal cavity by introducing a simple technical device, namely, by making a seromuscular suture between the stomach and the bowel before the lumina of these viscera were opened.** Finally, the "walling off" of the exposed stomach and of the selected loop of jejunum from the rest of the peritoneal cavity still further minimized the occurrence of peritonitis, **so that now peritonitis very seldom occurs.**

3. Hemorrhage.

Hemorrhage to-day is of infrequent occurrence. If it occurs, it may come:

a. From the suture-line of the anastomosis.

b. From the gastric or duodenal ulcer which was not removed.

c. From the mucosa of the stomach.

a. The most frequent cause of hemorrhage is bleeding from the suture-line of the anastomosis. The reason for this is that not all the blood-vessels were ligated or caught by the suture. This, especially, may occur when each individual blood-vessel is not ligated separately but is caught in the continuous suture which penetrates either the mucosa or the entire thickness of the stomach.

This condition may be remedied in two ways: Either the surgeon ligates the blood-vessels with a threaded needle, penetrating the mucosa after the seromuscular layer is incised (Haberer), or he releases the clamps holding the stomach before the mucosa is sutured and then clamps each bleeding vessel individually (Enderlen).

b. Bleeding from a gastric or duodenal ulcer which was not resected when the gastro-enterostomy was performed has been recorded by some surgeons. However, it is rather an infrequent occurrence.

c. Bleeding from the mucosa has been reported several times. Some surgeons blamed the use of stomach-clamps applied on the stomach while the gastro-enterostomy was performed. It occurred, however, just as frequently in cases in which clamps were not used and, therefore, **the clamps cannot be blamed for this condition.** Some believe that it is due to the change in the mutual relationship between the intragastric and intra-abdominal pressure (Spasokukotzki).

4. **Inanition.**

In the early days of gastro-intestinal surgery, the surgeons did not know how to find one of the upper loops of the jejunum and, for this reason, they sutured to the stomach any loop which they considered as an upper jejunal loop. Consequently, errors were very frequent, and cases were reported, even by the most eminent surgeons, in which the autopsy revealed that the stomach was sutured either to a lower loop of the ileum or even to the transverse colon. In such cases, the greater portion of the small bowel was eliminated from participation in the digestive action of the alimentary tract, and the patients, after recovering surgically, succumbed in a short time (two to three months) with symptoms of starvation.

This demonstrated very conclusively the necessity of elaborating a method of locating one of the upper loops of the jejunum.

Different methods of doing this were suggested, but they were not reliable until A. Wölfler advised searching for the **duodeno-jejunal plica.** The method which he suggested is employed with slight modification to-day. (The description of this method can be read in Chapter III, under the name "Wölfler-Socin rule".)

This obviated the occurrence of inanition. The surgeons would usually use a loop of the bowel 16 to 24 inches away from the duodeno-jejunal junction, bring it in front of the transverse colon, and suture it to the anterior stomach-wall. However, occasionally, difficulties were encountered.

In some cases, the mesojejunum was very short, and it was either difficult or even impossible to bring the jejunum in front of the transverse colon. Cases were described in which the jejunum compressed the colon and produced intestinal obstruction. In other cases the suture-line between the stomach and the jejunum was under so great a tension that it gave away, thus producing a fatal peritonitis.

It was a stroke of genius when Courvoisier, in 1883, suggested over-coming this difficulty **by making one opening in the transverse meso-colon and another in the gastrocolic ligament, and by bringing a loop of the jejunum behind the colon into the lesser peritoneal cavity and from there again into the general peritoneal cavity, and by then suturing the loop of the jejunum to the posterior wall of the stomach.**

In this manner it became possible to make an anastomosis between the stomach and a loop of the jejunum irrespective of whether its mesentery was long or short. **Thus, Courvoisier is the originator of the posterior gastro-enterostomy.**

The operation, however, did not appeal to the surgeons, until Von Hacker, in 1885, introduced two essential improvements in the Courvoisier method. He made a longitudinal slit in the transverse mesocolon, instead of the transverse slit which was used by Courvoisier with a possible injury to the important branches of the middle colic artery. He showed that it was not necessary to cut the gastrocolic ligament, but that the **posterior wall of the stomach can be pushed down from the lesser into the greater peritoneal cavity, and thus the anastomosis can be accomplished below the transverse mesocolon.**

This method, namely, the **Von Hacker's variety of posterior gastro-enterostomy,** was generally accepted by the profession, and it began to compete successfully with the older method, anterior gastro-enter-ostomy.

While this method was frequently used, facts were accumulating which showed that it should be preferred to anterior gastro-enterostomy, so that **finally it replaced anterior gastro-enterostomy and has now become the operation of choice.**

These facts will be discussed more fully when another complication of gastro-enterostomy, namely the regurgitant vomiting ("vicious circle"), is analyzed.

5. **The Vicious Circle.**

This term was coined by Mikulicz.

This was one of the most dreaded complications of gastro-enterostomy. It was not as frequent a complication as some others. However, it took more time to learn how to overcome this than many other complications of gastro-enterostomy.

The first incidence of a "vicious circle" occurred in the second case of gastro-enterostomy performed on a patient operated upon by Billroth.

According to the rapidity of its clinical manifestations it is differentiated thus:

a. Acute Vicious Circle.

It is this type of uncontrollable vomiting which, if not relieved surgically, leads to death in a few days.

b. Chronic Vicious Circle.

This term was coined by Finsterer. To this group belong the cases in which the vicious circle lasts for months.

c. Late Vicious Circle.

This term was coined by Brunzel. It is applied to those cases of vicious circle in which the symptoms appear for the first time many months or even years after the gastro-enterostomy was performed.

As mentioned above, the term "vicious circle", was coined by Mikulicz. He thought that there was only one way for its formation, namely, that the food passed through the stomach into the afferent loop, then passed backward into the jejunum, duodenum, pylorus, and then into the stomach, then again from the stomach into the afferent loop of the jejunum, duodenum, and so on. He also considered another possibility, namely, that the food passed from the stomach through the pylorus, duodenum, afferent loop of the jejunum into the stomach, then again through the pylorus, and so forth.

This explanation is correct for some cases. However, in many cases the persistent vomiting occurred even when the pylorus was cut transversely and both severed ends were closed entirely. This showed that the term "vicious circle", is not correct, and that the name "regurgitant vomitus", which is used in English-speaking countries, is more appropriate. **Evidently, there is not a single cause which produces the regurgitant vomitus.** Many other causes, according to investigators, are responsible for this condition, namely:

A. Spur-formation.

Some surgeons consider this as one of the causes of vicious circle. Different technical errors may produce a spur:

a. A short length of the suture-line between the stomach and the jejunum. Under such circumstances, both ends of the intestine hang vertically down. Thus, a spur may be formed. The size of this spur may be increased by traction of the mesentery. In order to remedy the abrupt hanging down of the jejunum, Hadra, in 1891, advised suturing the jejunum to the wall of the stomach on each side of the gastro-jejunal opening by a seromuscular suture.

b. Improper site for the suture.

If the portion of the jejunal wall lying very close to its mesenteric border is utilized for anastomosis with the stomach, then the possibility of a spur-formation at the site of the anastomosis is increased. For this reason, it is considered best to make the seromuscular suture one-sixth of an inch away toward the inner side of the antimesenteric border, to make the incision leading into the bowel on the antimesenteric border, and to make the anterior seromuscular suture-line one-sixth of an inch lateral to the antimesenteric border.

The correction of these faults, **however, did not eliminate the occurrence of regurgitant vomiting.**

This proves that if spur-formation may be the cause of regurgitant vomiting in some cases, there are, however, many other causes which may produce it.

B.   Some believed that placing the stomach and a loop of the jejunum in an antiperistaltic direction may produce regurgitant vomiting, and for this reason advised placing them in the isoperistaltic direction (**Wőlfler-Lűcke-Rockwitz method**).

C.   Recently, it was suggested by Kasper Blond that the cause of vicious circle in many cases is a temporary spasm of the stoma. This theory has many followers.

D.   However, the majority of surgeons believe that technical errors may be the predisposing factor, and that the deciding factor is **that the food is entering the afferent instead of the efferent loop.** For this reason, many ingenuous methods have been devised to prevent the passage of the food from the stomach into the afferent loop. It must be admitted that probably, the greatest help in this direction is afforded by nature itself, namely by the peristaltic movements of the bowel, which produce a suction-action into the efferent loop and thus, so to speak, invite the passing of the food from the stomach into this loop.

This is the reason why, in spite of the fact that so many technical errors are made, the food usually passes into the efferent loop, and cases of regurgitant vomiting are rare compared to the great number of gastro-enterostomies performed.

However, in order to diminish the possibility of the food passing in the wrong direction, many surgeons tried to constrict the afferent loop. Thus Wőlfler, in 1883, placed a circular purse-string around the mouth of the afferent loop and moderately constricted its lumen.

Von Hacker, in 1892, narrowed the mouth of the afferent loop in a manner similar to that of Wőlfler with the difference only that instead of making a purse-string, as Wőlfler did, he introduced a few interrupted sutures, thus producing folds of mucosa which projected into the lumen of the afferent loop thereby diminishing it.

T. Kocher, in 1894, suggested the following method: A loop of jejunum was placed transversely on the lowermost portion of the stomach. In this manner the afferent loop of the jejunum lay behind the efferent loop. A seromuscular suture was made between the stomach and the efferent loop of the jejunum. Then an incision was made through the entire thickness of the stomach-wall and of the wall of the efferent loop of the jejunum [on the jejunum the length of the incision was about half of the circumference of the bowel] and the lips were sutured together. Thus, an anastomosis was made between the stomach and the efferent loop of the jejunum.

The objection to all these methods of constricting the afferent loop is that if the narrowing is not considerable, the food can still pass into the lumen of the afferent loop. If the lumen is markedly constricted, it prevents a free flow of the bile and pancreatic juice from the afferent into the efferent loop.

A decisive step forward in the prevention of the development of regurgitant vomiting was the **method of Doyen:**

An opening was made in the gastrocolic ligament, and the great omentum was carried through this into the bursa omentalis. The transverse colon was then sutured to the anterior wall of the stomach immediately above the greater curvature. Then, one of the proximal jejunal loops was sutured to the anterior wall of the stomach by a seromuscular suture for a length of 10 to 12 cm. in an oblique direction, so that the proximal portion of the loop was placed higher than the distal portion. Then, an anastomosis was made between the stomach and the sutured loop of the jejunum for a length of four cm. The openings in the stomach and in the jejunum were placed in the center of the sutured seromuscular line. **In this manner, the afferent loop lay higher than the efferent loop.**

In order to diminish still further the possibility of food passing into the proximal loop of the jejunum, the latter was constricted by inserting a few Lembert sutures, so that longitudinal mucous folds were formed, which diminished the lumen of the afferent loop of the jejunum.

Thus, Doyen initiated the idea of making an ascending and a descending loop rather than a right and a left loop, an idea, which was further developed later by Czerny and his school (Petersen), and which ultimately made regurgitant vomiting a rare occurrence.

Lauenstein, in 1891, proposed supplementing anterior gastro-enterostomy by an entero-anastomosis between the afferent loop of the jejunum and **any other** jejunal loop situated distal to the gastro-jejunal stoma.

This supplementary entero-anastomosis prevents the occurrence of regurgitant vomitus, since in case the food passed into the afferent instead of the efferent loop it meets in its further advancement the stoma between these two loops. Then it changes its direction, and instead of passing further in the afferent loop against the peristaltic waves, passes into the efferent loop where its passage is facilitated by the isoperistaltic movements of this loop.

Jaboulay, in 1892, suggested supplementing gastro-enterostomy by a duodeno-jejunostomy, making a lateral intestinal anastomosis between the duodenum and the efferent loop of the jejunum a few inches away from the gastro-jejunal stoma.

The idea is the same as that of Lauenstein. Its advantage over the method of Lauenstein is that in the latter method of entero-anastomosis, the loop of the bowel used for this purpose could be at a considerable distance from the gastro-jejunal stoma, and thus an intestinal exclusion of a loop of a bowel of a considerable length might be produced.

Braun, in 1893, suggested making the entero-anastomosis between the two jejunal loops at a distance of about four inches away from the gastro-jejunal stoma (Fig. 209).

The suggestion of Lauenstein passed nearly unnoticed. However, the method of Jaboulay and that of Braun attracted the attention of the profession, and surgeons began to use them, at first, merely as a supplementary operation only for such cases in which after completion of the gastro-enterostomy symptoms of vicious circle appeared. Later, instead of doing Braun's entero-anastomosis as a re-operation, **it became a routine procedure to make the entero-anastomosis a regular step in every case of anterior gastro-enterostomy (Wőlfler-Braun method).**

This supplementary step, namely Braun's entero-anastomosis **is the most frequently employed method in cases in which anterior gastro-enterostomy is performed.** However, several other methods have been proposed in order to avoid the occurrence of the regurgitant vomitus.

Thus, Wőlfler suggested cutting a loop of the jejunum transversely and implanting the distal end of the severed loop into the anterior wall of the stomach, and the open end of the proximal loop into the lateral side of the distal loop.

This suggestion was carried out by Roux and is known as "Roux's Y gastro-enterostomy". Another name for this method is **"The second method of Wőlfler".**

Chaput utilized this idea in the following manner: A loop of the jejunum was cut transversely and both ends were closed blindly. Then, a lateral anastomosis was made between the stomach and the distal loop, and another lateral anastomosis between the proximal and the distal loops of the jejunum.

Witzel suggested his method: An anterior gastro-enterostomy was performed and this was supplemented by a Witzel type of gastrostomy. A rubber tube was passed then through the gastrostomy channel into the lumen of the stomach and then farther on through the stoma into the efferent loop. The patient was fed through the rubber tube, which assured the passage of the food into the efferent loop. After a few days the rubber tube was removed. This method is called **"gastro-enterostomy with a gastrostomy"** ("gastro-enterostomia cum gastrostomia").

Sonnenburg suggested, in 1894, the following method:

An incision was made along the free border of the jejunum for a distance of two and-one-half to three inches. Hemorrhage from the lips of this incision was checked by buttonhole-sutures which penetrated the entire thickness of the jejunal wall.

Another incision was made on the stomach the length of which was slightly less than that on the jejunum, and the lips of this incision were also sutured by buttonhole sutures: The ends of the thread were left long in at least three places. Then another incision was made about two cm. distal from the first incision on the jejunum, the length of which was about one-half of an inch. The ends of the thread left long on the stomach were introduced into the lumen of the jejunum through the large jejunal opening and then brought outside through the smaller jejunal opening. The threads were drawn tight, so that the stomach around its opening was wedged into the lumen of the efferent loop of the jejunum. A sero-muscular suture was made between the stomach and the jejunal wall surrounding the larger jejunal-opening. The ends of the thread from the stomach protruding through the smaller jejunal opening were cut short, and this opening was closed in the usual manner.

Thus, the stomach was wedged into the efferent loop of the jejunum, thereby making impossible the escape of food into the proximal jejunal loop.

In 1900, Walter Petersen, assistant in the surgical clinic of Prof. Czerny, at Heidelberg, gave his explanation of the causes of regurgitant vomiting. This was, in fact, the expression of thought of his master, Czerny, in Germany, and of Doyen, in France. He showed that regurgitant vomiting occurred just as frequently in the operation of posterior as of anterior gastro-enterostomy. **Regurgitant vomiting was a rare occurrence only in those clinics in which the usual operation was a posterior gastro-enterostomy with a very short loop.** Since usually the duodeno-jejunal junction lies at a higher level than the most dependent portion of the stomach, and since the stoma of the gastro-enterostomy is usually situated on the most dependent part of the stomach, the afferent loop always has an ascending direction and the efferent loop a descending direction from the stoma. Food will pass according to the law of gravity into the efferent loop.

In the case of an anterior gastro-enterostomy, the afferent loop should always be a long one, otherwise, it will compress the colon and produce an intestinal obstruction. If a long loop is taken, then there will be no ascending or descending loop, but a right and a left loop. The food will have a tendency to pass into the efferent loop, but if any, even the slightest, obstruction of the efferent loop occurs, the food will pass through the stoma into the afferent loop which may become distended and compress the efferent loop, and thus produce symptoms of regurgitant vomiting.

This makes it clear that since a short loop is an essential condition for the elimination of a vicious circle, and since a short loop can be used only in the case of a posterior gastro-enterostomy, **the posterior gastro-enterostomy should be the operation of choice.**

To recapitulate:

To obviate the occurrence of the regurgitant vomiting it is necessary to fulfil the following requirements:

   a. The **posterior** gastro-enterostomy should be the operation of choice.
   b. The stoma should be placed as **low as possible,** so that it will lie lower than the duodeno-jejunal junction.
   c. The loop should be taken as **close as possible** to the duodeno-jejunal junction without undue tension. Then, the afferent loop will be the ascending and the efferent the descending loop.
   d. All other technical errors, such as spur-formation should be eliminated.

As an indirect, but quite a convincing, proof of the correctness of the belief of the importance of having a short loop, is the fact that since surgeons began to use this **"short or no loop method"**, the occurrence of vicious circle has become very rare.

Although the introduction of a very short loop eliminated nearly entirely the occurrence of the regurgitant vomiting, this does not prove that the vomiting is due to the formation of an ascending and a descending loop. We believe that by the usual method of performing a posterior gastro-enterostomy with a short loop, it is impossible to make an ascending and a descending loop. Evidently something else occurs which actually eliminates the possibility of the regurgitant vomiting.

However, there are cases in which it is impossible to perform a posterior gastro-enterostomy. These occasions are:

   a. A very short transverse mesocolon.
   b. A very vascular transverse mesocolon so that it is impossible to find an avascular area of sufficient size.
   c. A very thickened transverse mesocolon, so that it is difficult to see the exact arrangement and distribution of the blood-vessels.
   d. Adhesions between the posterior wall of the stomach and the posterior abdominal wall, so that it is difficult to deliver the posterior gastric wall into the greater peritoneal cavity.
   e. Pathological changes of the posterior stomach-wall which makes it unsuitable for a gastro-intestinal anastomosis.

Under such conditions, it is necessary to perform an anterior gastro-enterostomy, which means that a long loop of jejunum should be taken, and hence there is a possibility of the development of the symptoms of regurgitant vomiting. In order to exclude this possibility several methods were proposed, the details of which have been described above and the best of which is the Wölfler-Braun method.

Thus, we may recapitulate:

Of all the methods of gastro-enterostomy, posterior gastro-enterostomy by a short or no-loop method is the operation of choice.

If this cannot be done, then **an anterior gastro-enterostomy with entero-anastomosis (Wölfler-Braun method)** should be performed.

6. **Post-operative gastro-jejunal ulcer.**—This complication occurs from time to time. The first case was reported, in 1897, by Berg. Denk, in 1920, collected from the literature to that date, 309 cases. This complication is usually observed in the first six months after the gastro-enterostomy was performed. Some estimate this incidence as low as two per cent. and others as high as thirty per cent. On the average, the occurrence is about four per cent.

In some cases this complication is the result of faulty technic, being due to careless suturing of the mucosa, so that the acid gastric contents pour onto the muscularis, thus producing ulcers.

However, in many instances this complication is due to the unsatisfactory selection of cases. In persons living the "high tension" life, and in neurotics whose medical treatment did not relieve them, this complication is more frequently met with than in the asthenic, phlegmatic type of patients.

In the last few years, Kasper Blond suggested a theory the essence of which is that in the neurotic or the "sthenic" type of people very frequently a spasm of the stomach involving the gastro-jejunal stoma occurs after a gastro-enterostomy has been performed, thus compressing either the gastric lip or the jejunal lip of the stoma. This produces a temporary ischemia of the lips, and they become then easy victims of the digestive action of the gastric juice with an ensuing gastro-jejunal peptic ulcer.

Many investigators believe in the correctness of this theory, and they advise the prescribing of tincture of belladonna for this type of patient for a short time after the gastro-enterostomy has been performed.

7. **Internal strangulation of the bowel.**—This was one of the earliest complications following the performance of posterior gastro-jejunostomy.

Von Hacker suggested, as early as 1885, the elimination of this complication by suturing the stomach to the edge of the opening in the transverse mesocolon before performing the gastro-jejunostomy.

This original maneuvre of Von Hacker was later changed by many surgeons who performed the gastro-enterostomy first and then sutured the edges of the opening in the transverse mesocolon to the wall of the stomach.

Lewis L. McArthur modified this method by suturing first the posterior wall of the stomach to the lower edge of the opening in the transverse mesocolon, then performing the posterior gastro-enterostomy, and then suturing the anterior edge of the opening in the mesocolon to the posterior wall of the stomach. **We consider this procedure the best.**

Some surgeons advocated suturing the edges of the mesocolon to the jejunum. In this manner the gastro-jejunal suture-line was thrown into the lesser peritoneal cavity. Others sutured the posterior wall of the stomach to the lips of the mesocolon at a distance of one-fourth of an inch away from the edges of the mesocolon, and then sutured these edges to the jejunum, thus peritonizing the gastro-jejunal suture-line.

The last two methods are unsafe, since cases have been recorded in which adhesions have been formed and extended from the edges of the transverse mesocolon, compressing the soft wall of the jejunum and producing an intestinal obstruction. The same adhesions, if they should compress the strong stomach-wall, would not be able to produce an obstruction.

8. **Retrograde intussusception of the small bowel through the stoma into the stomach, or progressive intussusception of the stomach into the jejunum through the stoma.**

The first case of retrograde intussusception was published by Steber, in 1917. Since that time up to-date more than thirty such cases have been reported There is no doubt that many cases that were diagnosed as an acute form of vicious circle actually were cases of invagination which occurred a few days after the operation was performed. Many cases of "chronic vicious circle" were actually cases of invagination which would from time to time spontaneously reduce, then re-appear, etc. This group of symptoms occurs after either anterior or posterior gastro-enterostomy has been performed. It has occurred as early as the sixth post-operative day and as late as 15½ years after the operation. The average time for the appearance of this condition is seven years.

The **symptoms** of this condition are those of a high intestinal obstruction. A bloody vomiting together with symptoms of a high intestinal obstruction, and a history of a previously performed gastro-enterostomy, make the diagnosis highly probable.

The etiological factors producing this condition are not clear. In the last few years many believe in the correctness of the theory suggested by Kasper Blond, namely, that this condition, as also the origin of the gastro-jejunal peptic ulcer, is due to temporary spasm of the jejunum.

The operative treatment of this condition is described in the last part of this chapter.

All cases of invagination through the gastro-jejunal stoma can be subdivided into two classes:

> **a. Ascending** invagination.
> **b. Descending** invagination.

a. The ascending invagination is the variety in which the jejunum enters into the lumen of the stomach; the majority of cases described are of this variety. The variations of this type which have been observed are:

> 1. Invagination of the afferent loop.
> 2. Invagination of the efferent loop.
> 3. Invagination of both afferent and efferent loops.

b. Descending invagination is the variety in which the stomach is invaginated into one of the jejunal loops. There are also two varieties of this form:

> 1. Invagination of the stomach into the afferent loop.
> 2. Invagination of the stomach into the efferent loop.

9. The gastro-jejuno-colic fistula.—The first who observed and operated for a gastro-jejuno-colic fistula was Kaufmann. Brock, in 1924, was able to report 216 cases of gastro-colic fistula, 91 of which were of a post-operative origin. The diagnosis of this condition is easily established, both clinically and roentgenologically. The treatment of this condition is purely surgical.

The operative management may be:

a. Conservative.

This consists in the disengagement of the stoma and closure of the stomach, the wall of the colon and of the jejunal-wall (if the jejunum is involved).

b. Radical.

This consists in resection of the fistula, including a part of the stomach-wall, and a portion of the colon and of the afferent and efferent loops of the jejunum (if the jejunum was involved).

10. Gastro-enterostomy disease.

Many surgeons, particularly of Continental Europe, have described a condition following gastro-enterostomy which is characterized by a variety of symptoms, of which one or another may be predominant in the individual patient. These symptoms consist of pain in the epigastric region, regurgitant vomiting (mostly of bilous contents), and belching.

There is no doubt that several other pathological conditions have appeared as sequelæ of gastro-enterostomy, such as peptic gastro-jejunal ulcer, regurgitant vomiting, retrograde invagination of the jejunum through the stoma into the stomach, spasm of the stoma (which includes the stomach-wall and the loops of the jejunum, either the afferent or the efferent or both of them), have been confused with gastro-enterostomy disease. Nevertheless, if all cases due to the above mentioned causes be excluded, there still are left a number of cases which exhibit the above enumerated symptoms and in which on re-operation no changes are found in the stoma.

These cases are cured by a mere **degastro-enterostomy.** They usually occur in patients upon whom gastro-enterostomy should not have been performed at all (such as cases of functional disorders of the stomach, or cases in which the surgeon expected to find a gastric or a duodenal ulcer, and not finding this, made a "prophylactic gastro-enterostomy"). **The presence of gastro-enterostomy disease in the greatest majority of cases is not a sign of poor surgical technic but of an improper indication for a gastro-enterostomy.**

However, some investigators (Pribram) believe that even if the indications for gastro-enterostomy were correct and the ulcers healed, the patient may develop "gastro-enterostomy disease" if the pylorus remains patent. In this fact they see the reason why a gastro-enterostomy should not be employed for the treatment of gastric or duodenal ulcer, instead of which they advocate the performing of a partial gastrectomy.

SITE OF THE STOMA.

In the early days of gastro-enterostomy there were numerous discussions as to where the stoma should be placed, whether on the body or on the antrum of the stomach.

Investigations carried out by Georg Kelling, in 1900, and which were confirmed later by several other investigators, showed that if the stoma is placed on the body of the stomach, the flow of the contents through the stoma is continuous, whereas, if it is placed in the antrum, the flow is intermittent.

Since the chief indication for the performance of a gastro-enterostomy is to secure a good drainage of the gastric contents, it is evident, that it is better to place the stoma at a point where the drainage will be continuous and where the stomach will make no great effort to evacuate the food. **For this reason the stoma should be placed on the body of the stomach.** As a rule, **it should be placed on the healthy portion of the wall of the stomach and always proximal to the site of the ulcer.**

HOW FAR FROM THE CURVATURES SHOULD THE STOMA BE PLACED?

There were numerous discussions as to whether the stoma should be placed closer to the lesser or to the greater curvature. The majority of surgeons agree that it should be placed as close to the greater curvature as is possible, since it then affords the best drainage with but little effort.

This gives the stomach more rest than if the stoma is placed higher up, and rest of the stomach will accelerate the healing of the ulcers.

On the bowel, the opening should be made on the anti-mesenteric border. (This suggestion was first made by Hahn.)

However, some surgeons believe that the opening of the bowel should be placed somewhat closer to the mesenteric border.

WHAT SHOULD BE THE LENGTH OF THE INCISION ON THE STOMACH AND ON THE JEJUNUM?

There have been different opinions as to this. Some consider that it should be as long as four inches and some as short as one and a-half inches. In order to facilitate the passage of the contents of the stomach into the bowel, the size of the **exit** from the stomach should be equal to the size of the **entrance** into the bowel. The size of the **entrance** into the bowel is represented by the size of the diameter of an upper jejunal loop, namely it is about one and a-half inches. However, the opening of the stomach should be larger than one and a-half inches, since the mouth of the afferent loop is also connected with the opening in the stomach. On deciding on the size of the incision on the stomach it should also be considered that the newly formed stoma has a tendency to contract. For these reasons, it seems advisable **to make the length of the stoma between two-and-a-half and three inches.**

HOW SHOULD THE STOMACH AND JEJUNUM BE PLACED—IN THE ISOPERISTALTIC OR IN THE ANTIPERISTALTIC DIRECTION?

This is quite a debatable subject even today. Some surgeons consider that the stomach and the loop of the jejunum should be placed in an iso-peristaltic direction. Others consider that they should be placed in an antiperistaltic direction. Many consider it immaterial in whch way they are placed. Wőlfler, in his first operation, placed them in an antiperistaltic direction, and later on, due to frequent occurrences of the vicious circle, he suggested placing them in an isoperistaltic direction, and this method is known, as already mentioned, as the **Wőlfler-Lűcke-Rockwitz method.**

It seems to us that in the case of an anterior gastro-enterostomy it is immaterial whether the stomach and the jejunum are placed in an iso-peristaltic or in an antiperistaltic direction for the following reasons:

The works of Halsted, Mall and many other investigators on **reverse peristalsis** showed conclusively that the peristaltic waves do not depend on the continuity of the segments of the bowels, but that they do depend on the intrinsic nervous apparatus located in the wall of the bowel itself.

Therefore, no matter how the jejunum may be placed in relation to the stomach, the movement of the food going into the **efferent** loop will always be facilitated by peristaltic movements, and in the **afferent** loop will always be hindered by antiperistaltic waves. **The main thing is to place the jejunum in relation to the stomach in such a manner as to secure the passage of the food from the stomach into the efferent loop and not into the afferent loop.**

How to accomplish this has already been discussed and will again be presented under the "Technic of anterior gastro-enterostomy" and of the "Technic of posterior gastro-enterostomy."

However, in performing anterior gastro-enterostomy we believe that it is best to place the stomach and jejunal loop in the isoperistaltic direction **(Wőlfler-Lücke-Rockwitz method)** not because the placing of the bowel will influence in one or another way the possibility of regurgitant vomiting, but because it eliminates an unnecessary twist of the jejunal loop.

In performing a posterior gastro-enterostomy, the distal end of the loop of the jejunum is attached to a point of the stomach on the greater curvature, and the proximal end of the loop is attached on the posterior wall of the stomach closer to the lesser curvature. The exact course of the jejunum-loop differs somewhat depending on which method is employed. However, we wish to state that in the most commonly used methods, such as **Mayo's or Moynihan's, the loop does not lie either in the iso- or in the antiperistaltic direction in relation to the stomach.**

WHICH INSTRUMENTS SHOULD BE USED FOR DIVIDING THE TISSUES, A KNIFE, SCISSORS OR THE THERMOCAUTERY?

As long ago as 1900, Georg Kelling proved experimentally that the incisions made by a knife afford the fastest healing, next were those made by scissors, and that the slowest healing follows incisions made by the thermocautery. Since that time these results have been corroborated by many other investigators.

WHAT SUTURE MATERIAL SHOULD BE USED FOR GASTRO-ENTEROSTOMY?

There are no unanimous views on this subject. Some surgeons use a soluble material only, such as plain or chromic catgut, for all the layers of the stomach and bowel. Others use only insoluble material, such as silk or the Pagenstecher celloidin linen-thread. **In our work, we use the Pagenstecher linen for suturing the serous or seromuscular layers, and plain or chromic catgut for suturing the mucosa or the entire thickness of the stomach or intestinal wall.**

IN HOW MANY LAYERS SHOULD THE STOMACH BE SUTURED TO THE BOWEL?

The oldest method consisted in sewing the lips of the stomach-opening and that of the jejunum by an over-and-over suture which was not reinforced by any other layer of sutures. However, very soon this method was replaced by suturing in two tiers, the first, an over-and-over and the second, a seromuscular suture.

This method has stood the test of time and should be considered as a good method of suturing.

However, in recent years some experimentators have shown that the **firmest union chiefly depends on a strict approximation of similar layers (serosa to serosa, muscularis to muscularis, and mucosa to mucosa).**

For this reason we believe it is better **in cases of gastro-enterostomy to use three layers in preference to two layers, since in all cases in which suturing of the stomach is involved exact approximation of the mucosa is of paramount importance.**

We will describe in detail the technic of posterior gastro-enterostomy with a short or "no-loop" **(Von Hacker-Petersen-Mayo method)** and of anterior gastro-enterostomy with an entero-anastomosis **(Wőlfler-Braun method).**

The other methods will not be described in detail. Those who are familiar with these two methods will have no difficulty in acquiring the technic of the other methods.

I. POSTERIOR GASTRO-ENTEROSTOMY.

(Von Hacker-Petersen-Mayo method).

Step 1. The abdomen is opened by:

    a. A paramedian left rectus incision, or

    b. A transverse left transrectus incision.

Step 2. The transverse colon with the omentum are grasped by the left hand and drawn upward. This brings the transverse colon outside of the abdominal cavity and places the transverse mesocolon on the stretch. The first loop of the jejunum is then located in the manner described in Chapter III under the "Wőlfler-Socin method" (Fig. 199). A segment of the jejunum, the length of which is four inches and which starts three or four inches away from the duodeno-jejunal junction, is grasped (Fig. 200). The contents of this segment are "milked out" and the loop is compressed axially by an intestinal clamp, tight enough to prevent the escape of intestinal contents when the bowel is opened, but not tight enough to shut off the blood-supply to that part of the bowel which forms the fold (Fig. 201). **The clamp is placed so that the blades are directed to the left shoulder and the handles to the right hip-joint.**

Step 3. An opening is made in the transverse mesocolon, the direction of which is perpendicular to the long axis of the transverse colon. This incision is made to the left of the main stem of the middle colic artery in the space which is rather poor in blood-supply and which is surrounded by the left branch of the middle colic artery and by the ascending branch of the left colic artery ("arteria magna Riolani") (Fig. 201). This "avascular area" is most suitable for the incision in the mesocolon. The incision is made in the following manner: A portion of the mesocolon in the "avascular area" is grasped by an Allis forceps, and half an inch away from the first forceps another Allis forceps grasps the transverse mesocolon, which is cut between the two forceps by scissors. The incision is continued upward by the scissors and downward by the knife. [Care should be taken

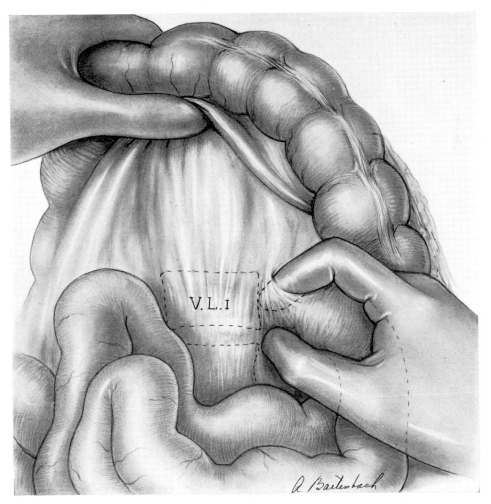

FIG. 199. POSTERIOR GASTRO-ENTEROSTOMY.
Location of the first jejunal loop by the Wölfler-Socin method.

not to cut the "arteria magna Riolani" when cutting the mesocolon upward and not to reach the base of the transverse mesocolon when cutting downward, in order to avoid injuring the branches of the superior mesenteric artery.]

Step 4. The tip of the little finger of the surgeon's left hand is placed on the anterior wall of the stomach on a vertical line drawn downward from the right side of the cardia to the greater curvature at a distance of about one and one-half inches above this curvature. The tips of the rest of the bent fingers of the surgeon's left hand are placed on the anterior wall of the stomach in such a manner that the index-finger will rest on the greater curvature and will be approximately two and a half inches to the

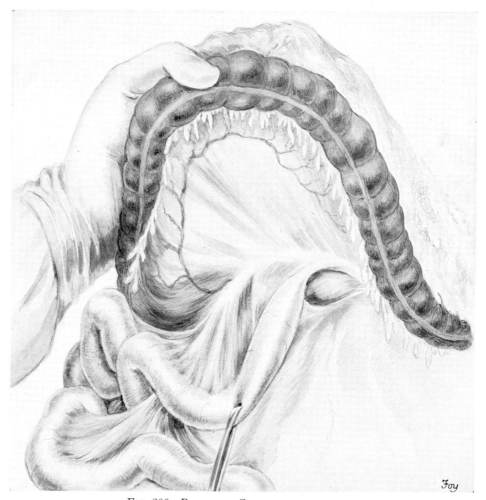

FIG. 200. POSTERIOR GASTRO-ENTEROSTOMY.
A loop of jejunum is grasped at a distance of four inches from the
duodeno-jejunal junction.

left from the vertical line extending from the right side of the cardia downward (Fig. 202). With the bent fingers of the left hand the stomach is pushed downward through the opening in the transverse mesocolon. In this manner the posterior wall of the stomach is protruded into the general peritoneal cavity, and is grasped by two Allis forceps at two points, one corresponding to the point on the posterior wall which is pushed by the index-finger, and the other by the little finger of the surgeon's left hand. Thus, two Allis forceps grasp the ends of the contemplated line of incision (Fig. 202). The posterior half of the edge of the opening in the transverse mesocolon is sutured to the stomach by interrupted or continuous sutures, which penetrate the seromuscular layer only. In case of interrupted

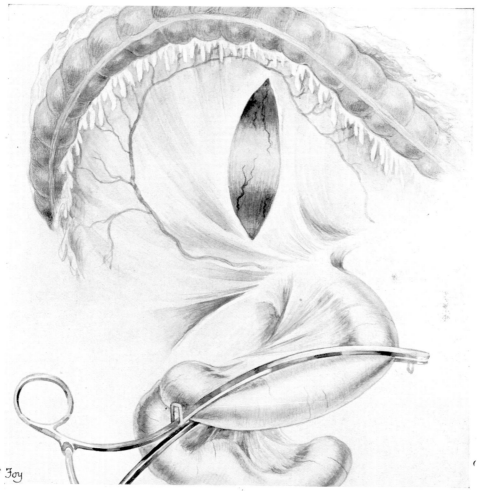

FIG. 201. POSTERIOR GASTRO-ENTEROSTOMY.
A loop of the jejunum is clamped axially; a slit is made in the transverse mesocolon.

sutures, each stitch should be at a distance of half an inch from the next one. Approximately six or seven sutures will be inserted (Fig. 203). [It is more convenient to do this suturing of the posterior part of the mesocolon to the stomach at this stage of the operation than after the gastro-enterostomy is completed. This was first suggested by L. L. McArthur.] A stomach-clamp is now placed on the stomach-fold in such a manner that the tips of the blades will be directed toward the right hip-joint and the handles toward the left shoulder-joint (Fig. 204). **Then the clamp holding the jejunal fold is turned in such a manner that the handles are directed toward the left shoulder-joint and the blades toward the right hip-joint.** Thus, the stomach and the jejunal clamps are laid side-by-side. The handles of both

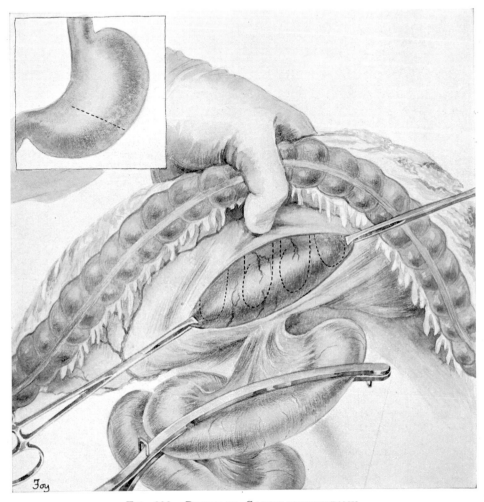

FIG. 202. POSTERIOR GASTRO-ENTEROSTOMY.
The posterior wall of the stomach protrudes into the greater peritoneal cavity.

clamps are directed now to the left shoulder-joint and the tips of the blades to the right hip-joint (Fig. 204). [As may be seen, the handles will lie on the assistant's side and the blades on the surgeon's side. This is an important technical point, since the assistant holds the clamps, and it is more convenient for him to hold its handles on his side than to lean over the body of the patient and hold it on the surgeon's side.] Another point worthy of notice is, that **the highest point of the stomach-incision is sutured to the proximal end of the jejunum, and the lowermost point of this incision is sutured to the distal end of the jejunum.** Also note that the direction of the incision on the stomach will exactly tally with the normal position of the first loop of the jejunum. The majority of surgeons inter-

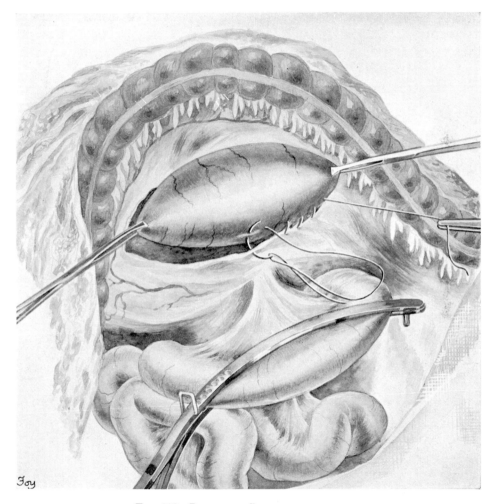

FIG. 203. POSTERIOR GASTRO-ENTEROSTOMY.
Suturing the posterior wall of the stomach to the posterior lip of the transverse mesocolon.

pret this mutual position of the stomach and jejunum as anti-peristaltic. **We believe, however, that it is neither anti- nor iso-peristaltic, since the incision on the stomach is made perpendicularly to the direction of its peristaltic waves.**

Step 5. The adjoining blades are attached to each other by an artery-clamp, grasping the rubber tubing which covers the blades. Laparotomy sponges are laid around the clamps so as to "wall off" the operative field from the rest of the peritoneal cavity. **In this manner, the instruments are covered with laparotomy sponges and only two folds, that of the stom-**

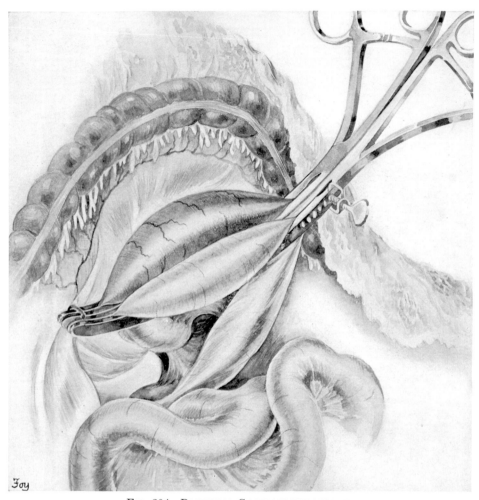

FIG. 204. POSTERIOR GASTRO-ENTEROSTOMY.
The folds of the stomach and of the jejunum are laid side by side. The tips of the blades are directed to the right hip-joint.

ach and of the jejunum are left exposed. [In our work we use the Lane clamp, which is shown on the pictures.]

Step 6. A continuous sero-serous suture with a straight needle is made between the folds of the stomach and the jejunum (**Dupuytren** or **Cushing type**). It starts from the assistant's and runs to the surgeon's side (Fig. 205, upper half). The short end of the thread is clamped by a

straight artery-forceps of the Kocher type and is placed under a towel
[no instruments should be left uncovered]. If the Dupuytren type of suture
is selected, the direction of the needle should always be from the surgeon's
right to his left hand. Each third stitch is locked, or, still better, a back-
stitch is made after each three ordinary stitches. As soon as the sero-
serous suture-line is completed for the length of about three inches, the

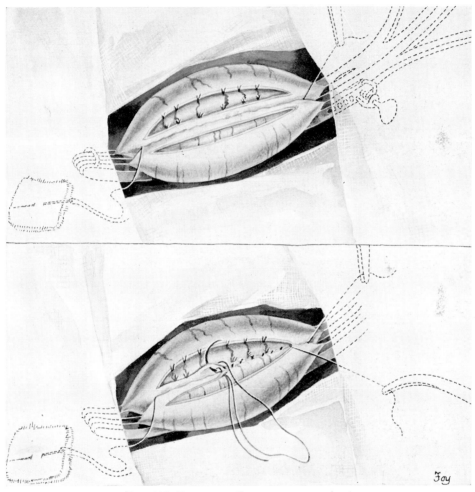

FIG. 205. POSTERIOR GASTRO-ENTEROSTOMY.
UPPER HALF. Sero-serous suture is inserted; a seromuscular incision is made.
LOWER HALF. Suturing the seromuscular lips to each other.

last stitch is then locked, or a last back-stitch is made, and the straight
needle is then inserted into a piece of gauze (so that it will not be lost)
and is placed with the gauze under a towel on the surgeon's side. **By adopt-
ing this technic, no instruments, needles or threads are left exposed. Everything except the two folds of the viscera are covered with towels. It is**

also worthy of note, that the beginning of the sero-serous suture is clamped with a straight forceps and the end of it is threaded on a straight neeedle.

Step 7. The seromuscular layers of the jejunum and stomach are now incised. On the jejunum, the incision should be at a distance of about one-eighth of an inch, and on the stomach, of about one-fourth of an inch

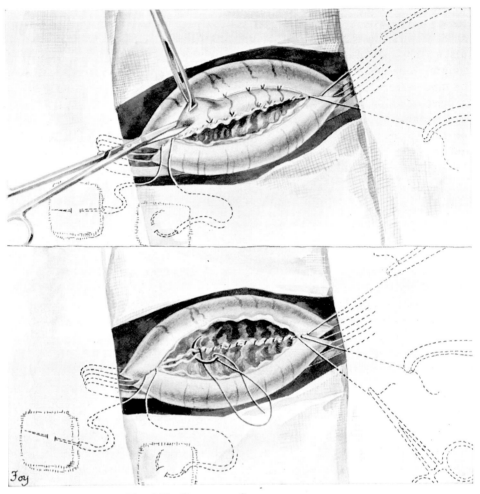

FIG. 206. POSTERIOR GASTRO-ENTEROSTOMY.

UPPER HALF. The lumen of the jejunum is opened; the scissors are in position to cut the mucosa of the stomach.

LOWER HALF. Suturing the mucosa of the posterior lips to each other.

from the suture-line (Fig. 205, upper half). [The reason for making the seromuscular incision on the stomach farther from the suture-line than on the jejunum is, that the seromuscular layer of the stomach contracts much more than does that of the jejunum.] **The incision is made on the jejunum by the right hand and on the stomach by the left hand. In this**

way the surgeon does not have to change the position of his body. All the blood-vessels running in the mucosa are ligated at symmetrical points (Fig. 205, upper half). Thus, the occurrence of a post-operative hemorrhage is greatly minimized (Haberer). Another continuous row of sutures which unites the seromuscular lips is now begun. It is made with a **curved** needle and starts also from the assistant's side and runs toward the surgeon's side (Fig. 205, lower half). The short end of this thread is clamped by a **curved** artery-forceps and is laid under the towel on the assistant's side. When the seromuscular suture-line reaches the surgeon's side, the last stitch is locked (and, of course, each third stitch should be locked while making this seromuscular suture-line or, still better, a back-stitch should be made after each three ordinary stitches). The needle is then inserted on a piece of gauze and is laid under a towel on the surgeon's side (Fig. 206, upper half). **Thus, we will have so far, the straight artery-forceps lying on the assistant's side attached to the thread which made the sero-serous suture, and the curved artery-forceps, lying on the assistant's side, attached to the thread which made the seromuscular-seromuscular suture.**

Step 8. The mucosa on the jejunum is opened by a knife, held in the right hand, slightly lateral to the line of the previously made seromuscular incision, because the mucous lip should be slightly wider than the seromuscular lip. On the stomach, it is not advisable to cut by the knife, since the mucosa is very tough and if the knife is not sharp as a razor (and that is usually the case) it slides between the seromuscular and the mucous layer and does not cut through the mucosa. The mucosa of the stomach is opened in the following manner: It is grasped by an Allis forceps and drawn up so that a cone is formed which is snipped with scissors (Fig. 206, upper half). The lumen of the stomach is thus opened. The mucosa is then cut by scissors, and care should be taken to make the mucous lip wider than the previously made seromuscular lip. The reason for this is that the mucosa has a great tendency to contract, and if cut on the same plane as the sero-muscular layer, it will contract to such an extent that it will retract beyond the seromuscular lip, and in suturing the mucosa of the stomach to the mucosa of the jejunum the line of suture will be under a great tension. **The length of the incision in the mucosa should be slightly shorter than that of the seromuscular incision.** The suturing of the mucosa starts from the assistant's side (Fig. 206, lower half). The thread is clamped by a mosquito artery-forceps, which is placed under the towel. Then an over-and-over mucosa-mucosa suture is made, taking each bite one-eighth of an inch from the other. Each third stitch is locked, or a back stitch is made after each three ordinary stitches. When the suture-line is completed in its entire circumference, the thread on the needle is tied to the beginning of the same thread which was clamped by the mosquito-forceps on the assistant's side, and the ends are cut short. The curved needle on the surgeon's side is then grasped and suturing of the anterior seromuscular lip is continued until it is entirely sutured anteriorly (Fig. 207, upper half). Then it is tied to the short end of the thread, which was clamped with a curved clamp on the assistant's side and the ends are cut short. The straight needle on the surgeon's side is then taken, and the serosa-serosa suture of the anterior lip is continued until the assistant's side is reached (Fig. 207, lower half). The threaded needle is

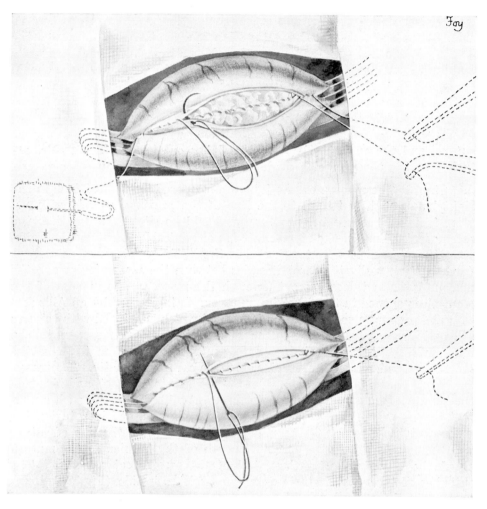

FIG. 207. POSTERIOR GASTRO-ENTEROSTOMY.
UPPER HALF. The mucosa is sutured; suturing of the muscular lips begun.
LOWER HALF. Suturing of the serosa.

then tied to the short end of the assistant's side and the ends are cut short. [The clamps are removed from the bowel and the stomach-fold, either after completion of the mucosa-mucosa suturing or after the serosa is sutured to the serosa.]

Step 9. The edges of the anterior half of the transverse mesocolon are sutured to the stomach by a continuous suture or by several interrupted sutures which penetrate the seromuscular layer of the stomach only (Fig. 208). If interrupted sutures are used, they lie at a distance of half an inch from each other and at about one-fourth of an inch away from the suture-

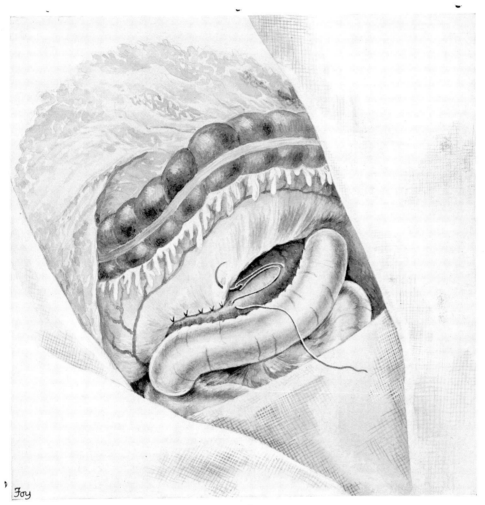

FIG. 208. POSTERIOR GASTRO-ENTEROSTOMY.
Suturing the edge of the transverse mesocolon to the stomach-wall.

line. Six to seven such sutures are usually required on the anterior half of the transverse mesocolon.

When the stomach drops back after completion of the operation, the anastomosed loop of the jejunum will acquire its original position, that is, the position which it held before the gastro-enterostomy was performed.

II. ANTERIOR GASTRO-ENTEROSTOMY WITH ENTERO-ANASTOMOSIS.

(Wőlfler-Braun Method) (Fig. 209).

Step 1. The abdomen is opened in the same manner as Step 1 of "Posterior Gastro-enterostomy".

Step 2. The first loop of the jejunum is located according to the

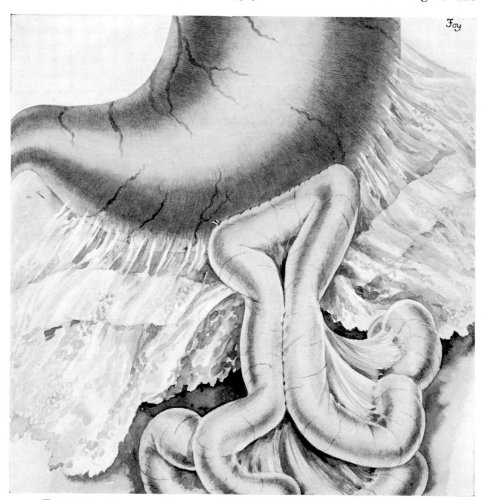

FIG. 209. ANTERIOR GASTRO-ENTEROSTOMY WITH ENTERO-ANASTOMOSIS.
Wőlfler-Braun method.

Wőlfler-Socin method, and is grasped at a distance of 16 to 24 inches away from the duodeno-jejunal junction. Its contents are "milked out", and a fold four inches long is clamped axially by an intestinal clamp, strong enough to prevent the escape of the intestinal contents when the bowel is opened, but not enough to shut off the blood supply to that part of the bowel which constitutes the fold. **The clamp is applied in such a manner that the handles lie to the left of the patient, that is, on the assistant's side.**

Step 3. A fold of the anterior wall of the stomach, the length of which is four inches, is grasped by a stomach-clamp very close to and parallel with its greater curvature. **This fold should be on the body of the stomach, not on the antrum. This clamp also is placed in such a manner that the handles lie to the left of the patient, that is, on the assistant's side.**

Step 4. Both clamps are laid side-by-side in such a manner that the handles lie on the assistant's side and the tips of the blades on the surgeon's side. [This is an important technical point, since it is more convenient for the assistant to hold the handles lying on his side than to lean over the body of the patient and hold them on the surgeon's side.] As may be seen, **in this method of placing the clamps, the stomach and the loop of the jejunum lie in an iso-peristaltic direction (Wőlfler-Lűcke-Rockwitz method).**

Step 5. As Step 5 in "Posterior Gastro-enterostomy".

Step 6. As Step 6 in "Posterior Gastro-enterostomy" (Fig. 205).

Step 7. As Step 7 in "Posterior Gastro-enterostomy" (Fig. 206).

Step 8. As Step 8 in "Posterior Gastro-enterostomy" (Fig. 207).

Step 9. Two folds of the jejunum are grasped each starting four inches away from the gastro-jejunal stoma, and one of which is on the afferent and the other on the efferent loop. The length of each fold is four inches. The contents of the loops are "milked out", and each fold is then clamped by an intestinal clamp. A lateral intestinal anastomosis connecting these two folds is made precisely in the same manner as described in the Chapter "Lateral Intestinal Anastomosis".

Steps 1 to 8 constitute Wőlfler's anterior gastro-enterostomy, and Step 9 constitutes **Braun's entero-anastomosis,** and is used to prevent the occurrence of regurgitant vomiting.

III. GASTRO-ENTEROSTOMY WITH A TRANSVERSE JEJUNAL INCISION.

This operation was first performed by Socin, and in recent times the interest in it has been revived by Moise, who elaborated the technic of its performance.

Step 1. The abdomen is opened.

Step 2. The first loop of the jejunum is located by the Wőlfler-Socin method. At a distance of 4 to 5 inches from the duodeno-jejunal junction two crushing-clamps are placed on the jejunum perpendicularly to its long axis and embracing only two-thirds of its circumference. The clamps lie very close to each other (Fig. 210). The bowel is cut between the clamps. Thus, but two-thirds of the circumference of the bowel are divided. The clamps are laid away from each other in opposite directions (Fig. 211).

Step 3. An opening in the transverse mesocolon is made precisely as in Step 3 of "Posterior gastro-enterostomy".

Step 4. The posterior wall of the stomach is pushed down through the opening in the transverse mesocolon, and a fold of it is grasped by an Allis forceps at each end. The posterior lip of the transverse mesocolon is sutured to the gastric fold.

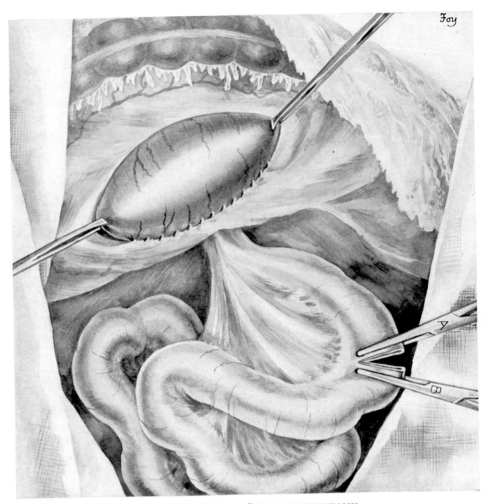

FIG. 210. POSTERIOR GASTRO-ENTEROSTOMY.
(Socin-Moise method).
The jejunum is cut transversely between two clamps for two-thirds of its circumference.

Step 5. A seromuscular suture is made between the stomach and the bowel (Fig. 211).

Step 6. An intestinal clamp is placed on the two limbs of the bowel at a distance of about six inches below the open portion of the bowel

(Fig. 211). The crushed part of the wall of the bowel is cut off by making an incision beneath the blades of the two crushing-clamps (Fig. 211).

Step 7. An opening is made through the entire thickness of the stomach-wall. The anastomosis is completed in the usual manner (Fig. 212).

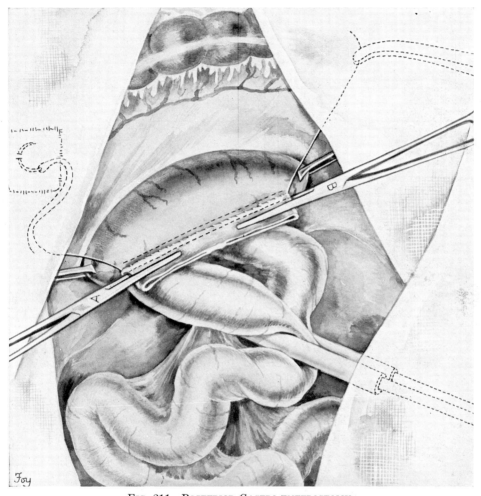

FIG. 211. POSTERIOR GASTRO-ENTEROSTOMY.
(Socin-Moise method).
A seromuscular suture connects the posterior wall of the stomach with the jejunum.

Step 8. The edges of the slit in the mesocolon are sutured to the stomach as described in Step 9 of posterior gastro-jejunostomy.

IV. SCHIASSI METHOD OF GASTRO-ENTEROSTOMY WITH SECTION OF THE VAGI AND SYMPATHETIC NERVES.

This operation consists of the following steps:

a.   Division of the terminal branches of the right and left vagi nerves of the stomach.

b.   Division of the sympathetic fibers which take their origin from the celiac plexus.

c.   Performance of a posterior gastro-enterostomy.

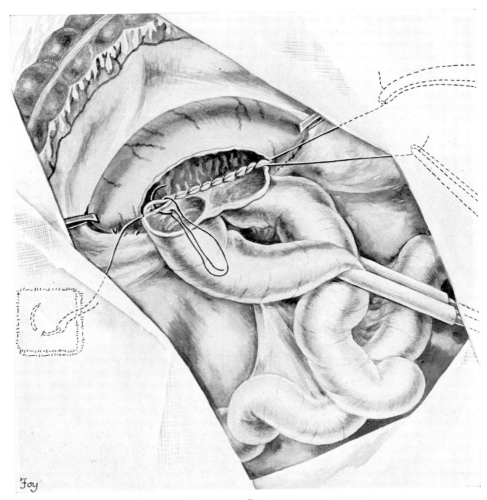

FIG. 212. POSTERIOR GASTRO-ENTEROSTOMY.
(SOCIN-MOISE METHOD).
Suturing the posterior wall of the stomach to that of the jejunum.

The reason for performing **a** and **b** is to prevent the transmission of any psychic irritations to the duodenum after the gastro-enterostomy has been performed. This operation is indicated for the surgical treatment of **gastric and duodenal ulcer, particularly the latter.**

Step 1. The abdomen is opened.

Step 2. The gastro-hepatic ligament is divided for a length of two inches along a line which runs parallel to and one-third of an inch above the margin of the lesser curvature (Fig. 213). The vertical portion of the pyloric artery serves as a landmark for this incision, since the gastro-hepatic ligament is cut one inch to the left and one inch to the right of the

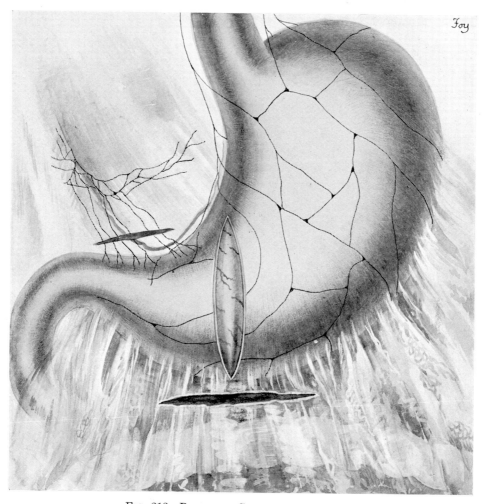

FIG. 213. POSTERIOR GASTRO-ENTEROSTOMY.
Supplemented by section of nn. vagi and sympathici (Schiassi method).
(Schiassi, Annals of Surgery, Vol. 81). (See text).

artery, which is in the meantime ligated. [N.B. This incision cuts the six sympathetic filaments which run from the celiac sympathetic plexus to the pylorus and the first part of the duodenum.] The lips of the divided gastro-hepatic ligament are sutured.

Step 3. The gastro-colic ligament is cut for a length of two inches in that portion which connects the antrum with the transverse colon (Fig. 213). The posterior wall of the antrum is turned anteriorly, and a seromuscular incision is made on the posterior wall of the stomach starting at the angular notch above and reaching the great curvature below. The incised seromuscular layer is sutured by several interrupted sutures or by a continuous suture (Fig. 214).

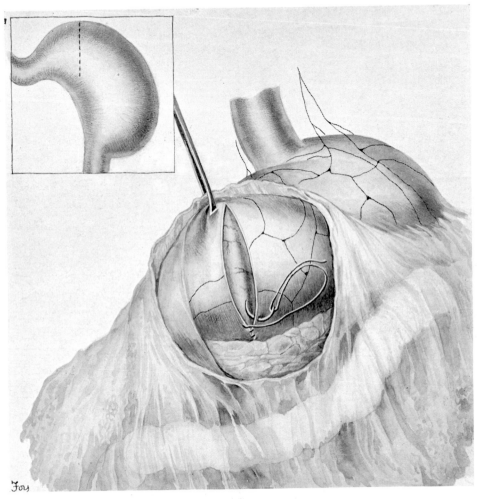

FIG. 214. POSTERIOR GASTRO-ENTEROSTOMY.
Supplemented by section of nn. vagi and sympathici (Schiassi method).

Step 4. The stomach is returned to its original position, and the opening in the gastro-colic ligament is closed by a few interrupted sutures.

Step 5. A seromuscular vertical incision is made on the anterior gastric wall extending from the angular notch of the lesser curvature to the great curvature and corresponding to the vertical incision on the posterior wall (Fig. 213). The lips of the seromuscular incision are sutured by a few interrupted sutures or by a continuous suture (Fig. 215). These two vertical incisions cut the branches of the right and left vagus nerves.

Step 6. A posterior gastro-enterostomy is now performed. The final view will be as in Fig. 215.

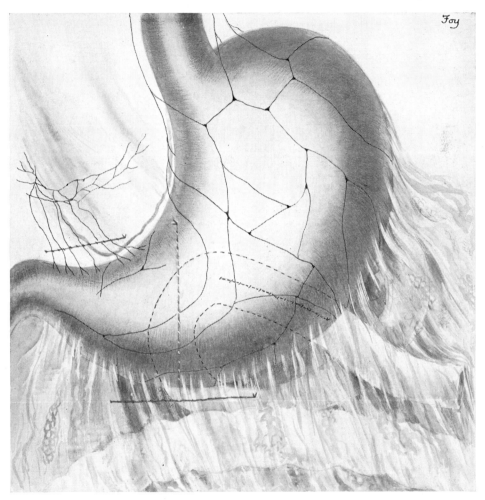

FIG. 215. POSTERIOR GASTRO-ENTEROSTOMY.
Supplemented by section of nn. vagi and sympathici (Schiassi method).

V. DEGASTRO-ENTEROSTOMY.

This consists in undoing a previously made gastro-enterostomy opening.

Indications.

1. **Gastro-jejunal peptic ulcer,** not yielding to medical treatment.

2.   **Gastro-jejuno-colic fistula.**

3.   **Gastro-enterostomy disease.**

The technic of this operation is as follows:

Step 1. The omentum with the transverse colon are lifted by the left hand, thus putting the transverse mesocolon on the stretch.

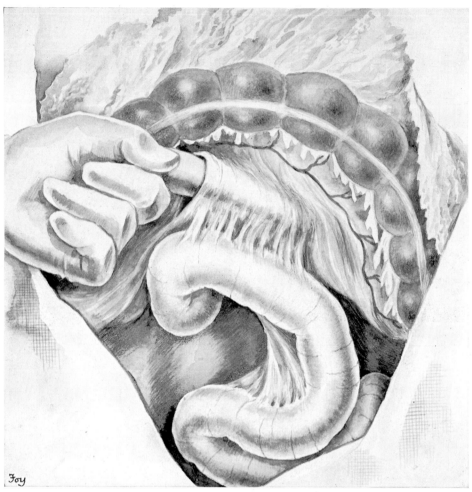

FIG. 216. DEGASTRO-ENTEROSTOMY.
Separation of the mesocolon from the stomach by the index-finger.

Step 2. The mesocolon is cut at any convenient place at a distance of about one-fourth of an inch from the suture-line between it and the stomach. [Care should be taken not to cut large branches of the middle colic artery.] The left index-finger is then introduced into the opening thus made, and under its guidance the mesocolon is gently separated from the stomach for its entire circumference (Fig. 216).

Step 3. The jejunal loop is caught and pulled down. This brings further down a portion of the posterior wall of the stomach. The contents of each jejunal loop adjoining the stoma are "milked out", and an intestinal clamp is placed transversely on each of these jejunal loops, on the proximal, just a little away from the duodeno-jejunal junction, and on

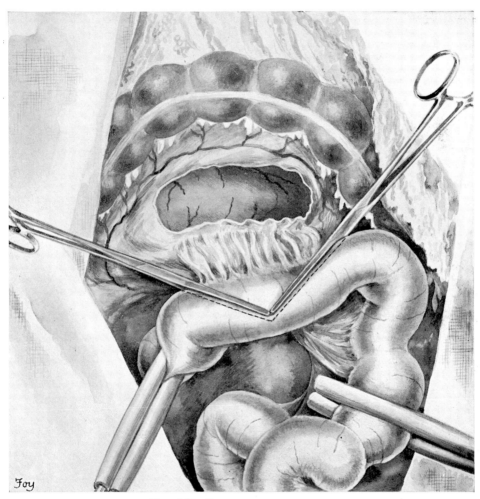

FIG. 217. DEGASTRO-ENTEROSTOMY.
Two crushing clamps are placed on the jejunum; the proximal and distal jejunal loops are clamped by two intestinal clamps.

the distal, about five inches away from the stoma (Fig. 217). Two Kocher or Ochsner clamps are then placed on the jejunum, one on each loop in such a manner that the tips of the blades look downward and inward. The tips should meet each other, and each tip should reach a point midway between the mesenteric and the free border of the jejunal loop which is attached to the stomach (Fig. 217).

Step 4. The jejunum is cut immediately distal to each clamp (Fig. 218). In this manner, the opening connecting the stomach with the jejunum is closed by the clamps, thus preventing the escape of the stomach-contents. The jejunal opening is now closed in a transverse direction (Fig. 219).

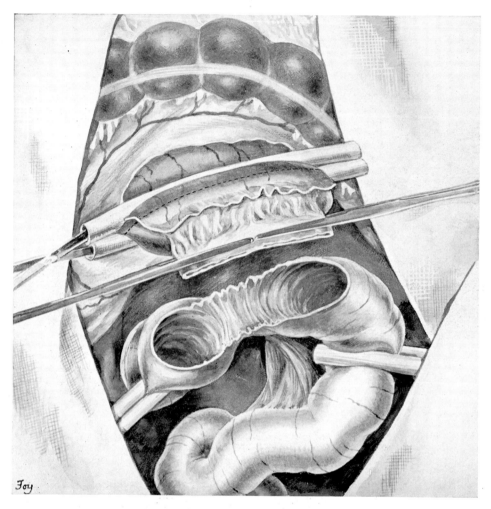

FIG. 218. DEGASTRO-ENTEROSTOMY.
The opening into the stomach is closed by two crushing clamps thus preventing escape of the stomach-contents.

Step 5. The ulcerated portion of the stomach is excised and this opening is then closed (Fig. 219).

Step 6. The opening in the mesocolon is closed.

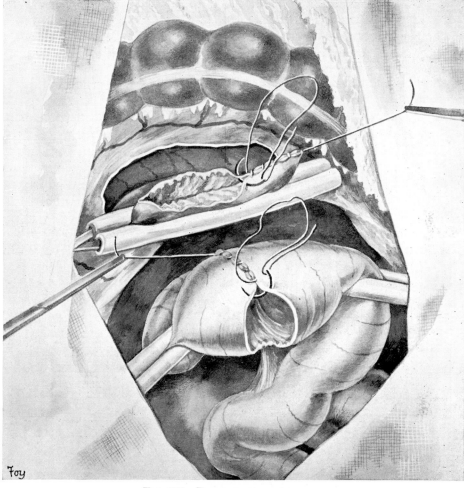

FIG. 219. DEGASTRO-ENTEROSTOMY.
Closure of the jejunal and gastric openings.

VI. REDUCTION OF A RETROGRADE INVAGINATION OF THE JEJUNUM INTO THE STOMACH.

Step 1. The abdomen is opened.

Step 2. The jejunum is pulled downward until the reduction is complete. If, however, the invagination is not corrected by this maneuver, then:

Step 3. An incision in the anterior wall of the stomach is made, and the left index-finger is introduced into its lumen. The invaginated portion of the bowel is pushed downward by the finger of the left hand, and with the right hand the jejunum is pulled downward until the reduction is accomplished.

Step 4. The opening in the anterior wall of the stomach is closed.

Hardly any supplementary procedures are required for preventing a future occurrence of invagination, since records from the literature show that only once has re-invagination taken place.

ASEPTIC METHODS OF GASTRO-ENTEROSTOMY.

All that has been said about the different "aseptic methods" of intestinal anastomosis in Chapter VII may be repeated here. For this reason, we refer the reader to the historical part of Chapter VII. However, we would like to emphasize here only a few points:

1. "The **ideal** aseptic methods," such as Postnikow's, Bastianelli's and Boari's, should never be used either in intestinal or in gastro-intestinal anastomosis on account of possible complications, such as failure of making an opening either in the stomach or in the jejunum, or in both.

2. The "**relatively** aseptic methods", such as are performed by using "basting-suture methods" or "closed clamps methods", are excellent for intestinal suturing only, particularly when the large bowel is involved in the suturing, **but should never be used in stomach work,** since in these methods **the mucosa of the stomach is not sutured to the mucosa of the bowel,** and this may readily produce a postoperative jejunal ulcer. This as a rule, is worse than the original gastric or duodenal ulcer for the relief of which the original operation was performed. For this reason, we may say that **"aseptic methods" are contraindicated in all surgery in which suturing of the stomach is involved.**

BIBLIOGRAPHY.

A. Angerer. Invagination nach Gastroenterostomie.
Zbl. f. Chir. 59:1572-1574; y. 1932.

I. Back. A new technique in gastro-jejunostomy.
Lancet, 2:802-803; y. 1933.

D. C. Balfour. The sequelæ of gastro-enterostomy. The indications for disconnecting the anastomosis and the technic of the operation.
Annals of Surgery, 82:421-428; y. 1925.

D. C. Balfour. Results of gastro-enterostomy for ulcer of the duodenum and stomach.
Ann. Surg. 92:558-562; y. 1930.

A. E. Barker. A case of gastro-enterostomy for cancer of the pylorus and stomach: good recovery: a new method of suture.
Brit. Med. Journ. I:292-294; y. 1886.

M. Bass. Experimentelle und klinische Untersuchungen mit einer vereinfachen Methode der De-Gastroenterostomie beim Ulcus pepticum jejuni und der Fistula gastrocolica nach dem Verfahren von Hesse.
Arch. f. klin. Chir. 172:226-239; y. 1932.

C. Bauer. Dauerresultate, Fehler und Gefahren der Gastroenterostomie als Behandlungsmethode und Ulcuskrankheit.
Deutsche Zeitschr. f. Chir. 235:45-57; y. 1932.

C. Beck. Gastro-enterostomy by a plastic flap.
Journ. Am. Med. Ass. 62:909-910; y. 1914.

P. Bernay. La sténose transitoire de la bouche de gastro-entérostomie.
Lyon méd. 152:273-276; y. 1933.

A. D. Bevan. Gastro-enterostomy disease.
Surg. Clin. of North America, 8:469-480; y. 1928.

K. Blond. Die Beziehungen des sogenannten Circulus Vitiosus nach Gastroenteroanastomose zum Ulcus pepticum jejuni postoperativum. Ein Beitrag zur spasmogenen Ulcusgenese.
Arch. für klin. Chir. 135:281-339; y. 1925.

K. Blond. Experimenteller Beitrag zur aufsteigenden Invagination in den operierten Magen.
Arch. f. klin. Chir. 153:53-61; y. 1928.

H. Braun. Über die Gastroenterostomie und gleichzeitig Entero-anastomose. Bericht über die Verhandlungen der Deutschen Gesellschaft für Chirurgie, XXI Kongress.
Beilage zum Zbl. für Chirurgie, p. 102; y. 1892.

A. Brenner. Zur Technik der Gastroenterostomie.
Wien. klinisch. Wchnschr. 5:375-376; y. 1892.

J. E. Briggs & L. R. Whitaker. On electrosurgical method for aseptic gastro-enterostomy.
New England Journ. of Med. 201:6-10; y. 1929.

H. F. Brunzel. Ueber den Spätcirculus nach vorderer Gastroenterostomie.
Deutsch. Zeitschr. f. Chir. 135:555-564; y. 1916.

E. Bundschuh. Ueber den Circulus vitiosus nach Gastroenterostomie.
Bruns Beiträge zur klin. Chir. 119:62-85; y. 1920.

Cannon and Blake. Gastroenterostomy and pyloroplastik.
Annals of Surg. 41:686-711; y. 1905.

Chaput. Étude sur la gastroenterostomie.
Presse méd. 2:225-228; y. 1894.

Chaput. Un nouveau bouton anastomotique pour les opérations intestinales.
Bull. et mém. de Soc. de chir. 21:746-762; y. 1895.

V. Chlumsky. Ueber die Gastroenterostomie.
Bruns Beiträge zur klin. Chir. 20:231-274; and 487-544; y. 1898.

C. S. Collivadino. Resultados alejados de la gastro-enterostomia en las ulceras gastroduodenales.
La Semana méd. I:1088; 1152; 1242; y. 1932.

L. G. Courvoisier. Gastro-enterostomie nach Wölfler bei inoperablem Pyloruscarcinom.
Zbl. f. Chir. 10:794-797; y. 1883.

H. Donovan. Jejunostomy and Witzel's operation in the treatment of vicious circle vomiting.
   Brit. Med. Journ. I:609-610; y. 1932.

E. Doyen. Contribution a l'étude de la chirurgie de l'estomac et de l'intestin.
   Arch provinc. de Chir. I:22-76; y. 1892.

G. Duran. Nota previa sobre una rara dificultad en la busca del ansa anastomotica para gastroenterostomia.
   Med. ibera, I:269-273; y. 1932.

J. L. Faure. Sur un nouveau procédé de gastro-enterostomie: La gastroenterostomie par invagination.
   Congres franç. de chir. Paris, XI:421-431; y. 1897.

A. H. Ferguson. Gastroenterostomy.
   Am. Journ. of Surg. 18:211-219; y. 1905.

R. J. Ferreira. Da sutura suspensiva systhematica da alca afferente do jejuno, como meio seguro para evitar o "Circulus vitiosus" no curso da gastroenterostomia transmesocolica posterior, vertical, inferior o marginal.
   Rev. brasil. de med. e pharm. 6:371-388; y. 1930.

H. Finsterer. Chronischer circulus vitiosus nach Gastroenterostomie.
   Bruns Beitr. z. klin. Chir. 81:341-360; y. 1912.

I. I. Genkin. Gastroenterostomie bei Situs viscerum inversus totalis.
   Deutsch. Zeitschr. f. Chir. 241:124-126; y. 1933.

A. Gridnev. Einige Bemerkungen zur Auswahl der Gastroenterostomiemethoden.
   Zbl. f. Chir. 57:3048-3050; y. 1930.

G. M. Gurewitsch. Über Blutungen nach Gastroenterostomie.
   Arch. f. klin. Chir. 147:518-529; y. 1927.

H. Haberer. Zur Vermeidung von Nachblutungen nach Magenoperationen. Bemerkung zu dem Aufsatz von Flörcken.
   Zbl. f. Chir. 60:2568; y. 1933.

Von Hacker. Zur Casuistik und Statistik der Magenresectionen und Gastroenterostomieen.
   Arch f. klin. Chir. 32:616-625; y. 1885.

Hadra. Discussion in "Freie Vereinigung der Chirurgen Berlin's".
   Deutsche med. Wchnschr. 17:1138; y. 1891.

Hadra. Ueber Gastroenterostomie. (Krankenvorstellung).
   Berl. klin. Wchnschr. 29:75; y. 1892.

J. B. Hall. A new route for posterior gastro-jejunostomy.
   Brit. Med. Journ. II:895-897; y. 1903.

A. Hammesfahr. Die Gastroenterostomie mit Gastrostomie nach Rutkowsky.
   Zbl. f. Chir. 30:601-603; y. 1903.

C. Henschen. Uber die Invaginationen im Bereiche des Magens, insonder-
heit die gastroduodenalen Mageninvaginationen.
Arch. f. klin. Chir. 148:730-790; y. 1927.

E. Hertel. Die Gastroenterostomie und ihre Fehlerquellen.
Bruns Beiträge zur klin. Chir. 142:157-220; y. 1928.

H. Hilarowicz. Zur Frage der sogenannten Degastroenterostomisation.
Zbl. f. Chir. 56:1551-1555; y. 1929.

H. M. Hinrichsen. Über Gastro-Colische Fisteln nach Gastroenterostomie.
Arch. f. klin. Chir. 171:149-156; y. 1932.

Jaboulay. La Gastro-entérostomie. La Jejuno-Duodénostomie. La Résection du Pylore.
Arch. Provinc. de Chir. Paris, I:1-22; y. 1892.

H. Jansen. Einige Bemerkungen zur Degastroenterostomie.
Arch. f. klin. Chir. 151:706-711; y. 1928.

E. L. Jenkinson. Importance of size of stomach and stoma in gastro-
enterostomies.
Journ. Am. Med. Ass. 102:354-357; y. 1924.

C. Johnsen. Magenulcus und Gastroenterostomie.
Zbl. f. Chir. 55:2314-2315; y. 1928.

W. Katz. Die Gastroenterostomia posterior retrocolica verticalis.
Bruns Beitr. zur klin. Chir. 71:672-690; y. 1911.

G. Kelling. Studien zur Chirurgie des Magens.
Arch. für klin. Chir. 62:1-42; y. 1900.

H. Klose & P. Rosenbaum. Beiträge zur Magenchirurgie. Vergleichende
experimentelle Untersuchungen über die Magennähte.
Arch. f. klin. Chir. 124:15-27; y. 1923.

Th. Kocher. Zur Technik und zu den Erfolgen der Magenresection.
Corr.-Bl. f. Schweiz. Aerzte. 23:682-694; 713-724; y. 1893.

F. H. Lahey. Excision of the stoma for Gastro-jejunal ulcer.
Surg. Clin. of North America, 8:35-43; y. 1928.

C. Lauenstein. Zur Anlegung der Magendünndarmfistel.
Zbl. f. Chir. 15:472-475; y. 1888.

C. Lauenstein. Zur Indikation, Anlegung und Funktion der Magendünndarmfistel.
Zbl. für Chir. 18:776-779; y. 1891.

R. Leriche. Considerations générale sur le traitement des ulcères duodeno-
gastriques.
Gaz. d. hôp. 101:1489-1493; y. 1928.

Lindner. Ueber Witzel's Gastroenteroanastomose und Gastrostomose.
Zbl. f. Chir. 27:1112-1113; y. 1900.

P. MacLean. Zur Kenntniss der postoperativen Magen-Kolonfistel.
Bruns Beitr. z. klin. Chir. 155:525-534; y. 1932.

O. Madariaga y H. Madariaga. Gastrectomia vs. Gastroenterostomia.
Vida nueva, 20:185-191; y. 1927.

K. H. Martzloff & G. R. Suckow. Wound healing in anterior gastroenterostomy following various methods of suture; experimental study in dogs.
Arch. of Surg. 26:345-381; y. 1933.

Masnata. Nuovo processo di gastroenterostomia.
Il Policlinico. II:465; y. 1904.

Mattoli. La Gastroenterostomia.
Societ. editric. Dante Alighieri, Rome 1903.

Wm. Mayo. A review of 500 cases of gastro-enterostomy, including pyloroplasty, gastroduodenostomy and gastrojejunostomy.
Annals of Surgery; 42:641-655; y. 1905.

Wm. Mayo. The technique of gastrojejunostomy.
Annals of Surg. 43:537-542; y. 1906.

Theo. McGraw. Upon the use of the elastic ligature in the surgery of the intestine.
Journ. Am. Med. Ass. 16:685-694; y. 1891.

Theo. McGraw. Gastro-enterostomy by the elastic ligature.
New York Med. Journ. 73:132-139; y. 1901.

P. E. McMaster. Effects of diverting gastric contents to the lower intestinal levels.
Arch. of Surg. 28:825-836; y. 1934.

R. W. McNealy & M. E. Lichtenstein. Evolution and present technique of gastrojejunostomy.
Surg. Gyn. & Obst. 60:1003-1015; y. 1935.

T. S. Moise, C. D. Haagensen & E. C. Vogt. A method for gastro-enterostomy with a transverse jejunal incision.
Surg. Gyn. & Obst. 44:824-828; y. 1927.

T. S. Moise. Gastro-enterostomy with transverse jejunal incision; preliminary clinical report.
Surg. Gyn. & Obst. 47:383-392; y. 1928.

A. Monprofit. De la Gastro-entérostomie antérieure en Y.
Arch. prov. de Chir. 12:457-466; y. 1903.

B. Moynihan. The direction of the jejunum in the operation of gastroenterostomy.
Annals of Surg. 47:481-485; y. 1908.

P. Niehans. Aseptische Methode der Gastrojejunostomie und der laterolateralen, termino-terminalen, termino-lateralen Enteroanastomose durch intrainstrumentelle Einkerbung isoperistaltisch aufeinander gequetschter Magen oder Darmteile.
Schweiz. Med. Wochenschr. 57:544-547; y. 1927.

W. Noetzel. Gastroenterostomia retrocolica posterior mit Entero-anastomose zwischen der abführenden Jejunumschlinge und dem Querkolon.
Zbl. fűr Chir. 53:2657-2658; y. 1926.

V. Pauchet. Que faire aux anciens gastro-enterostomisés non guéris?
Clinique, Paris. 23:331-340; y. 1928.

V. Pauchet & P. L'Helias. Anastomose au bistouri diathermique sans
ouverture de la muqueuse en chirurgie gastro-intestinale.
Arch. méd. belges 83:745-747; y. 1930.

V. Pauchet. Indications de la gastro-entérostomie.
Gaz. d. hôp. 104:169 and 323; y. 1931.

V. Pauchet. Ulcus anastomatique.
Tech. chir. 25:257-288; y. 1933.

V. Pauchet. Indications de la gastro-entérostomie.
Tech. chir. 26:81-107; y. 1934.

Perret. Technique d'un procédé nouveau strictement aseptique d'Entero-
anastomose et de Gastro-jejunostomie.
Schweiz. Med. Wchnschr. 57:533-539; y. 1927.

W. Petersen. Anatomische und chirurgische Beiträge zur Gastro-Enterostomie.
Bruns Beiträge zur klin. Chir. 29:597-616; y. 1900-1901.

A. Podres. Gastroenterostomia und Enteroanastomosis, ein neues verein-
fachtes Verfahren.
Arch. f. klin. Chir. 57:358-369; y. 1898.

P. Postnikow. Die zweizeitige Gastroenterostomie.
Zbl. f. Chir. 19:1018-1021; y. 1892.

B. O. Pribram. Zur Frage: Die Gastroenterostomie als Krankheit.
Zbl. f. Chir. 52:238-241; y. 1925.

H. Puhl. Die anatomischen Grundlagen des Schmerzrezidivs nach Gastro-
jejunostomie wegen Magenduodenalgeschwűrs.
Arch. f. klin. Chir. 176:38-85; y. 1933.

C. E. Rees. Anterior gastro-enterostomy by short loop method.
Surg. Gyn. & Obst. 60:1125-1127; y. 1935.

H. Richter. Hat sich fűr die operative Behandlung des Ulcus pepticum
ventriculi resp. duodeni die Magenresektion als die beste Methode
bewahrt?
Chirurg, I:270; y. 1929.

G. Rocchi & U. Stoppato. Die neue Ruggi'sche Methode der doppelten
Verbindungsöffnung zwischen Jejunum und Magen bei der Gastro-
enterostomie.
Zbl. f. Chir. 38:955-956; y. 1911.

C. Rockwitz. Die Gastro-enterostomie.
Deutsche Zeitschr. für Chir. 25:502-564; y. 1886-1887.

M. Rutkowski. Zur Technik der Gastroenterostomie.
Zbl. f. Chir. 26:1057-1059; y. 1899.

N. Sawkoff. La Gastro-entérostomie est la méthode de choix dans la traitement des ulceres de l'estomac et du duodenum. Travail base sur 700 cas personnels.
Rev. de Chir. 66:353-366; y. 1928.

A. Schachner. Gastrectomy versus gastro-enterostomy in Gastro-duodenal Ulcers.
Am. Journ. of Surg. 8:81-86; y. 1930.

N. Schilling. Intussusception through gastro-enterostomy stoma.
Ann. Surg. 95:958; y. 1932.

F. Schroeter. Über Gastroenterostomie.
Deutsche Zeitschr. f. Chir. 38:296-312; y. 1894.

A. A. Segal. The vicious circle after gastroenterostomy and its treatment.
Sovetsk. Khir. I:206-221; y. 1931.

Matteo Selmi. La Gastro-Enterostomia.
Bologna, Presso N. Zanicelli; y. 1909.

J. P. Shearer & E. M. Pickford. Intussusception of the small intestine into stomach through a gastro-enterostomy stoma.
Annals of Surgery, 87:574-577; y. 1928.

A. N. Simin. Eine neue Methode der Anlegung von Gastroenteroanastomose.
Russki Wratsch; y. 1908 (No. II) also in Zbl. f. Chir. 35:915-916; y. 1908.

A. Socin. Zur Magenchirurgie.
Correspondenz-Blatt für Schweizer Aerzte, 14:513-517; y. 1884.

R. Solé & R. Acosta. Mal resultado alejado en dos enfermos gastro-enterostomizados por ulcera.
La Semana méd. 2:456-458; y. 1927.

A. Stanischeff. Gastroenterostomia anterior obliqua.
Zbl. f. Chir. 55:3267-3268; y. 1928.

F. Starlinger & W. Richter. Zur Heilungsdauer der Anastomosennaht nach Magendarmvereinigung.
Wien. klin. Wchnschr. 44:962-966; y. 1931.

W. Sykoff. Eine einfache Methode zur Gastro-enterostomie.
Arch. f. klin. Chir. 56:418-424; y. 1898.

I. Tansini. Per una semplificazione della tecnica della gastro-enterostomia e della resezione gastrica.
Gazz. d. osp. 49:720-724; y. 1928.

M. Thalheimer. De la degastro-enterostomisation.
Journ. de Chir. 30:385-393; y. 1927.

L. Torraca. Klemmung der anastomotischen Ansa am mesokolischen Einschnitt in einem Falle von Gastro-enterostomia posterior.
Zbl. für Chir. 59:652-656; y. 1932.

R. C. Webb. Disconnecting gastroenterostomy stomatas.
Surg. Gyn. & Obst. 33:681-686; y. 1921.

F. W. White & I. R. Jankelson. Late intussusception of bowel into stomach after gastro-enterostomy.
New England Journal of Med. 199:1189-1193; y. 1928.

O. Witzel & C. Hoffman. Die Gastroenterostomosis, Gastrostomosis und ihre Verbindung zur Gastroenterostomosis externa.
Deutsche Med. Wochenschr. 26:301-303; and 325-327; y. 1900.

A. Wölfler. Gastro-enterostomie.
Zbl. für Chir. 8:705-708; y. 1881.

A. Wölfler. Zur Technik der Gastro-enterostomie und ähnlicher Operationen, mit Demonstration von Präparaten.
Verhandl. der Deutsch. Gesellschaft für Chir. 12:21-25; y. 1883.

M. B. Zamoshchin. Retrograde invagination of small intestines into stomach through gastro-enterostomy stoma.
Novy Khir. Arkhiv. 30:263-267; y. 1934.

CHAPTER XVIII.

GASTRO-DUODENOSTOMY.

Definition.

This is the establishment of an artificial communication between the lumen of the stomach and that of the duodenum.

Historical.

This operation was first performed on a human being by Péan, in 1879, Rydygier, in 1880, and Billroth, in 1881, as one of the steps of pylorectomy.

Kocher, in 1890, while performing a partial gastrectomy, implanted the severed duodenum into the anterior wall of the remaining portion of the stomach, and in the following two cases of gastrectomy implanted it into the posterior wall of the stomach. He coined the expression "gastro-duodenostomy".

Jaboulay, in 1892, conceived the idea of making a gastro-duodenostomy **as an operation per se and not as a mere step in gastrectomy.** He suggested that this operation be used instead of gastro-jejunostomy in all cases of pyloric stricture or obstruction, in which pyloroplasty is contra-indicated. He considered it a more physiological procedure than gastro-jejunostomy and free of such complications as regurgitant vomiting ("vicious circle"). He advised suturing the anterior wall of the stomach to the second (descending) portion of the duodenum (Fig. 220, a). It was first performed by him on a human in 1894, **and he is quite justly considered as the originator of this operation.**

Villard, on April 20, 1897, performed his first case of this type of gastro-duodenostomy, and he coined the expression **"subpyloric gastro-duodenostomy"** (**"Gastro-duodenostomie sous-pylorique"**).

Julius Schnitzler, of Vienna, performed gastro-duodenostomy several times. His first case was done on August 18th, 1899. His associate, E. Klein, reported this first case of Schnitzler in 1900, and he coined for this type of gastro-duodenostomy the name **"lateral gastro-duodenostomy."**

However, neither Jaboulay nor Schnitzler mobilized the second portion of the duodenum, and the technic of the performance of this operation in the manner as employed by Jaboulay, Villard and Schnitzler was not easy.

Henle, in 1898, reported a case of gastro-duodenostomy which was performed by Mikulicz according to the plan of Henle. The stomach was united with the pars superior duodeni (Fig. 220, d).

418

Kocher greatly facilitated the technic of gastro-duodenostomy by mobilizing the second portion of the duodenum, which made its technic a simple procedure (Fig. 220, b). His article was published in January, 1903. His technic is that of the lateral gastro-duodenostomy of Schnitzler (Klein) or of the subpyloric gastro-duodenostomy of Jaboulay (Villard).

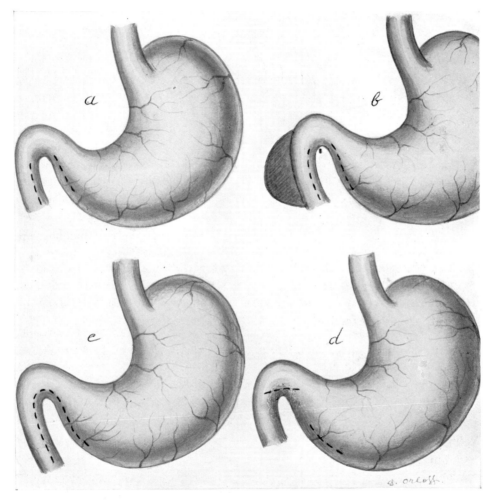

FIG. 220. DIFFERENT TYPES OF GASTRO-DUODENOSTOMY.
a. Jaboulay method;   b. Kocher method;   c. Finney method;   d. Henle method.

Finney, in July, 1902, published his method of gastro-duodenostomy (Fig. 220, c), which he quite correctly calls **pyloroplasty,** since in his method the incision is made not only through the stomach and the duodenum but also through the pyloric ring, whereas, in the methods of Jaboulay, Henle and Kocher, the pyloric ring is left intact.

All these methods, with the exception of the Finney method, are now very seldom used. For this reason, we shall describe here only two methods:

1. **The Method of Kocher,** (since it carries the very important feature of mobilization of the second part of the duodenum, which is of great importance in performing a partial gastrectomy by the Billroth 1 method).

2. **The Method of Finney.**

Indications.

The indications are the same as for a gastro-jejunostomy.

The *advantages* of a gastro-duodenostomy over a gastro-jejunostomy are:

1. Gastro-duodenostomy eliminates the occurrence of regurgitant vomiting.

2. No ulcers are formed at the site of the new stoma (nevertheless, this might occasionally occur).

3. The duodenum is retained as a part of the alimentary tract, whereas, in case a gastro-jejunostomy has been performed, the duodenum is transformed into an excretory duct conveying bile and pancreatic juice.

The *disadvantages* of gastro-duodenostomy are:

1. It is technically more difficult to perform.

2. In all methods of gastro-duodenostomy the stoma is not located on the most dependent portion of the stomach.

1.   KOCHER'S GASTRO-DUODENOSTOMY.

This operation is actually a lateral gastro-duodenostomy. The characteristic feature of it is the mobilization of the second portion of the duodenum.

Technic.

Step 1. The abdomen is opened by a longitudinal or transverse incision.

Step 2. The parietal peritoneum which covers the anterior surface of the hilum of the right kidney is cut longitudinally at a distance of about one and-a-half inches away from the right border of the second portion of the duodenum. This enables the surgeon to introduce the index-finger of his left hand behind the duodenum and lift it from the structures lying back of it (Fig. 221). However, it is not advisable to carry the separation to the left of the vena cava inferior. Not only the duodenum, but also the most lateral portion of the head of the pancreas is lifted. No blood-vessels are injured.

Step 3. A fold of the second portion of the duodenum is clamped axially by an intestinal clamp, and a fold of the anterior stomach-wall very close to the greater curvature is also clamped axially by an intestinal (or stomach) clamp. An anastomosis is made between these folds precisely

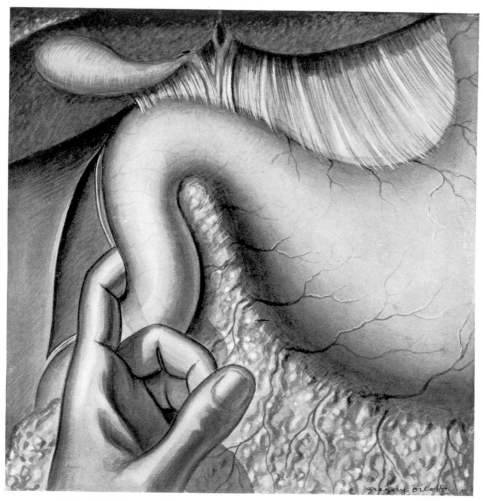

FIG. 221. KOCHER METHOD OF MOBILIZATION OF THE DUODENUM.

as described in the lateral intestinal anastomosis [N.B. In his original description, Kocher does not mention the use of clamps.]

2. THE METHOD OF FINNEY.

This method was described in 1902.

Step 1. A suture is inserted into the upper end of the anterior surface of the pylorus (point A, Fig. 222, insert), another into the anterior wall of the stomach at the greater curvature and about five inches below the first suture (Fig. 222, insert, point B), and a third is passed through point C on the anterior wall of the second portion of the duodenum at a distance of five inches from the point A (point C, Fig. 222). These three sutures are used as traction-sutures. They should be of catgut and they penetrate the seromuscular layer only.

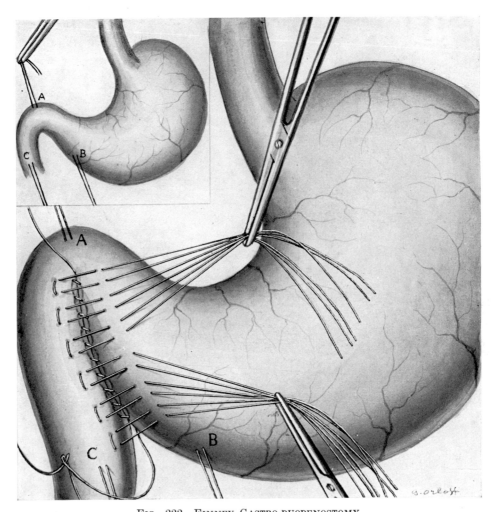

FIG. 222. FINNEY GASTRO-DUODENOSTOMY.
INSERT. Guy sutures inserted.
MAIN PICTURE. Seromuscular continuous sutures inserted; a series of mattress-sutures are made.

Step 2. The guy-suture A is drawn upward, the guy-sutures B and C downward. The adjacent portions of the stomach and duodenum are then laid side-by-side. A continuous seromuscular suture is inserted, connecting the adjacent portions of the stomach and duodenum (Fig. 222).

Step 3. A number of interrupted seromuscular mattress-sutures are inserted connecting the anterior wall of the stomach with that of the duodenum (Fig. 222). The distance between each two consecutive sutures is one-fourth of an inch. The bite of each mattress-suture on the duodenal side is inserted about one-fourth of an inch away from the seromuscular suture-line, and on the stomach about one-half of an inch away from the

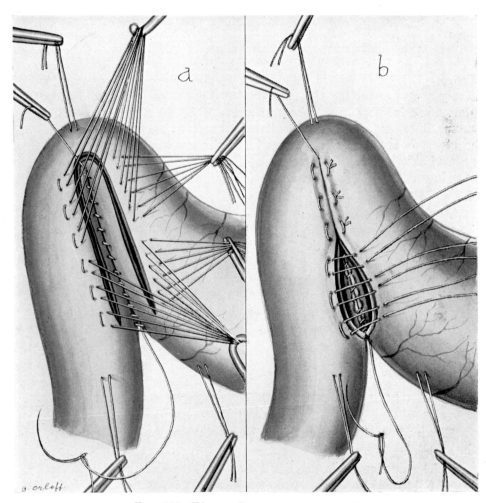

FIG. 223. FINNEY GASTRO-DUODENOSTOMY.
a. Horse-shoe incision which penetrates the stomach and the duodenal walls.
b. The posterior lips are united by a continuous suture; the mattress-sutures are tied.

same line (Fig. 222). The ends of each mattress-suture are not tied now, but the free ends of the upper half of the series of sutures are grasped by one clamp and the free ends of the lower half of the series are grasped by another clamp.

Step 4. At the point where the threads cross the seromuscular suture-line which connects the stomach with the duodenum, they are lifted by two hooks, the upper half by one hook which pulls them upward and the lower by another hook which pulls them downward (Fig. 223, a).

Step 5. A horse-shoe incision is made through the entire thickness of the gastric and duodenal walls, the vertical limbs of which stop one-fourth of an inch above the lower end of the seromuscular suture-line. The incision is made on the duodenal side at a distance of about one-eighth of an inch, and on the stomach side at a distance of about one-fourth of an inch, from the seromuscular suture-line (Fig. 223, a). [The making of the incision is technically simple on the stomach and on the duodenum. However, it is more difficult at the pyloric ring, since if we will apply the same pressure in cutting the first part of the duodenum as in cutting the pylorus, one is liable **to cut the posterior wall of the first part of the duodenum.** In order to prevent this, it is best to cut first the anterior wall of the stomach up to the highest point and then to do the same on the duodenal side. Then a tissue-forceps, the blades of which are directed to the pylorus, is inserted and the anterior wall of the pylorus is cut between the separated blades.]

Step 6. The scar-tissue upon either side of the incision is excised. The redundant edges of the mucous membrane of the stomach are cut away in order to prevent the formation of a valve-like fold of this membrane.

Step 7. A continuous through-and-through suture is inserted on the posterior lips of the incision (Fig. 223, b).

Step 8. The ends of each mattress-suture are tied serially (Fig. 223, b).

Step 9. A continuous seromuscular suture reinforces the anterior suture-line.

3. THE GOULD MODIFICATION OF FINNEY'S GASTRO-PYLORO-DUODENOSTOMY.

This modification differs from the original method of Finney in two points:

1. The duodenum is mobilized according to the method of Kocher (Fig. 221); and
2. Intestinal clamps are used both on the stomach and on the duodenum. The operation is then performed precisely in the same manner as was described in "Lateral Intestinal Anastomosis".

The Gould modification is technically easier to perform than the original Finney gastro-duodenostomy. However, there is only one drawback to this method, namely, that while applying an intestinal clamp on the duodenum the ampulla of Vater may be caught in the clamp and injured.

Technic.

Step 1. The duodenum is mobilized by Kocher method (Fig. 221).

Step 2. Intestinal clamps grasp a fold on the duodenum and another on the stomach. The fold on the duodenum is about three inches long and the clamp holding it lies in such a manner that the tip of the inner jaw

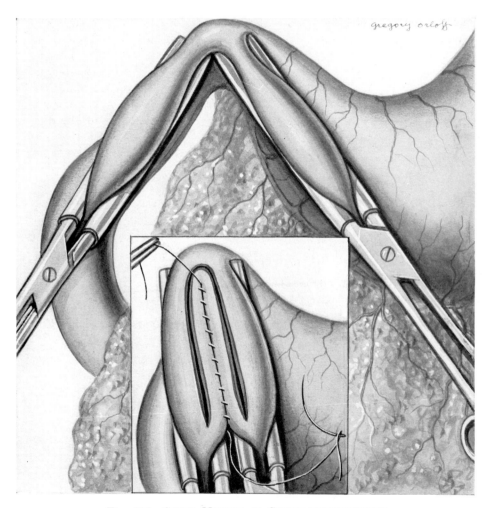

FIG. 224. GOULD METHOD OF GASTRO-DUODENOSTOMY.
MAIN PICTURE. Clamping a fold of the stomach and of the duodenum.
INSERT. The folds of the stomach and the duodenum laid side by side; a seromuscular suture is inserted.

rests against the lower border of the pyloric sphincter. The other clamp is placed on the stomach in a similar manner, so that the tip of the inner jaw of the latter touches that of the duodenal clamp at the pylorus (Fig. 224).

Step 3. The clamps are laid side-by-side, and a row of seromuscular sutures, three inches long, is inserted beginning at the pyloric angle (Fig. 224, insert).

Step 4. A horse-shoe incision is made in the same manner as described in the Finney gastro-pyloro-duodenostomy (Fig. 224, insert).

Step 5. A through-and-through suture is inserted in the posterior lips starting at the pyloric angle. These posterior lips form the posterior wall of the newly formed stoma. The suture is continued over the lateral lips which form the anterior wall of the newly formed stoma. This anterior suture-line is reinforced by a seromuscular suture which is made with the same thread that was used for making the seromuscular suture on the posterior lip.

BIBLIOGRAPHY.

J. M. T. Finney. A new method of pyloroplasty.
Bullet. of the Johns Hopkins Hospit. 13:155-161; y. 1902.

E. R. Flint. Gastro-duodenostomy; further experiences.
Lancet I:12-13; y. 1927.

Gould. Operations upon the intestines and the stomach. pp. 222-236; Saunders Co., Publishers; 1905.

A. Henle. Ein Fall von Gastroduodenostomie.
Zbl. für Chir. 25:753-756; y. 1898.

Jaboulay. La gastro-enterostomie. La Jéjuno-Duodénostomie. La Résection du Pylore.
Arch provinc. de Chir. I:1-22; y. 1892.

Jaboulay. De la Gastro-duodénostomie.
Archives Provinciales de Chirurgie, I:551-554; y. 1892.

E. Just. Zur Frage der Gastroduodenostomie lateralis.
Deutsche Zeitschr. f. Chir. 230:399-404; y. 1931.

E. Klein. Ein Sanduhrmagen in Folge von Salzsäureverätzung. (Gastroduodenostomie).
Wien. klin. Rundschau, 14:85-89; y. 1900.

T. Kocher. Ueber eine neue Methode der Magenresektion mit nachfolgender Gastro-Duodenostomie.
Arch. f. klin. Chir. 42:542-544; y. 1891.

T. Kocher. Mobilisierung des Duodenum und Gastroduodenostomie.
Zbl. f. Chir. 30:33-40; y. 1903.

C. Nicoladoni. Horizontale Gastroduodenostomie.
Zbl. f. Chir. 29:609-610; y. 1902.

W. F. Rienhoff Jr. Infra-papillary gastro-duodenostomy by mobilization with retromesenteric displacement of duodenum and jejunum.
Annals of Surgery, 95:183-197; y. 1932.

J. Schnitzler. Zur Gastroduodenostomia lateralis.
Zbl. f. Chir. 30:287-289; y. 1903.

E. Villard. Gastroduodenostomie sous-pylorique.
Revue de Chir. 22:495-520; y. 1900.

E. Villard. Gastroduodénostomie sous-pylorique.
Lyon Médical, 98:577-578; y. 1902.

CHAPTER XIX.

GASTRECTOMY.

Definition.

The term gastrectomy consists of two Greek words γαστήρ, stomach and ἐκτομή, removal. It means removal of the stomach.

Nomenclature.

There is some confusion in terminology. Some use different terms for the very same procedure. The names most commonly used are:

1. **Sphincterectomy,** when only the pyloric sphincter is removed (Fig. 225).

2. **Pylorectomy,** when the pylorus is removed (Fig. 225).

3. **Partial gastrectomy,** when the pylorus and part of the body of the stomach is removed up to the Hartmann or to the Mikulicz line (Fig. 225).

4. **Subtotal gastrectomy,** when the pylorus and the greater part of the body are removed up to the Mayo line (Fig. 225).

5. **Total gastrectomy,** when the entire stomach is removed, leaving on the proximal end the cardia and on the distal end the first portion of the duodenum (Fig. 225).

6. **Annular gastrectomy** (or "sleeve resection"), when the middle portion of the body of the stomach is removed (Fig. 225, insert).

7. **Fundusectomy,** when the fundus is removed (Fig. 235).

Indications.

1. **Carcinoma of the stomach.**—This is an absolute indication, provided that the case is operable in the mechanical sense.

2. **Large callous ulcers of the stomach.**—The majority of surgeons consider this as an indication for gastrectomy. However, there are surgeons who employ some other operation for callous gastric ulcer, such as mere excision of the ulcer, or excision with a gastro-enterostomy, or a mere jejunostomy.

3. **Duodenal ulcer.**—Many surgeons, particularly in Germany, are performing gastrectomy for the treatment of duodenal ulcer.

METHODS EMPLOYED.

The great number of different methods described can be classified into two groups:

1. **Billroth I.**—This method is characterized by the removal of a portion of the stomach and by reëstablishment of the continuity of the gastro-intestinal tract **by suturing the remaining portion of the stomach to the duodenum** (Fig. 226).

2. **Billroth II.**—This method is characterized by the removal of a portion of the stomach and by reëstablishment of the continuity of the gastro-intestinal tract by suturing **the stomach to the jejunum** (Fig. 227).

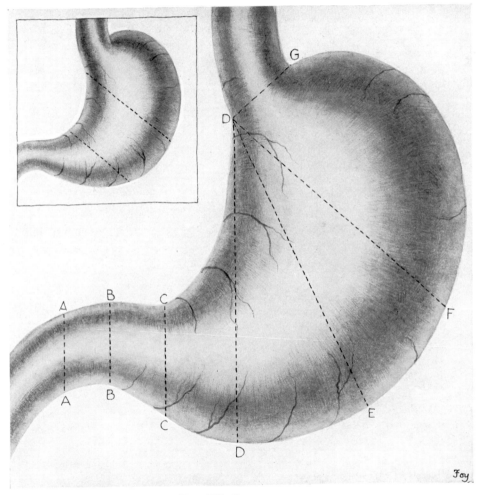

FIG. 225. GASTRECTOMY.

SPHINCTERECTOMY. Removal of the portion of the stomach between the lines AA and BB;

PYLORECTOMY. Removal of the portion of the stomach between AA and CC.

PARTIAL GASTRECTOMY. Removal of the portion of the stomach between AA and DD (HARTMANN LINE) or DE (MIKULICZ LINE).

SUBTOTAL GASTRECTOMY. Removal of a portion of the stomach up to DF (MAYO LINE).

TOTAL GASTRECTOMY. Removal of the entire stomach between AA and DG.

SLEEVE RESECTION. See insert.

There are described a few modifications of the Billroth I operation, and numerous modifications of the Billroth II.

BILLROTH I AND ITS MODIFICATIONS.

Billroth I.—This operation consists of a resection of a portion of the

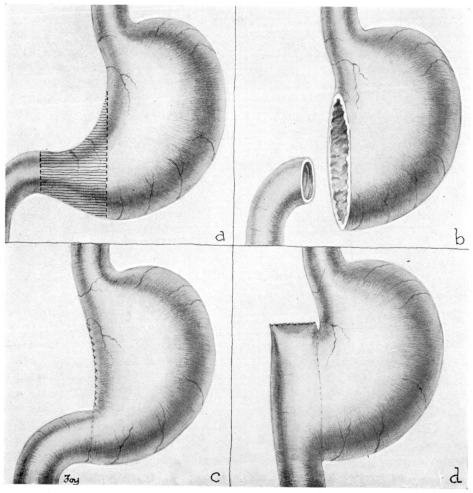

FIG. 226. BILLROTH I AND ITS MODIFICATIONS.
a. The portion of the stomach between the dotted lines is to be removed;   b. This portion of the stomach is removed;   c. Final view of Billroth I;   d. Kocher (Haberer-Finney) modification of Billroth I.

stomach, plus blind closure of the upper portion of the stomach-stump, plus end-to-end gastro-duodenostomy (Fig. 226, a, b, c).
Its Modifications.

1. **Kocher's side-to-end gastro-duodenostomy.**—This consists in a resection of a portion of the stomach, plus blind closure of the stomach-

stump, plus side-to-end gastro-duodenostomy, anterior or posterior. This method is obsolete.

2. **Kocher's end-to-side gastro-duodenostomy.**—This consists in a resection of a portion of the stomach, plus blind closure of the duodenal stump, plus implantation of the stomach-stump into the lateral wall of the second part of the duodenum (Fig. 226, d). This method was suggested by Kocher, in December, 1902, in the following words:

"One can, if he employs such an operation [gastro-duodenostomy], come across those cases in which, after resection of the pylorus, it may be advisable to close blindly the severed duodenum, and perform a lateral gastro-duodenostomy between the stomach and the descending part of the duodenum." Von Haberer, in 1922, being unaware of Kocher's description, suggested this method as a new operation. It is known in Europe as **Haberer's modification of Billroth I.** Finney, in 1923, suggested this method again. He refers to Haberer's work. However, he does not mention Kocher's article, evidently having been unaware of it. It is known in the United States as the **Haberer-Finney modification of Billroth I.**

A far greater number of methods have been described at different times by different men for variations of the Billroth II method. They did not know that the particular method had already been described, and claimed that they had discovered "a new method". Numerous charges and counter-charges were made by many for the right to claim the priority of one or another modification, and the most interesting part of the controversies is that many participated in these charges except the originators of the methods. We will discuss this more in detail in the historical part of gastrectomy.

Historical.

The first thesis on the removal of a portion of the stomach was written by Daniel Paul Carl Theodore Merrem, of Giessen, in 1810. In this article, he states that pylorectomy was first performed by an American surgeon of Philadelphia, who performed several pylorectomies on dogs and who, in spite of the fact that they all died, advised its use in suitable cases in human beings. Finney believes that the surgeon referred to is John Jones, who was, before coming to Philadelphia, the first professor of Surgery in King's College of New York, afterwards the College of Physicians and Surgeons and later Columbia University. Merrem performed three pylorectomies on dogs, of which two survived. After removal of the pylorus he sutured the remaining portion of the stomach into the duodenum by the invagination method, which was at that time the method of reëstablishing the continuity of the intestinal tract.

Ruggero Torelli is probably the man to whom should belong the credit for being the first who resected a portion of the stomach in a human being. It was, however, only a resection of the anterior stomach-wall which was incarcerated in a fissure of a ventral hernia. It was not a gastrectomy as we understand it now, in which the essential element of the operation is the removal not only of the portion of the anterior but also of the posterior wall including both curvatures. He performed the operation on September 14, 1865. After removal of a portion of the anterior gastric wall, he closed this opening in the stomach with sutures. The patient recovered. However, this was not a deliberately planned operation. It was carried out because of the force of circumstances. In 1876, Gussenbauer and Winiwarter reported seven cases of pylorectomy on dogs, of which two survived the operation. Kaiser, of the Czerny clinic, in 1876 and 1877, repeated the experiments of Gussenbauer and Winiwarter and reported the results in 1878. He made an annular resection of the stomach on five dogs. He was more fortunate than Gussenbauer and Winiwarter, since of the five dogs, four survived the operation. Czerny and Kaiser also performed five total gastrectomies, of which four dogs died and one survived. The latter was the famous "Czerny dog" which lived five years after the operation and later was killed and examined by the great physiologist Ludwig. In 1877, Billroth performed a gastrorrhaphy on a human, and in reporting the case he wrote, "Es ist von dieser Operation zur Resektion eines Stückes carcinomatos degenerirten Magens nur noch ein kűhne Schritt zu machen". ("From this operation to resection of a piece of a carcinomatously degenerated stomach it is necessary only to make one bold step.") He, evidently did not know, that a portion of the stomach had already been resected twelve years previously to this statement by Ruggero Torelli. However, this in no way diminishes the great services of Billroth, who spoke of a **deliberately planned removal of a portion of a carcinomatous stomach, thus introducing for the first time the surgical treatment of cancer of the stomach.**

Péan, on April 9, 1879, performed the first pylorectomy on a human being. The operation lasted two and a half hours. The patient died on the fifth post-operative day. No autopsy was made because of refusal of the relatives. This type of pylorectomy (pylorectomy plus gastro-duodenostomy) is known in France as **"Péan's operation".** The next case of pylorectomy was performed by Rydygier on November 16, 1880. The operation lasted four hours and the patient died four hours after the operation.

On January 29, 1881, Billroth operated upon a woman, 43 years of age, for cancer of the stomach. The operation lasted one and a half hours. The patient recovered. **This is the first case of a successfully performed pylorectomy on a human being.** He reëstablished the continuity of the gastro-intestinal tract by suturing the remaining portion of the stomach to the duodenum. This type of operation is known as the **Billroth I operation** (Fig. 226).

After the first case, several other cases were reported by different surgeons, for the most part in Germany and Austria. At that time, they did not know how to mobilize the duodenum. For this reason, they could not make an extensive gastric resection on account of the inability to suture the remaining portion of the stomach to the duodenum. Extensive gastric resections became possible only after the Billroth II method had been developed. It is interesting to note that this, the "Billroth II method", was not introduced for the purpose of overcoming the difficulties encountered in performing the Billroth I method. Billroth had a case of a very weak patient, and he was afraid that the patient might not be able to stand an operation of such magnitude as gastrectomy in one stage. Therefore, he decided to perform as a first stage the gastro-enterostomy, and a few days later, as the second stage, a pylorectomy. After completing the anterior gastro-jejunostomy, which was the usual type of gastro-enterostomy at that time, he found the patient to be in fairly good condition. He, therefore, proceeded with the operation. He removed a portion of the stomach between the duodenum and the site of the anastomosis, and closed blindly both the duodenal and the stomach ends. This operation was performed on January 15, 1885, and on February 20, 1885, Billroth reported the case at a meeting of the Royal Medical Society in Vienna. In the very same year, Von Hacker reported this case, and describing the technic of Billroth, wrote, that the continuity of the gastro-intestinal tract can be **reëstablished by suturing the lower part of the open end of the remaining portion of the stomach to a loop of jejunum. Therefore, if credit should be given to any man for introducing a "Modification of the Billroth II Method", it should be given first of all to Von Hacker.** Krönlein, of Zürich, was the first man who actually carried out the suggestion of Von Hacker. On November 24, 1887, he performed a partial gastrectomy, closed blindly the duodenum and reëstablished the continuity of the gastro-intestinal tract by making an end-to-side gastro-jejunostomy antecolica, using for anastomosis the entire length of the stomach-stump. As we may see, this operation differs from Polya's operation only in this respect, that Krönlein brought the jejunum in front of the colon, whereas in Polya's method this was placed retrocolically. In order to avoid making a large stoma between the stomach and the jejunum, Von Eiselsberg, in a case of gastrectomy performed on April 2, 1888, closed blindly the upper portion of the stomach-stump and sutured the lower end of it to the jejunum, which also was brought antecolically. This method was much later rediscovered, with the difference only that the jejunum was placed retrocolically, and this is called, by several other men, quite erroneously, as the "Finsterer-Hoffmeister's modification of Polya" (Fig. 228, insert).

The first who placed a loop of the jejunum retrocolically for partial gastrectomy was Roux, who performed a gastrectomy in the following manner: Partial gastrectomy, plus blind closure of the duodenal stump, plus blind closure of the stomach-stump, plus gastro-jejunostomy retrocolica in a "Y" form. The first who performed gastrectomy in the manner which is now commonly known as the "typical Billroth II method" was Braun, who did it in 1894. His method differs from the original Billroth II method in this respect, namely, that whereas in the original Billroth II method the loop of the jejunum was placed antecolically, he placed it retro-colically. Therefore, his method is a "partial gastrectomy, plus blind closure of the duodenal stump, plus closure of the stomach-stump, plus gastro-jejunostomy retrocolica posterior" (Fig. 227, b). Reichel, in 1908, published a method that he had been practicing since 1907, namely a partial gastrectomy, plus blind closure of the duodenal stump, plus end-to-side

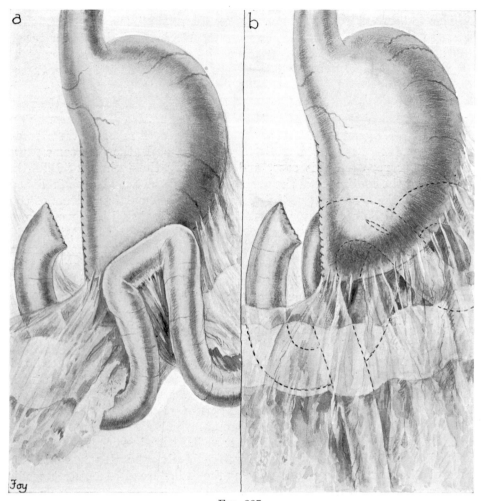

FIG. 227.
a. "Original" Billroth II.
b. Braun modification of Billroth II.

gastro-jejunostomy retrocolica (Fig. 228). As already mentioned, this method differs from the operation performed by Krönlein, in 1887, only in this respect, that he placed the loop retrocolically. Polya, in 1911, de-scribed a procedure which is identical with the operation described by Reichel in 1908 (Fig. 228). Stumpf, in 1908, described the method of partial gastrectomy as used by Hoffmeister, of Stuttgart. Hoffmeister began this method in 1905, and it consisted of a partial gastrectomy, plus blind closure of the duodenal stump, plus closure of the upper end of the stomach-stump, plus end-to-side gastro-jejunostomy retrocolica inferior. This is the operation which, as mentioned before, was done in 1888 by Von Eiselsberg, with the difference only that Hoffmeister placed the loop retro-

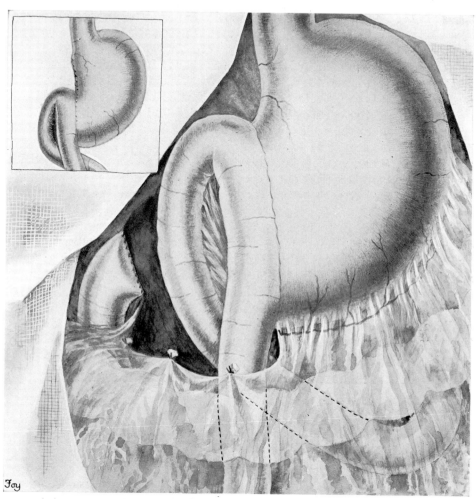

FIG. 228. MODIFICATION OF BILLROTH II.
INSERT. "Billroth II retrocolica oralis inferior" (known as the "Hoffmeister-Finsterer method").
MAIN PICTURE. "Billroth II retrocolica oralis" (known as the "Polya method").

colically. Sasse, of Frankfurt on the Main, in 1909, published a report of twelve cases in which he closed the upper end of the stomach and sutured the lower end of it to the jejunum which was brought behind the colon. He also did not mention the names of his predecessors in this method, evidently being convinced that he was the originator of the method.

A. von Bergmann, of Riga, performed several partial gastrectomies after 1900 in the following manner: A partial gastrectomy, plus blind closure of the duodenal stump, plus end-to-side gastro-jejunostomy retrocolica, utilizing either the entire length of the opening of the stomach or only its lower end. He also does not mention any names connected with the method, evidently being convinced that he was the originator of the method. As may be seen, he antedated Hoffmeister. **He, however, introduced a very helpful technical improvement, namely, the making of a seromuscular suture between the jejunum and the stomach before the portion of the stomach was removed.**

Burk, in 1911, published the work done at Hoffmeister's clinic and mentioned that Hoffmeister usually sutured the lower end of the stomach to the jejunum brought retrocolically, but that in some cases he used the entire length of the open end of the stomach. If, however, he could not bring the jejunum retrocolically, he took a long loop of the jejunum and brought it in front of the colon and supplemented it with a Braun's entero-anastomosis. **Thus, what is known as the Balfour modification of Polya's method has been described not only before Balfour described his modification of Polya, but even before Polya described his method.**

Finsterer, in 1913, described his new method. It consisted of a partial gastrectomy, plus blind closure of the duodenal stump, plus blind closure of the upper end of the stomach-stump, plus end-to-side gastro-jejunostomy retrocolica. As may be seen, there is nothing new in his "new method". **Summarizing all that is written above, we may say, that with the exception of one name, in addition to that of Billroth, namely von Hacker, there is no justification for using any other name in the different modifications of the Billroth II method.** Narath suggests using descriptive topographical names for all the variations of the Billroth II method.

THE BILLROTH II METHOD AND ITS MODIFICATIONS.

1. **Billroth II (original).**

    This consists of a resection of the stomach, plus blind closure of the duodenum, plus blind closure of the stomach-stump, plus gastro-jejunostomy antecolica anterior (Fig. 227, a). This method is obsolete.

2. **Typical Billroth II (Braun's modification).**

    This consists of a resection of the stomach, plus blind closure of the duodenum, plus blind closure of the stomach-stump, plus gastro-jejunostomy retrocolica posterior (Fig. 227, b). This variation is now known as the "typical Billroth II method", and is used quite frequently.

3. **Resection by the Billroth II antecolica oralis.**

    This consists of a resection of the stomach, plus blind closure of the duodenal-stump, plus end-to-side gastro-jejunostomy antecolica, plus entero-anastomosis (Fig. 229).

4. **Resection by the Billroth II antecolica oralis inferior.**

    This consists of a resection of the stomach, plus blind closure of the duodenum, plus closure of the upper part of the stomach-stump, plus end-to-side gastro-jejunostomy antecolica, plus entero-anastomosis.

5. Resection by the Billroth II retrocolica oralis.

This consists of a resection of the stomach, plus blind closure of the duodenum, plus end-to-side gastro-jejunostomy retrocolica (Fig. 228).

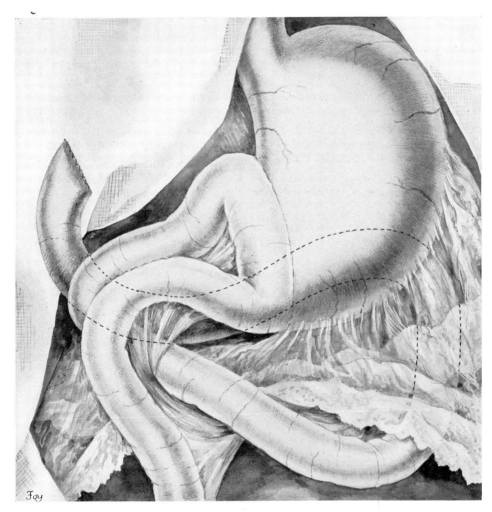

FIG. 229. MODIFICATION OF BILLROTH II.
Billroth II antecolica oralis with enteroanastomosis" (known as the "Balfour method").

6. Resection by the Billroth II retrocolica oralis inferior.

This consists of a resection of the stomach, plus blind closure of the duodenum, plus closure of the upper end of the stomach, plus end-to-side gastro-jejunostomy retrocolica (Fig. 228, insert). The names in "3", "4", "5" and "6" were suggested by Narath, of Heidelberg.

As many of these modifications are familiar to surgeons by the names of different men who are justly or unjustly connected with the method, we attach a table, taken from the excellent monograph of G. Cavina on Gastrectomy.

TABLE I. BILLROTH I AND ITS MODIFICATIONS.

1. **End-to-end.**—Péan (1879) ; Rydygier (1880) ; Billroth (1881). These three authors performed what is known as the "typical Billroth I" operation.

Variations:—Goepel (1923) ; Horsley (1926) ; Babcock (1926) ; Von Haberer (1927).

Gastrectomy with incision of the lesser curvature:—Schmieden (1921) ; Luquet et Pauchet (1923) ; Schoemaker (1929).

2. **Side-to-end.**—Posterior variation: Kocher (1895). **Anterior variation:** Kustscha-Lissberg (1925) ; Pototschnig (1930).

3. **End-to-side.**—Von Haberer (1922) ; Finsterer (1923) ; Winkelbauer (1927).

4. **Side-to-side.** Alessandri, Oliani (1924) ; Leriche (1927).

TABLE II. BILLROTH II AND ITS MODIFICATIONS.

1. **Side-to-side**
    - **anterior**
      - antecolica—Billroth II (1885) ; Schiassi "Y" method (1913) ;
      - retrocolica—Dubourg (1898).
    - **posterior**
      - antecolica—v. Eiselsberg (1899) ;
      - retrocolica—Braun (1894) ;
      - v. Hacker (1894).
    - **marginal** V. Mikulicz (1887).

2. **Side-to-end**—posterior, retrocolic—Roux "Y" method (1893).

3. **End-to-end**—retrocolica; Rydygier "Y" method (1904) ; Moszkowicz (1908) ; Soresi (1921).

4. **End-to-side**
    - **total oralis**
      - antecolica—Krönlein (1887) ; Balfour; Moynihan II.
      - retrocolica—Reichel (1907) ; Polya (1911) ; Sasse (1911) ; Moynihan I. ("Y" method).
    - **partial oralis inferior oralis** (idea of V. Hacker 1885).
      - antecolica—v. Eiselsberg (1888) ; Cunéo "Y" method (1909).
      - retrocolica—Hoffmeister (1905) ; Wilms (1911) ; Finsterer (1911).
    - **Superior oralis**—Schmieden (1921).

TOTAL GASTRECTOMY.

The first case of a total gastrectomy was performed on a human by Phineas S. Conner, of Cincinnati, and the report thereof read before the Cincinnati Academy of Medicine, on November 3, 1884. The patient expired on the table after total removal of the stomach, but before the cardiac end of the esophagus was sutured to the bowel. After this, several unsuccessful attempts at performing a total gastrectomy were made. The first successful total gastrectomy was done by Carl Schlatter, of Zürich, at that time assistant of Prof. Krönlein, on September 6th, 1897. He closed the duodenum blindly and sutured the cardiac end of the esophagus to the jejunum placed in front of the colon. The patient lived more than a year and died from carcinoma. The second successful case of a total gastrectomy was done by Charles Brook Brigham, in 1898. There are two distinct views as to what constitutes a total gastrectomy.

a. Krönlein believed that a gastrectomy was total if the entire stomach was removed, so that on the proximal part was left the abdominal portion of the esophagus and on the distal the first portion of the duodenum.

b. Billroth believed a gastrectomy to be total, if the cardia and the distal portion of the pylorus were still left in situ.

To perform a gastrectomy, in the meaning of Billroth, is mechanically easier, and secondary anemia usually does not follow the operation. In case of a total removal of the stomach in the meaning of Krönlein, the patient frequently loses appetite, pepsin-hydrochloric acid digestion is disturbed, and very frequently he develops marked symptoms of secondary anemia to which he succumbs unless liver-treatment is instituted. The explanation why these symptoms do not ensue in all cases of total gastrectomy in the Krönlein sense is, that occasionally some gastric mucosa is found in the abdominal portion of the esophagus. **If even a very small amount of gastric mucosa is left, the physiological functions of the stomach are not disturbed.** Up to the year 1928, Finney collected from the literature 122 cases of total gastrectomy, of which 67 were performed in the manner of Krönlein and 55 in the manner of Billroth.

TECHNIC OF GASTRECTOMY.

The technic varies, depending on:
    a. The cause for the gastrectomy.
    b. The seat of the pathology.

a. If the gastrectomy is performed on account of the presence of a gastric or duodenal ulcer, some surgeons do not ligate the right and the left gastro-epiploic arteries, since a part of the blood-supply to the great omentum takes its origin from these two arteries and after they are ligated the great omentum looses its luster. If, however, the gastrectomy is performed on account of carcinoma of the stomach, these blood-vessels are ligated.

b. Some surgeons begin the dissection from the point where the pathological portion is located. They perform first the most difficult part of the operation. If they have been able to separate this pathologically changed portion from the surrounding viscera, then they know that the case is mechanically operable and they proceed with the further steps of the removal of the stomach.

The other group of surgeons proceed precisely in a reversed order. They begin at first the separation of the healthy tissues, thus making the stomach more movable, and this facilitates the removal of the diseased portion of the stomach.

PARTIAL GASTRECTOMY BY THE BILLROTH II METHOD (RETROCOLICA ORALIS METHOD).

This method is also known as the **Polya method.** However, as men-

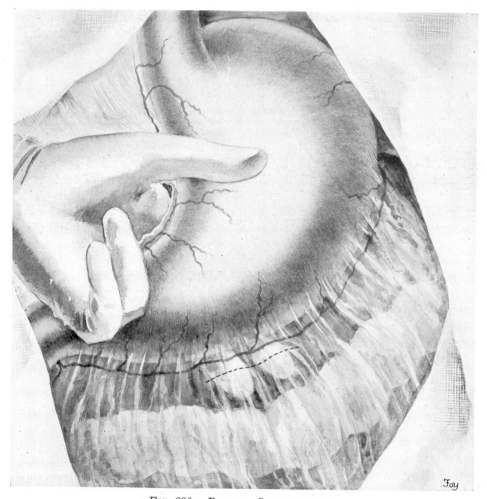

FIG. 230. PARTIAL GASTRECTOMY.
Division of the gastrocolic ligament. Two fingers separate the gastrocolic ligament from the transverse mesocolon.

tioned already in the historical part of this chapter, it had been employed by several surgeons long before Polya described it.

Step 1. Division of the gastro-hepatic and the gastrocolic ligaments (Fig. 230).

The gastro-hepatic ligament is torn by the index and middle fingers

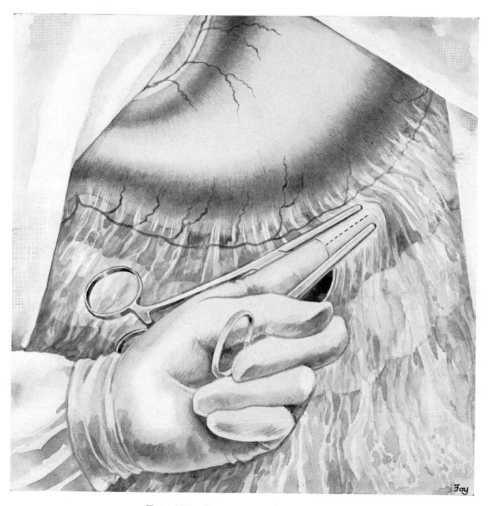

FIG. 231. PARTIAL GASTRECTOMY.
Division of the gastrocolic ligament.

of the left hand. These two fingers then pass behind the stomach until the gastrocolic ligament is reached, **which will lie in front of the fingers,** while the transverse mesocolon with its important middle colic artery **will lie behind the fingers** (Fig. 230). The gastrocolic ligament is then divided in sections between two clamps for the desired length (Fig. 231).

The two fingers which lie behind the gastrocolic ligament in the bursa omentalis serve to prevent injury to the middle colic artery.

[Alternate method of division of the gastrocolic ligament (Fig. 144).

The gastrocolic ligament is grasped by two tissue-forceps and cut **very carefully** between them.   The index-finger of the left hand is inserted

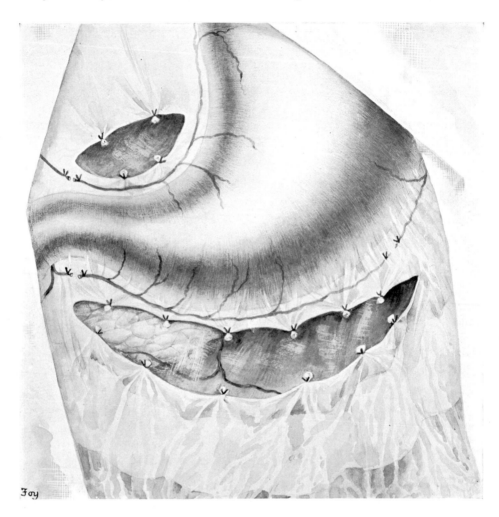

FIG. 232. PARTIAL GASTRECTOMY.
The gastrocolic and gastro-hepatic ligaments divided. The right and left gastro-epiploic arteries and the right gastric artery are divided and ligated.

into the opening and gently separates the gastrocolic ligament (which lies in front of the finger) from the transverse mesocolon (which lies behind the finger). The gastrocolic ligament is then clamped in succession by artery-forceps and is cut between each two of them precisely as described in the previous method.]

Step 2. Ligation of the right gastro-epiploic artery.

A curved forceps holding a thread, passes between the artery and the lower border of the first portion of the duodenum. Another thread is carried through the same opening and the artery is ligated by these two threads at a distance of three-fourths of an inch from each other. The artery is cut between them, leaving the **larger stump** on the duodenal side. The ends of the thread are cut short (Fig. 232).

Step 3. The left gastro-epiploic artery is ligated in the same manner as the right (Fig. 232).

Step 4. The right gastric artery is ligated by passing two threads with a curved forceps just above the upper margin of the first portion of the duodenum. The artery is then divided between the two ligatures (Fig. 232).

Step 5. The opening in the gastro-hepatic ligament, which was made in Step 1 of this operation, is now enlarged by dividing the ligament between the clamps (Fig. 232).

Step 6. A Payr enterotribe clamps the first portion of the duodenum and an artery-forceps clamps the pylorus very close to the Payr clamp (Fig. 233, insert). A laparotomy sponge is placed behind the pylorus. The first portion of the duodenum is cut between the Payr and the arterial clamps very close to the former ("shave it off"). It is cut by a knife, or still better by a Paquelin cautery. If it has been cut by a knife, the exposed mucosa of the duodenum on the blade is disinfected by iodine and alcohol. The open end of the duodenum is closed by the "over the clamp" method (Fig. 114), and is sutured to the pancreatic capsule, thus causing it to lie retroperitoneally.

Step 7. Ligation of the left gastric artery (Fig. 233, main picture).

The divided portion of the stomach is drawn to the left and is used as a handle. The left gastric artery is now ligated precisely in the same manner as described in the ligation of the other vessels of the stomach. **The branches close to the stomach are ligated, if the gastrectomy is done for an ulcer, and far away from the stomach, just distally from the origin from the celiac artery, in case the gastrectomy is done for carcinoma of the stomach.** The proximal end of the left gastric artery is ligated first by a double ligature and then more distally by a single one.

Step 8. An opening is made in the transverse mesocolon, precisely in the same manner as described in posterior gastro-jejunostomy. The first loop of the jejunum is located and is brought through the opening in the mesocolon to the posterior wall of the stomach, so that the proximal end of the jejunum is brought to a point close to the lesser curvature and the distal end close to the greater curvature of the stomach. Each end of the jejunum is attached to the stomach by an interrupted suture. A sero-

serous suture is then made between these two viscera (Fig. 234). A seromuscular incision is then made on the jejunum and on the stomach. The
blood-vessels lying in the mucosa of the stomach are ligated (Fig. 234).
A seromuscular suture is made between the lips of the jejunum and
stomach. The seromuscular surface **of the anterior wall of the stomach is
now cut,** and the blood-vessels in the mucosa are ligated.

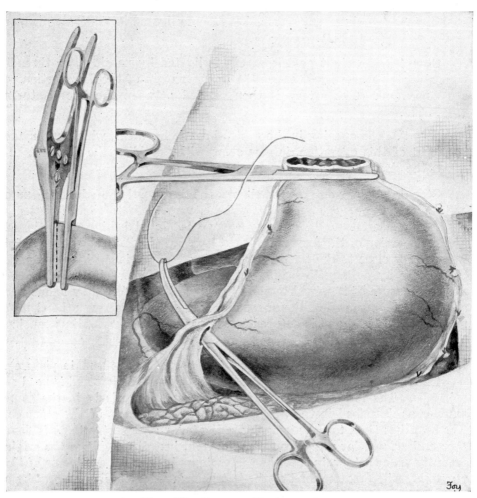

FIG. 233. PARTIAL GASTRECTOMY.
INSERT. Division of the pyloro-duodenal junction.
MAIN PICTURE. Ligation of the left gastric artery.

Step 9. An intestinal clamp is placed on the stomach and another on
the jejunum **behind** the seromuscular suture-line, and a Payr clamp grasps
the stomach just distal to the exposed mucosa (Fig. 234, insert). [This
will prevent the soiling of the operative field when the portion of the
stomach is removed].

Step 10. The stomach is cut away just below the Payr clamp (Fig. 234, insert). While doing this the outer lip of the stomach is caught by a few Allis forceps so as to prevent slipping of the outer stomach-lip behind the intestinal clamp.

Step 11. An incision is made through the mucosa of the jejunum. The length of this incision is a trifle shorter than that of the seromuscular

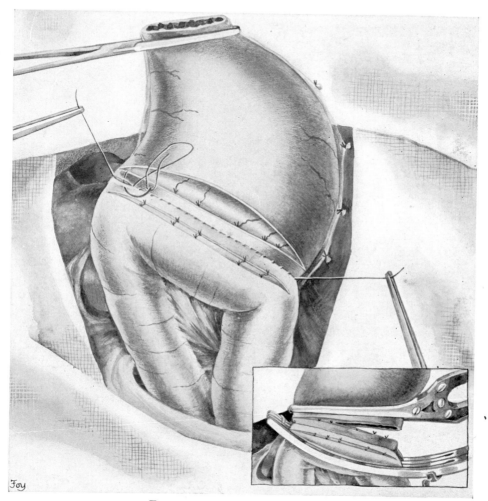

FIG. 234.   PARTIAL GASTRECTOMY.
Suturing the stomach to a jejunal loop brought retrocolically.

incision (one-fourth inch shorter on each end). The opening of the stomach is sutured to the opening of the jejunum in the same manner as described in the technic of posterior gastro-enterostomy.

Step 12. The edges of the opening of the mesocolon are sutured to the stomach, if it is possible to bring the stomach down without undue tension.

If, however, this is not possible, the mesocolic slit is sutured to both limbs of the jejunum.

FUNDUSECTOMY (FIG. 235).

This is the removal of the greater portion of the fundus of the stomach. The theoretical ground for this operation, as propounded by its

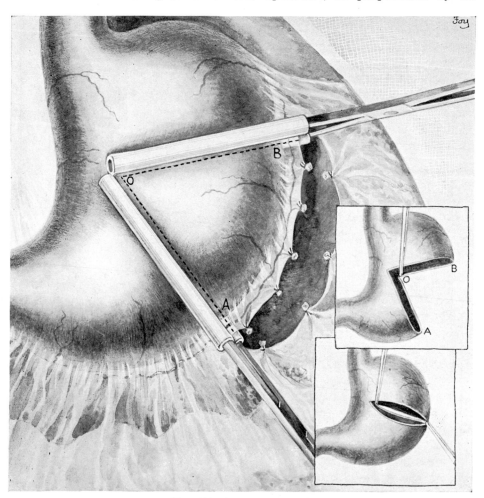

Fig. 235. Fundusectomy.
MAIN PICTURE. The clamps are applied in a proper position.
UPPER INSERT. A portion of the fundus is removed.
LOWER INSERT. Closure of the opening in the stomach.

originator F. G. Connell, is that it is better to remove the "acid-bearing area" (that is, the fundus) which contains the acid-secreting glands, than to remove the "ulcer-bearing area" (that is the pyloro-antral region), which is mainly the motile portion of the stomach. The technic, according to its originator, is as follows:

Step 1. Ligation of the gastrocolic and the gastrosplenic ligaments between points A and B.

Step 2. The stomach is clamped at a right angle by two stomach-clamps placed so that the tips of the blades will meet one inch below the lesser curvature.

Step 3. The stomach is cut along the lines AO and BO.

Step 4. One Allis forceps grasps the posterior wall at O, and another the posterior wall at A and B, and the lips of the posterior wall are then sutured to each other.

Step 5. The lips of the anterior wall are sutured to each other, and the openings in the gastrocolic and gastrosplenic ligaments are closed.

This procedure seems to be a logical one. However, too few cases have been reported thus far in order to decide definitely whether it will become a commonly used operation.

TECHNIC OF BILLROTH I.

(This is the "Original Péan-Billroth" operation).

Step 1. As Step 1 in Partial gastrectomy by Billroth II.

Step 2. As Step 2 in Partial gastrectomy by Billroth II.

Step 3. As Step 3 in Partial gastrectomy by Billroth II.

Step 4. As Step 4 in Partial gastrectomy by Billroth II.

Step 5. As Step 5 in Partial gastrectomy by Billroth II.

Step 6. Mobilization of the duodenum (by the Kocher method) and division of the first portion of the duodenum.

The posterior parietal peritoneum is grasped in front of the hilum of the right kidney by two Allis forceps and cut by scissors. The left index-finger is inserted into the opening thus made and separates the posterior parietal peritoneum from the connective tissue in an upward and downward direction. The separated parietal peritoneum is then cut in a vertical direction. The index-finger is then inserted behind the duodenum and lifts the latter. This constitutes what is known as the "mobilization of the duodenum". The retroperitoneal space is closed, if it is possible. An arterial or a Payr clamp is placed on the first portion of the duodenum and an artery-clamp on the pylorus. A laparotomy sponge is placed behind the pylorus. The first portion of the duodenum is divided between these arterial clamps very close to the clamp on the duodenal side of the pyloroduodenal junction ("shave it off"). It is cut by a knife, or still better by the Paquelin cautery.

Step 7. Ligation of the left gastric artery.—This is done as in Step 7 of partial gastrectomy by the Billroth II method.

Step 8. An arterial clamp with a four inch blade grasps the stomach immediately distal to the line to be removed and embracing that portion which adjoins the greater curvature. Another arterial clamp grasps in the same manner the portion of the stomach adjoining the lesser curvature (Fig. 236). The two clamps lie then in such a manner that they form a straight line and embrace the entire circumference of the stomach. A seromuscular suture-line is made between the duodenum and the portion of the stomach grasped by the clamp which embraces the greater curvature. This suture-line is made at a distance of one-sixth of an inch from the clamp on the duodenum and one-third of an inch from the clamp on the stomach. A Payr clamp grasps the stomach proximal to the two straight

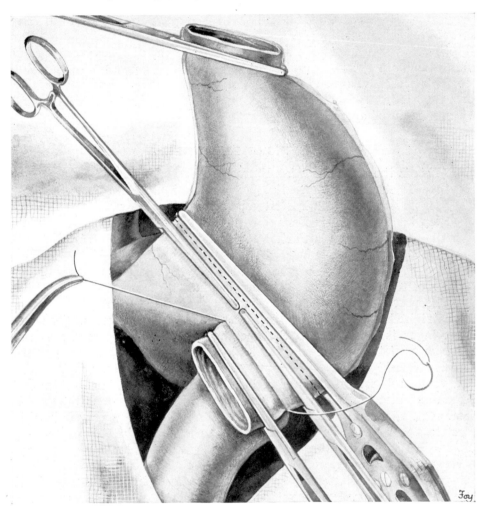

FIG. 236. PARTIAL GASTRECTOMY BY BILLROTH I METHOD.
Seromuscular suturing of the stomach to the duodenum.

arterial clamps, and the stomach is "shaved off" just beneath the Payr clamp, between it and the two arterial clamps (Figs. 236 and 237, upper half). If it is cut by a knife, the cut surface of the stomach is disinfected by iodine and alcohol.

Step 9. An intestinal clamp covered with rubber tubing is applied to

the stomach behind the suture-line. **No clamp is applied to the duodenum.**
The upper portion of the stomach is closed in the following manner: A
short cut of about half an inch is made beneath the arterial clamp. This
opening is then closed. Another cut of half an inch is made beneath the
arterial clamp and closed with the same thread. This cutting and suturing
procedure is continued until the upper half of the stomach is closed (Fig.

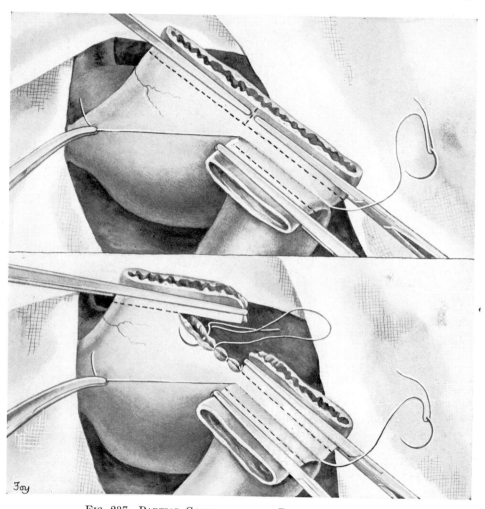

FIG. 237. PARTIAL GASTRECTOMY BY BILLROTH I METHOD
UPPER HALF. The dotted line shows the line of incision.
LOWER HALF. Alternate cutting and suturing of the portion of the stomach adjoining
the lesser curvature.

237, lower half). The seromuscular layer of the stomach and that of the
duodenum, is now incised by a knife below the arterial clamp (Fig. 238).
The blood-vessels of the exposed mucosa of the stomach are ligated (Fig.
238). The seromuscular lips of the stomach and of the duodenum are

sutured to each other by a continuous row of sutures. Then the mucosa of the duodenum and that of the stomach are cut below the crushing-clamps in their entire circumference, and the mucosa of the stomach is sutured to that of the duodenum on the posterior lip and this is continued onto the anterior lip. After the mucosa is sutured in its entire circumference, a seromuscular suture is inserted between the anterior lip of the

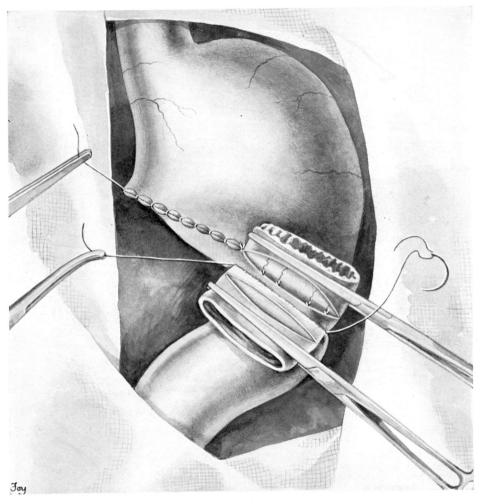

FIG. 238. PARTIAL GASTRECTOMY BY BILLROTH I METHOD.
The portion of the stomach adjoining the lesser curvature is closed; suturing of the duodenum to the portion of the stomach adjoining the greater curvature.

stomach and that of the duodenum. After this the serous suture which attached the posterior lips of the stomach and the duodenum to each other is continued onto the anterior lip of the stomach and that of the duodenum. This is further continued upward to cover the upper portion of the stomach-stump (Fig. 239). The upper and the lower angles of junction between the stomach and the duodenum are reinforced by a V-suture (Fig. 239, insert).

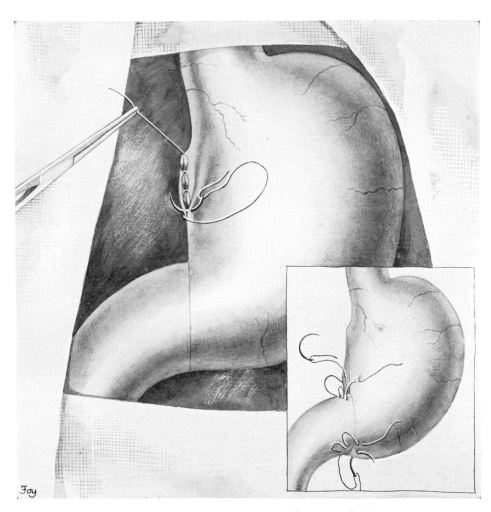

FIG. 239. PARTIAL GASTRECTOMY BY BILLROTH I METHOD.
The suturing of the stomach to the duodenum is completed. The seromuscular suture-line reinforces the over-and-over suture of the upper portion of the stomach.
INSERT. Reinforcing the angles at each end of the gastro-duodenal junction.

TECHNIC OF TOTAL GASTRECTOMY.

A total gastrectomy offers more technical difficulties than does a partial or a subtotal. The stomach should be separated from its attachment to the spleen by cutting the gastro-splenic ligament (and great care should be taken not to injure the splenic artery and vein). The methods of reëstablishment of the continuity of the alimentary tract are the same as in partial gastrectomy, namely, the cardia can be sutured to the duodenum or to the jejunum.

The mortality-rate in total gastrectomy is much higher than in partial gastrectomy, and particularly in those cases in which a total gastrectomy has been performed in the Krönlein manner, in which, on the proximal side is left only the abdominal portion of the esophagus which **lacks**

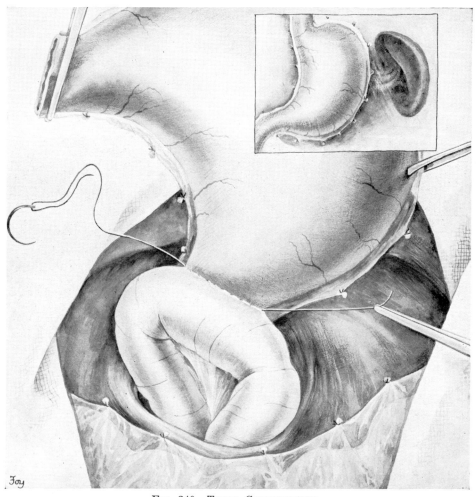

FIG. 240. TOTAL GASTRECTOMY.
INSERT. The gastro-splenic ligament is divided.
MAIN PICTURE. Suturing of the jejunum to the posterior wall of the cardiac end of the stomach.

the peritoneal covering and which, therefore, makes the suture-line between the abdominal portion of the esophagus and the duodenum or the jejunum very unsafe. In order to overcome this difficulty, Goepel, of Leipzig, suggested forming a seromuscular tube from the uppermost portion of the stomach (or the lowermost portion of the cardia), retracting it backward in the form of a cuff for a distance of three-fourths of an inch, then cutting the mucous tube so that it projects beyond the seromuscular cuff for a distance of half an inch, and then suturing the mucous tube to the entire thickness of the wall of the opened end of the duodenum by a through-and-through suture. Then the cuff is replaced in its previous position as a seromuscular tube. The edges of this seromuscular tube are

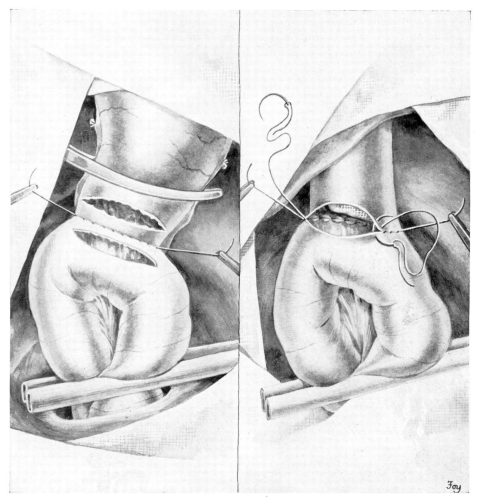

FIG. 241. TOTAL GASTRECTOMY.
LEFT HALF. The jejunum is incised; the stomach is opened;
RIGHT HALF. The posterior lips are sutured; suturing of the anterior lips begun.

now sutured to the serous surface of the duodenum.

The same suggestion of suturing two hollow viscera, one of which is covered with and the other lacks a serous covering, was described by Felix Mandl and Max Gara, of Vienna, about the same time and independently of Goepel.

Technic.

Steps 1 to 7 are the same as Steps 1 to 7 in partial gastrectomy with this difference only, that the gastro-splenic ligament is cut and the greater curvature of the stomach is freed from its connections with the surrounding structures through its entire length (Fig. 240, insert).

Step. 8 A seromuscular suture-line unites the posterior surface of

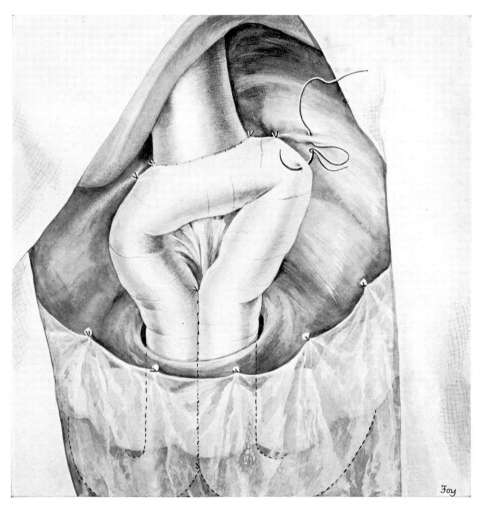

FIG. 242. TOTAL GASTRECTOMY.
Suturing of the jejunum to the diaphragm.

the cardiac end of the stomach to a loop of jejunum brought retrocolically (Fig. 240). A soft-bladed clamp grasps the cardiac end of the stomach about one inch distal from the seromuscular suture-line. An intestinal clamp covered with rubber tubing grasps both jejunal loops at a distance of four inches from the seromuscular suture-line (Fig. 241, left half).

The posterior wall of the cardia and the anterior wall of the jejunum are incised (Fig. 241, left half) and suturing of the posterior lips is begun. After this is completed the stomach is removed by making an incision through the anterior wall of the cardia. A piece of gauze is placed in the cardiac end of the stomach (so as to prevent contamination of the wound). The thread, which sutured the posterior lips by an over-and-over suture,

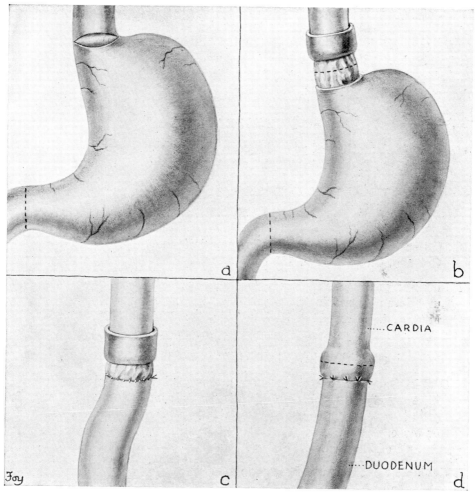

FIG. 243. TOTAL GASTRECTOMY. (GOEPEL METHOD).
a. Seromuscular incision of the cardiac end of the stomach; b. Reflection of the cuff; c. Suturing of the cardia to the duodenum; d. Serous layer of the cardia covers the cardio-duodenal suture-line.

is suturing now the anterior lips (Figs. 241, right half) (the piece of gauze should be removed from the cardia before suture of the anterior lips is completed). The sutured anterior lip is now reinforced by a seromuscular suture.

Step 9. The jejunum is attached to the diaphragm by three sutures, at each side of the cardio-jejunal junction (Fig. 242), in order to diminish the tension on the cardio-jejunal line of anastomosis.

If after total removal of the stomach it is decided to unite the cardia with the duodenum, the Goepel method, as just mentioned, may be advantageously employed: A seromuscular circular incision is made at the lowermost portion of the cardiac end of the stomach (Fig. 243, a). The seromuscular flap is reflected in the form of a cuff for a distance of three-fourths of an inch. The mucous layer of the cardia is cut transversely so as to leave a tube of mucosa protruding one-half an inch beyond the cuff (Fig 243, b). The mucous tube is sutured to the duodenum by an over-and-over suture (Fig. 243, c). The peritoneal cuff is sutured to the duodenum (Fig. 243, d).

BIBLIOGRAPHY.

W. Babcock. A method of partial gastrectomy with telescopic anastomosis.
Surg. Gyn. & Obst. 42:403-415; y. 1926.

W. H. Barber. Annular gastrectomy. Further observations on the cause of its failure.
Annals of Surg. 98:161-167; y. 1933.

H. H. Berg. Misserfolge nach Magenoperationen.
Chirurg, 4:318-333; y. 1932.

H. Biesenberger & W. F. Wieser. Technische Fehler bei Magenoperationen und deren Vermeidung.
Mitt. a. d. Grenzgeb. d. Med. u. Chir. 42:29-56; y. 1930.

T. Billroth. Offenes Schreiben an Herrn Dr. L. Wittelshöfer.
Wien. Med. Wchnschr. 31:161-165; y. 1881.

J. C. Bloodgood. Ultimate results and actual functional results after different types of operations for gastric and duodenal ulcer, for gastric cancer and for hour-glass stomach after an interval of 5 years or more.
Annals of Surg. 92:574-596; y. 1930.

G. Cavina. Tecnica della Resezione Gastrica.
Bologna, 1932.

D. Chamberlain. A new method of approach in gastric surgery.
Brit. Med. Journ. I:343; y. 1929.

F. G. Connell. Fundusectomy. A new principle in the treatment of gastric or duodenal ulcer.
Surg. Gyn. & Obst. 49:696-701; y. 1929.

F. G. Connell. Resection of the fundus of the stomach for peptic ulcer.
Annals of Surg. 96:200-203; y. 1932.

P. S. Conner. "Report of complete resection of the stomach" at the meeting of the Cincinnati Academy of Medicine, Nov. 3, 1884.
Medic. News, Phila. 45:578; y. 1884.

J. B. Deaver & A. P. C. Ashhurst. Surgery of the upper abdomen.
2nd Ed. y. 1921. Philadelphia, P. Blakiston's Son & Co.

R. Demel. Die technische Durchführung der Magenresektion an der Klinik Eiselsberg.
Arch. f. klin. Chir. 172:1-28; y. 1933.

H. B. Devine. Gastric exclusion.
Surg. Gyn. & Obst. 47:239-243; y. 1928.

J. Ducuing, C. Soula & R. Fränkel. La gastrectomie totale chez l'homme.
Journ. de Chir. 44:175-210; y. 1934.

G. Egidi. Sulla resezione dello stomaco per via superiore.
Policlinico (sez. prat.) 36:1769; y. 1929.

A. F. von Eiselsberg. Ueber die Magenresektionen und Gastroenterostomieen.
Arch. f. klin. Chir. 39:785-844; y. 1889.

A. Eiselsberg. Zur Benennung der Magenresektion.
Wien. Med. Wochenschr. 79:516-520; y. 1929.

Enderlen. Zur Geschichte der Gastrectomia totalis.
Zbl. f. Chir. 58:954-955; y. 1931.

J. M. T. Finney. A new method of gastro-duodenostomy, end-to-side, with illustrations.
Tr. South. Surg. Ass. 36:576-588; y. 1923.

J. M. T. Finney & W. F. Rienhoff, Jr. Gastrectomy.
Arch. of Surg. 18:140-162; y. 1929.

R. Finochietto. Gastrectomia por ulcera. Tecnica de la anestesia local.
Rev. de cir. Buenos Aires. 10:514-518; y. 1931.

H. Finsterer. Local anæsthesia; methods and results in abdominal surgery.
New York 1923.

H. Finsterer. Erfahrungen mit der Magenresektion nach Billroth I und deren Modifikation nach Haberer.
Arch für klin. Chir. 135:650-667; y. 1925.

H. Finsterer. Technique de la gastrectomie.
Bull. et mém. Soc. de chir. de Paris, 24:100-117; y. 1932.

H. Finsterer. Kolongangrän nach Magenresektionen.
Zbl. f. Chir. 60:1285-1287; y. 1933.

M. Flesch-Thebesius. Die Verwendung der Duodenalsonde zur Behandlung der akuten Magenlähmung und zur Ernährung im Anschluss an Magenoperationen.
Arch. f. klin. Chir. 165:220-228; y. 1931.

T. Fohl & E. Schneider. Die Netzexstirpation bei der Magenresektion wegen Karzinom.
Deutsch. Zeitschr. f. Chir. 232:317-326; y. 1931.

E. Forgue. La fermeture du bout duodénal dans la gastrectomie; ses conditions et ses améliorations techniques. Les instruments de Hültl et de von Petz; l'appareil du professeur Mario Donati.
Rev. de Chir. 51:564-588; y. 1932.

R. Friedrich. Die Bedeutung der Infektion für die Magennaht. Der "intersuturale Raum" auf Grund tierexperimenteller Untersuchungen.
Arch. f. klin. Chir. 181:1-23; y. 1934.

G. K. Gerekke. Errors in gastric surgery.
Vratchebnoe Delo. 16:661-664; y. 1933.

R. Goepel. Zum Einmanschettierungsverfahren.
Zbl. f. Chir. 52:1702-1706; y. 1925.

G. Gohrbandt. Zur Technik des Duodenalverschlusses.
Zbl. f. Chir. 60:1815-1817; y. 1933.

S. M. Goldhamer. Pernicious anæmia syndrome in gastrectomized patients.
Surg. Gyn. & Obst. 57:257-260; y. 1933.

C. Gussenbauer & A. von Winiwarter. Die Partielle Magenresection.
Arch. f. klin. Chir. 19:347-380; y. 1876.

H. Haberer. Terminolaterale Gastroduodenostomie bei der Resektionsmethode nach Billroth I.
Zbl. f. Chir. 49:1321-1326; y. 1922.

H. Haberer. Betrachtungen über unsere Misserfolge nach Resektion wegen Magen—und Duodenalgeschwüren.
Zbl. f. Chir. 57:66-76; y. 1930.

H. Haberer. Meine Technik der Magenresektion.
Münch. med. Wchnschr. 80:915-921; y. 1933.

H. Haberer. Zur Vermeidung von Nachblutungen nach Magenoperationen. Bemerkung zu dem Aufsatz von Florcken.
Zbl. f. Chir. 60:2568; y. 1933.

Von Hacker. Zur Casuistik und Statistik der Magenresektionen und Gastroenterostomieen.
Arch. f. klin. Chir. 32:616-625; y. 1885.

T. Hernando y Ortega. La gastrectomía (sus indicaciones, técnicas y resultados).
Siglo méd. 91:601-612; y. 1933.

E. Hesse. Fehler, Gefahren und unvorhergesehene Komplikationen in der Chirurgie des Magens und Zwölffingerdarms.
Ergebnisse d. Chir. u. Orthop. 25:154-305; y. 1932.

H. Hilarowicz. Zur Technik der totalen Magenexstirpation.
Zbl. f. Chir. 58:2613-2617; y. 1931.

W. Himmelmann. Über innere Einklemmung nach Magenoperationen.
Chirurg, 5:906:913; y. 1933.

S. Judine. De quelques difficultes de la Gastrectomie large et des moyens de les surmonter.
Presse med. 41:2079-2081; y. 1933.

M. Kirschner. Meine Technik der Resektion beim chronischen Magen-Duodenalgeschwürs. Vorbemerkungen und Technik der gewöhnlichen Resektion.
Chirurg, 4:417-421; y. 1932.

E. Klein. Left vagus section and partial gastrectomy for duodenal ulcer with hyperacidity.
Annals of Surg. 90:65-68; y. 1929.

T. Kocher. Ueber eine neue Methode der Magenresektion mit nachfolgender Gastro-Duodenostomie.
Arch. f. klin. Chir. 42:542-544; y. 1891.

T. Kocher. Zur Technic und zu den Erfolgen der Magenresektion.
Corr.-Bl. f. Schweiz. Aerzte, 23:682-694 and 713-724; y. 1893.

T. Kocher. Mobilisierung des Duodenum und Gastroduodenostomie.
Zbl. f. Chir. 30:33-40; y. 1903.

Krönlein. Fall von traumatischer narbiger Pylorusstenose. Resectio pylori und Gastroenterostomie.
Korr.-Bl. für Schweiz. Aerzte, 18:317-318; y. 1888.

E. Kustscha-Lissberg. Zur chirurgischen Behandlung des Magen und Zwölffingerdarm.
Deuts. Zeitsch. f. Chir. 191:1-28; y. 1925.

H. Garcia Lagos. Tratamiento de las ulceras del estomago.
Prensa med. argentina, 20:2067-2074; y. 1933.

F. H. Lahey. A method of dealing with the proximal jejunal loop in posterior Polya anastomosis.
Surg. Gyn. & Obst. 57:227-230; y. 1933.

P. LeGac. Technique de la gastrectomie; la succession des différents temps. Quelques détails.
Rev. de Chir. 51:435-459; y. 1932.

R. Leriche. Sur un nouveau type d'anastomose gastro-duodénale après gastrectomie dans le cas de mésocolon court.
Lyon Chir. 24:44; y. 1927.

R. Leriche. Considérations générales sur le traitement des ulcères duodéno-gastriques.
Gaz. d. hôp. 101:1489-1493; y. 1928.

W. Lobenhoffer. Ueber totale Magenresektionen.
Münch. med. Wchnschr. 81:241-243; y. 1934.

H. Madariaga & O. Madariaga. Gastrectomia vs. Gastroenterostomia.
Vida nueva, 20:185-191; y. 1927.

W. J. Mayo. Radical operations on the stomach with especial reference to mobilization of the lesser curvature.
Surg. Gyn. & Obst. 36:447-453; y. 1923.

D. Merrem. Animadversiones quædam chirurgicæ experimentis. Animalibus sactis illustratæ.
Gissæ, 1810.

J. Mikulicz. Beiträge zur Technik der Operation des Magencarcinoms.
Arch. f. klin. Chir. 57:524-532; y. 1898.

J. Miyagi. Unsere Erfahrungen mit der Resektion des Kardiakrebses.
Arch. f. klin. Chir. 149:187-193; y. 1928.

A. Monprofit. La Gastrectomie. Histoire et méthodes opératoires. Paris, 1908.

A. Narath. Zur Geschichte der zweiten Billrotschen Resectionsmethode am Magen. Benennung der einzelnen Ausführungsarten.
Deutsch. Zeitschr. f. Chir. 136:62-136; y. 1916.

E. Neuber. Technique of gastric resection.
Surg. Gyn. & Obst. 45:204-208; y. 1927.

Pachon & Carvalho. Sur l'extirpation totale de l'estomac (quoted by Monprofit).

G. T. Pack. Indications for two-stage resection of carcinoma of the stomach.
Surg. Clin. of North Amer. 13:517-523; y. 1933.

V. Pauchet. Indications de la gastrectomie pour ulcus gastrique, duodénal, jejunal.
Gaz. d. hôp. 104:1053-1056; y. 1931.

Péan. De l'ablation des tumeurs de l'estomac par la gastrectomie.
Gaz. des. Hôp. 52:473-475; y. 1879.

E. Polya. Zur Stumpfversorgung nach Magenresektionen.
Zbl. f. Chir. 38:892-894; y. 1911.

G. Pototschnig. Gastro-duodenostomia latero-terminalis anterior bei der Resektionsmethode nach Billroth I.
Zbl. f. Chir. 57:2717-2719; y. 1930.

Reichel. Discussion in "Verhandl. d. Deutsch. Gesellsch. f. Chir." 37:211-213; y. 1908.

H. Richter. Hat sich für die operative Behandlung des ulcus pepticum ventriculi resp. duodeni die Magenresektion als die beste Methode bewährt?
Chirurg, 1:270; y. 1929.

W. Rieder. Spätresultate bei ausgedehnter Magenresektion wegen Ulcus Ventriculi und duodeni.
Zbl. f. Chir. 61:198-203; y. 1934.

A. M. Romeo. Zulla resezione della stomaco.
Catania, 1886, p. 11. (Quoted by Monprofit).

B. Rossi. La tecnica della resezione gastrica.
Clin. Chir. 30:1-25; y. 1927.

Roux. Chirurgie Gastro-intestinale.
Rev. de Chir. 13:402-403; y. 1893.

Rydygier. Ueber Magenresection mit Demonstration Von Präparaten.
Arch. f. klin. Chir. 26:731-743; y. 1881.

Rydygier. Zur Geschichte der circulären Pylorectomie.
Deutsche Zeitschr. f. Chir. 60:588-590; y. 1901.

C. Schlatter. Ueber Ernährung und Verdauung nach vollständiger Entfernung des Magens—Esophago-Enterostomie beim Menschen.
Bruns Beitr. z. klin. Chir. 19:757-776; y. 1897.

V. Schmieden. Über die Excision der Magenstrasse.
Zbl. f. Chir. 48:1534-1538; y. 1921.

E. Schwarz. Über die Totalexstirpation des Magens.
Zbl. f. Chir. 53:578-584; y. 1926.

L. Serrada y Díaz. La Gastrectomia; sus indicaciones, técnicas y resultados.
Siglo méd. 91:565-587; y. 1933.

P. F. Shapiro & B. N. Berg. Return of gastric acidity after subtotal gastrectomy and double vagotomy.
Arch. Surg. 28:160-179; y. 1934.

J. Piñeiro Sorondo. La cirugía de la úlcera gastro-duodenal ante la fisiologia.
Día. méd. 2:397; y. 1930.

F. Starlinger. Das Ruckfallsgeschwür nach Magenresektion wegen Ulcus Ventriculi oder duodeni.
Arch. f. klin. Chir. 162:564-573; y. 1930.

A. Strauss. Longitudinal resection of the lesser curvature.
Journ. Am. Med. Ass. 82:1765-1770; y. 1924.

L. Stropeni. La fisio-patologia dell'ulcera gastro-duodenale come fondamento per la scelta del metodo chirurgico di cura (gastro-enterostomia, resezione gastrica, duodeno-pilorectomia anteriore).
Clin. Chir. 36:653-665; y. 1933.

R. Stumpf. Beitrag zur Magenchirurgie.
Bruns Beiträge z. klin. Chir. 59:551-641; y. 1908.
(Describes Hoffmeister Method).

E. J. Uhlhorn. Total exstirpationen des Magens.
  Arch. f. klin. Chir. 144:593-611; y. 1927.

A. Winkelbauer. Erfahrungen mit der infrapapillären terminolateralen Methode nach Billroth I.
  Arch. f. klin. Chir. 160:439-448; y. 1930.

PART IV.

CHAPTER XX.

SURGERY OF THE GALL-BLADDER AND BILIARY PASSAGES.

A. ANATOMY OF THE GALL-BLADDER AND BILIARY PASSAGES.
VARIATIONS IN THE COURSE OF THE CYSTIC AND HEPATIC
ARTERIES AND OF THE CYSTIC, HEPATIC AND
COMMON BILE-DUCTS.

The gall-bladder is a pear-shaped sac which is on the average 8 to 12 cm. long and 4 to 5 cm. in its widest portion and, when not distended, contains about 40 to 50 c. cm. of fluid. It consists of three portions: the fundus, the body, and the neck, the latter being continued into the cystic duct. The wall of the gall-bladder consists of three layers: the tunicæ serosa, muscularis and mucosa. The mucosa is plicated in numerous folds, which become longitudinal in the neck, and finally form a spiral-shaped fold—the **spiral valve (Heister valve),** which reaches the cystic duct and occasionally continues into it.

The fundus of the gall-bladder usually lies free and projects in front of the anterior border of the liver. The body is attached to the substance of the liver (the "bed of the gall-bladder"). The visceral peritoneum, which covers the liver, passes onto the inferior and lateral surfaces of the gall-bladder, binding it down to the liver-substance. This peritoneum covers nearly the entire gall-bladder with the exception of its superior surface, where it is attached to the liver. Occasionally it surrounds the gall-bladder entirely, and thus the gall-bladder may be surrounded as it were by a meso-gall-bladder.

TOPOGRAPHICAL ANATOMY.

Holotopic Considerations.

The gall-bladder is situated in the right half of the epigastrium.

Skeletotopic Considerations.

The fundus of the gall-bladder lies at the point where the lateral border of the right rectus muscle crosses the cartilage of the eighth or ninth right rib.

Syntopic Considerations.

The **upper** surface of the body of the gall-bladder lies in contact with the substance of the liver. The **lower** surface of the fundus rests on the

463

right colic flexure (hepatic flexure of the colon), and the lower surface
of the body rests on the pars superior duodeni.

Abnormalities.

The gall-bladder is occasionally absent. Occasionally, there are two
separate, independent gall-bladders.

Cystic Duct.

The cystic duct is usually S-shaped and joins the main hepatic duct
at an acute angle, thus forming the common bile-duct. This is, however,
true only in 75 per cent. of all cases. In the rest of the cases there are
variations which will be discussed later. The average length of the cystic
duct is 4.6 cm., the length ranging usually from one and a half to eleven
centimeters. **The main hepatic duct** is formed by the union of the right
and left hepatic ducts, each of which is an excretory duct for the corresponding lobe of the liver. The hepatic duct runs as an unpaired trunk for
a few centimeters when it is joined by the cystic duct to form the common
bile-duct. However, in some cases the right and the left hepatic ducts join
each other in the substance of the liver, forming there the main hepatic
duct, so that outside of the liver, there is seen only the main hepatic duct.

The average length of the main hepatic duct is about 4.5 cm., being
in some cases as short as 2 cm. and in others as long as 9 cm. **The
common bile-duct** is formed by the union of the cystic and the main hepatic
ducts. After it is formed, it runs along the outer border of the gastro-
hepatic ligament, and is subdivided into the **supraduodenal, retroduodenal,**
and **intraduodenal** portions. In its retroduodenal portion the common bile-
duct usually lies in the substance of the pancreatic tissue and occasionally
in a deep grove or in a shallow furrow on the posterior surface of the
pancreas. The average length of the common bile-duct, according to
Langenbuch, is 8 cm. Most frequently the pancreatic duct **(Wirsungian
duct)** joins the common bile-duct in the wall of the duodenum, namely, in
the diverticulum duodeni **(ampulla Vateri)**. However, quite frequently
the Wirsungian duct joins the common bile-duct outside of the duodenum.
In such cases, they enter the ampulla Vateri by a common opening.

In some cases these two ducts run independently of each other,
although in very close proximity, and independently penetrate the ampulla
Vateri. Each then has its own opening, these being separated from each
other by a transverse mucous fold. In some cases the accessory pancreatic
duct **(ductus Santorini)** joins the common bile-duct, whereas the Wirsungian duct runs the entire length separately.

The **diverticulum duodenale** (or **ampulla Vateri**) is a hollow cone-like
sac, which lies in the submucous layer of the duodenum. The size of the
ampulla Vateri is, according to Opie, 3.9 by 2.5 mm. In its base lies either
the common opening of the common bile-duct and of the Wirsungian duct,
or their separate openings. In the apex of the cone lies a small opening—

the porus papillaris, through which the mixed bile and pancreatic juice leave the ampulla and enter the lumen of the bowel.

The surgical significance of the course of the common bile-duct and of its close relationship to the pancreas and to the Wirsungian and Santorini ducts is twofold: First, it is a difficult procedure to attack the intrapancreatic portion of the common bile-duct. Second, there is an intimate relationship between diseases of the biliary tract and of the pancreas. Any inflammation of the pancreas may compress the pancreatic portion of the common bile-duct, the walls of which are very soft, and thus produce stagnation of the bile. Any inflammation of the gall-bladder or of the biliary passages may find its way into the Wirsungian duct and produce disturbances of the pancreas. It has been proved many times that the injection of staining-paste through the gall-bladder will reach the Wirsungian duct before it enters the lumen of the duodenum through the porus papillaris.

VARIATIONS OF THE BILIARY DUCTS AND THEIR SURGICAL SIGNIFICANCE.

a. Cystic duct.

In the majority of cases the cystic duct joins the main hepatic duct at an acute angle (Fig. 244, A). However, in many cases the method of union of the cystic and hepatic ducts is different. One of the earliest writers on this subject, Ernst Ruge, of the Körte clinic, classified all the variations of union of the cystic and hepatic ducts into three types:

Type I—Angular union (Fig. 244, A).

Type II—Parallel course, in which the cystic duct, before opening into the hepatic duct, runs parallel to it for a shorter (Fig. 244, B) or longer distance (Fig. 244, C), ranging from two to six or seven cm. In the majority of cases the parallel portions are long rather than short. The parallel portions of the cystic and hepatic ducts are bound by connective tissue, so that in many cases they can be separated from each other by sharp dissection only, and even then with great difficulty. When the parallel branches of the cystic and hepatic ducts are very long, then they may join each other behind the duodenum in the pancreatic tissues, and in some cases they may join each other even within the wall of the duodenum (Fig. 244, D).

Type III—Spiral type.

In this type of union the cystic duct, before joining the hepatic, passes in front of or behind the latter and courses either on its anterior surface (Fig. 244, E) or on its posterior surface (Fig. 244, F), or continues spirally to the left and opens on the left side of the hepatic duct (Fig. 244, G) or even on the anterior surface of this duct, thus making one-fourth, one-half, or even a complete circle. The frequency of the different types of union of the cystic and hepatic ducts differs according to different investigators.

	Number of cases (total)	Normal Angular	Parallel	Spiral
Ruge	43	14(33%)	12(29%)	17(38%)
Kunze	39	20(51%)	19(49%)	—(0%)
Descomps	50	40(80%)	6(12%)	4(8%)
Eisendrath	100	75(75%)	17(17%)	8(8%)
Total	232	149(64%)	54(23½%)	29(12½%)

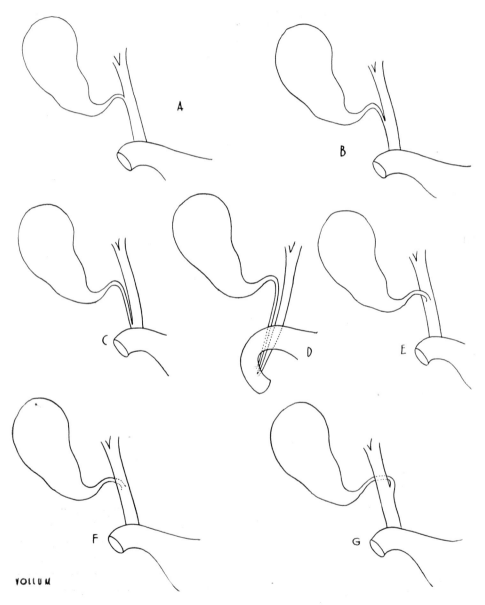

VOLLUM

FIG. 244. VARIATIONS IN THE COURSE OF THE CYSTIC DUCT.

The surgical significance of cystic duct variations lies in the fact that it is very easy to injure the cystic, hepatic and the common bile-duct by removing the gall-bladder and that a large portion of the cystic duct may be left behind. A few months after a cholecystectomy has been performed it may dilate and give the same symptoms as the original gall-bladder, similar to attacks of appendicitis after an incomplete appendectomy has been performed.

b. Hepatic Duct. Occasionally, the right and the left hepatic ducts join each other in the substance of the liver, and outside of the liver they then present themselves as a single main hepatic duct. In some cases, there are three hepatic ducts, which form the main hepatic duct (Fig. 245, A). Cases have been observed with five hepatic ducts before they united to form the main hepatic duct.

Occasionally, the main hepatic duct is absent. In these cases the cystic duct and two hepatic ducts join each other at a common angle, thus forming at once the common bile-duct.

The surgical significance of this variation is, that if the surgeon wants to drain the main hepatic duct through the cystic duct he will insert a drain into one of the hepatic ducts, thus producing only a partial drainage. Further: If the drainage of the hepatic duct has been made with the intention of diverting temporarily the flow of bile into the common bile-duct after suturing the latter, this aim will not be accomplished.

ACCESSORY BILE-DUCTS.

The presence of accessory bile-ducts is not uncommon. Flint in 200 dissected cases found it 29 times, *i.e.* in 14.5 per cent.

These accessory bile-ducts are tributaries either of the right hepatic duct (Fig. 245, A), or of the main hepatic duct (Fig. 245, B), or of the common bile-duct (Fig. 245, C) and even of the cystic duct. They are, on the average, of a fairly good size, being approximately about half of the size of the right or of the left hepatic ducts. However, they may be as large as the size of the right or left hepatic duct or so small as to admit only a bristle into the lumen.

In about thirty per cent. of all cases, the accessory duct is a tributary of the right hepatic or of the upper end of the main hepatic duct, and this is of no surgical significance. In about thirty-five per cent. the accessory duct is a tributary of the lower part of the main hepatic duct, and in about thirty-five per cent. it enters close to the site of union of the cystic and the main hepatic ducts. This is of great surgical significance, since the duct may be easily clamped by the surgeon while performing a cholecystectomy.

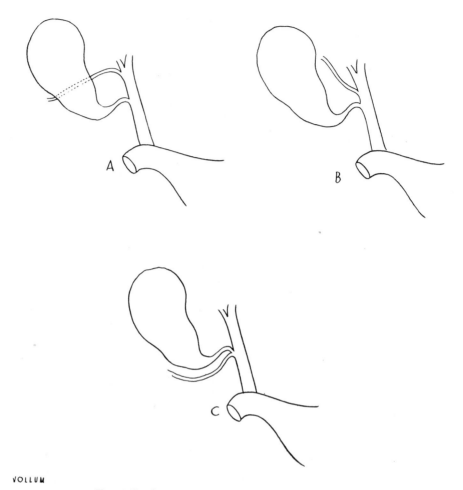

VOLLUM

FIG. 245. ANOMALIES OF THE BILIARY PASSAGES.

BLOOD-VESSELS.

Normal Arrangement.

The hepatic artery takes its origin from the celiac artery and runs retroperitoneally to the right until it reaches the right gastro-pancreatic ligament which it penetrates, and then turns upward. Before turning upward it gives off the gastro-duodenal artery and a little higher the right gastric artery. Then it breaks into its two terminal branches, the right and the left hepatic arteries, each of which runs to the corresponding lobe of the liver. From the right hepatic artery arises the cystic artery, which runs to the gall-bladder and breaks there into two branches, the anterior and the posterior, which give the blood-supply to the corresponding surfaces of the gall-bladder (Fig. 246, A).

VARIATIONS IN THE BLOOD-SUPPLY.

a. The **right hepatic artery** usually takes its origin from the main hepatic artery. However, occasionally it springs from the aorta, the right gastric, the right renal or the superior mesenteric artery.

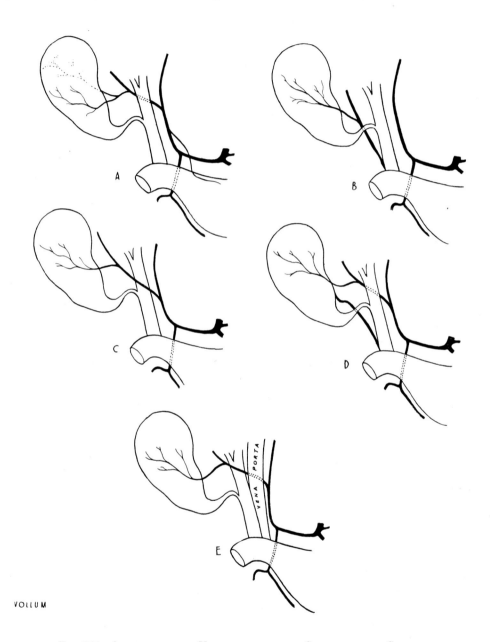

VOLLUM

FIG. 246. ANOMALIES AND VARIATIONS IN THE COURSE OF THE CYSTIC AND HEPATIC ARTERIES.

The normal arrangement of the branches of the hepatic artery is seen in Fig. 246, A.

The different variations are shown in pictures 246, 247, and 248. According to Flint, based on the dissection of 200 cadavers, the frequency of anomalies of the arteries is:

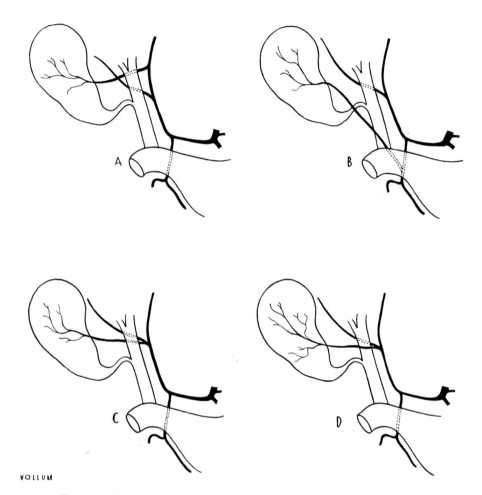

VOLLUM

FIG. 247. ANOMALIES AND VARIATIONS IN THE COURSE OF THE CYSTIC AND HEPATIC ARTERIES.

The right hepatic artery sprang from the main hepatic in 79 per cent.
"   "   "   "   "   "   " superior mesenteric in 21 per cent.

The right hepatic artery before it reached the liver ran **behind** the common hepatic duct in 86 per cent. (Fig. 246, A), and in **front** of it in 14 per cent. (Fig. 246, C).

Two **right** hepatic arteries were present in 3½ per cent., and in each case one took its origin from the main hepatic artery and the other from the superior mesenteric artery (Fig. 246, D).

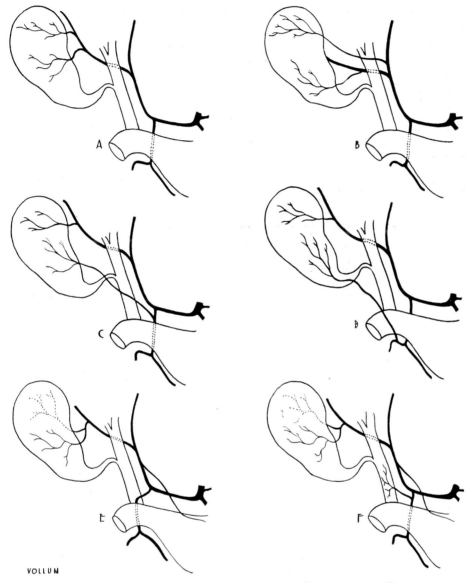

VOLLUM

FIG. 248. ANOMALIES AND VARIATIONS IN THE COURSE OF THE CYSTIC AND HEPATIC ARTERIES.

Two **left** hepatic arteries were present in two cases, both taking their origins from the main hepatic, one passing in **front** and the other **behind** the common hepatic duct. In four cases, the main hepatic or the right hepatic artery also passed behind the portal vein.

b. The **cystic artery** sprang from the right hepatic artery in 98 per cent. (Fig. 246, A), from the left hepatic artery in 1.5 per cent. (Fig. 247, A), and from the gastro-duodenal artery in 0.5 per cent (Fig. 247, B).

The cystic artery ran along the **right side** of the common hepatic duct, or **behind** it, in 84 per cent. and in **front** of the common hepatic duct in 16 per cent.

An accessory cystic artery was present in 15.5 per cent. It arose from the **right** hepatic artery in 51.6 per cent. (Fig. 248, A), from the **left** hepatic artery in 9.7 per cent. (Fig. 248, B), from the **gastro-duodenal artery** in 35.5 per cent. (Fig. 248, C), and from the **pancreatico-duodenal artery** in 3.2 per cent. (Fig. 248, D).

If it takes its origin from the gastro-duodenal or from the pancreatico-duodenal artery (and that occurs in nearly 39 per cent.) it is easily liable to injury in choledochotomy operations.

Whenever there was an accessory cystic artery it invariably crossed in front of the bile-ducts.

THE SURGICAL SIGNIFICANCE OF ABNORMALITIES OF BILE-DUCTS AND BLOOD-VESSELS.

Many difficulties may be encountered by the surgeon in performing operations on the biliary tract.

In removing the gall-bladder, particularly from below, he is liable to injure the hepatic duct (Fig. 244, E, F, G) or the arteries (Fig. 246, B, D; Fig. 247, B; Fig. 248, C, D). If he clamps the cystic duct far from the point where it joins the hepatic duct, and in many cases even if he cuts close to what appears to him as the point of junction of the cystic with the main hepatic duct, he will leave behind a large cystic duct which will in a few months become distended enough **to form practically a new gall-bladder.** These patients may have attacks of cholecystitis after the gall-bladder has been removed just the same as, occasionally, patients have attacks of appendicitis after appendectomy has been performed. In the latter case, this is the fault of the surgeon who could remove the entire appendix if he would bear in mind that a portion of it occasionally lies under the serous surface of the cecum. This is not true, however, in the removal of the gall-bladder, since the removal of the spiral cystic duct with a turn of 180° or even of 360°, would offer such great difficulty that it would probably be the wisest thing not to attempt the removal of the spiral cystic duct in its entire length, but merely to cut it off at the point where the neck of the gall-bladder joins the cystic duct.

Anomalous blood-vessels running **behind or below the cystic duct** are also a source of danger (Fig. 246, D; Fig. 247, B; Fig. 248, C, D).

The cystic, or the right hepatic artery when it crosses in front of the common bile-duct is also a source of danger when choledochotomy is performed (Fig. 247, B; Fig. 248, C). The same is true when the gastro-duodenal artery makes a curve in front of the common bile-duct, (Fig.

248, E), just as well as in those anomalous cases in which the cystic artery takes its origin from the gastro-duodenal (Fig. 248, C), the superior pancreatico-duodenal (Fig. 248, D) or the superior mesenteric artery and crosses in front of the common bile-duct.

The drainage of the hepatic and common bile-ducts is by no means a simple procedure in the "long parallel type" of union of the cystic and main hepatic ducts.

Removal of stones from the cystic duct of the spiral type, when the stones lie in that portion of the duct which is situated **behind the main hepatic duct, will result in opening of two ducts instead of one** (Fig. 244, F, G). All these possibilities have to be kept in mind by a surgeon before he starts any kind of work on the gall-bladder or on the biliary passages.

B. SURGICAL PROCEDURES ON THE BILIARY TRACT.

I. CHOLECYSTOTOMY (CHOLECYSTENDESIS).

This is an operation in which the gall-bladder is opened and closed at the same sitting. It has usually been performed for the removal of gall-stones. Van der Wiel, in 1687, was probably the first who performed it on a living human being. Later it was entirely forgotten until Meredith performed it in 1883. After opening the gall-bladder and the removal of the stones he closed the gall-bladder. Some surgeons considered this operation as an "ideal cholecystotomy". However, now there can hardly be found any surgeon who would consider this operation ideal. **Whenever the gall-bladder is deliberately opened it should be drained. This means that cholecystotomy should never be performed.**

II. CHOLECYSTOSTOMY.

The first deliberately planned cholecystostomy for the removal of stones was done by Jean Louis Petit, in 1743.

Thudichum, in 1859, suggested a two-stage cholecystostomy. In the first stage the gall-bladder was sutured to the abdominal wall, and in the second stage it was opened. As a "one stage" operation, this was first performed by an American surgeon, Bobbs, in 1867, when he thought that he had opened an ovarian cyst. Kocher was the first who, in 1878, performed successfully and deliberately a cholecystostomy in one stage.

Definition. The term "cholecystostomy" consists of 3 Greek words: χολή, bile; κύστις, cyst; and στόμα, mouth. It signifies an artificial fistula of the gall-bladder, connecting the latter with the outside world.

Indications.

1. Gall-stones, with severe infection of the gall-bladder.

2. Any pathology of the gall-bladder usually requiring cholecystectomy, but associated with pathology of the common bile-duct which cannot be taken care of at the time of the operation. In such a case it would be unwise to remove the gall-bladder on account of a possible future need for

it should it become necessary to side-track the common bile-duct by performing a cholecysto-enterostomy.

3. In feeble patients in whom cholecystectomy is indicated, but which on account of their weakness must be postponed until some other time.
Technic.
Abdominal Incision.

Different incisions are used for work on the gall-bladder. We use in our work the Courvoisier or Kausch incision (Fig. 36, 1 and 3).

Step 1. The abdomen is opened, and the right side of the patient's back is placed in an elevated position either by a sand-bag or by lifting the side of a specially-constructed table (Fig. 249). This simple change

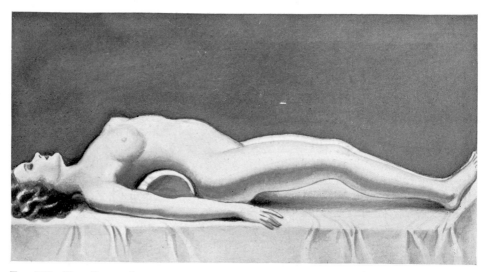

FIG. 249. THE RIGHT SIDE OF THE CHEST IS ELEVATED. (WHEELOCK ELLIOT METHOD).

in the position of the patient was introduced by Wheelock Elliot, of Boston. **This brings the liver to the surface of the skin and facilitates all operations on the gall-bladder and liver.**

Step 2. The round ligament of the liver is grasped by an artery-forceps and handed to the assistant who pulls it slightly in the direction of the left shoulder-joint of the patient. The biliary region is "walled off" from the rest of the peritoneal cavity by placing three laparotomy pads moistened in warm normal salt-solution. One pad is laid in the pouch between the inferior surface of the right lobe of the liver and the upper pole of the right kidney (Morison pouch), another, in front of the stomach, and the third, below the stomach in front of the small bowel.

In order to prevent the loops of the small bowel from appearing in the operative field, we have used for many years the following simple procedure. Before placing the third laparotomy pad, **we pick up the** omentum and spread it carefully over the small bowel. Then only do we place in front of it the third laparotomy pad.

This simple procedure eliminates entirely the troublesome feature of the small bowel appearing constantly in the operative field.

By placing the three laparotomy pads in the above described manner, the entire abdominal cavity is "walled off" from the operative field.

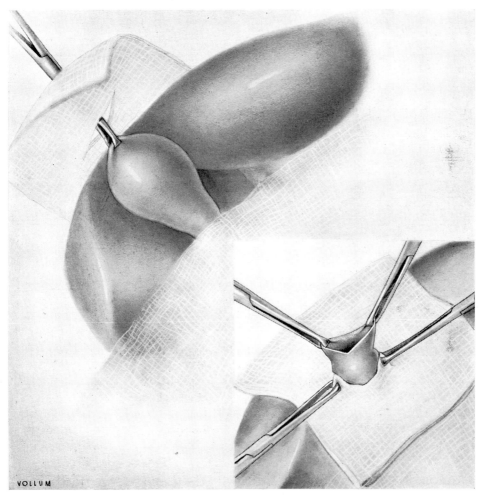

FIG. 250. CHOLECYSTOSTOMY.
MAIN PICTURE. Covering the gall-bladder with gauze.
INSERT. The gall-bladder is opened.

Step 3. A moist laparotomy sponge with an opening in it, the length of which is one inch, covers the gall-bladder in such a manner that the opening corresponds to the place in the gall-bladder where the incision is contemplated (Fig. 250). The sponge is attached to the wall of the gall-bladder by two Allis forceps, and the wall of the exposed portion of the gall-bladder is grasped by two vulsella after which the contents of the gall-bladder are aspirated by a syringe attached to a fine needle.

Step 4. The wall of the gall-bladder is snipped with scissors between the two vulsella for a distance of half-an-inch. The vulsella are reapplied

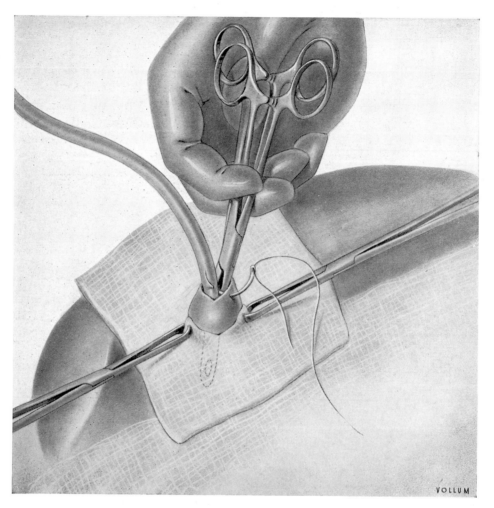

FIG. 251. CHOLECYSTOSTOMY.
Immobilization of the catheter by a transfixing suture.

by catching the lips of the opening in the gall-bladder (Fig. 250, lower insert).

A scoop is introduced into the gall-bladder and all the stones are removed. The cystic, hepatic and common bile-ducts are then palpated to ascertain whether any stones are present in them.

If there are any stones, an attempt should be made to "milk" them back into the gall-bladder. [We should not be misled by mistaking a calcified lymphatic gland for an intra-biliary stone.] If very small particles of stones ("sand") are present, it is best to introduce a piece of gauze and remove them by it.

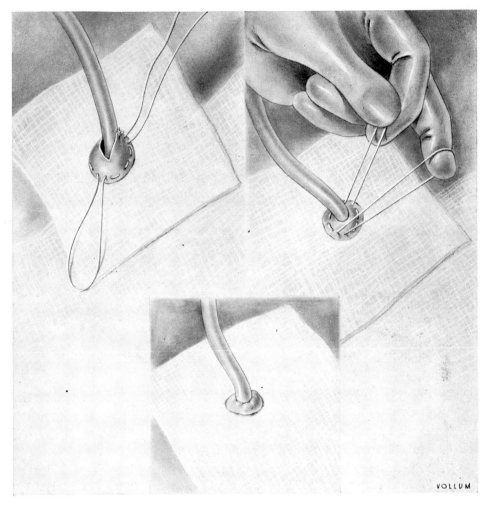

FIG. 252. CHOLECYSTOSTOMY.
LEFT UPPER INSERT. Purse-string suture is inserted.
RIGHT UPPER INSERT. Showing the method of invagination of the catheter.
LOWER INSERT. The catheter is fixed in its final position.

Step 5. A rubber tube with a diameter of about eight millimeters (about one-third of an inch) is introduced into the lumen of the gall-bladder for a distance of one inch. The rubber tube is fixed to the wall of the gall-bladder by a transfixing suture (Fig. 251).

Step 6. A purse-string suture is inserted into the gall-bladder precisely in the same manner as in the Stamm method of gastrostomy, leaving one loop and two long ends (Fig. 252, left upper insert). The purse-string is then tied in the same manner as described in the Stamm method of gastrostomy. This will invert the serous edges of the gall-bladder, which will facilitate the future spontaneous closure of the opening when there is no longer need for a drain (Fig. 252, lower insert).

The wall of the gall-bladder should not be fixed to the parietal peritoneum, since fixation causes a dragging pain and occasionally, due to pulling of the gall-bladder, causes kinks in the common bile-duct which may result in an obstruction of the duct.

III. CHOLECYSTECTOMY.

The first cholecystectomy on a human being was performed by Langenbuch, in 1882. On animals it was done as early as in the 17th century. Zambecarri, of Italy, performed it successfully on a dog in 1630.

In Switzerland it was first performed on a human by Courvoisier in 1885, in France, by Thiriar, in 1885, and in the United States by Ohage, in 1887.

Definition.

The term "cholecystectomy" consists of three Greek words: χολή, bile; κύστις, cyst; and ἐκτομή, excision. It signifies removal of the gall-bladder.

Indications.

1. Primary carcinoma of the gall-bladder.
2. Chronic and subacute cholecystitis (in acute cases, the operation should be postponed until the acuteness "cools off").
3. Gangrene of the gall-bladder.
4. Chronic empyema of the gall-bladder due to stricture of the cystic duct.
5. Benign tumors of the gall-bladder.
6. Multiple ulcerations of the gall-bladder.
7. "Strawberry" gall-bladder. [Some surgeons do not consider a "strawberry" gall-bladder as a pathological condition and they advise leaving it alone.]
8. Calcification of the gall-bladder.

Cholecystectomy should not be performed as the first of a series of operative steps in the case of stricture of the common duct, or in the presence of stones in this duct. The pathology of the common bile-duct must first be corrected, since if anything should happen to this duct at the time of its repair after the removal of stones, the surgeon may utilize the gall-bladder for anastomosis with the gastro-intestinal tract. **Only after the common bile-duct pathology has been corrected may the surgeon perform cholecystectomy.**

Technic.

Step 1. Abdominal Incision. Various incisions are used (Figs. 36, 37). We prefer either the Courvoisier or the Kausch incision (Fig. 36, 1 and 3). In the case of stout patients the Sprengel incision (Fig. 36, 2) gives additional room.

The position of the patient is the same as in all cases of gall-bladder surgery and has been already described.

Step 2. After the abdomen is opened the gall-bladder and the surrounding viscera should be examined.

First, the stomach should be explored, especially along the anterior and posterior surfaces of the lesser curvature, since in 80 to 90 per cent. of all the cases of ulcer of the stomach the ulcer is situated close to the lesser curvature. If an ulcer is present there the surgeon should decide as to the pathology of which organ is responsible for the patient's condition.

If both organs are pathologically altered to about the same degree, **the gall-bladder should be removed first and the pathology of the stomach should be corrected at some future time.** However, if the operation on the stomach has been deferred, it should never be resumed without checking up, both clinically and roentgenologically, whether the ulcer of the stomach is still present, since cases have been encountered in which a **gastric ulcer, definitely demonstrated at the time of the first operation, healed after the gall-bladder and the appendix had been removed.**

After the stomach has been examined, the liver should be "rotated". This consists in making the inferior surface face anteriorly. This is accomplished by grasping the anterior border of the liver with the hand covered by moist gauze and drawing the liver upward. The newly acquired position of the liver can be sustained by holding the border of the liver by the hand and by catching with an artery-forceps the round ligament of the liver. This rotation of the liver can be made still more pronounced by passing the hand of the surgeon between the liver and the diaphragm, so that a suction of air takes place. However, this maneuvre should never be tried in the case of an acute condition of the gall-bladder, on account of the possibility of infecting the subdiaphragmatic space, with the subsequent formation of a subphrenic abscess. After "rotation" is done, the gall-bladder should be "walled off" by three laparotomy pads as described above.

Next the cystic, hepatic and common bile-ducts should be examined. The index-finger of the right hand is placed along the lower border of the gall-bladder and is carried in a upward, medial and backward direction until it reaches the foramen epiploicum ("foramen of Winslow"). The common bile-duct is palpated by keeping the index-finger of the right hand in the foramen of Winslow with the thumb of this hand resting on the ventral surface of the anterior wall of the foramen (Fig. 253). [It should be kept in mind that the common bile-duct lies in the most lateral portion of the anterior wall of the foramen of Winslow. It should also be kept in mind that a calcified gland or glands may be present lying close to the common bile-duct, and these should not be mistaken for intrabiliary stones.]

If stones are found in the common bile-duct their removal from this duct should be undertaken first, and only after this is successfully done

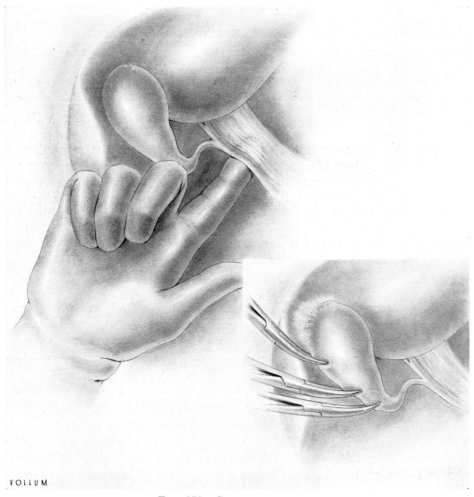

VOLLUM

FIG. 253. CHOLECYSTECTOMY.
MAIN PICTURE. Palpation of the anterior wall of the foramen of Winslow.
INSERT. Clamping the wall of the gall-bladder.

should the gall-bladder be removed. We should always remember that **until it is decided whether the gall-bladder should be removed or not, no forceps should clamp its wall.**

The removal of the gall-bladder can be done from below or from above. The operation from below is neater. However, due to the frequency of anomalies in the course of the blood-vessels and of the biliary ducts, it is safer to remove the gall-bladder from above.

a. Removal of the gall-bladder from above.

Step 3. The wall of the gall-bladder is grasped by an artery-forceps close to the fundus and is put on a stretch by pulling the forceps. With another artery-forceps the lower border of the gall-bladder is grasped

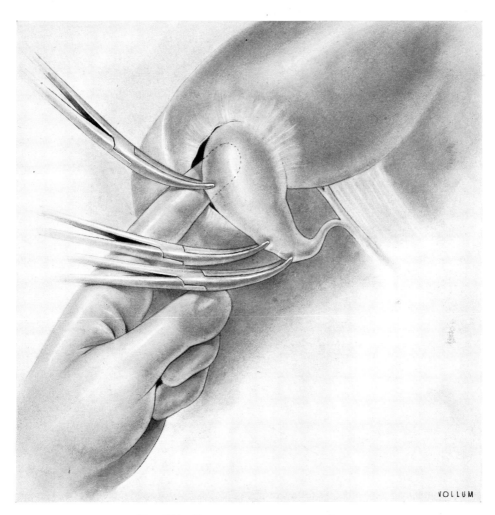

FIG. 254. CHOLECYSTECTOMY FROM ABOVE.
Separation of the gall-bladder from its bed.

about one inch or an inch and-a-half below the first forceps (Fig. 253, lower insert).

A fold connecting the proximal portion of the gall-bladder with the duodenum [this is present in 12 to 25 per cent. of all cases] is exposed. It is grasped close to the gall-bladder by a surgical tissue-forceps and is torn down to the neck of the gall-bladder. Usually this is accomplished very easily. If it cannot be pulled readily, then its edge is snipped by scissors and it is separated by the index-finger of the right hand, covered with a piece of gauze. **However, before cutting or separating this fold from the**

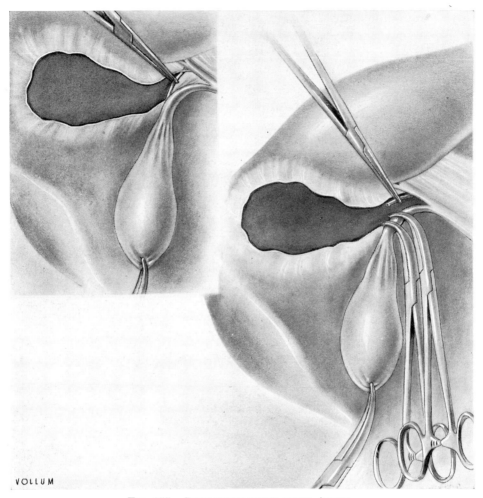

Fig. 255. Cholecystectomy from Above.
Upper insert. Clamping the cystic artery.
Main picture. The cystic artery is cut; clamping the cystic duct.

gall-bladder it should be palpated, since in anomalous cases a blood-vessel may traverse it in the direction toward the gall-bladder.

After this fold has been severed, the portion of the gall-bladder close to the neck is exposed and the wall of the gall-bladder in this region is grasped by a third artery-forceps. **By slight pulling with the three artery-forceps the entire gall-bladder is now well exposed.**

Step 4. The upper forceps attached to the fundus of the gall-bladder is gently pulled forward. Thus, the peritoneal fold which connects the gall-bladder with the liver will become stretched, and the outline of the gall-bladder wall will be clearly seen. This stretched peritoneum is then cut close to the wall of the gall-bladder for a length of one inch. The

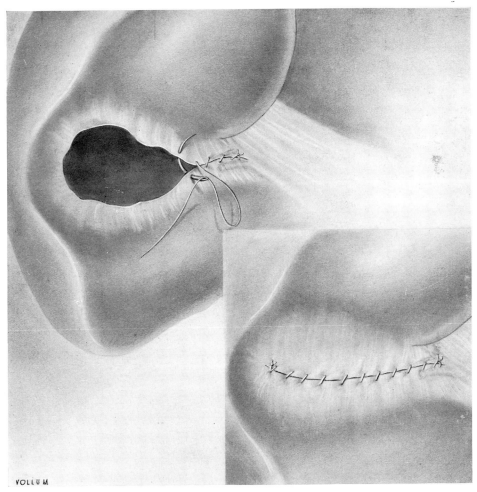

FIG. 256. CHOLECYSTECTOMY FROM ABOVE.
Peritonization of the bed of the gall-bladder.

index-finger of the left hand is introduced behind the gall-bladder and separates it from its liver-bed (Fig. 254). While doing this the gall-bladder is gently pulled away from the liver. This will bring into marked relief the peritoneum which connects the wall of the gall-bladder with the liver. The peritoneum is then cut close to each side of the wall of the gall-bladder. **When approaching the neck of the gall-bladder a peritoneal fold will be**

seen. This should be clamped by an artery-forceps, since in it runs the cystic artery (Fig. 255, left insert). This fold is cut between the artery-forceps and the wall of the gall-bladder. Now the three forceps attached to the gall-bladder are gently pulled upward. This will expose the cystic duct and the place where it joins the hepatic duct in order to form the common bile-duct.

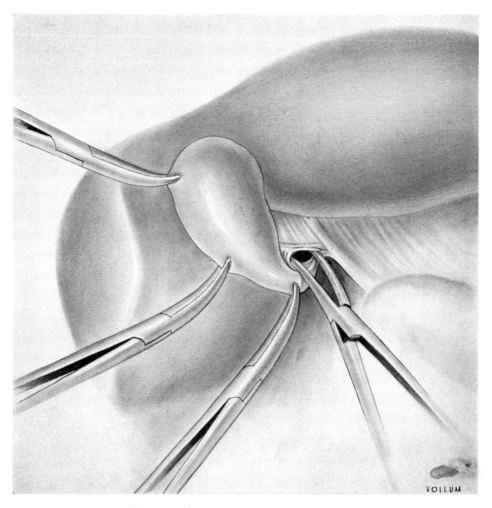

FIG. 257. CHOLECYSTECTOMY FROM BELOW.
Separation of the cystic duct from the artery.

The cystic duct is now clamped by a curved artery-forceps placed half an inch from its point of junction with the hepatic and common bile-ducts. Another curved artery-forceps clamps the duct, which is then cut between the two clamps (Fig. 255). The open end of the duct is disinfected by tincture of iodine and alcohol and then ligated by plain catgut No. 1. The ends of the thread are cut short.

It is not advisable to ligate the cystic duct either very close to or too far from its junction with the hepatic duct. In the first case, the surgeon is liable to injure the hepatic or the common bile-duct, and in the other

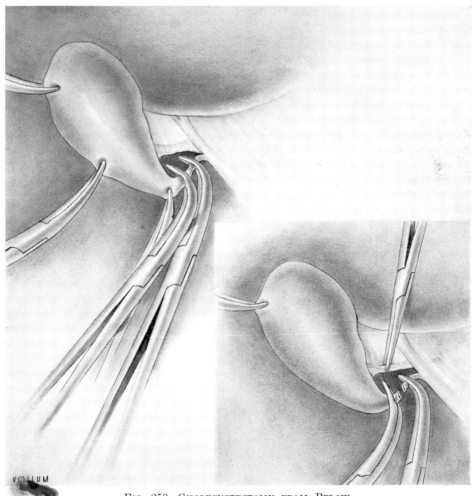

VOLLUM

FIG. 258. CHOLECYSTECTOMY FROM BELOW.
MAIN PICTURE. Clamping the cystic duct.
INSERT. Division of the cystic duct and clamping the cystic artery.

case, the remaining cystic duct may expand and become, so to speak, a new gall-bladder.

Step 5. The lips of the peritoneal folds are sutured together so as to cover the bed of the gall-bladder (Fig. 256).

b. Removal of the gall-bladder from below.

Step 3. As Step 3 in "Removal of the gall-bladder from above".

Step 4. With a curved forceps the peritoneum is torn anteriorly between the cystic duct and the cystic artery (Fig. 257). There is generally no danger either of tearing the duct or the artery, since they usually slide away. A curved forceps is then introduced into the slit thus produced between the cystic duct and artery. The jaws of the clamp are then spread sufficiently to separate the cystic duct from the cystic artery for a distance

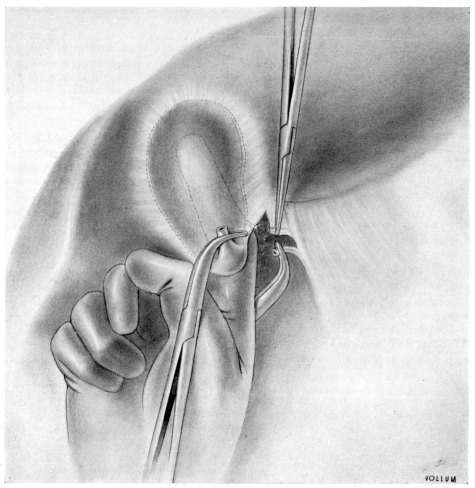

FIG. 259. CHOLECYSTECTOMY FROM BELOW.
The cystic duct and artery are cut; separation of the gall-bladder from the liver.

of one inch (Fig. 257). A curved forceps then clamps the cystic duct one-fourth of an inch away from its point of junction with the hepatic duct. This forceps is placed in such a manner that its convex surface faces the common duct (Fig 258). Another curved forceps clamps the cystic duct one-fourth of an inch distal from the first clamp, and the duct is cut between these two forceps (Fig. 258, lower insert). The clamp attached to the distal end of the severed cystic duct is then gently pulled. This will put the peritoneal folds connecting the gall-bladder with the liver on the stretch. An artery-forceps then clamps the peritoneal fold in which the cystic artery runs (Fig. 258). This fold is then cut distal to the artery-forceps, between it and the wall of the gall-bladder. The index-

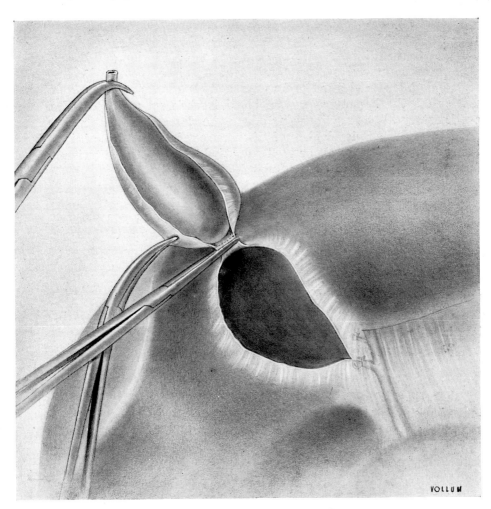

FIG. 260. CHOLECYSTECTOMY FROM BELOW.
A forceps clamps the peritoneal fold from which hangs the gall-bladder.

finger of the right hand is introduced behind the gall-bladder and separates it from the bed of the liver (Fig. 259). The peritoneal folds which extend between the gall-bladder and the bed of the liver are then put on a stretch and cut by scissors. These manipulations are continued until only a very small fold is left connecting the fundus of the gall-bladder with the liver. An artery-forceps then clamps this fold (Fig. 260), which is cut distal to the clamp, thus freeing the gall-bladder from any connections with the liver. The clamp attached to this peritoneal fold enables the surgeon to hold the liver conveniently while the next step is being performed. The cystic artery and the duct are now ligated.

Step 5. The lips of the peritoneal folds are sutured together so as to cover the bed of the gall-bladder.

In case a ligature slips from the cystic artery, the supposed location of this artery should not be grasped blindly. The following should then be done: A finger is introduced into the foramen of Winslow and the anterior wall of this foramen is put on the stretch. A Spivack non-crushing arterial forceps is introduced into the foramen and clamps its anterior wall. This will arrest the hemorrhage. The blood is then sponged out, when the cystic artery will be readily seen and may be clamped by an artery-forceps and ligated. The Spivack clamp is then removed. There is no injury done either to the blood-vessels or to the duct which form the anterior wall of foramen of Winslow, since the Spivack clamp does not damage either the intima of the blood-vessels or the endothelium of the duct.

The question of drainage has aroused considerable controversy:

The opponents of drainage (followers of the "ideal cholecystectomy") give the following objections to drainage:

1. Placing of the drainage-tube on the stump of the cystic duct prevents the accumulation of serum and the sealing of the stump, thus inviting a leakage of bile from the cystic duct with the formation of a biliary fistula.

2. The drainage-tube weakens the anterior abdominal wall, thus inviting the future development of a postoperative ventral hernia.

3. Drainage increases the length of time of confinement to bed.

4. Drainage facilitates the formation of adhesions, thus increasing the future morbidity of the patient.

For these reasons, many surgeons, particularly in Germany, after removing the gall-bladder close the abdomen completely: They are doing an "ideal cholecystectomy". This procedure was inaugurated in Germany as long ago as 1913. However, the objections raised by the opponents of drainage may now nearly all be eliminated. Thus:

1. There is no necessity for placing the drainage-tube on the stump of the cystic duct. If bile escapes from the cystic duct it accumulates in the most dependent portion, which is the innermost portion of the Morison pouch. **For this reason, we place the drain in the innermost portion of the pouch so that it does not touch the stump of the cystic duct at all.**

2. **It is not necessary to bring the drainage-tube out through the original abdominal incision.** We usually pass the drainage-tube through a small stab-wound situated midway between the last rib and the iliac crest in the anterior axillary line, and close completely the original abdominal incision. This eliminates the objection that the drain prolongs the

time of confinement to bed and tends to the formation of post-operative ventral hernia.

3. The objection that the drain produces adhesions and increases the morbidity is valid.

This objection is probably the only valid objection suggested by the opponents of drainage. However, the followers of drainage consider

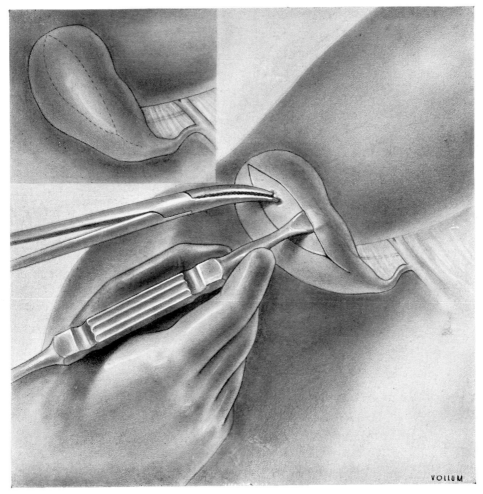

FIG. 261. SUBSEROUS CHOLECYSTECTOMY.
"Shelling out" the gall-bladder from its serous covering.

drainage for this reason as of paramount importance, since bile should always be considered septic and as long as there is seepage of bile from the liver it should be drained. Seepage of bile comes not only from the cystic duct from which a ligature has slipped off, but also from the accessory extrahepatic bile-ducts (which were described in the subchapter

"Variations of bile-ducts"), and also from the accessory bile-ducts which directly connect the liver-substance with the gall-bladder and which were torn during the process of removal of the gall-bladder. **As, in the usual methods of removing the gall-bladder, there is no way of preventing tears of the small accessory ducts which directly connect the liver-bed with the gall-bladder, there is nothing else left for the surgeons but to drain, or as**

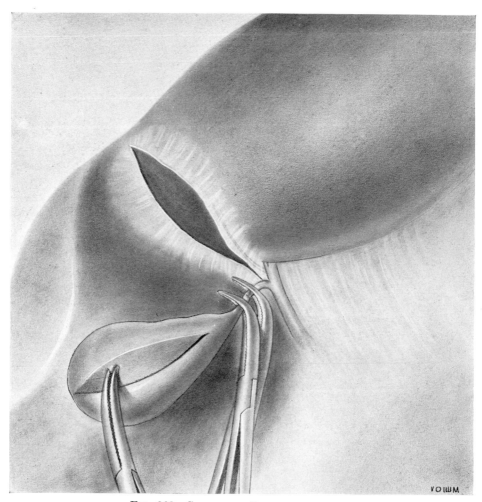

FIG. 262. SUBSEROUS CHOLECYSTECTOMY.
The gall-bladder is "shelled out"; the cystic duct is clamped.

an alternative to employ those methods which will prevent leakage of bile from the liver.

Two procedures have been suggested to prevent the leakage of bile:

1. **Subserous cholecystectomy,** in which the serous layer of the gall-bladder is incised and the musculo-mucous layer is shelled out;

2. **Mucoclasis (Pribram operation),** in which the mucosa and all or a part of the muscularis are destroyed either by the thermocautery or by diathermy.

1.   SUBSEROUS CHOLECYSTECTOMY.

The term, "subserous cholecystectomy" was coined by Witzel in 1906.

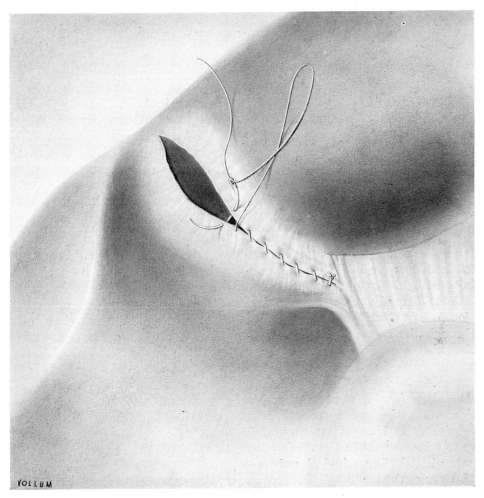

FIG. 263. SUBSEROUS CHOLECYSTECTOMY.
Suturing the leaflets of the serosa layer of the gall-bladder to each other.

However, Courvoisier, Langenbuch and others performed it long before Witzel described it. This may be seen in their writings.

Technic.

Step 1. The serosa on the inferior surface of the gall-bladder is incised in the form of a racquet from the fundus to the cystic duct (Fig. 261, insert). The line of cleavage between the serosa and the muscularis is found, and the serosa is separated from the muscularis along this line until the musculo-mucous wall is shelled out from its serous covering (Fig. 262). The cystic duct is then clamped by two forceps and the gall-bladder is cut between them. The cystic duct is now ligated.

Step 2. The leaflets of the serosa are sutured to each other (Fig. 263).

This method is superior to mucoclasis. However, it is not always possible to perform it. Then the following method is used by some surgeons:

2. MUCOCLASIS (PRIBRAM OPERATION).

This operation was described by Pribram in 1928. At the time of the first publication of his method he had performed it on 200 patients. He advocated destroying the mucous membrane of the gall-bladder, without removal of the gall-bladder by sharp instruments such as knives, so that the bed of the gall-bladder was left intact. He called this operation **mucoclasis.** He advised using the thermocautery for destroying the mucosa of the gall-bladder after ligation of the cystic duct and artery, with subsequent suturing of the remaining seromuscular layer by a serous approximation.

However, in a following paper on the same subject, published on April 27, 1929, he advocated the use of diathermy instead of the thermocautery, in order to destroy the inner surface of the gall-bladder by electrocoagulation. He used an electrode of 1 by 2 cm. in size and advised pressing the electrode against the mucosa **with only slight pressure** so as not to burn through the entire thickness of the wall of the gall-bladder and injure the substance of the liver. P. L. Mirizzi and F. A. Olmedo, in November, 1931, published their results in an article entitled "Mucoclasis of Pribram", reporting thirteen cases in which they electrocoagulated the mucosa and muscularis by diathermy and reduced the thickness of the wall by two-thirds. All the patients recovered. Pop, of Cluj University (Rumania), published, in 1931, the report of 36 cases of mucoclasis as performed mostly by himself in the clinic of Prof. Jacobivici. He mentioned in this paper that Pribram had already performed 310 operations with 9 deaths (2.9 per cent. mortality). In his 36 cases there was not a single death. He used the thermocautery in the earlier operations, and electrocoagulation by diathermy in the later cases.

Albertin, in 1933, published an additional 10 cases of obliteration of the gall-bladder by the Pribram method without a single death.

Thorek, in November 1933, and in July, 1934, published 75 cases of electrocoagulation without a single death. **He emphasized that not only the mucosa and the muscularis, but even the serosa and also the liver-bed, should be electrocoagulated.**

Thorek Technic.*

Step 1. The abdomen is opened, the surrounding structures are examined, and the gall-bladder is walled off from the rest of the peritoneal cavity.

Step 2. The gall-bladder is grasped by an artery-forceps at the

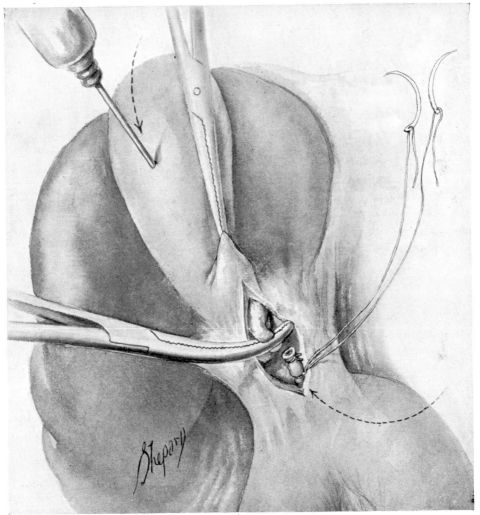

FIG. 264. MUCOCLASIS OPERATION.
(THOREK TECHNIC).

fundus. A needle, connected with a syringe, is inserted into the gall-bladder and the bile is aspirated. An artery-forceps clamps the wall of the gall-bladder as soon as the needle is removed so as to occlude the hole produced by the latter. At the same time the surgeon may use this artery-

*Dr. Thorek operated 143 cases by electrocoagulation without a single death (Personal communication).

forceps as a holder. The artery-forceps which was placed at the beginning of the operation is now removed (Fig. 264).

Step 3. The cystic duct and artery are now isolated, cut, and the ends ligated separately, precisely in the same manner as has been described in the technic of "Cholecystectomy from below" (Fig. 264).

Step 4. The gall-bladder is opened by a knife, scissors or diathermy-

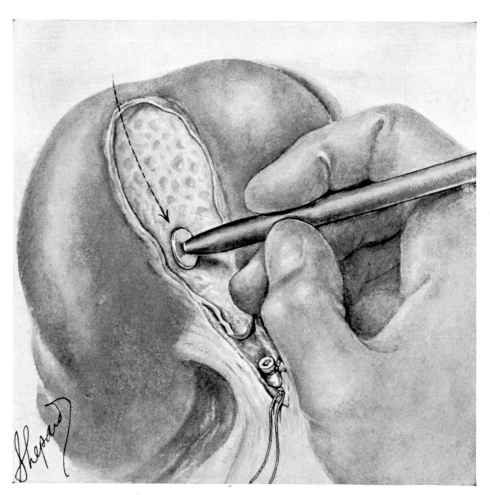

FIG. 265. MUCOCLASIS OPERATION.
(THOREK TECHNIC).

knife along its entire length up to 1 cm. from the divided distal end of the cystic duct.

Step 5. An electrode of the size of 1 by 2 cm. is applied to the mucosa of the gall-bladder, so as to electrocoagulate the entire thickness of the mucosa and muscularis. The electrode should not press **too lightly on the**

mucosa nor too heavily; in the former case there will be no electrocoagulation, and in the latter case the liver may be damaged (Fig. 265).

Step 6. The remnants of the gall-bladder wall are sutured to each other by their serous surfaces. In this way the gall-bladder is entirely obliterated.

Step 7. The abdomen is closed in tiers.

Several objections have been raised against the method of Pribram:

1. **Opening of the lumen of the gall-bladder.** Even after all its contents have been aspirated it is still hazardous to open an infected gall-bladder.

2. Electrocoagulation of the inner layer of the wall of the gall-bladder eliminates only one possible source of seepage of bile, by occluding the numerous small bile-ducts running from the liver-bed to the gall-bladder. It will not preclude the possibility of escaping of the bile either through the cystic duct (if the ligature slipped by accident) or through the large accessory ducts, if they were present and inadvertently cut.

There seems to be a growing sense of disappointment in the results obtained from a cholecystectomy. Many consider the gall-bladder not only as a mere reservoir for bile, but they attach to it an important physiological function. They believe that as long as possible the gall-bladder should not be removed. For this reason, Pribram lately suggested, instead of using cholecystectomy, making a small opening in the neck of the gall-bladder, removing the stones (if they are present), and then performing cholecysto-choledochostomy, an operation which was already performed by Wolff, in 1909. In all the cases that he reported thus far the results have been gratifying. The description of this method will be found under cholecysto-choledochostomy.

Some other surgeons advised performing a cholecysto-gastrostomy or cholecystoduodenostomy instead of a cholecystectomy, thus producing "internal drainage of bile". The technic of these procedures will be given below.

IV.   CYSTICOTOMY.

Definition. This is the opening and closure of the cystic duct at the same sitting.

Indications.

There are hardly any indications for the performance of this operation. However, it was often used in the pioneer days of biliary surgery for removal of stones in the cystic duct or for hydrops of the gall-bladder due to the obstruction of the cystic duct by stones. This operation was first performed by Lindner, in 1891.

After the cystic duct was exposed it was incised, the stones removed, the opening closed by two rows of catgut sutures, and the gall-bladder drained. Surgeons today prefer to perform a cholecystectomy. With the latest trend in surgery in preserving the gall-bladder, it is highly probable that cholecystogastrostomy and cholecystocholedochostomy will be performed for the cases in which formerly cysticotomy was done.

V. HEPATICOTOMY.

This consists in the opening and closure of the hepatic duct at the same sitting. It is usually performed for the removal of stones.

The first hepaticotomy was performed by Kocher, in 1889, unintentionally. He removed a stone, making an incision of a structure that he believed to be the gall-bladder. The autopsy showed that the opened viscus was the hepatic duct.

Usually, after the opening in the duct is closed, the abdominal cavity is drained. This operation is technically difficult on account of poor accessibility of the hepatic duct. The best thing to do in the case of a stone in the hepatic duct is to "milk" it into the gall-bladder or into the common bile-duct.

VI. HEPATICOSTOMY.

This is an artificial communication between the lumen of the hepatic duct and the outside world. It was first performed by Knowsley Thornton in 1888. This can be accomplished by opening the hepatic duct and suturing its edges to the anterior abdominal wall. In the case of a moderately distended hepatic duct, this is hardly possible. In the case of a very dilated hepatic duct it can be easily executed, and this is the manner in which Knowsley Thornton performed it.

VII. CHOLEDOCHOTOMY AND CHOLEDOCHOSTOMY.

Definition. This consists in incising the common bile-duct and closing it at the same sitting with (choledochostomy) or without draining the duct (choledochotomy). Langenbuch was the first who suggested it, in 1884; Kŭmmell was the first to perform it in the same year. Knowsley Thornton was the first who successfully performed it, in 1889. In case the common bile-duct is closed without drainage it is called choledochotomy, and if a drain is placed, one end of which lies in the common bile-duct and the other is brought outside of the abdominal cavity, it is called choledochostomy.

Indications. This operation is usually done for the removal of impacted stones, which may lie either in:

a. The supraduodenal portion.

b. The retroduodenal portion.

c. The intraduodenal portion of the common bile-duct where the duct traverses the thickness of the duodenal wall.

d. The diverticulum duodeni (ampulla of Vater).

According to the location of the stone there are described:

a. The supraduodenal choledochotomy or choledochostomy **(Langenbuch operation).**

b. The retroduodenal choledochotomy or choledochostomy **(Haasler operation)**.

c. The transduodenal choledochotomy or internal choledochoduodenostomy **(Kocher operation)**.

d. The duodeno-choledochotomy or ampullary choledochotomy **(McBurney operation)**.

a. THE SUPRADUODENAL CHOLEDOCHOSTOMY (LANGENBUCH OPERATION).

Step 1. The position of the patient, the abdominal incision, and the "walling off" of the biliary region are precisely the same as in other operations on the gall-bladder and on the biliary passages, and have been already described.

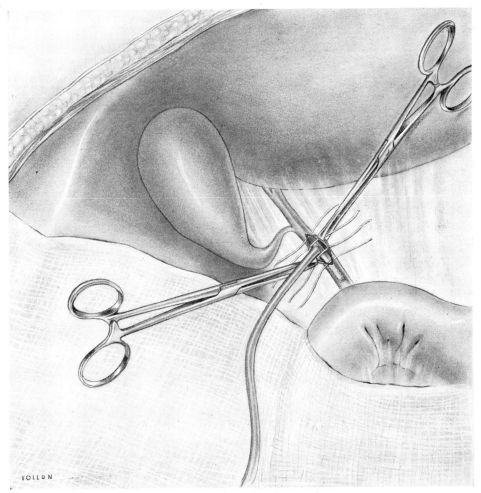

FIG. 266. SUPRADUODENAL CHOLEDOCHOSTOMY. (LANGENBUCH OPERATION).

Step 2. The index-finger of the left hand is inserted into the foramen of Winslow and the duct is palpated between the thumb and this finger. The stone is located and steadied with the thumb and the finger. The wall of the common bile-duct is cut over the stone which is squeezed out.

The edges of the lips of the incised wall of the common bile-duct are grasped by two vulsellum forceps. An L-shaped tube is introduced into the duct and the other end is brought outside the abdominal cavity. The common bile-duct is closed snugly around this tube (Fig. 266). A soft rubber tube is placed to the right of the common bile-duct and the other end of it is also brought outside of the abdominal cavity. [N.B. There is quite a divergence of opinion as to whether the common bile-duct should be drained after it is incised. Some place a rubber catheter for drainage of the hepatic duct only. Some drain only the common bile-duct; some place a T-tube, draining both the hepatic and the common bile-duct; some use an L-shaped tube. Some do not use a drain in the common bile-duct at all, being satisfied with placing a drain extrabiliary.]

b.   RETRODUODENAL CHOLEDOCHOSTOMY (HAASLER OPERATION).

This was suggested by Haasler, in 1898. The characteristic feature of this procedure is that the second part of the duodenum is mobilized by the Kocher method and the posterior wall of the duodenum is turned anteriorly (Fig. 221).

This portion of the duct is either covered by pancreatic tissue or lies in a groove within the pancreas. The gland must for this reason either be cut or separated bluntly. After the duct is exposed, it should be incised, the stone removed and the duct sutured. A drain should be left in the surrounding tissues.

c.   TRANSDUODENAL CHOLEDOCHOSTOMY OR INTERNAL CHOLEDOCHO-DUODENOSTOMY (KOCHER OPERATION) (FIG. 267).

(Kocher operation) (Fig. 267).

This operation was first performed by Kocher, in 1894, and was described by him as "Internal Choledocho-duodenostomy". It consists in incising the anterior wall of the second part of the duodenum and then the posterior wall, until the duct is exposed lying intramurally, and then in opening the common bile-duct.

This is usually done for removal of stones impacted in the third part of the common bile-duct, that is, in the portion of the duct which traverses the wall of the duodenum.

Technic.

Step 1. The abdominal incision, the position of the patient, and the rotation of the liver are the same as usual in operations on the gall-bladder and biliary passages.

Step 2. The mobilization of the duodenum by the Kocher method and the bringing of the duodenum to the surface of the skin are done in the manner already described.

Step 3. The duodenum is steadied with two fingers of the left hand which hold its wall close to the impacted stone. The anterior wall of the duodenum is cut, and a vulsellum grasps each lip of the wound. A finger is inserted into the lumen of the duodenum and its posterior wall is palpated. If the stone lies close to the ampulla, an attempt is made to extricate it through the ampulla. If the surgeon fails to do this (and that

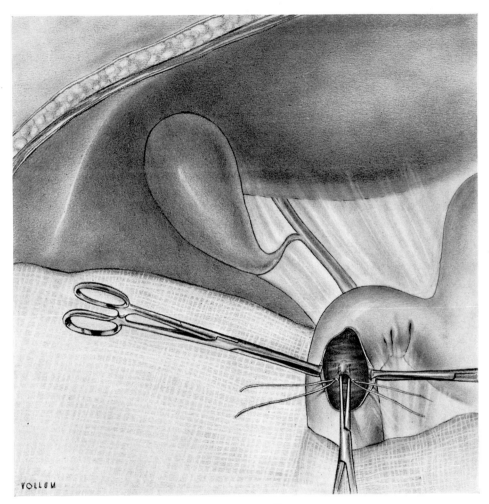

FIG. 267. TRANSDUODENAL CHOLEDOCHOSTOMY.
(KOCHER OPERATION).

happens most frequently), **then the posterior wall of the duodenum and the duct over the stone are cut.**

Two catgut sutures are inserted, one on each lip, which include all the substance between the mucosa of the posterior wall of the duodenum and the stone. Each suture thus includes part of the posterior wall of the duodenum and the anterior wall of the duct. These two sutures are used as traction-sutures and facilitate the removal of the stone. After the latter is removed, **it is important not to suture the lips, that is, to leave them open.** Thus, a **choledocho-duodenostomy has been performed.** If, however, in order to remove the stone the incision of the posterior wall is continued upward and reaches the retroduodenal portion of the duct, then

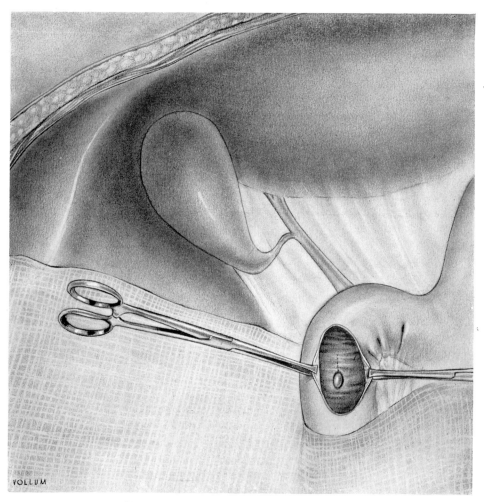

FIG. 268. AMPULLARY CHOLEDOCHOSTOMY.
(MCBURNEY OPERATION).

the lips of the open posterior wall of the duodenum should be sutured to the lips of the opened common bile-duct. Otherwise, leakage of bile and of intestinal contents into the free peritoneal cavity or into the retro-peritoneal space will ensue.

Step 4. The anterior wall of the duodenum is sutured in layers. The first is through-and-through and the second seromuscular. The seromuscular suture-line is covered by omentum.

Step 5. The abdomen is closed without drainage.

We must emphasize again, that as the third part of the common bile-duct lies in the thickness of the duodenal wall, in the Kocher operation **the posterior wall of the duodenum is cut into, but not through.**

d. AMPULLARY CHOLEDOCHOSTOMY (McBURNEY OPERATION) (FIG. 268).

This consists in opening the anterior wall of the duodenum in order to expose the ampulla Vateri and then in cutting through the lip of the opening (porus duodeni) followed by the extraction of the stone.

After the stone is removed, **the incised lip of the ampulla is not sutured (otherwise stricture of the porus duodeni may ensue),** but the incised anterior wall of the duodenum is, of course, sutured.

VIII. RECONSTRUCTION OF THE BILIARY TRACT.

Numerous procedures have been described to reëstablish the flow of bile into the alimentary tract in case the permeability of the duct has been lost from any cause, or to make new channels for the flow of bile into the alimentary tract. These numerous methods can be grouped into several classes:

1. **Reconstruction of the biliary tract by excision or by plastic methods.**

    A.   **Excision of the constricted portion of the bile-duct with end-to-end anastomosis of the divided ends.**

            a.   **Direct end-to-end anastomosis.**

            b.   **Indirect end-to-end anastomosis.**

    B.   **Plastic reconstruction of the biliary tract:**

    a.   Incision of the anterior wall of the bile-duct longitudinally with suturing of it transversely.

    b.   Longitudinal incision of the anterior wall of the constricted bile-duct with the introduction into its lumen of a portion of a catheter, and surrounding the opening with omentum.

    c.   Reconstruction of the biliary tract by a pedicle-flap made from the wall of an adjoining viscus of the gastro-intestinal tract or from the gall-bladder.

    d.   Reconstruction of the biliary tract by a flap of different structures not connected with their mother-tissue (fascia, veins, arteries, etc.) ("Free transplantation").

2. **Implantation of a portion of the biliary tract into some portion of the gastro-intestinal tract (stomach, duodenum, jejunum):**

            a.   Direct implantation.

            b.   Indirect implantation.

3. **Direct communication between the liver and some gastro-intestinal viscus.**

4.   **Implantation of an existing external biliary fistula into the gastro-intestinal tract, or the artificial formation of an external biliary fistula with subsequent implantation of it into the selected hollow viscus of the gastro-intestinal tract:**
> a.   Direct implantation.
> b.   Indirect implantation.

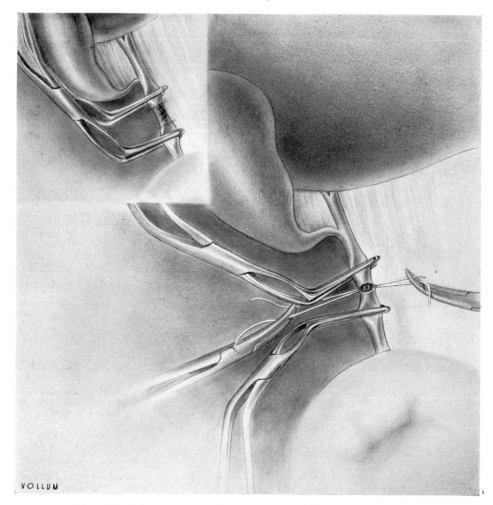

Fig. 269. Resection of a Portion of the Common Bile-Duct.

1.   **Reconstruction of the biliary tract.**

    A.   **Excision of the constricted portion with an end-to-end anastomosis.**

    a.   **Direct anastomosis.** In case of impermeability of the common bile-duct the constricted portion may be excised and the remaining portion sutured together.

The first end-to-end anastomosis of the common bile-duct was performed by Doyen, in 1892. He sutured the divided ends over a rubber tube. Kőrte, in 1898, sutured the ends of the divided duct without the use of prothesis. The technic, as it is used now, is as follows:

Step 1. The abdomen is opened, the patient placed in the proper

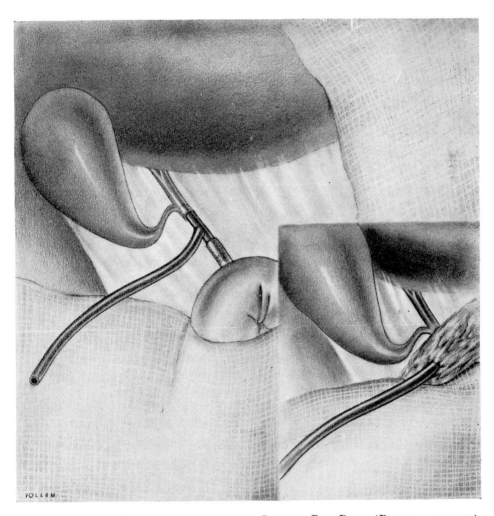

FIG. 270. INDIRECT RECONSTRUCTION OF THE COMMON BILE-DUCT (PROPPING METHOD).

posture, the operative field isolated, and the surrounding structures examined.

Step 2. The liver is rotated so as to make the constricted common bile-duct lie as superficially as is possible. Then the common bile-duct is separated from the other structures of the anterior wall of the foramen of Winslow. Two Spivack non-crushing forceps then clamp the common bile-duct, one proximally and the other distally from the site of the stricture (Fig. 269, insert).

Step 3. The stricture is excised.

Step 4. Four fine silk sutures are inserted, which unite the respective ends of the posterior lips of the divided duct (Fig. 269). The ends of these sutures are tied; those of the middle two threads are then cut short and those of the lateral two threads are left long. The non-crushing clamps are now disengaged. An L-shaped tube is inserted in such a manner that the short end of the tube lies in the hepatic duct, the long end of the horizontal portion in the common bile-duct, and the vertical portion is brought outside of the abdominal cavity.

Step 5. A suture is inserted, connecting the anterior lips of the duct on each side of the vertical end of the L-tube. The threads are tied and the ends are cut short.

The immediate and late results of end-to-end anastomosis are good. However, this method should never be employed if there is any tension after the ends are brought together.

b. **Indirect anastomosis of the ends of the divided common bile-duct** (Fig. 270).

This is usually done when the divided ends are far from each other (more than one-third of an inch). It was first performed by Verhoogen, in 1907. Propping, in 1909, performed an indirect anastomosis utilizing a T-tube as a bridge in order to connect the separated ends of the divided common bile-duct. The operation, as performed by Propping, is seen in Fig. 270. It is always better to follow the suggestion of Sullivan, namely, to cover the exposed part of the rubber tube with omentum.

The immediate results of the operation are good, but the late results (after 1 to 1½ years subsequent to the operation) are not good, since a stricture of the newly formed channel ensues. **Therefore, this method should not be used.**

B. PLASTIC RECONSTRUCTION OF THE BILIARY TRACT:

a. **Plastic reconstruction by a longitudinal incision of the anterior wall in the strictured portion and by suturing it in a transverse direction** (Fig. 271).

This method is analogous to the Heineke-Mikulicz method of pyloroplasty, and is best done either over a T-tube or over two tubes, one of which is inserted into the hepatic and the other into the common bile-duct.

The results of this method are good. **However, it can be used only in those rare cases in which the stricture is short.** If the latter is long, then it is not convenient to use this method, since the points most distant from each other, namely, the upper and lower ends of the stricture cannot be brought together.

b. **Plastic reconstruction by a longitudinal incision of the constricted bile-duct and surrounding the opened duct with omentum.**

The duct is opened longitudinally. A small portion of a rubber tube or of a catheter is inserted into its lumen and the distal end is brought outside the abdomen. The opening in the duct is covered with omentum or it may be left open. One lip of the duct is then sutured to the other over this rubber tube.

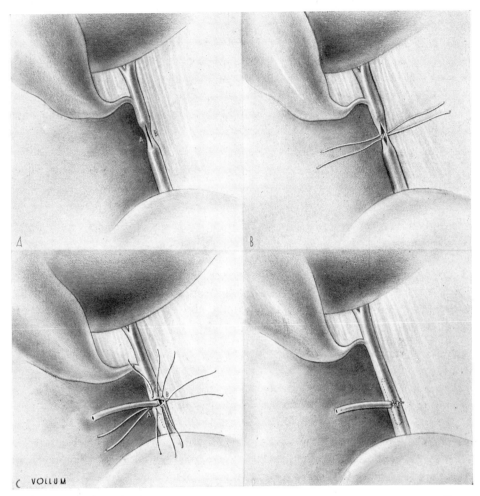

FIG. 271. PLASTIC RECONSTRUCTION OF THE COMMON BILE-DUCT BY CUTTING THE DUCT LONGITUDINALLY AND SUTURING IT TRANSVERSELY.

This method is good as long as the tube stays in. As soon as it drops off stricture ensues.

c. Reconstruction of the biliary tract by the formation of a pedicle-flap from the wall of an adjoining viscus of the gastro-intestinal tract or from the gall-bladder.

This consists in making a flap of the entire thickness of a portion of the anterior gastric wall or of the wall of the gall-bladder and in implanting it into the defect of the wall of the common bile-duct. To Kehr belongs the credit for introducing this method. It gives good results and should be considered as a good method.

d. Reconstruction of the biliary tract by flaps of different structures not connected with their mother-tissue, such as fascia, arterial tubes, venous tubes, etc. ("Free transplants").

This method has been used by many surgeons, both on the human and experimentally. The transplants were autogenous, homogenous and even heterogenous. **The results were unsatisfactory and for this reason we do not advise this method at all.**

2. Implantation of a portion of the biliary tract into a selected part of the gastro-intestinal tract (stomach, duodenum, jejunum).

The portion of the biliary tract selected for implantation may be the gall-bladder, the cystic, hepatic or the common bile-duct. The viscus into which it is implanted may be the stomach, duodenum or the jejunum. The anastomosis may be **direct** or **indirect.** In case of a direct anastomosis, this may be done by a suture method or by a mechanical device, such as the Murphy button, etc. [**We always prefer the suture method to any in which a mechanical device is employed.**]

a. Direct implantation of the biliary tract into the gastro-intestinal tract.

This is an artificial communication between the lumen of the gall-bladder or of the cystic, hepatic or common bile-duct and that of the stomach or of the bowel. The first cholecysto-enterostomy (it was cholecysto-colostomy) was performed by Winiwarter, in 1880, by a six stage method.

A Russian surgeon, Monastyrski performed a cholecysto-enterostomy (cholecysto-jejunostomy) **as a one stage** operation, in 1887, by a **suture** method. A cholecysto-jejunostomy by the "Y" method was first performed by Monprofit and reported in 1904.

The first cholecysto-duodenostomy was performed by Bardenheuer, in 1888. The first cholecysto-gastrostomy was performed by Gersuny, in 1892, and published by Wickhoff and Angelberger, in 1893. Cholecysto-choledochostomy was first performed by Wolff, in 1909. He did it as a side-tracking operation in case of a previously completely divided common bile-duct.

Pribram, in 1935, suggested the very same operation by making an anastomosis between the neck of the gall-bladder and the common bile-duct. The reason for using this operation, according to Pribram, is that in recent years a close study of the physiology of the gall-bladder showed that this organ should be preserved whenever possible and not removed. By making an anastomosis between the neck of the gall-bladder and the common bile-duct the gall-bladder is placed comparatively at rest, and this not only prevents a further development of the pathology of its wall but even an existing pathology may subside. Pribram reported eleven cases treated in this manner with gratifying results. As may be seen, Pribram's cholecysto-choledochostomy is identical with Wolff's, but it is done not as a side-tracking, but as an "internal drainage" operation.

The first lateral cystico-duodenostomy was performed by Mayo Robson, in 1898, and the first hepatico-duodenostomy by Kehr, in 1902. The first lateral choledocho-duodenostomy was performed by Riedel, in 1888.

CHOLECYSTO-GASTROSTOMY.

The first cholecysto-gastrostomy was performed in 1892 by Gersuny, and the report of this case was made by Wickhoff and Angelberger, in 1893. The object of the operation was to side-track the obstructed common bile-duct. For many years this operation served as one of the sidetracking type of operations.

Wayne Babcock, in 1920, advised using cholecysto-gastrostomy not only as a sidetracking operation, but also **for the treatment of a gastric or duodenal ulcer by neutralizing the high acidity of the stomach by the alkaline contents of the gall-bladder.**

The same operation for the surgical treatment of gastric or duodenal ulcer was advocated by Bogoras, in 1925, and it is known in Europe as the "Bogoras operation". DuBose, in 1931, advocated the performing of a cholecysto-gastrostomy not only as a sidetracking operation and for the treatment of gastric or duodenal ulcer, but also as an "internal drainage" operation, which should replace the external drainage of bile (cholecystostomy) and cholecystectomy.

Technic (Fig. 272).

Step 1. The abdominal incision and the exposure of the liver are the same as in all gall-bladder operations.

Step 2. A seromuscular suture running in a vertical direction is made between the fundus of the gall-bladder and the stomach for a distance of one and one-half inches. On the stomach, the suture-line is made on the antrum, one inch proximal to the pyloric canal.

Step 3. The stomach and the gall-bladder walls are incised for a distance of one inch. The line of incision on the stomach is at a distance of one-third of an inch from the suture-line, and on the gall-bladder one-sixth of an inch. The mucosa of the stomach is sutured to the mucosa of the gall-bladder by a continuous suture, using chromic catgut number 0. When the suturing of the mucous layer is completed, a seromuscular suture is made between the anterior lips of the gall-bladder and stomach.

Step 4. The suture-line is reinforced by covering it with a piece of omentum.

Another method of making an anastomosis between the gall-bladder and the stomach was described by Stubenrauch, in 1905. A flap of the anterior wall of the stomach was made (Fig. 273, A) and its free edge was sutured to the wall of the gall-bladder (Fig. 273, B). The gall-bladder was then opened so that its lumen communicated with that of the stomach, and the flap served as a bridge between these two lumina (Fig. 273, C). The

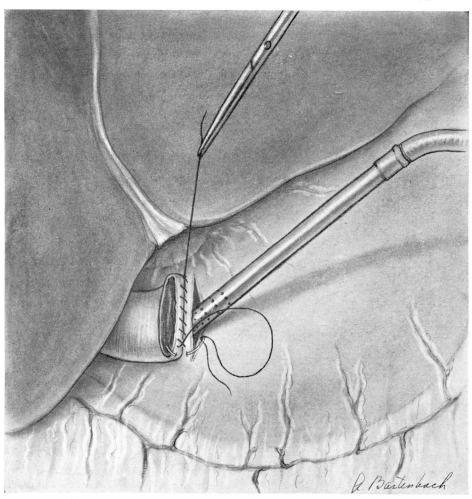

FIG. 272. CHOLECYSTOGASTROSTOMY BY THE SUTURE METHOD.

flap was then sutured in the form of a tube. Thus, a tubular communication between the lumina of the gall-bladder and stomach was established (Fig. 273, C).

One objection is raised against cholecysto-gastrostomy, namely, the possibility of an ascending cholangitis. Whereas there is unanimity of opinion that this is always present in dog experimentation, its occurrence in the human is much disputed. Some believe that it hardly ever occurs in the human, particularly when the anastomosis is made between the gall-bladder and the stomach and not between the gall-bladder and the jejunum. However, there are reports from several leading clinics that an ascending cholangitis was observed after performing this operation. In order to overcome this difficulty several procedures have been suggested:

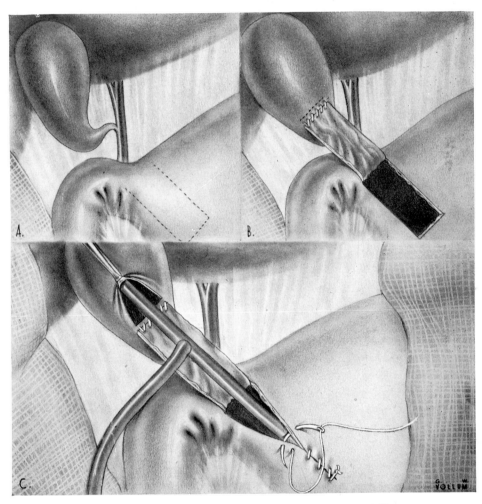

FIG. 273. CHOLECYSTOGASTROSTOMY BY THE STUBENRAUCH METHOD.

a. To make the anastomosis in such a manner that a portion of the gall-bladder shall lie in a channel of the Witzel type formed on the anterior wall of the stomach or of the duodenum (Lambret method).

b. To make the anastomosis between the gall-bladder and the stomach or the duodenum so that a portion of the gall-bladder traverses the thickness of the anterior wall of the stomach (or duodenum) similar to the Schnitzler type of gastrostomy **(Roeder technic, Spivack technic).**

c. To make an anastomosis between the gall-bladder and the common bile-duct **(Wolff-Pribram cholecysto-choledochostomy).**

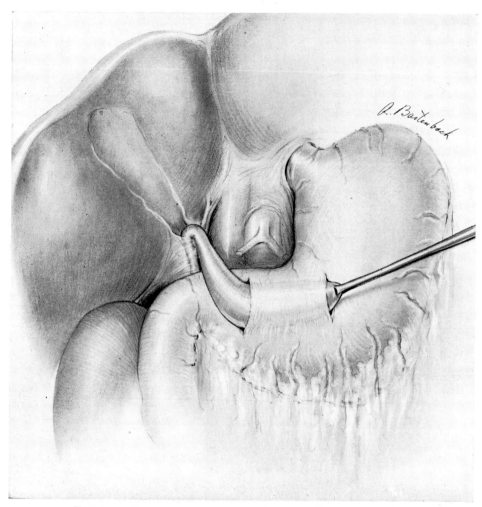

FIG. 274. CHOLECYSTOGASTROSTOMY BY THE SPIVACK METHOD.
A portion of the gall-bladder is placed in the thickness of the stomach-wall.

CHOLECYSTO-DUODENOSTOMY BY THE LAMBRET METHOD.

Step 1. A seromuscular continuous suture is made between the inferior surface of the gall-bladder and the anterolateral surface of the duodenum. If it is difficult to place them in this manner without tension then the duodenum should be mobilized by the Kocher method.

Step 2. The gall-bladder is placed on the anterior wall of the duodenum, and an anastomosis is made between the apex of the fundus and the innermost part of the anterior surface of the duodenum.

Step 3. The portion of the gall-bladder which lies on the anterior wall of the duodenum is covered by the duodenal wall by making a series of interrupted or continuous sutures so as to form some kind of a Witzel channel, with the exception of the place where the stoma is made.

Thus, the contents of the gall-bladder escape into the duodenum or into the stomach and the contents of the stomach or of the duodenum will not run in an opposite direction.

CHOLECYSTO-GASTROSTOMY BY THE SPIVACK METHOD.

Step 1. A seromuscular incision is made on the antrum of the stomach very close to the pylorus (Fig. 274). Another seromuscular incision is

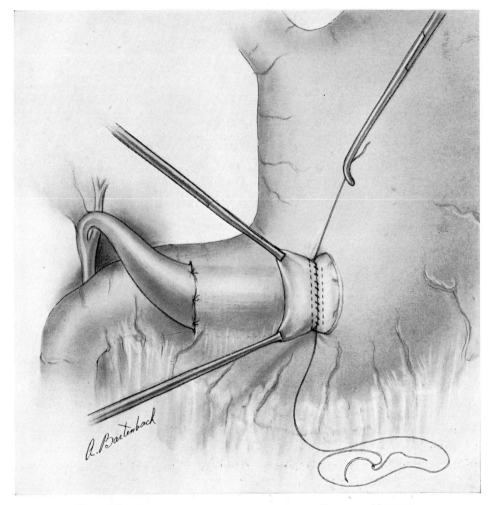

FIG. 275. CHOLECYSTOGASTROSTOMY BY THE SPIVACK METHOD.
Anastomosis between the stomach and the gall-bladder is begun.

made on the stomach one and a half inches proximal from the first, and the seromuscular layer of the wall of the stomach between these two incisions is undermined. The fundus (and, if necessary, a portion of the body) of the gall-bladder is drawn through this seromuscular channel (Fig. 274). A seromuscular suture is made between the anterior lip of

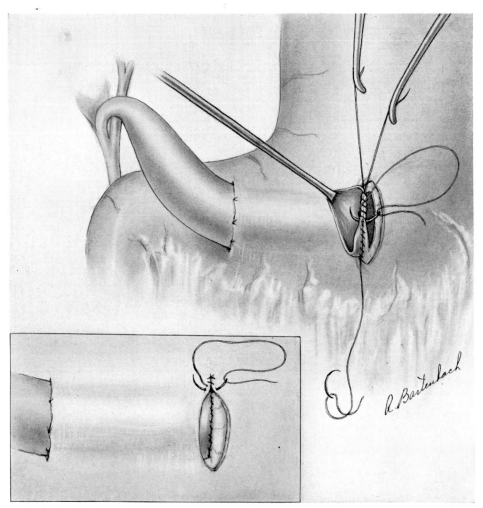

FIG. 276. CHOLECYSTOGASTROSTOMY BY THE SPIVACK METHOD.
MAIN PICTURE. Suturing the mucosa of the stomach to the entire thickness of the gall-bladder-wall.
INSERT. Suturing the lips of the stomach-wall to each other over the line of anastomosis.

the distal incision of the stomach (that is, the one lying closer to the pylorus) and the gall-bladder (Fig. 275).

Step 2. The cone of the gall-bladder is incised as is also the mucosa of the stomach. An anastomosis is made between these two structures

(Fig. 276), suturing the mucosa of the stomach to the entire thickness of the wall of the gall-bladder.

Step 3. The seromuscular lips of the stomach are sutured to each other, thus covering the site of the anastomosis between the gall-bladder and the stomach (Fig. 276, insert).

In this way, the gall-bladder traverses the thickness of the stomach-wall approximately in the same manner as the common bile-duct traverses the wall of the duodenum, and this prevents regurgitation of the gastric or of the duodenal contents into the biliary tract.

CHOLECYSTO-CHOLEDOCHOSTOMY BY THE WOLFF-PRIBRAM METHOD
(FIG. 277).

Step 1. The gall-bladder and the common bile-duct are well exposed. The neck of the gall-bladder is opened for a length of an inch, and all

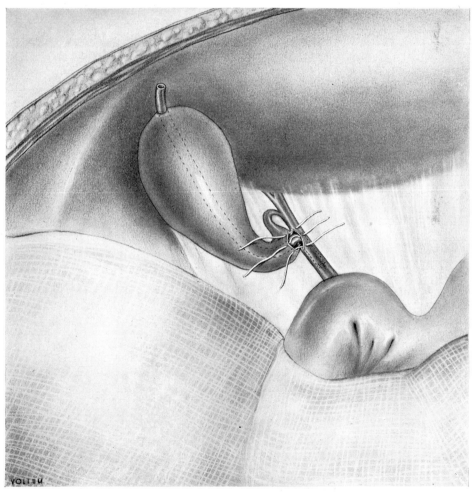

Fig 277. Cholecysto-choledochostomy.
(Wolff-Pribram method).

stones, if they are present, are removed from the gall-bladder. The common bile-duct is incised for an inch, and a lateral anastomosis is performed between the opening of the gall-bladder and that of the common bile-duct by one layer of interrupted buttonhole or mattress-sutures (Fig. 277). This layer is reinforced by covering it with the gastro-hepatic ligament.

This operation has the merit of giving good drainage of the gall-bladder without bringing it in direct communication with the alimentary tract. However, the disadvantage of this method lies in the technical difficulties, since the common bile-duct is narrow, unless it has had large stones in its lumen at some previous time.

Cholecysto-jejunostomy is performed in the same manner as a cholecysto-gastrostomy. **Whenever the cholecysto-gastrostomy can be performed, it should be given the preference to cholecysto-jejunostomy.**

b. Indirect Anastomosis between the Biliary and the Gastro-intestinal Tracts.

An indirect anastomosis is done only in those cases in which the direct anastomosis is impossible. This was first performed by Jenckel, in 1905, and published in 1910. He inserted one end of a rubber tube into the end of the divided hepatic duct and the other end into the lumen of the duodenum. Before entering the lumen of the duodenum, the rubber tube traversed for some distance the wall of the duodenum in a channel formed according to the Witzel type.

Sullivan, in 1909, published a report of his experiments on dogs. He performed a series of choledocho-duodenostomies in the same manner as just described (his report appeared **before** Jenckel published his report). The difference between Sullivan's and Jenckel's methods was that Sullivan did not perform a secondary operation for the removal of the rubber tube (which Jenckel did), but waited for the tube to pass into the duodenum, which actually took place in his experiments. Sullivan advised wrapping the rubber tube with traumatized omentum (Fig. 278).

The early and late results of this operation are unsatisfactory. For this reason, **indirect hepato-duodenostomy** or **choledocho-duodenostomy should be used only in those cases in which a direct anastomosis is impossible.**

3. Direct anastomosis between the liver-parenchyma and some portion of the gastro-intestinal tract (Hepatocholangio-gastrostomy and Hepatocholangio-enterostomy).

This consists in suturing the lips of the opened wall of the stomach or bowel to the lips of the incised capsule of the liver, thus establishing a direct communication between the substance of the liver and the lumen of the gastro-intestinal tract. This operation was first suggested by Langenbuch, in 1897, and carried out by Kehr, Maylard, Garré and others. **The results are very unsatisfactory, and for this reason this method should never be resorted to.**

4. **Implantation of an existing external biliary fistula into the gastrointestinal tract, or the artificial formation of an external biliary fistula with its subsequent implantation into some hollow viscus of the gastrointestinal tract.**

a.   **Direct Implantation.**

Czerny was the first who implanted, in 1902, an external biliary fistula

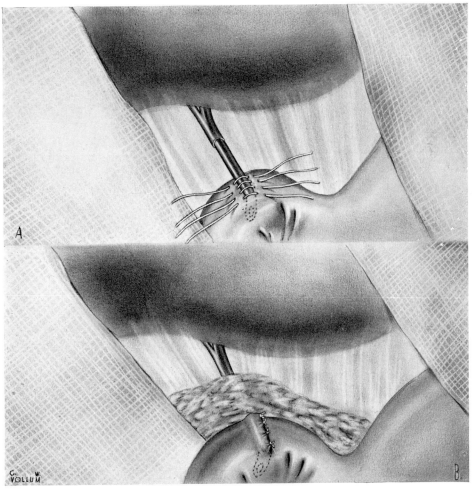

FIG. 278.   INDIRECT METHOD OF CHOLEDOCHO-DUODENOSTOMY.
OR HEPATO-DUODENOSTOMY.
(JENCKEL-SULLIVAN METHOD).

into the alimentary tract. Since that time several cases have been reported in which an external biliary fistula has been implanted into the stomach, duodenum, jejunum, and even into the common bile-duct. **The results of direct implantation of an external biliary fistula into the alimentary tract are excellent.**

b.   Indirect Implantation.

This consists in placing one end of a rubber tube into the distal end of the biliary fistula and the other end into the stomach or small bowel. Before this end of the rubber tube enters the lumen of the stomach or of the bowel it lies in a channel made of the anterior wall of the viscus in the form of a Witzel channel. **The results of indirect implantation are not good.**

It appears a promising procedure to form as the first stage an external biliary fistula, and as the second stage to implant this fistula into the stomach or bowel or the common bile-duct.

CONCLUSIONS

Among the numerous methods of repair of the biliary passages, the best is the direct suturing of the ends of the divided common bile-duct. The next best is direct anastomosis between the gall-bladder and the gastro-intestinal tract. Indirect anastomosis in general is not satisfactory, and should be done only when the previously mentioned satisfactory methods are difficult to employ.

BIBLIOGRAPHY.

R. Albertin. Suppression de la vésicule biliaire par la méthode de Pribram. Lyon Chirurgical, 30:207-214; y. 1933.

A. W. Allen & R. H. Wallace. Technique of operation on common bile-duct, with special reference to instrumental dilatation of papilla of Vater. Amer. Journ. of Surg. 28:533-561; y. 1935.

P. D. Amadon. Agenesis of gall-bladder, associated with pancreatitis. Report of a case.
Am. Journ. of Surg. 19:263-267; y. 1933.

L. Arnsperger. Die chirurgische Bedeutung des Icterus zugleich ein Beitrag zur Pathologie und Chirurgie der tiefen Gallenwege.
Bruns Beitr. z. klin. Chir. 48:673-779; y. 1906.

W. Wayne Babcock. Cholecystogastrostomy and cholecystoduodenostomy. Am. Journ. of Obst. & Gyn. 1:854-859; y. 1920.

D. C. Balfour. The technic of hepaticoduodenostomy, with some notes on the reconstructive surgery of the biliary ducts.
Annals of Surg. 73:343-347; y. 1921.

Bardenheuer. Anlegung einer Gallenblasen-Dünndarmfisteln.
Berlin. klin. Wchnschr. 25:877; y. 1888.

K. Barlos. Abnorme Lagerung der Gallenblase bei Zweilappung der Leber. Arch. f. klin. Chir. 164:280-285; y. 1931.

F. Barnstorf. Zur Agenesie der Gallenblase.
Frankfurt. Zeitschr. f. Pathol. 42:304-318; y. 1931.

M. G. Beaver & F. C. Mann. Some suggestions in experimental surgery; technic for opening and closing thorax; simple method for transplantation of ureter and common bile-duct into intestine.
Ann. of Surg. 95:620-623; y. 1932.

L. Bérard & P. Mallet-Guy. Les indications légitimes de la cholécystogastrostomie.
Lyon Chir. 27:5-16; y. 1930.

L. Bérard & P. Mallet-Guy. Résultat éloigné d'une cholécysto-gastrostomie pour un syndrome vésiculaire douloureux déterminé par un état pathologique de la voie biliaire principale (vésicule intolerante).
Lyon méd. 145:573-577; y. 1930.

L. Bérard & P. Mallet-Guy. L'étude expérimentale des anastomoses de la vésicule biliaire; revue critique.
Lyon Chir. 30:17-36; y. 1933.

F. Bernhard. Experimentelle und klinische Untersuchungen über das Zustandekommen des Hydrops der Gallenwege oder der sog.
Weissen Galle.
Arch. f. klin. Chir. 178:495-502; y. 1933.

F. Bernhard. Die spontanen inneren Gallenfisteln und ihre operative Behandlung.
Deutsch. Zeitsch. f. Chir. 242:493-506; y. 1934.

F. Bernhard. Die Früh-und Spätergebnisse der Cholecystogastrostomie, der Cholecystoduodeno-und Choledochoduodenostomie bei 128 Fällen.
Deutsche Zeitschr. f. Chir. 242:736-756; y. 1934.

N. Bogoras. Über Cholecystogastrostomie bei dem Magenulcus. Eine neue Operationsmethode zur Behandlung des Magenulcus.
Arch. f. klin. Chir. 134:42-50; y. 1925.

E. A. Boyden. Problem of double ductus choledochus (an interpretation of an accessory bile-duct found attached to pars superior of duodenum).
Anat. Rec. 55:71-93; y. 1932.

Budde. Beiträge zur Kenntniss der Topographie der normalen A. hepatica und ihrer Varietäten sowie der Blutversorgung der Leber.
Deutsche Zeitschr. f. Chir. 86:18-40; y. 1906.

Büngner. Zur Anatomie und Pathologie der Gallenwege und des Pancreas.
Wien. med. Presse. 43:1784-1786; y. 1902; also abstract in Zbl. f. Chir. 29:1252-1253; y. 1902.

C. Clavel & Chabannes. Recherches sur l'anatomie comparée des voies biliaires dans les deux sexes et sur leur abord chirurgical.
Ann. d'anat. pathol. 10:895-903; y. 1933.

H. M. Clute & N. W. Swinton. Exploration of common duct in gallstone surgery.
Surg. Gyn. & Obst. 59:906-912; y. 1934.

F. G. Connell. Liver deaths (so called) : rapid high temperature deaths.
Ann. Surg. 100:319-327; y. 1934.

O. Copello & L. O. Zemo. A propósito de la anestesia esplácnica en cirugía
hepato-biliar.
Bol. y. trab. de la Soc. de cir. de Buenos Aires, 14:53-57; y. 1930.

H. Costantini. A propos du traitement de l'ouverture dans les voies
biliaires des kystes hydatiques du foie.
Rev. de Chir. Paris, 53:69-81; y. 1934.

L. G. Courvoisier. Casuistisch-Statistische Beiträge zur Pathologie und
Chirurgie der Gallenwege.
Leipzig, 1890.

G. Crile. Pathologic physiology of the liver and gall-bladder; five points
in surgery of the gall-bladder and the ducts.
South. Surg. 3:171-180; y. 1934.

R. A. Cutting. Principles of preoperative and postoperative treatment.
Amer. Journ. of Surg. 11:145; 375; 575; 12:165; 343; 561; 13:131;
333; 589; 14:507; 703; y. 1931.

J. B. Deaver. Congenital absence of gall-bladder and extrahepatic ducts.
Am. Journ. of Dis. of Children, 46:356-358; y. 1933.

P. Delbet. Sur certaines particularités des voies biliaires.
Soc. de Chir. de Paris, 31:1126-1130; y. 1905.

P. Descomps. Six cas d'anomalies des voies biliaires.
Bull. de la Soc. anat. 4:328-331; y. 1910.

P. Descomps. Recherches d'anatomie chirurgicale sur les artères de l'abdomen, le tronc coeliaque.
Paris, G. Steinheil; y. 1910.

E. Desmarest. De la cholécystectomie sous-séreuse sans drainage.
Journ. de Chirurgie, 30:641-649; y. 1927.

G. Doberauer. Zur drainagelosen Gallenoperation.
Wien. klin. Wchnschr. 46:549-551; y. 1933.

E. Doyen. Quelques opérations sur le foie et les voies biliaires.
Arch. Provinc. de Chir. 1:149-178; y. 1892.

F. G. DuBose. Gall-bladder function with special reference to cholecysto-
gastrostomy and the absence of ascending cholangitis.
Annals of Surg. 93:736-744; y. 1931.

S. de Dziembowski. Sur la valeur des opérations anastomosantes dans la
chirurgie des voies biliaires.
Bull. et mém. Soc. de chirurg. de Paris, 23:545-563; y. 1931.

D. N. Eisendrath. Anomalies of the bile ducts and blood vessels.
Journ. Am. Med. Ass. 71:864-867; y. 1918.

D. N. Eisendrath. Operative injury of the common and hepatic bile ducts.
Surg. Gyn. Obst. 31:1-18; y. 1920.

S. Eiss & J. H. Whaley Jr. Changes in biliary system after cholecystectomy; causes of recurrence of gall-bladder symptoms.
Ann. of Surg. 101:921-926; y. 1935.

Enderlen. Zur Cholecystogastrostomie.
Deutsche Zeitschr. f. Chir. 234:787-790; y. 1931.

J. F. Erdmann. Common duct injuries and reconstruction.
Southern Surgeon, 4:180-196; y. 1935.

Fedoroff. Einige Richtlinien in der Gallenwegschirurgie.
Deutsche Zeitschr. f. Chir. 240:695-706; y. 1933.

E. R. Flint. Abnormalities of the right hepatic, cystic, and gastroduodenal arteries, and of the bile-ducts.
Brit. Journ. of Surg. 10:509-519; y. 1922-23.

H. Flörcken. Die Operation bei Steinverschluss des Ductus choledochus.
Med. Klin. 30:194-195; y. 1934.

R. S. Fowler. Cholecystectomy without drainage.
Annals of Surg. 93: 745-748; y. 1931.

J. M. Frawley & S. H. Mentzer. Rudimentary gall bladder and congenitally absent common duct; report of a case.
Californ. & West. Med. Journ. 33:607; y. 1930.

R. Friedrich. Die Peritonealisierung der Cysticoduodenostomie (Gleichzeitig tierexperimenteller Beitrag zur Theorie "die Gallenblase der Druckregulatur des Gallengangssystems". Mortalitätsstatistik der Operationen an den tiefen Gallenwegen).
Arch. f. klin. Chir. 179:262-279; y. 1934.

A. Fullerton. A modification of the operation of cholecystenterostomy.
Brit. Med. Journ. I:995; y. 1922.

Gatewood & S. E. Lawton. Effect of cholecystenterostomy on biliary tract.
Surg Gyn. & Obst. 50:40-44; y. 1930.

A. Gentile. Cholecystogastrostomy and hepatitis; experimental study.
Arch. of Surg. 30:449-475; y. 1935.

O. Goetze. Die Entstehung, Verhütung und Beseitigung postoperativer hoher Gallengangstenosen.
Deutsche Zeitschr. f. Chir. 229:171-191; y. 1930.

E. A. Graham. How shall we estimate operative risk and diminish mortality in patients with disease of the biliary tract?
Proc. Calif. Acad. of Med. pp. 1-13; y. 1931-32.

E. A. Graham. Clinical application of some recent knowledge of biliary tract.
Harvey Lect. 1933-1934; pp. 176-203; y. 1935.

G. J. Heuer. Factors leading to death in operations upon gall-bladder and bile-ducts.
Ann. of Surg. 99:881-892; y. 1934.

C. G. Heyd. "Liver deaths" in surgery of the gallbladder.
Journ. Americ. Med. Ass. 97:1847-1848; y. 1931.

O. Hoche. Über Umgehungs-und plastische Operationen im Bereich der Gallenwege.
Arch. f. klin. Chir. 176:621-627; y. 1933.

E. Horgan. Reconstruction of the biliary tract.
McMillan Co., Publishers; y. 1932.

K. Hutter. Zur Anlegung innerer Gallenblasenfisteln.
Arch. f. klin. Chir. 146:332-362; y. 1927.

S. Hybbinette. Quelques suggestions de l'expérience dans le traitement des fistules biliaires post-opératoires complètes.
Acta chir. Scandinav. 69:327-336; y. 1932.

L. Jacques. Secondary plastic repair of common duct; new aid in finding proximal stump.
Surg. Gyn. & Obst. 52:1151-1153; y. 1931.

A. Jenckel. Beitrag zur Chirurgie der Leber und der Gallenwege.
Deutsche Zeitschr. f. Chir. 104:1-121; y. 1910.

A. Jentzer. Die Cholecystogastrostomie.
Schweiz. med. Wchnschr, 14:542-546; y. 1933.

E. S. Judd & V. G. Burden. Benign stricture of the bile ducts.
Arch. of Surg. 11:459-472; y. 1925.

H. Kehr. Die Hepato-Cholangio-Enterostomie.
Zbl. f. Chir. 31:185-189; y. 1904.

R. Kennon. Double gall-bladder opening by two cystic ducts into common bile-duct.
Brit. Journ. of Surg. 20:522; y. 1933.

H. Kment. Operations-und Dauererfolge nach Eingriffen an den Gallenwegen.
Bruns Beitr. zur klin. Chir. 150:534-573; y. 1930.

W. König. Die Chirurgie der Gallenwege.
Zbl. f. Chir. 61:2968-2980; y. 1934.

H. Kuntzen. Über plastischen Ersatz der extrahepatischen Gallengänge.
Zbl. f. Chir. 62:1021-1025; y. 1935.

H. Kunze. Beiträge zur Anatomie und Chirurgie der Gallenausführungsgänge.
Bruns Beitr. z. klin. Chir. 72:491-504; y. 1911.

O. Lambret. Du drainage interne de la vésicule biliaire. Cholecystoduodenostomie a trajet intraparietal.
La Presse Médical. 35:1089-1091; y. 1927.

Langenbuch. Chirurgie der Leber und Gallenblase.
Stuttgart, Enke Publishers; y. 1897.

W. E. Lee & H. P. Totten. Primary carcinoma of the common bile-duct.
Ann. of Surg. 99:930-938; y. 1934.

E. Leo. La colecistectomia ideale. Modo semplice di realizzare la peritoneizzazione, l'emostasi e la colestasi del moncone cistico e della loggia epatica.
Arch. ital. di chir. 30:655-684; y. 1931.

G. Lusena. Colecisto-gastrostomia extraperitoneale.
Arch. ed atti d. Soc. ital. di chir. 36:969-972; y. 1930.

W. A. Mackey. Cholecystitis without stone; investigation of 264 operated cases from clinical, radiological, and pathological aspects. Attempt to determine factors of service in estimating prognosis.
Brit. Journ. Surg. 22:274-295; y. 1934.

P. Mallet-Guy. L'angiocholite ascendante après les anastomoses de la voie biliaire principale; son traitement par l'exclusion duodénale.
Rev. de chir. 52:175-206; y. 1933.

W. J. Mayo. Restoration of the bile passage after serious injury to the common or hepatic ducts.
Surg. Gyn. & Obst. 22:1-6; y. 1916.

W. J. Mayo. Surgery of the hepatic and common bile-ducts.
Lancet, I:1299-1302; y. 1923.

W. J. S. McKay. Preoperative preparation of patients with jaundice due to gall bladder disease.
Med. Journ. of Australia, 2:591-595; y. 1930.

E. P. McNamee. Intrahepatic gallbladder.
Amer. Journ. of Roentgen. 33:603-610; y. 1935.

G. L. McWhorter. Experimental suture of common bile-duct with new methods of anastomosis. Results two and one-half years after the operation.
Surg. Clin. of North America, 12:163-168; y. 1932.

E. Melchior. Zur Kenntnis des übermässigen äusseren Gallenflusses nach Gallenoperationen.
Med. Welt, 7:483-485; y. 1933.

E. Melchior. Courvoisier'sches und Pseudo-Courvoisier'sches Phänomen.
Zbl. f. Chir. 61:2606-2608; y. 1934.

P. L. Mirizzi & F. A. Olmedo. La mucoclasia de Pribram.
Revista de Cirugia de Buenos Aires, 10:681-685; y. 1931.

P. L. Mirizzi & F. A. Olmedo. Präparation des Cysticus innerhalb der subserösen, dränagelosen Cholecystektomie. Spezielle Technik zum Vernähen der erweiterten Cysticusstümpfe.
Deutsche Zeitschr. f. Chir. 235:775-781; y. 1932.

P. L. Mirizzi. Colecisto-duodenostomía valvular. Técnica personal.
Bol. y. trab. de Soc. de cir. de Buenos Aires, 18:1319-1327; y. 1934.

P. L. Mirizzi. Colédoco-duodenostomía interna transduodenal (técnica personal).
Bol. y trab. de la Soc. de cir. de Buenos Aires, 18:1328-1334; y. 1934.

N. D. Monastyrski. Zur Frage der chirurgischen Behandlung der vollständigen Undurchgängigkeit des Ductus choledochus.
Chirurgitschesky Vestnik, 1888; also abstract in Zbl. f. Chir. 15:778-779; y. 1888.

A. Monprofit. Une nouvelle méthode de cholécystentérostomose:
La cholécystentérostomie en Y.
Arch. Provinc. de Chir. 13:380-383; and 449-453; y. 1904.

L. Moskowicz. Die Technik der Transduodenalen Choledocho-Duodenostomie.
Zbl. f. Chir. 54:2015-2019; y. 1927.

B. Moynihan. A case of simple stricture of the common bile duct treated by a plastic operation.
Brit. Med. Journ. II:1390-1391; y. 1905.

Th. Naegeli. Zur Frage des Choledochusersatzes bei narbiger Schrumpfung oder grossen Defekten.
Zbl. f. Chir. 51:727-728; y. 1924.

T. G. Orr. Biliary infection following cholecystoduodenostomy.
Kansas City Southwest Clin. Soc. Monthly Bull. 6:26-30; y. 1930.

V. Pauchet & A. Hirchberg. A propos de quelques observations de chirurgie des voies biliaires accessoires. (Drainage et cholecystectomie).
Technique opératoire. Discussion et deductions.
Rev. de Chir. 52:75-109; y. 1933.

V. Pauchet. Les quatre opérations les plus courantes du traitement des affections des voies biliaires d'après notre dernière statistique.
Tech. Chir. 25:227-252; y. 1933.

W. L. Peple. Unusual if not a unique operation upon the gall-bladder.
Virgin. Med. Monthly, 58:238-240; y. 1931.

A. Pop. Die Pribram'sche "Mukoklase" bei den Erkrankungen der Gallenblase.
Zbl. f. Chir. 58:3194-3197; y. 1931.

H. L. Popper. Über postoperative Pancreatitis nach Operationen am Gallensystem.
Deutsche Zeitschr. f. Chir. 236:124-136; y. 1932.

G. Pototschnig. Anzeigestellung und Ergebnisse der Choledocho-Duodenostomia externa.
Deutsche Zeitschr. f. Chir. 244:288-297; y. 1935.

B. O. Pribram. Mukoklase und drainagelose Gallenchirurgie.
Zbl. f. Chir. 55:773-779; y. 1928.

B. O. Pribram. Zur Technik der Mukoklase.
Zbl. f. Chir. 56:1054-1055; y. 1929.

B. O. Pribram. Der Costalschnitt bei Operationen der Gallenwege.
Deutsche Zeitschr. f. Chir. 225:446-450; y. 1930.

B. O. Pribram. Die Cholecysto-Choledochostomie. Einiges über die Ursachen der Rezidivbeschwerden, die Funktion der Gallenblase und Versuche zu ihrer Erhaltung bei Gallenoperationen.
Zbl. f. Chir. 60:2003-2012; y. 1933.

K. Propping. Regenerierung des Choledochus nach Einlegen eines T-Rohres.
Bruns Beitr. zur klin. Chir. 83:369-378; y. 1913.

W. Rieder. Schnittführung bei Operationen an den Gallenwegen unter besonderer Berücksichtigung der postoperativen Hernien.
Zbl. f. Chir. 59:583-588; y. 1932.

W. Rieder. Anomalien des Gallengangssystems und ihre chirurgische Bedeutung.
Chirurg, 4:516-522; y. 1932.

P. Rio Branco. Essai sur l'Anatomie et la médicine opératoire du Tronc Coeliaque et de ses Branches de l'Artère Hépatique en particular.
Paris, Steinheil; y. 1912.

C. A. Roeder. Modified cholecystogastrostomy.
Ann. of Surg. 94:311-313; y. 1931.

E. Ruge. Beiträge zur Chirurgischen Anatomie der grossen Gallenwege. (Ductus hepaticus, cysticus, choledochus und pancreaticus).
Arch. f. klin. Chir. 87:47-78; y. 1908.

R. Saldaña. Aportación a la anomalía de la rama derecha de la arteria hepática en cirugía biliar.
Arch. de med. cirug. y especialid. 37:847-850; y. 1934.

J. Schnitzler. Algunas nociones fundamentales acerca de la cirugía de las vías biliares.
Rev. med. german-iber.-amer. 4:348-353; y. 1931.

V. I. Schrager, A. C. Ivy & J. E. Morgan. A method for the plastic reconstruction of the common bile duct.
Surg. Gyn. & Obst. 54:613-620; y. 1932.

C. W. Sharples. Liver deaths following operation of biliary tract.
West. Journ. of Surg. 42:337-343; y. 1934.

R. V. B. Shier. Common duct stone.
Canad. Med. Ass. Journ. 31:385-389; y. 1934.

G. Sicca. Deviazioni chirurgiche interne della bile. (Casi clinici).
Annal. ital. di chir. 13:201-218; y. 1934.

E. Siegmund. Ueber die Gefahren bei operativen Eingriffen an den Gallenwegen und Mittel zu deren Bekämpfung mit besonderer Berücksichtigung der cholämischen Blutungen.
Deutsche Zeitschr. f. Chir. 230:353-371; y. 1931.

F. G. Slaughter & H. H. Trout. Duplication of the gall-bladder; case report with a review of the literature.
Am. Journ. of Surg. 19:124-125; y. 1933.

R. Solé. La infiltración anestésica del plexo solar en cirugía hepatobiliar.
Bol. y trab. de la Soc. de la cir. de Buenos Aires, 14: 24-49; y. 1930.

K. Speed. Two cases of intrahepatic gall-bladder.
Surgic. Clin. of North America, 14:851-858; y. 1934.

E. M. Stanton. The immediate causes of death following operations on the gall bladder and ducts.
Amer. Journ. of Surg. 8:1026-1032; y. 1930.

W. J. Stater. Transplantation of gall-bladder; preliminary report.
New England Journ. Med. 204:1101-1102; y. 1931.

W. A. Steel. Internal drainage of the gall-bladder as a routine operative procedure.
Surg. Gyn. & Obst. 44:393-395; y.1927.

H. L. Stewart & M. M. Lieber. Hepatic changes associated with decompression of obstructed biliary passages.
Arch. of Pathology, 18:30-41; y. 1934.

V. Stubenrauch. Ueber plastische Anastomosen zwischen Gallenwegen und Magendarmcanal zur Heilung der completen äusseren Gallenfistel.
Arch. f. klin. Chir. 79:1015-1030; y. 1906.

A. G. Sullivan. Reconstruction of the bile ducts.
Journ. Am. Med. Ass. 53:774-777; y. 1909.

I. M. Talman. Recidive von Koliken nach Operationen an den Gallenwegen.
Arch. f. klin. Chir. 175: 472-546; y. 1933.

S. Teneff. La funzionalita epatica in rapporto all'intervento ed all'anestesia, nelle malattie chirurgiche in genere, nelle affezioni e nel drenaggio delle vie biliari (richerche clinico-sperimentali).
Arch. ital. di chir. 39:221-300; y. 1935.

M. Thorek. Cholecystoelectrocoagulectomy without drainage in treatment of gall-bladder disease.
Illin. Med. Journ. 64:425-439; y. 1933.

M. Thorek. Electrosurgical obliteration of the gall-bladder.
Arch. of Physic. Therapy, 16:207-218; y. 1935.

M. Trautmann, H. J. Robbins & C. C. Stewart. An experimental study of the operation of cholecystenterostomy.
Surg. Gyn. Obst. 44:612-616; y. 1927.

C. Trinchera. Sul comportamento della cistifellea dopo interruzione del dotto cistico (Indagini sperimentali e considerazioni cliniche).
Clin. Chir. 36:181-208; y. 1933.

D. Vallone. Le modificazioni anatomiche e batteriologiche delle vie biliari dopo le colecistoenteroanastomosi sperimentali.
Ann. ital. di chir. 10:158-189; y. 1931.

J. R. Verbrycke Jr. Cholecystectomy without drainage. Report of 86 consecutive cases without mortality.
Med. Journ. and Record. 126:705-708; y. 1927.

O. M. Walter & A. Neiman. Case report of intra-hepatic gall-bladder in adult with review of literature.
Illin. Med. Journ. 60:478-480; y. 1931.

M. Walters. Successful resection of ampulla of Vater, including portion of duodenum with choledochoduodenostomy for carcinoma of ampulla of Vater.
Surg. Gyn. & Obst. 55:648-651; y. 1932.

A. G. Watkins & G. P. Wright. Congenital atresia of the bile ducts.
Lancet, I:1066-1068; y. 1933.

M. Wickhoff & F. Angelberger. Casuistische Mittheilungen.
Wien. klin. Wochenschr. 6:325-327; y. 1893.

H. Wildegans. Heilungsergebnisse nach Anastomose zwischen Gallenwegen und Magendarmkanal.
Chirurg, 2:991-995; y. 1930.

Wilms. Bildung eines künstlichen Choledochus durch ein einfaches Drainrohr.
Berlin. klin. Wchnschr. 49:536-537; y. 1912.

A. von Winiwarter. Ein Fall von Gallenretention bedingt durch Impermeabilität des Ductus Choledochus. Anlegung einer Gallenblasen-Darmfistel.
Prag. med Wochenschr. 7:201; y. 1882.

O. Witzel. Zur Gallenblasenexstirpation.
Zbl. f. Chir. 33:865-869; y. 1906.

H. Wolff. Die Cysto-Choledochostomie: eine neue Gallenwegverbindung.
Zbl. f. Chir. 41:231-235; y. 1914.

CHAPTER XXI.

SURGERY OF THE LIVER.

I. ROUTES FOR EXPOSURE OF THE INFERIOR, ANTERIOR, SUPERIOR AND POSTERIOR SURFACES OF THE LIVER.

Different incisions are used for this purpose depending upon which surface is to be approached.

a. Approach to the Inferior and Anterior Surfaces.

For approaching these surfaces various abdominal incisions are used such as those of Courvoisier, Kausch, Mayo Robson, Bevan, Kehr, Langenbuch, Kocher, König-Perthes, Czerny-Perthes, Don, Pochhamer and others which were described in Chapter II.

b. Approach to the Superior Surface.

This was described in Chapter II.

c. Approach to the Posterior Surface.

This was described in Chapter II.

II. SUTURE OF THE LIVER.

Suture of the liver is used for the purpose of:

A. Checking hemorrhage.

B. Partial hepatectomy.

A. CHECKING HEMORRHAGE.

In case of a hemorrhage from the liver two important tasks confront the surgeon:

a. He should prevent the occurrence of a sudden gush of blood from the injured liver after the abdomen is opened.

b. He should permanently control the bleeding after the abdomen is opened.

a. When hemorrhage of the liver occurs the blood fills the abdominal cavity and acts as a tampon, which compresses the liver and finally checks the hemorrhage. As soon as the abdomen is opened, this pressure disappears and profuse bleeding may ensue. For this reason, as soon as the abdomen is opened a finger is immediately introduced into the foramen of Winslow and its anterior wall is grasped between the index-finger and the thumb, thus compressing the hepatic artery and the portal vein **(method of Hogarth Pringle)**. In order to have enough room in the operative field it is advisable to replace the fingers in the foramen of Winslow by blood-vessel forceps. These forceps should not crush either the intima of the blood-vessels or the endothelial lining of the common bile-duct. The

Spivack clamp serves this purpose. After the clamps are applied the blood is sponged out and the operative field becomes clear. Now it is necessary to use some measure to permanently check the bleeding.

b. Permanent control of the bleeding.

Different procedures are used to accomplish this. Of all the methods employed, three are most commonly used, namely, **suturing, packing**, and a **combination of packing and suturing of the wound.** It is best to pack the wound with iodoform-gauze and to suture the Glisson capsule over it, and then to bring the gauze out of the abdominal cavity. This method was very much recommended by M. Kousnetzoff and J. Pensky.

B. RESECTION OF THE LIVER.

Historical.

The liver was considered as a "noli me tangere" ("do not touch me") organ until 1870, when Bruns removed a portion of the liver in a soldier wounded in the Franco-Prussian war. In the later eighties he performed a partial hepatectomy for echinococcosis of the liver, and also for a case of carcinoma of the liver. He cut with the cautery, thus checking the hemorrhage, but if this persisted he tied the individual blood-vessels with silk ligatures. Lins, of Germany, removed a solid tumor from the liver in 1887. In Italy the first resection of the liver was performed by Loreta for echinococcosis of the liver, and published in 1888. Kőnig, in 1889, in Germany, and Keen, in the United States, in 1891, resected a portion of the liver. Hochenegg, in 1890, removed a portion of the liver for carcinoma, and being unable to suture the hepatic lips to each other, he sutured the lips of the Glisson's capsule of the liver to the peritoneum **(thus being the first who produced a marsupialisation of the liver),** and packed the wound with iodoform-gauze. However, all these cases of resection of the liver were rather sporadic.

The technic of resection of the liver was placed on a firm basis after Michael Kousnetzoff and Julius Pensky, both from the surgical clinic of Prof. Grube, of Kharkoff, published the results of their experiments in the St. Petersburg Surgical Review, in 1896. They performed their experiments on dogs and rabbits, and Mikulicz applied their method to the human with good results. Their conclusions were as follows:

1. A ligature of the liver tied slightly does not guarantee sufficiently against primary and secondary hemorrhage. **In order to check the hemorrhage completely, the ligature should be tied very snugly.**

2. The stump of the liver should be left in the peritoneal cavity and should not be extraperitonealized.

3. The use of blunt needles prevents pricking of the wall of the intrahepatic blood-vessels, and, therefore, only blunt needles should be used for suturing the liver.

4. The application of ligatures to isolated hepatic blood-vessels is possible, since the walls of these blood-vessels offer great resistance.

This method actually solved the problem of hemorrhage and made possible resection of the liver.

Later, other surgeons modified the technic of suturing of the liver; however, the essential elements are the same as those of the original Kousnetzoff and Pensky method.

1. KOUSNETZOFF AND PENSKY METHOD.

Straight and curved needles with blunt points are used. For suture-material, heavy silk No. 5 is used. The technic, as described by these surgeons is as follows:

The needle, threaded with a double silk thread, enters on the upper surface, about 1 cm. away from the plane in which the liver will be cut,

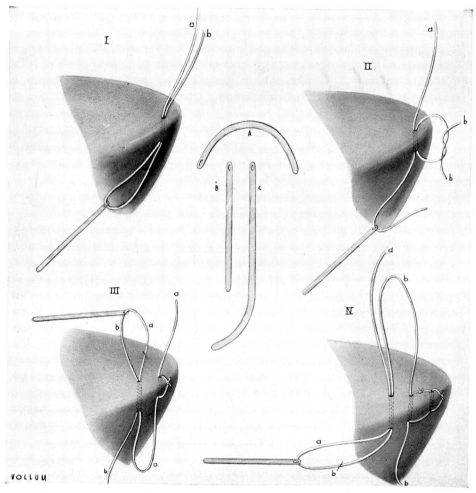

Fig. 279. Suturing of the Liver
(Kousnetzoff-Pensky method).

and reappears on the lower surface. Thus, the free ends of the thread are situated on the upper surface, and the needle with two threads is seen on the lower surface. The thread **b** is cut, close to the eye of the needle (Fig. 279, I), and the ends of the thread **b** are tied to each other (Fig. 279, II). The remaining part of thread **b** on the lower surface is made longer by traction. This is done at the expense of the thread **a** on the upper surface. This traction is continued until thread **a** on the upper surface is only about 5 cm. long. Then the needle is passed through the liver from below upward. Thread **a** is cut on the upper surface close to the eye of the needle (Fig. 279, III). The two free ends of thread **a** are tied to each other on the upper surface. Thread **a** is drawn away from the eye of the needle so as to make thread **b** on the lower surface only about 5 cm. long, and the needle is then passed from the upper to the lower surface of the liver. This procedure is repeated as often as necessary (Fig. 279, IV). [As may be seen, two threads are passing continually through the thickness of the liver, one compressing the tissue to the left and the other to the right.] The ends of the thread should be tied **gradually and very tightly**, so that they crush the liver-parenchyma and compress the vessels. After this "mass ligature", is completed, the liver should be resected 1 cm. distal from the suture-line. Usually, after tight ligation there is no bleeding from the individual vessels. However, if any individual blood-vessel bleeds it should be caught by an arterial clamp and ligated.

Kousnetzoff and Pensky demonstrated definitely that the blood-vessels of the liver are not more friable than those of any other organ.

2.   AUVRAY MODIFICATION OF THE KOUSNETZOFF-PENSKY "MASSIVE LIGATURE METHOD."

This method was described by Maurice Auvray, of the Terrier clinic of Paris, in 1897. It consists of a series of mattress-sutures, which resemble the Kousnetzoff and Pensky suture, from which they differ only in the method of application. Auvray used a specially-constructed needle, which is a combination of a Reverdin and an Emmet needle (Fig. 280). He used two silk sutures No. 5; the length of each thread was from twenty-five to thirty cm. His technic was as follows:

The threads, lying very close to each other, penetrate the liver from the upper surface to the lower. The ends of each thread intertwine with each other so that each lies within the loop of the other (Fig. 280, I). The Auvray needle passes from the upper surface to the lower. Thread **B** is passed through the eye of the needle and brought out on the upper surface of the liver. Thread **A** is slowly and gradually tied by one knot with thread **B** on the upper surface of the liver, until the parenchyma of the liver between O and O^1 is crushed. Then the second knot is made (Fig. 280, II). The Auvray needle is then passed from below upward in the furrow produced by the crushed parenchyma of the liver. Thread

B is passed through the eye of the needle and brought out on the lower surface of the liver. The Auvray needle penetrates the liver from the upper surface to the lower at point O", a distance of 1 cm. away from O'. Thread B is passed through the eye of the needle and is brought out on the upper surface of the liver. The ends of threads A and B are tied to each other gradually and snugly, so that the liver is crushed between

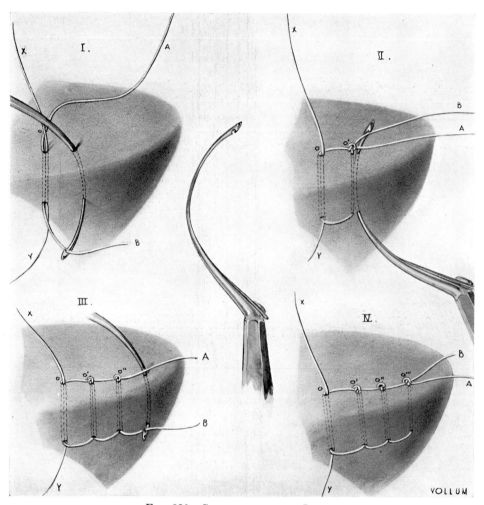

FIG. 280. SUTURING OF THE LIVER.
(AUVRAY METHOD).

the points O' and O", and then the second knot is made. This maneuvre is repeated as often as necessary (Fig. 280, III, IV). The same procedure is done with thread XY in the opposite direction. After the suturing is completed, the liver is resected, and if there are any bleeding vessels they should be caught individually by artery-forceps.

3. HOUGH METHOD.

This is performed as follows: A definite number of sutures are passed from one surface of the liver to the other. The free ends on the upper surface are tied to each other successively, that is, the first thread to the second, then one free end of the knot of the second thread is tied to the

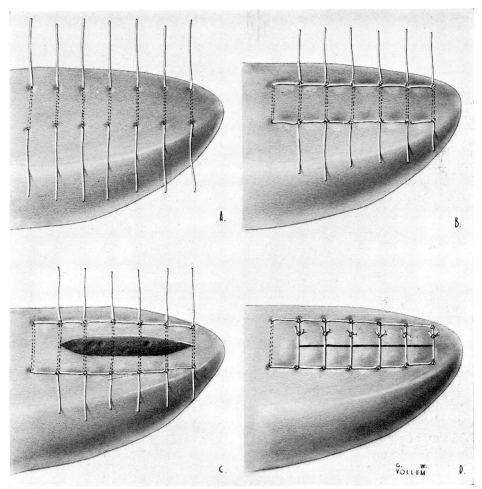

FIG. 281. SUTURING OF THE LIVER.
(HOUGH METHOD).

third thread, etc., so that actually a continuous buttonhole suture is formed on the upper surface of the liver. The same procedure is done on the lower surface. After that the portion of the liver lying to the periphery of these button-hole sutures is excised and one of the free ends of each knot on the upper surface is tied to the corresponding free end of each knot of the lower surface. After all the knots are tied the picture will be as shown in Fig. 281.

As may be seen, there will be knots on the upper surface and on the lower surface, and also knots produced by tying the strands of the upper surface of the liver to the strands of the lower surface of the liver. This is an excellent method of suturing, and we believe it is much simpler than any other method described.

III. OPERATIONS FOR ABSCESS OF THE LIVER.

Of the different types of abscess of the liver the amebic form is that most frequently met with. The amebic abscess may be either single or multiple. It is not always treated surgically. In some cases the intramuscular injection of emetine hydrochloride, followed by the oral administration of ipecacuanha, gives excellent results. The surgical treatment may be as follows:

        a. Aspiration of the abscess.

        b. Incision and drainage of the abscess.

a. Aspiration of the Abscess.

This consists in emptying the abscess once or, if necessary, repeatedly, with or without washing out of the cavity by some antiseptic fluid, such as Dakin's solution. Although, generally such "closed methods" are considered non-surgical, nevertheless, experience shows that this method has reduced the mortality from 50 per cent. to 5 per cent., **and it should be considered as a method of choice.**

The objection to the "closed method" lies in the supposed danger of secondary infection. However, this is groundless, since from 80 to 90 per cent. of all amebic abscesses contain sterile pus, and the *endamoeba histolytica* is embedded in the wall of the abscess cavity.

Aspiration is done by means of a large-caliber needle connected with a large glass syringe or by a Potain aspirator. The needle may be attached to a rubber tube which is connected with any kind of a suction-apparatus. It is not advisable to wash out the emptied cavity with an antiseptic solution. **This surgical intervention should always be followed by an intramuscular injection of emetine** (0.06 gm. of emetine for the first 6 days, 0.03 gm. of emetine for the following 4 days, and 0.06 gm. of emetine once a week for 4 more weeks, always intramuscularly and followed by the oral administration of ipecacuanha).

b. Incision and Drainage of the Abscess.

This method carries a great risk of secondary infection, and for this reason it is indicated only under definite conditions, as follows:

    1. Cases in which aspiration and emetine have not given relief.

    2. In case the abscess is located in the left lobe of the liver (this occurs only in 20 per cent. of all cases; in 80 per cent. it is localized in the right lobe of the liver), when aspiration carries some dangers of injury to the large blood-vessels.

    3. In case the abscess has ruptured into the pleural or peritoneal cavity.

Technic.

Step 1. The incision depends upon the location of the abscess. In the majority of cases the abscess is located on the postero-superior surface of the liver. Therefore, a right side abdominal or thoraco-abdominal incision with resection of one or two ribs will be sufficient. [Extreme care should be taken in case of a rib-resection not to open the pleural cavity.]

Step 2. The parietal peritoneum is sutured to the capsule of the liver at a distance of an inch and a half from the abscess. If it cannot be sutured all the way circularly, then the peritoneal cavity should be "walled off" from the abscess and not sutured at all.

Step 3. The liver-substance is opened over the abscess by diathermy and the pus evacuated. A finger is introduced into the cavity to discover whether any other abscess-cavities are present. Some surgeons advise scraping of the wall of the abscess, since the *endamoebæ histolyticæ* are usually situated in the wall. However, many surgeons, highly authorative on the subject of surgery of tropical diseases, do not advise scraping, but using emetin intramuscularly postoperatively. A rubber tube is placed in the cavity.

IV. SURGICAL TREATMENT OF ECHINOCOCCUS OF THE LIVER.

The various operative procedures as practised to-day can be divided into three groups:

1. Resection of the portion of the liver which contains the echinococcus.

2. Incision of the hydatid cyst with drainage in one or two stages.

3. Enucleation of the cyst.

1. Resection of the portion of the liver containing the cyst.

This is an ideal method. It became possible only after suture of the liver had been placed on a safe basis. However, it is not always possible to employ this method on account of the inaccessibility of the cyst. The technic of its execution is exactly as described in "Resection of the Liver."

2. Incision of the hydatid cyst with drainage in one or two stages.

a. One Stage Method.

Step 1. The abdomen is opened in the manner described previously for exposure of the liver.

Step 2. The cyst is "walled off" from the rest of the peritoneal cavity. **The abdominal wall should be carefully protected from a possible contamination by the contents of the cyst.** The fluid is carefully aspirated, and 300 to 400 c.cm. of one per cent. solution of formol is injected into the cystic cavity and kept there for five minutes to kill the scolices (suggestion of Quénu and Dévé).

Step 3. A one inch incision is made through the liver-tissue and the wall of the cyst. Each lip of the wall of the cyst is caught by an Allis forceps. A suction-apparatus is introduced to aspirate the formol. The incision is then enlarged. A finger is introduced into the cavity for its examination; daughter cysts may bulge into the cavity. If so, they should be broken by the finger.

Step 4. The endocyst is caught by a forceps and gently drawn out. **The entire endocyst should be removed.**

Step 5. The cavity is packed with gauze. The lips of the incised wall of the cyst are sutured to the parietal peritoneum, the posterior sheath of the rectus muscle, and to the entire thickness of the muscle. The laparotomy pads, which were "walling off" the peritoneal cavity from the cyst, are removed gradually while the liver is sutured to the anterior abdominal wall.

Step 6. The pack in the cavity of the cyst is removed and replaced by a rubber tube and gauze.

Step 7. The abdomen is closed in layers with the exception of the portion through which the gauze projects.

b.   Two Stage Operation.

First Stage.

Step 1. The abdomen is opened as in the previous operation. As an additional precaution it is advisable to "wall off" the cyst from the peritoneal cavity and to protect the anterior abdominal wall, just as in the previous operation.

Step 2. The liver around the cyst is sutured to the parietal peritoneum. The wound is packed with gauze.

Step 3. The abdomen is closed.

Four days later the second stage is performed:

Second Stage.

Step 1. The abdomen is reopened through the original incision.

Step 2. The contents of the cyst are aspirated; 300 to 400 c. cm. of a one per cent. solution of formol is introduced into the cavity. The cyst is incised after the formol solution has been there for five minutes. The endocyst is removed. A rubber drain wrapped in gauze is placed in the cavity of the cyst, and is brought outside of the abdominal cavity.

Step 3. The abdominal wall is closed.

Some surgeons prefer the "one stage method" to the "two stage method", and others *vice versa*. Moynihan gives preference to the one stage method because it gives more room for the operation, and in case of careful "walling off" of the cyst from the rest of the peritoneal cavity the danger of contamination is slight.

3.   **Enucleation of a Hydatid Cyst.**

This consists in a complete enucleation of the cyst with blind closure of the regular liver-gap, and closure of the abdomen without drainage.

The first enucleation was performed by Knowsley Thornton, in 1883. However, he removed the endocyst only. In France, this method is known as the "Delbet operation". However, Delbet performed it the first time only in 1895. The priority, therefore, belongs to Knowsley Thornton. In Russia and in the rest of Continental Europe, with the exception of France, it is known as the "Bobrow method". However, Bobrow described it only in 1898. J. P. Buckley, in 1913, described a **total enucleation** in which not only the endocyst but also the ectocyst was removed.

The enucleation method should be employed only for "clean cases", that is, those in which the contents of the sac have not suppurated. For suppurative cases, the "incision and drainage method" as a one or two stage operation should be employed.

Technic.

Step 1. The abdomen is opened. The area around the cyst is "walled off" from the rest of the peritoneal cavity.

Step. 2. The contents of the cyst are aspirated; 300 to 400 c. cm., of a one per cent. solution of formol are injected. Five minutes later, the cyst is incised and the contents evacuated.

Step 3. An artery-clamp grasps the endocyst and removes it from the ectocyst. [Many surgeons, who are very competent in this particular field of surgery, do not consider it important to remove the ectocystic wall.]

Step 4. Several sutures are passed within the cavity of the cyst catching the ectocystic wall on one side and suturing it to the opposite wall, thus eliminating the "dead spaces".

Step 5. The edges of the incised liver are sutured to each other.

Step 6. The abdominal wall is closed in layers without drainage.

V.   OPERATIONS FOR ASCITES DUE TO CIRRHOSIS OF THE LIVER.

The numerous operations which are used for drainage of ascites due to cirrhosis of the liver may be classed in two groups:

A.   **Operations which diminish the flow of blood to the obstructed portal vein.**

B.   **Operations which drain directly or indirectly the ascitic fluid.**

A.   OPERATIONS WHICH DIMINISH THE FLOW OF BLOOD TO THE
OBSTRUCTED PORTAL VEIN.

As is well known, the portal and systemic venous systems have a definite anastomosis with each other, namely:

a. Between a vein in the round ligament of the liver, which is a tributary of the left branch of the portal vein, and the superior epigastric vein of the anterior abdominal wall.

b. Between the left gastric and both azygos veins through the esophageal plexus.

c. Between the inferior mesenteric and the internal iliac vein by means of the middle and inferior hemorrhoidal plexuses.

d. Between the pancreatic and the lumbar veins.

These normal connections become greatly exaggerated in the case of portal obstruction. The aim of all the operations of this group is to increase these vascular connections by forming adhesions between the abdominal viscera, which drain the blood into the portal vein, and the abdominal parieties, which drain the blood into the venæ cavæ (superior and inferior), or to make a direct anastomosis between the large veins of the portal and systemic system, such as between the inferior vena cava and the vena porta **(Eck fistula),** or between the inferior vena cava and the superior mesenteric vein **(Bogoras operation).**

The vascular connections between the systemic and portal systems are increased by forming adhesions:

a. Between the omentum and the anterior abdominal wall.

b. Between the liver and the spleen with the vault of the diaphragm or the anterior abdominal wall.

c. Between the gall-bladder, or even the bowel, and the anterior abdominal wall.

a. FIRST TALMA OPERATION (DRUMMOND-MORISON OPERATION).

This operation was suggested by Talma in his course on "Pathology of the Liver", in the year 1887. It was first performed by Van der Meulen in 1889, and by Schelkly in 1891, in both cases at Talma's suggestion, and published by Talma's student, Dr. Th. Lens, in 1892. It consisted in suturing the great omentum to the inner surface of the peritoneum (as done by Van der Meulen), or by supplementing this with suturing of the gall-bladder to the anterior abdominal wall (operated so by Von Eiselsberg at the suggestion of Talma on March 7th, 1896), or by placing the spleen in front of the rectus muscle between it and the skin in the sac thus formed (operated in this way by Narath at the suggestion of Talma, on July 2nd, 1896). Talma himself had his first opportunity of operating for ascites only in 1898. David Drummond and Rutherford Morison performed this operation on Sept. 3rd, 1894, and on October 22nd, 1895, prior to their publication of the method on Sept. 19th, 1896. However, to Talma and his pupils belong the priority both in performing and in publishing the method.

Technic.

Step 1. The abdomen is opened. The fluid is evacuated very slowly until the abdominal cavity is dry. The diaphragmatic surfaces of the liver and spleen are vigorously scrubbed with gauze. The peritoneal surface of the diaphragm lying opposite the scrubbed surfaces of the liver and spleen are also scrubbed with gauze.

Step 2. The omentum is sutured either to the inner surface of the parietal peritoneum, or is placed in a sac formed between the outer surface of the peritoneum and either the posterior sheath of the rectus muscle or the rectus muscle itself.

Step 3. The abdomen is closed.

b. SECOND TALMA OPERATION (SCHIASSI TECHNIC).

Step 1. A rectangular musculo-cutaneous incision is made in the following manner: The vertical limb starts at the left midclavicular line about one inch below the costal margin, and is continued in a vertical direction downward for six inches. At the upper end of this incision another incision runs in a direction perpendicular to the midline (Fig. 282, insert).

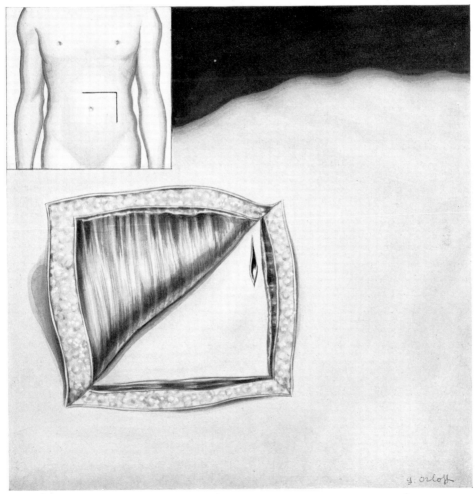

FIG. 282. SURGICAL TREATMENT OF ASCITES (SCHIASSI MODIFICATION OF THE
TALMA OPERATION).
INSERT. Skin-incision viewed from the front.
MAIN PICTURE. The flap is reflected (view from the left side).

The abdominal wall is incised down to the peritoneum. Thus, the rectus muscle is split longitudinally in one direction and cut transversely in another direction. The musculo-cutaneous flap is reflected to its base (Fig. 282).

Step 2. A small opening is made in the peritoneum at the medial end

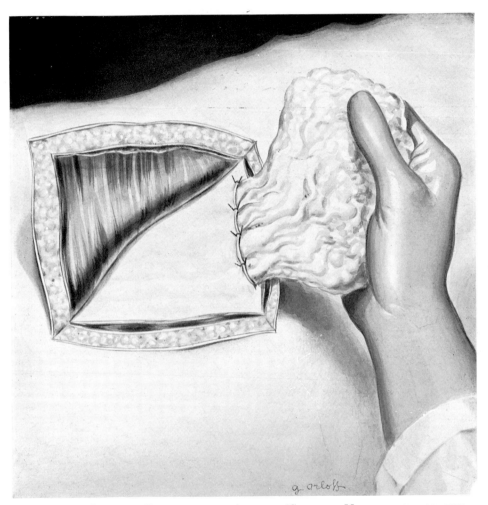

FIG. 283. SURGICAL TREATMENT OF ASCITES (SCHIASSI MODIFICATION OF THE TALMA OPERATION).
Suturing the posterior surface of the omentum to the peritoneal lip.

of the transverse incision and the fluid is **gradually evacuated** (Fig. 282). The transverse opening of the peritoneum is enlarged laterally for two-thirds of the length of this horizontal incision. The omentum is drawn outside until it entirely covers the exposed peritoneum. The omentum is lifted and its posterior surface is sutured by interrupted sutures to the inferior lip of the peritoneum (Fig. 283). The upper surface of the omentum is sewed to the superior lip of the transverse peritoneal incision (Fig. 284). The free margin of the omentum is sutured to the peritoneum along the base of the musculo-cutaneous flap (Fig. 284).

Step 3. A vertical incision is made through the peritoneum to the

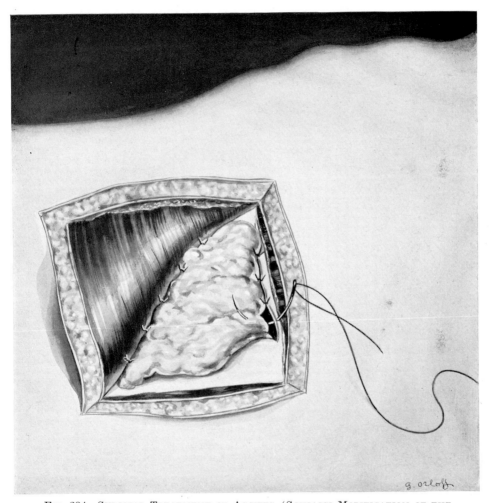

FIG. 284. SURGICAL TREATMENT OF ASCITES (SCHIASSI MODIFICATION OF THE TALMA OPERATION).
Suturing of the anterior surface of the omentum to the peritoneal lip. The edge of the omentum is already sutured to the base of the musculo-cutaneous flap.

left of the lateral end of the transverse peritoneal incision (Fig. 285). The length of this incision is about five inches. The spleen is brought into the wound. A roll of gauze is introduced into the abdominal cavity and placed between the upper pole of the spleen and the diaphragm. The free end of this gauze is brought outside of the abdominal cavity. Another roll of gauze is placed between the lower pole of the spleen and the diaphragm and its free end is also brought outside the abdominal cavity through the lower end of the incision (Fig. 285).

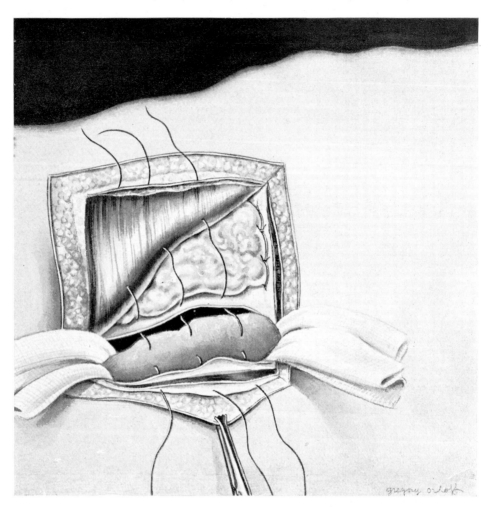

FIG. 285. SURGICAL TREATMENT OF ASCITES (SCHIASSI MODIFICATION OF THE TALMA OPERATION).
A splenopexy is done.

Step 4. Fixation of the spleen to the anterior abdominal wall.

A large curved needle, threaded with catgut No. 5, penetrates the entire thickness except the skin of the left lip of the anterior abdominal wall, two inches away from the opening. Then it passes through the capsule of the spleen including some of its parenchyma. Then it runs in an opposite direction, grasping the peritoneum and the entire thickness of the musculo-cutaneous flap, with the exception of the skin (Fig. 285).

These sutures are placed at a distance of one and a half inches apart. The number of sutures depends on the size of the spleen. **These sutures are not tied at this time.** [Instead of penetrating the entire thickness of the abdominal wall, these transfixing sutures may grasp the peritoneum and the transversalis fascia only.]

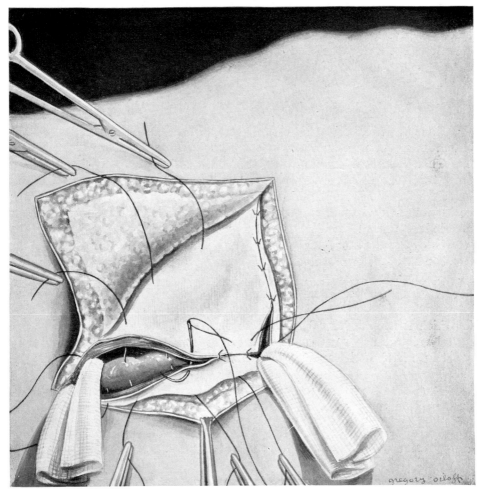

FIG. 286. SURGICAL TREATMENT OF ASCITES (SCHIASSI MODIFICATION OF THE TALMA OPERATION).
Suturing the anterior abdominal wall.

Step 5. Suturing of the anterior abdominal wall in layers (Fig. 286).
The peritoneum, with the posterior sheath of the rectus muscle, the muscle itself, and the anterior sheath, are sutured in layers, leaving untied sutures only at the upper and lower ends of the incision where the gauze makes its exit from the abdominal cavity. **Then the sutures which**

fix the spleen to the anterior abdominal wall are tied. The skin-sutures are now inserted, leaving again a few skin-sutures untied at the place of exit of the gauze rolls. A few days later, when the gauze is removed, all the untied sutures at the upper and lower end of the incision are tied.

c. SECOND TALMA OPERATION (NARATH TECHNIC).

This is an omentopexy supplemented by a splenopexy in which the spleen is placed in front of the left rectus muscle.

Step 1. As Step 1 of the previous operation.

Step 2. The skin and superficial fascia are retracted from the anterior sheath of the left rectus muscle so that a sac is formed. The omentum and spleen are brought outside of the abdominal cavity and placed in the sac.

Step 3. The abdomen is closed, care being taken not to compress the omentum or the pedicle of the spleen (the gastro-splenic ligament).

This operation differs from the Schiassi operation in this respect only, that Narath places the omentum and spleen in front of the rectus muscle, whereas, in the Schiassi method the omentum is placed behind the rectus muscle and the spleen remains in the abdominal cavity.

d.   Splenectomy is used by some surgeons for the purpose of diminishing the degree of obstruction of the portal vein with or without the Talma operation.

If the spleen is normal in size about one-seventh of the blood of the portal vein is contributed by the splenic vein. The larger the spleen becomes (and its enlargement is a rule in cases of cirrhosis of the liver in which ascites develops), the more the splenic vein contributes to the portal vein, and in very large spleens the blood of the splenic vein may constitute half of the amount of the blood-supply of the portal vein. For this reason, splenectomy deprives the portal vein of a very important tributary. **However, splenopexy is far less dangerous, particularly in weakened patients, than splenectomy, and gives no worse results. Therefore, it should be given preference to splenectomy.**

e. DIRECT ANASTOMOSIS BETWEEN THE PORTAL VEIN AND THE INFERIOR VENA CAVA (ECK FISTULA).

This operation has been performed a number of times, but several objections have been raised against its use:

1. It is hazardous to sidetrack the entire blood of the portal vein, which carries all the blood of the small and large bowels with their toxins, without the benefit of the filtrating and detoxicating influences of the liver.

2. The technical difficulties of its execution.

We believe that this operation will probably never be of great appeal to the surgeon.

f. IMPLANTATION OF THE SUPERIOR MESENTERIC VEIN INTO THE INFERIOR VENA CAVA (BOGORAS OPERATION).

This was first performed in 1912 and published in January, 1913, by N. A. Bogoras, of Tomsk, Russia. The superior mesenteric vein is cut at the lower end of the meso-ileum and its distal (aboral) end is implanted into the vena cava inferior.

Technic.

Step 1. Abdominal section through a right pararectal incision six inches in length which starts three inches above the level of the umbilicus.

Step 2. The ascitic fluid is drained. The terminal portion of the ileum is drawn outside the abdominal cavity and the terminal meso-ileum is exposed. The superior mesenteric vein in this locality is exposed. It is easy to find this because it lies close to the artery which can be seen or felt pulsating. The vein is exposed for a distance of about two inches. A ligature is applied to the proximal end of the exposed vein, care being taken to leave several veins proximal to the point of ligation, so as not to divert the entire amount of blood of the small intestines from the portal circulation. A blood-vessel clamp is placed transversely on the superior mesenteric vein at a distance of about two inches distal from the ligature, and the vein is cut close to the ligature. The bowels are replaced and the vein hangs free upon the inferior surface of the meso-ileum.

Step 3. The parietal peritoneum of the posterior abdominal wall is cut in front of the inferior vena cava, the anterior wall of which is exposed for two inches. Part of the anterior wall is caught axially with an arterial non-crushing clamp. A small opening is made in the fold of the inferior vena cava. Four sutures, placed at equal distance from each other, unite the circumference of the open end of the superior mesenteric vein with the opening of the vena cava. These sutures penetrate the entire thickness of the wall of each blood-vessel. The ends are left long and are used as traction-sutures. A row of continuous sutures is placed between each two traction-sutures, care being taken not to produce a purse-string action.

Step 4. The edges of the incised parietal peritoneum of the posterior abdominal wall are resutured.

It should be mentioned that although this operation is technically difficult and can be done only by a skilful surgeon, nevertheless, it is easier than one would think from observing the size of the superior mesenteric vein in the cadaver, since in the presence of portal obstruction all the intestinal veins become greatly enlarged. **Several reports have been published in which this method was employed with gratifying results.** However, we do not believe that this procedure will be frequently adopted.

In 1926, Flerow suggested a new method, which consists in the ligation of the left gastric **artery**, the right and left gastro-epiploic **arteries**, and the inferior mesenteric **vein**. The aim of this procedure is evident: By ligation of the several arteries carrying the blood-supply to the stomach, the veins of the stomach will receive their blood-supply mainly from the portal vein by a reverse flow of blood from this vein. By ligation of the inferior mesenteric vein, the amount of blood running to the portal vein is still further diminished, thus lessening the engorgement of that vein. Several cases have been reported in which this operation was performed with good results.

Recently, E. Holman suggested a new method of treatment of ascites due to hepatic cirrhosis, which consisted in the ligation of the **splenic artery** followed by splenopexy. The expectation is that the venous blood will, under such conditions, change its direction, and will flow from the portal vein into the splenic, thus diminishing the degree of obstruction.

However, in the only case reported the results were unsatisfactory. Further reports will be necessary before the value of this operation can be established. As may be seen, the Holman suggestion is based upon the Flerow principle.

B. OPERATIONS WHICH DRAIN THE ASCITIC FLUID DIRECTLY OR INDIRECTLY.

Various procedures are employed for this purpose, of which we shall describe only a few:

a. ASPIRATION METHOD.

This is the oldest and simplest method. Two complications may arise in performing it, namely, injury of a large blood-vessel of the anterior abdominal wall, and puncturing of a bowel with the possibility of peritonitis or the developing of a fecal fistula. However, the main objection to this method is that the fluid constantly accumulates, and puncture necessarily becomes a frequent procedure.

b. IMPLANTATION OF THE SAPHENOUS VEIN INTO THE PERITONEAL CAVITY (RUOTTE OPERATION).

This operation consists in the implantation of the great saphenous vein into the peritoneal cavity. The ascitic fluid runs into the saphenous vein and farther on into the femoral vein, thus entering the general blood circulation. The back-flow of blood from the femoral vein into the free peritoneal cavity is prevented by the valves in the vein which allow the blood or any fluid to run in one direction and prevents it from running in the opposite direction. The operation was first performed by Ruotte, in 1907.
Technic.

Step 1. A skin-incision is made on the anterior surface of the thigh, starting at a point three centimeters lateral to the pubic spine, and four centimeters below it. This incision is carried in a downward and slightly medial direction for a distance of ten centimeters. The long saphenous vein is exposed for the same distance from its mouth, and is cut at a distance of ten centimeters from the femoral vein. Its distal end is ligated (Fig. 287).

Step 2. The anterior wall of the abdomen is cut through its entire thickness for a length of three centimeters slightly above the Poupart ligament. The peritoneum is cut for a length of two centimeters only (Fig. 288). The ascitic fluid is gradually withdrawn.

Step 3. A subcutaneous canal is formed between the upper and lower skin-incisions, and the portion of the saphenous vein which is connected

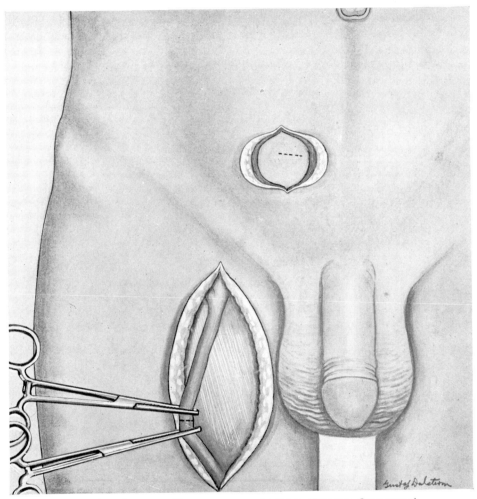

FIG. 287. SURGICAL TREATMENT OF ASCITES (RUOTTE OPERATION).
Exposure and clamping of the great saphenous vein.

with the femoral vein is brought through it (Fig. 288, B). The edge of the vein is bevelled, and the lips of the opened peritoneum are sutured to the open end of this vein, thus forming an anastomosis between the peritoneal cavity and the venous system (Fig. 288, B).

Step 4. The wound is closed in the usual manner. No drain should be placed.

Several cases have been reported by different authors who have used this method. Most of the reports were commendatory. **However, some cases are recorded in which either the anastomosis became occluded, or in which the entire portion of the saphenous vein between the femoral vein and the peritoneum became obliterated, so that it was necessary to resort to other methods for overcoming the ascites.**

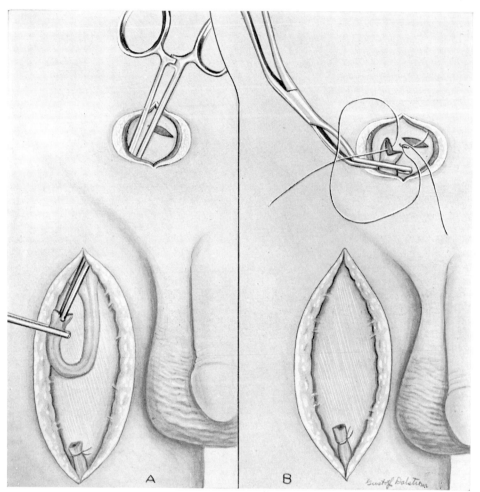

FIG. 288. SURGICAL TREATMENT OF ASCITES (RUOTTE OPERATION).
A. The great saphenous vein is cut; its proximal end is caught and ready to be drawn through a subcutaneous canal.
B. Suturing the great saphenous vein to the lip of the peritoneal opening.

c. OPENING OF A NEW LYMPHATIC PATHWAY (KALB OPERATION)
(FIG. 289).

This operation is based on the idea that the best method of handling the ascites is to drain it into the subcutaneous tissues. By this procedure two things will be accomplished; namely, the patient will not lose the albuminous portion of the ascitic contents, which will be reabsorbed, and the ascitic fluid will disappear from the abdominal cavity.

Technic.

Step 1. Abdominal section is made through a midline incision extending from the umbilicus downward for 4 to 5 inches. After the opening has been made the fluid is slowly evacuated.

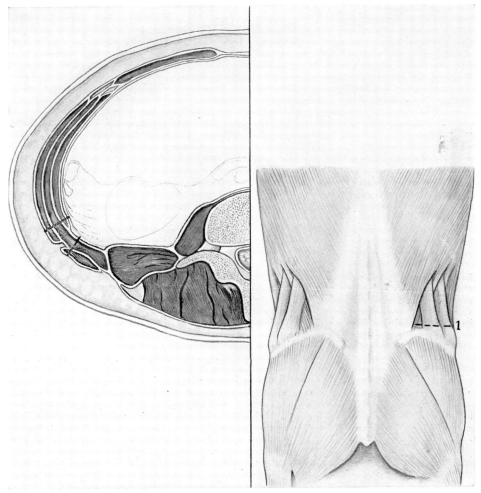

FIG. 289. SURGICAL TREATMENT OF ASCITES (KALB OPERATION).
(See text).
1. Petit triangle.

Step 2. An incision is made to the left of the sigmoid in the left lumbar region, and another to the right of the cecum in the right lumbar region, at the space which forms the Petit triangle. The peritoneum and the muscles of these regions are excised (part of the latissimus dorsi medially, part of the external oblique muscle laterally, and part of the internal oblique and transversus abdominis muscles at the floor of the triangle) **so that only the subcutaneous tissue and the skin are left intact.** The size of the excised portion is about that of a silver dollar.

Step 3. The abdomen is closed in the usual manner.

Several cases have been reported by different surgeons in which this technic has been used with good results.

VI. HEPATOPEXY.

Definition.

This term consists of two Greek words: ἦπαρ, liver and πηγνύναι, to fasten. It signifies "fastening of the liver".

Indications.

A movable liver which has become partially or totally displaced from its bed.

General remarks.

The first reported case of a movable liver was encountered by the great German anatomist Laurent Heister on the dissecting-table, in 1754. The first hepatopexy for **partial hepatoptosis** was performed by Billroth, in 1884, and for **total hepatoptosis** by Michl, of Prag, in 1887. To the latter is usually given the credit of being the first surgeon who performed hepatopexy. In France, for many years the credit for priority has been erroneously given to Gérard-Marchant, who performed the operation for the first time only in 1891. He was preceded not only by Billroth and Michl but also by Tcherning, who performed hepatopexy for partial hepatoptosis in 1886, and by Langenbuch who performed this operation in 1890, for total hepatoptosis.

The treatment depends on whether the hepatoptosis is partial or total. [By **partial hepatoptosis** is understood a condition in which the upper surface of the liver has not lost its contact with the diaphragm. The lower portion becomes enlarged, forms a flap, and this part actually becomes movable and responsible for symptoms. Under the name of **total hepatoptosis,** or **wandering liver,** or **hepar migrans,** is understood a condition in which the liver has lost its contact with the diaphragm and does not lie in the right hypochondrium only, but descends and lies in the lumbar or even in the iliac region.] In the case of total hepatoptosis, the treatment is surgical only, while in the case of partial hepatoptosis medical treatment should be attempted at first. Surgery in the latter cases should be resorted to only after medical treatment has failed.

Numerous procedures have been suggested differing from each other in the position of the abdominal incision, in the method of fixation of the liver, in the use of different suture-material, in various types of needles employed, etc.

Abdominal Incisions in Hepatopexy.

Transverse incisions running below and parallel to the right costal arch are most frequently employed for this operation. However, longitudinal incisions, such as the midline, midrectal and right pararectal, are used quite frequently.

In many cases, a transverse incision starting at the lumbar region and reaching the midline is employed. As a matter of fact, this is the earliest type of incision, because the surgeons started the operation with an erroneous diagnosis of a movable kidney. Poppert used a flap incision of a " Λ " shape, the vertical part of which is a right pararectal incision and the oblique limb runs parallel to the right costal arch.

The suture-material used is silver-wire, catgut or silk. The needles which are used are either ordinary large curved needles, penetrating the tissue by the eye instead of the point, or specially devised needles of the type of Kousnetzoff and Pensky or Auvray. The depth of the bite through the liver-tissue also varies: Some surgeons (Bobrow) passed the thread through the entire thickness of the liver, others (Langenbuch, Gérard-Marchant) only through the entire thickness of the anterior edge of the liver, some advised piercing the liver only for a depth of 2cm., etc.

METHODS OF FIXING THE LIVER IN ITS PROPER POSITION.

The numerous methods described may be classed into several groups:

A. **The formation of adhesions between the upper surface of the liver and the diaphragm or the parietal peritoneum of the anterior abdominal wall.**

B. **Anchoring of the liver to the anterior thoracic or abdominal wall by sutures.**

C. **Anchoring of the round ligament to the chest-wall or to the anterior abdominal wall.**

D. **Formation of a partition, either from the peritoneum or from the falciform ligament, which supports the liver and prevents its sliding from its bed into the lumbar or iliac region.**

E. **Excision of a part of the anterior abdominal wall (laparectomy).**

F. **A combination of the above mentioned methods.**

A. **Formation of adhesions between the superior surface of the liver and the diaphragm or the parietal peritoneum of the anterior abdominal wall.**

This is accomplished either by rubbing with gauze the adjoining surface of the liver and diaphragm or by scarification of the adjoining surfaces of these structures by a knife or a needle, or by the thermocautery, which is placed at some distance from the structures, or by inserting gauze between the adjoining surfaces of the liver and diaphragm or the anterior abdominal wall, which is removed several days later.

B. Anchoring of the liver to the anterior thoracic or abdominal wall by sutures.

In this group of operations the mattress-sutures pass either through the entire thickness of the parenchyma of the liver or through the superficial layer only. The number of sutures varies from one to nine. The free

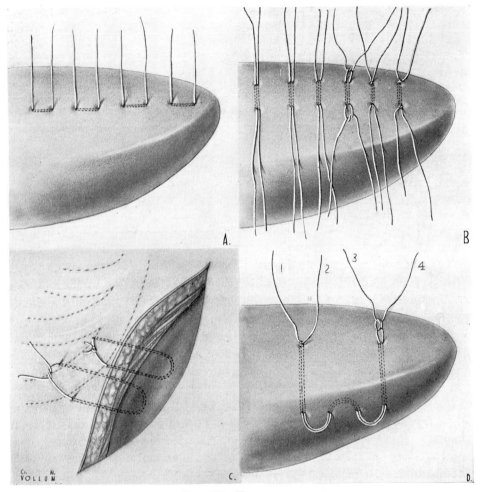

FIG. 290. HEPATOPEXY.
a. Cramer method;   b. Delagénière method;   c. Bobrow method;   d. Legueu method.

ends are brought outside either through the abdominal wall or through the lower end of the chest-wall.

1. **Cramer Method** (Fig. 290, A).

Three or four silk sutures are inserted into the substance of the liver at a distance of 3cm. from each other. The free ends are brought outside the anterior abdominal wall. The sutures are tied only after all have been inserted.

2. **Delagénière Method** (Fig. 290, B).

Six catgut double-threaded sutures are placed on the anterior surface of the liver parallel to each other and at a distance of one and one-half cm. from each other. At the sites of entrance and exit of each double thread, the individual thread is tied to its fellow. The knots so formed prevent hemorrhage from any tracks formed in the liver-parenchyma by the passage of the threads. The free ends of the threads are brought outside the anterior abdominal wall and tied to each other.

3. **Bobrow Method** (Fig. 290, C).

Two silk sutures penetrate the upper surface of the liver and are brought out through the chest-wall and fixed to the cartilage of the ninth rib.

4. **Legueu Method** (Fig. 290, D).

A Reverdin needle penetrates the liver from the lower to the upper surface and draws two threads from above downward. Then the sutures pass along the lower surface of the liver, care being taken not to include the gall-bladder in them. The Reverdin needle passes then from the upper surface of the liver to the lower and brings the threads from below upward. The ends of the thread 1, 2, 3, and 4 are brought outside either through the abdominal or chest-wall, and 1 is tied to 2 and 3 to 4.

C. **Anchoring of the round ligament to the chest-wall or to the anterior abdominal wall.**

1. **Ramsay Technic.**

The round ligament of the liver is fastened to the seventh rib, and in addition to this the parenchyma of the right lobe is sutured to the anterior abdominal wall.

2. **Werelius Method.** (Figs. 291, 292).

The abdomen is opened. The superior surface of the liver and the corresponding surface of the diaphragm are rubbed with gauze so as to facilitate the formation of adhesions. The chest-wall is punctured **above** the cartilage of the ninth rib. The round ligament is brought through this opening outside the abdominal cavity onto the chest-wall and hooked around this cartilage and then brought back into the abdominal cavity through another small incision **below** the cartilage of the ninth rib. The two limbs of the round ligament which form a loop around the cartilage of the ninth rib are sutured to each other. The abdomen is then closed.

3. **Grosz Method.**

This is similar to the Werelius method with the difference only that the round ligament is cut across and the end of the proximal part is hooked around the cartilage of the ninth rib, as in the Werelius technic, and the two limbs are sutured to each other.

D. **Formation of a partition, either from the peritoneum or from the falciform ligament, which supports the liver and prevents its sliding from its bed into the lumbar or iliac region.**

Even as fixation of the uterus is considered incomplete unless the perineum is strengthened from below by perineorrhaphy, so some surgeons consider that no matter how strongly the liver is immobilized from above,

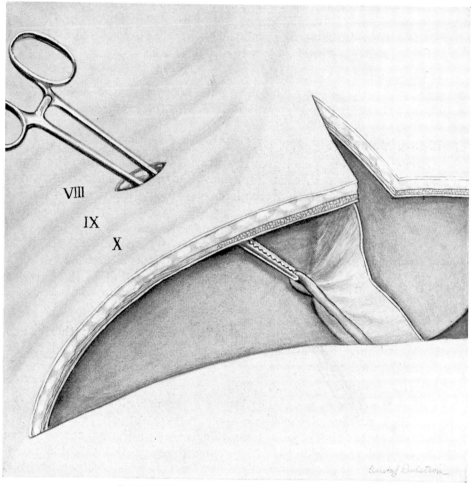

FIG. 291. HEPATOPEXY (WERELIUS METHOD).

An artery clamp enters the abdominal cavity through the eighth intercostal space and grasps the round ligament.

some kind of a partition should be built below the lower edge of the liver which will prevent it from sliding downward.

1. **Péan Method.**

This method was suggested by Péan in June, 1896.

Step 1. A transverse abdominal incision is made below the costal arch and reaches the umbilicus. The liver is placed in its proper position. The parietal peritoneum, with the transversalis fascia of the upper lip, are made mobile by separating them from the superficially situated muscles, and are sutured to the parietal peritoneum of the posterior abdominal wall, thus producing a partition which will prevent downward sliding of the liver.

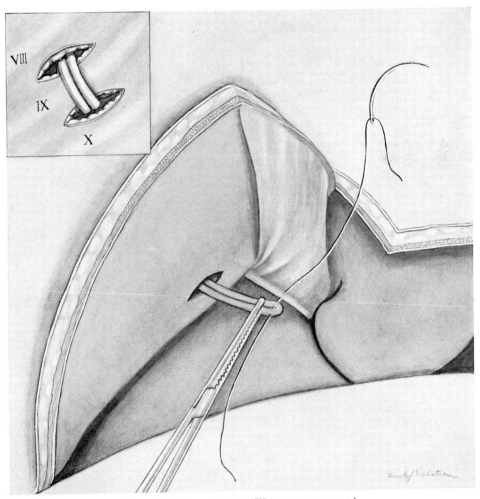

FIG. 292. HEPATOPEXY (WERELIUS METHOD).

INSERT. A portion of the round ligament is brought outside of the abdominal cavity. MAIN PICTURE. The round ligament is brought back into the abdomen and sutured to its beginning.

We believe that this method, supplemented by the artificial formation of adhesions between the liver and the diaphragm, and also by fixation of the liver by the aid of the round ligament, constitutes an excellent method of hepatopexy.

2. Franke Method.

This was described in 1895. A transverse incision is made parallel to and below the right costal arch. The peritoneum and the transversalis fascia of the upper lip are mobilized from the superimposed muscles. A series of sutures are passed which connect the anterior surface of the liver with the mobilized peritoneum and transversalis fascia and also the superimposed muscles of the upper lip, after which the knots are tied in front of the muscles. That portion of the peritoneum of the upper lip between the sutures and its free edge is turned behind the liver and sutured to its posterior surface. This method, with a slight modification was redescribed, in 1904, by A. Depage and L. Mayer of Brussels, and is known in France and Belgium as the Depage-Mayer method. However, priority belongs to Franke.

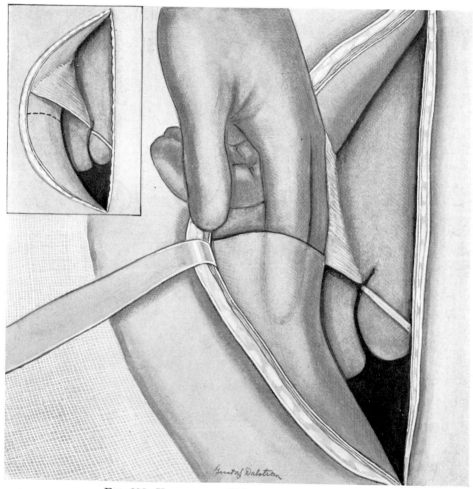

FIG. 293. HEPATOPEXY (FÖDERL-KAISER METHOD).
INSERT. A transverse incision is made in the posterior sheath of the rectus muscle.
MAIN PICTURE. A pocket is made between the rectus muscle and its posterior sheath.

3.   **Főderl-Kaiser Method** (Fig. 293).

This was published by Kaiser in 1922. The abdomen is opened by a midline incision which is made between the ensiform process and the umbilicus. The peritoneum and the transversalis fascia, situated behind the right rectus muscle, are cut transversely, and the lower lip is mobilized by separating it from the superimposed muscle so as to form a pocket. The liver is replaced in its normal position, and its lower edge is placed in this pocket. The peritoneal edge of the lower lip is sutured to the posterior surface of the liver, thus preventing the edge of the liver from slipping out of the pocket. The abdomen is closed in layers.

This method is a further improvement of a similar method which was described by Főderl, in 1908. However, the method, in reality is not new at all. As early as 1895, Rydygier employed a similar procedure for fixation of a movable spleen, a description of which is given in the Chapter on "Surgery of the Spleen".

4.   **Ellsworth Eliot Method.**

The abdomen is opened by a midline incision between the ensiform process and the umbilicus. The hepatopexy operation, as described by the originator, is as follows:

"The obliterated umbilical vein, forming a thick cord in the free edge of the falciform ligament, is then identified and drawn forward until it comes in contact with the parietal peritoneum. The hepatic extremity of the ligament then rests against the under surface of the right lobe of the liver in front of the transverse fissure. The lower or umbilical extremity is in close contact with the anterior parietal peritoneum, the two portions of the ligament now forming a right angle. In this position the round ligament is sutured to the anterior parietal peritoneum with chromic gut and the redundant falciform peritoneal reflection is spread out laterally and sutured to the contiguous portion of the parietal peritoneum with the same material. In this manner a shelf is formed for the under surface of the liver. The abdominal wound is then closed in layers".

E.   **Excision of a portion of the anterior abdominal wall (laparectomy)—**

Depage method.

This method was used for those cases in which hepatoptosis was only one feature of general splanchnoptosis. For this condition Depage considered hepatopexy only as a palliative procedure. He believed that general splanchnoptosis is largely due to a general weakening of the abdominal wall, and he remedied it by the excision of a part of this wall, diminishing the wall in two dimensions.

In several cases operated upon by this method the results were satisfactory. There was a relief of the symptoms of splanchnoptosis and no hernia formation followed. However, with the development of other methods of surgical treatment of splanchnoptosis, **the Depage method will hardly appeal to a modern surgeon.**

F.   A combination of the above mentioned methods.

Many surgeons are using not only one or another type of operation but a combination of some features from the different types. It seems to us that the best results are obtained by immobilizing the liver by forming adhesions between its upper surface and the diaphragm, reinforcing this by a suspension-operation with the aid of the round ligament which is attached either to the abdominal wall or still better to the chest-wall, and, finally, immobilizing the liver by forming a peritoneal partition below it. This operation is as follows:

Step 1. The abdomen is opened by a transverse incision running from the tenth right costal cartilage to the midline.

Step 2. The patient is placed in the Trendelenburg position. The upper surface of the liver and the diaphragm are vigorously rubbed with gauze. The liver is placed in its normal position. The round ligament is brought outside the abdominal cavity through a small incision made above the cartilage of the ninth rib, and then returned into the abdominal cavity through a small incision made below the cartilage of the same rib, so that the round ligament forms a loop around the cartilage of this rib. The two limbs of the round ligament are sutured to each other (Fig. 292).

Step 3. The peritoneum and the transversalis fascia of the upper lip are separated from the superimposed structures and sutured to the inferior surface of the liver, thus forming a pocket.

The operation thus performed produces fixation and suspension of the liver, and reinforcing this from below makes it analogous to fixation or suspension of the uterus with reinforcement of the pelvic floor by perineorrhaphy.

BIBLIOGRAPHY.

A. L. Abel. Primary carcinoma of the liver: with report of a case success-fully treated by partial hepatectomy.
Brit. Journ. of Surg. 21:684-700; y. 1933-1934.

M. Ascoli. Studio clinico sui tumori primitivi del fegato.
Policlinico (sez. chir.) 37:309-330; y. 1930.

M. Auvray. Étude expérimentale sur la résection du foie chez l'homme et chez les animaux.
Rev. de Chir. 17:319-331; y. 1897.

P. Barco. Sull'emostasi epática. Contributo sperimentale.
Annal. ital. di chir. 10:913-950; y. 1931.

J. A. Bargen & F. W. Rankin. Tests of hepatic function in carcinoma; their value in cases of neoplasm of colon with and without metastasis to liver.
Ann. Surg. 91:225-232; y. 1930.

Bariéty. Les ascites cirrhotiques; conception actuelle, traitement.
Paris méd. 1:33-36; y. 1934.

P. Bastianelli. Resezione di grosso tumore (Cancro nodulare del lobo destroepatico) ed affondamento ideale introperitoneale del fegato. Guarigione.
Arch. ital. di Chir. 34:207-212; y. 1933.

A. A. Bobrow. Ein Fall von Hepatopexie.
Zbl. f. Chir. 23:990; y. 1896.

A. A. Bobrow. Ueber ein neues Operationsverfahren zur Entfernung von Echinococcus in der Leber und anderen parenchymatosen Bauchorganen.
Arch. f. klin. Chir. 56:819-826; y. 1898.

N. A. Bogoras. The transplantation of the superior mesenteric vein into the inferior vena cava in cirrhosis of the liver.
Russki Vratch, 12:48-50; y. 1913.

F. K. Boland. Abscess of the liver.
Annals of Surg. 94:766-775; y. 1931.

C. J. Bond. On the treatment of hydatid disease by incision and evacuation of the cyst without drainage.
Brit. Med. Journ. I:795-796; y. 1891.

C. Bottcher. Ueber Hepatopexie.
Deutsche Zeitschr. f. Chir. 56:252-335; y. 1900.

T. Brugsch. Die Leber in der Chirurgie.
Arch. f. klin. Chir. 173:647-663; y. 1932.

J. P. Buckley. True total enucleation of two hydatid cysts from the same liver.
Brit. Med. Journ. II:725-727; y. 1913.

L. Caporale & G. Bertini. Ricerche sperimentali sulle suture di ferite del fegato e della milza mediante nastro di catgut.
Boll. e mem. Soc. piemontese di chir. 4:585-601; y. 1934.

G. Caprio. Resección del lóbulo izquierdo del ígado.
Bol. y trab. de la Soc. de cir. de Buenos Aires, 16:298-306; y. 1932.

L. Caravani. Chirurgia delle vie biliari.
Roma, R. Garroni, 1925.

K. Chaterjii. Tropical surgery and surgical pathology.
Wood & Co., Publishers, New York; y. 1927.

Chevallier. Technique de l'hepatopexie. (Procédé de Legueu).
Thèse de Paris, 1898.

A. Cioffi. Emostasi epática. Contributo sperimentale.
Ann. ital. di chir. 11:361-382; y. 1932.

Costantini. La thoraco-phréno-laparotomie sans pneumothorax dans le traitement chirurgical des Kystes hydatiques du foie à localisation supéro-postérieure.
Presse Méd. 33:1107-1109; y. 1925.

H. Delagénière. Cirrhose hépatique et hépatoptose. Hépatopexie et Cholecystostomie. Guérison.
Arch. prov. de Chir. 6:310-316; y. 1897.

A. Depage & L. Mayer. Über Hepatopexie.
Zbl. f. Chir. 31:112-114; y. 1904.

A. Depage. De l'intervention chirurgicale dans la splanchnoptose.
Bruxelles, 1893.

F. Dévé. Des greffes hydatiques postopératoires (pathogénie et prophylaxie).
Rev. de Chir. 26:533-559; y. 1902.

C. F. Dixon & G. T. Murphy. Primary idiopathic abscess of the liver.
Surg. Gyn. & Obst. 54:20-25; y. 1932.

M. Donati. Valeur diagnostique et pronostique des altérations anatomo-fonctionelles du foie dans la chirurgie des voies biliaires.
Bull. et mém. Soc. nat. de Chir. 61:139-147; y. 1935.

D. Drummond & R. Morison. A case of ascites due to cirrhosis of the liver cured by operation.
Brit. Med. Journ. II:728-729; y. 1896.

S. I. Duchinova. Über temporäre Abklemmung des Lig. Hepatoduodenale für blutlose Operationen an der Leber.
Vestnik Khirurgii, 5:34-56; y. 1925-1926.

Ecarius. Über subcutane Leberrupturen.
Arch. f. klin. Chir. 172:755-774; y. 1933.

E. L. Eliason. Congenital non-parasitic cyst of the liver.
Ann. Surg. 99:691-696; y. 1934.

E. Eliot. Hepatoptosis complicated by gastroptosis; a suggestion as to treatment.
Med. News, 85:913-917; y. 1904.

R. O. Eolian. Über Amöbenabscesse der Leber und des Subdiaphragmalraums.
Arch. f. klin. Chir. 163:137-146; y. 1930.

H. Eppinger & R. Leuchtenberger. Zur Pathogenese der Lebercirrhose.
Zeitschr. f. d. gesamm. exper. Med. 85:581-597; y. 1932.

Faure. L'appareil suspenseur du foie. L'hépatoptose et l'hépatopexie.
Thèse de Paris, 1892.

O. Föderl. Über "Hepatoptose".
Wien. klin. Wchnschr. 21:1657-1661; y. 1908.

W. Tejerina Fotheringham. Cirugía de la ascitis en los cirróticos.
La Semana méd. 2:871-876; y. 1929.

J. Frank. Incising and suturing the liver. A new method to reëstablish a continuity and for the control of hemorrhage.
Journ. Am. Med. Ass. 45:446-452; y. 1905.

F. Franke. Zur Technik der Hepatopexie.
Zbl. f. Chir. 23:775-779; y. 1896.

E. Fulde. Die bekannt gewordenen Ergebnisse der Radikaloperationen der Gallengangskrebse.
Zbl. f. Chir. 54:1481-1487; y. 1927.

C. Garré. Beitrage zur Leberchirurgie. Exstirpation eines Leber-Echinococcus mittelst Resection eines Teiles des rechten Leberlappens.
Bruns Beitr. z. klin. Chir. 4:181-196; y. 1888.

C. Garré. On resection of the liver.
Surg. Gyn. & Obst. 5:331-341; y. 1907.

L. Gioja. Sulla resezione del fegato con affondamento ideale intraperitoneale dell'organo.
Arch. ital. di Chir. 35:533-537; y. 1933.

Th. Glück. Ueber die Bedeutung der physiologisch-chirurgischer Experimente an der Leber.
Arch. f. klin. Chir. 29:139-145; y. 1883.

Th. Glück. Ueber Exstirpation von Organen.
Arch. f. klin. Chir. 28:604-609; y. 1883.

K. Goto. Untersuchungen über Vorkommen und Häufigkeit der angeborenen Leberspalten und ihre Beziehungen zu verschiedenen Krankheiten.
Ztschr. f. d. ges. Anat. (abt. 2); 16:357-378; y. 1931.

A. J. Graham. Subcutaneous rupture of the liver.
Ann. of Surgery. 86:51-61; y. 1927.

W. Grosz. Zur Technik der Operation der Hepato- und Gastroptosis.
Deutsch. Med. Wochensch. 53:196-197; y. 1927.

R. Hanser. Misbildungen der Leber.
Handb. der Spez. pathol. Anat. & Histol. (Teil I); 5:1-70; y. 1930.

S. W. Harrington. Amebic hepatic, subphrenic and pulmonary abscesses.
Arch. of Surg. 21:1146-1160; y. 1930.

S. N. Hayes. Treatment of hepatic abscesses of amoebic origin.
Indian Med. Gaz. 62:13-15; y. 1927.

C. Henschen. Die akuten, subakuten und chronischen Schwellungskrisen der Leber (akutes und chronisches Leberglaukom) und ihre chirurgische Behandlung.
Arch. f. klin. Chir. 167:825-905; y. 1931.

C. Henschen. Die Bedeutung der Leber in der Chirurgie.
Arch. f. klin. Chir. 173:488-646; y. 1932.

R. Herbst. Zur Klinik und Therapie der Subcutanen Leberruptur.
Deutsche Zeitschr. f. Chir. 241:602-614; y. 1933.

A. Herrmannsdorfer. Zur Wirkung der Talmaschen Operation bei Lebercirrhose.
Arch. f. klin. Chir. 173:682-684; y. 1932.

C. G. Heyd. Protective rôle of the liver in abdominal surgery.
Am. Journ. Obst. & Gyn. 19:203-210; y. 1930.

J. Hochenegg. Ein Beitrag zur Leberchirurgie.
Wien klin. Wchnsch. 3:223-225; y. 1890.

E. Holman. Implantation of spleen in abdominal wall for portal obstruction; a suggested operation for hepatic cirrhosis.
West. Journ. Surg. 41:255-261; y. 1933.

E. Höpfner. Des Ascites und seine chirurgische Behandlung.
Ergebnisse d. Chirurg. u. Orthop. 6:410-479; y. 1913.

F. S. Hough. "Communications" (Description of a new method of suturing the liver).
Iowa Med. Journ. 14:238-241; y. 1907-1908.

O. Kalb. Zur Ascitesdrainage.
Deutsche Zeitschr. f. Chir. 138:105-112; y. 1916.

W. W. Keen. Report of a case of resection of the liver for the removal of
a neoplasm, with a table of seventy-six cases of resection of the liver
for hepatic tumors.
Ann. of Surg. 30:267-283; y. 1899.

T. P. Kilner. Operative procedures in amebic abscess of liver based on
recent experiences.
Proc. Roy. Soc. Med. (Sect. Trop. Dis. & Parasit.) 25:10-14; y. 1931.

J. G. Knoflach. Zur Chirurgie der nicht parasitären Leberzysten.
Wien. klin. Wchnschr. 45:786-787; y. 1932.

Van Buren Knott. A new liver suture.
Ann. of Surg. 46:790-792; y. 1907.

M. Kousnetzoff & J. Pensky. Sur la Résection partielle du Foie.
Revue de Chir. 16:501-521 and 954-992; y. 1896.

K. P. Krasowitow. Ueber eine neue chirurgische Behandlungsmethode der
Ascites. (Description of Flerow method.)
Novy Chir. Arch. pp. 422-426; y. 1925.
Abstract in Zbl. f. Chir. 53:799; y. 1926.

W. W. Krestowski. The operative treatment of cirrhotic ascites by a direct
anastomosis between the portal system and inferior vena cava.
Vestnik Khir. 6:87-92; y. 1926.

A. P. Krymoff. Technic in fixation of mobile liver.
Vestnik Khir. (No. 64); 22:20-22; y. 1930.

C. Langenbuch. Chirurgie der Leber und Gallenblase.
Deutsche Chirurgie, Lief. 45c, 2 Hälfte.

Th. Lens. Hechting van het omentum majus aan den buikwand bij cirrhosis hepatis atrophica.
Nederlandsch. Tijdschrift voor Geneeskunde, 28(1st part) ; 645-650 ; y. 1892.
(Description of Talma operation.)

Levy-Neumand. Les ruptures traumatiques du foie.
Paris, Norbert Maloine, y. 1925.

A. Ludlow. Liver abscess. Report of one hundred operations.
Surg. Gyn. & Obst. 36:336-343 ; y. 1923.

F. L. Marting & B. Halpert. Topographic distribution of metastases in the liver from carcinomas primary in the gastro-intestinal tract.
Yale Journ. Biol. & Med. 6:541-543 ; y. 1934.

E. P. McNamee. Intrahepatic gall-bladder.
Am. Journ. Roentg. 33:603-610 ; y. 1935.

A. Messing & M. F. Ashley-Montagu. Note on a case of complete absence of the left lobe of the liver in a man.
Anat. Rec. 53:169-172 ; y. 1932.

H. W. Mills. Hydatid cysts of the liver.
Surg. Gyn. & Obst. 44:577-591 ; y. 1927.

H. G. Mogena. La Ascitis de la cirrosis hepática (Nuevas orientaciones patogénicas).
Arch. de med. cir. y especialid. 36:835-837 ; y. 1933.

Monprofit. Traitement Chirurgical de la cirrhose du Foie.
Paris, 1904.

F. Oehlecker. Leberveränderungen bei Verschluss des linken Astes der Pfortader.
Arch. f. klin. Chir. 173:663-681 ; y. 1932.

A. O'Malley. The surgical treatment of hepatic ascites.
Am. Journ. of the Med. Sciences. 131:873-883 ; y. 1906.

G. Pascale & A. G. Chiariello. Le epatiti croniche (Comprese le cirrosi).
Arch. ed atti. d. Soc. ital. di Chir. 39:478-567 ; y. 1933.

E. Payr & A. Martina. Experimentelle und klinische Beiträge zur Lebernaht und Leberresection (Magnesiumplattennaht).
Arch. f. klin. Chir. 77:962-998 ; y. 1905.

H. E. Pearse, Jr. & G. E. Ward. Electrosurgery as hemostatic instrument in operations upon the liver, kidney and spleen.
Am. Journ. of Surg. 10:540-546 ; y. 1930.

E. Ponfick. Experimentelle Beiträge zu Pathologie der Leber.
Virchow's Arch. 118:209-249 ; y. 1889.

J. Hogarth Pringle. Notes on the arrest of hepatic hemorrhage due to trauma.
Ann. of Surg. 48:541-549; y. 1908.

Quénu. Note sur le traitement opératiore des Kystes hydatiques du foie. Deux petites incisions dans l'ouverture des Kystes hydatiques du foie.
Bull. et Mém. de la Soc. de Chir. 30:953-959; y. 1904.

F. W. Ramsay. Fixation of the liver and both kidneys in a case of Glenard's disease.
Brit. Med. Journ. I:1152-1153; y. 1897.

L. Rogers. Amebic liver abscess; its pathology, prevention and cure.
Lancet, I:463-469 and 569-576; y. 1922.

L. Rogers. Recent advances in tropical medicine.
Blakiston Publishers, y. 1928.

M. Ruotte. Abouchement de la veine saphène externe au péritoine pour résorber les épanchements sciatiques.
Lyon Méd. 109:574-577; y. 1907.

E. Schepelmann. Klinische Erfahrungen mit meiner Methode der plastischen Ascitesdrainage.
Arch. f. klin. Chir. 106:663-688; y. 1914-1915.

B. Schiassi. Le développement chirurgical d'une double circulation complementaire dans le traitement de quelques maladies hepato-spleniques.
La Semaine Méd. 23:169-172; y. 1903.

B. Schiassi. Il valore odierno della operazione di Talma.
Riforma med. 48:1739-1741; y. 1932.

H. von Seemen. Subkutane Leberruptur mit Pfortaderverletzung—Operative Versorgung, Gefässnaht—Heilung.
Schweiz. med. Wchnschr. 65:83-84; y. 1935.

G. Segura. Consideraciones sobre el absceso hepático.
La Semana Méd. 34:799-804; y. 1927.

E. Simon. Zur Diagnose und Behandlung des Leberechinococcus.
Chirurg, 2:793-800; y. 1930.

G. Steinberg. Beitrag zur Chirurgie der Leber (Ueber einen chirurgisch behandelten Fall von Hæmangioendothelioma hepatis).
Bruns Beiträge z. klin. Chir. 158:303-308; y. 1933.

G. de Takats. Cholecystectomy for hyperacidity.
Surg. Gyn. & Obst. 40:221-223; y. 1925.

S. Talma. Chirurgische Oeffnung neuer Seitenbahnen für das Blut der Vena Porta.
Berl. klin. Wchnschr. 35:833-836; y. 1898.

J. Tandler. Zur Frage der Hepatoptose.
Wien. klin. Wchnschr. 21:1661-1664; y. 1908.

T. Tannahill. Operative treatment of cirrhosis of the liver.
Brit. Med. Journ. I:281-282; y. 1930.

F. Terrier & M. Auvray. Le foie mobile et son traitement chirurgical.
Rev. de Chir. 17:621-645; y. 1897.

J. Knowsley Thornton. Two cases of hepatotomy for hydatids.
Med. Times and Gazette, 1:89-90; y. 1883.

A. Tietze. Aufgaben der Leberchirurgie.
Bruns Beitr. zur klin. Chir. 140:320-326; y. 1927.

J. Tongern. Über Hepatopexie.
Inaug. Diss., Bonn, 1920.

F. I. Valker. Certain anatomic data on operations of liver and biliary
tract.
Vestnik Khir. (No. 52) ; 18:85-91; y. 1929.

A. Werelius. Hepatoptosis and hepatopexy.
Journ. Am. Med. Ass. 58:610-615; y. 1912.

C. L. Wilmoth. Amebic abscess of the liver. Method of treatment: Injection of cavity with iodized oil for definite localization.
Am. Journ. of Surg. 8:983-987; y. 1930.

CHAPTER XXII.

SURGERY OF THE SPLEEN.

I. DIFFERENT ROUTES FOR EXPOSURE OF THE SPLEEN.

The routes for exposure of the spleen are the same as for the liver, with this difference only that in the latter they are made on the right side, whereas for the spleen they are made on the left side.

II. SPLENOTOMY.

Definition.

This term consists of two Greek words: σπλήν, spleen, and τέμνειν, to cut. It signifies an incision of the spleen.

Indications.

    a. Abscess.

    b. Large single cyst. In the case of numerous cysts splenectomy is indicated.

Technic.

This operation can be done either as a one- or a two-stage operation.

One-stage Operation.

    Step 1. The abdomen is opened by one of the incisions already described.

    Step 2. The spleen is isolated from the rest of the peritoneal cavity by tampons the ends of which are brought outside of the abdominal cavity. Exploratory puncture by a needle is made to ascertain the location of the abscess. If pus is found, an incision through the capsule is made and the pus is evacuated. A roll of gauze with a rubber drain is introduced into the cavity in the spleen and the ends are brought outside the abdominal cavity. The abdomen is closed in layers, leaving openings at the upper and lower angles of the wound for the ends of the gauze rolls. A few days later, the tampons which "walled off" the spleen and lie in the abdominal cavity are removed. By this time, adhesions have been formed which prevent contamination of the general peritoneal cavity. A few days later, the tampon and rubber drain are removed from the cavity in the spleen. The majority of surgeons prefer the one-stage method.

III. SUTURE OF THE SPLEEN (SPLENORRHAPHY).

Indications.

Wound of the spleen. This method is suitable only for small wounds. In the case of a large wound, it is difficult to stop the bleeding by the suture method, and for this reason splenectomy should be given preference. The first successful splenorrhaphy for a wounded spleen was performed by Parlavecchio, in 1893.

Step 1. The abdomen is opened.

Step 2. A large piece of omentum is excised and tucked into the open wound in the spleen. This will act not only as a tampon but as an active

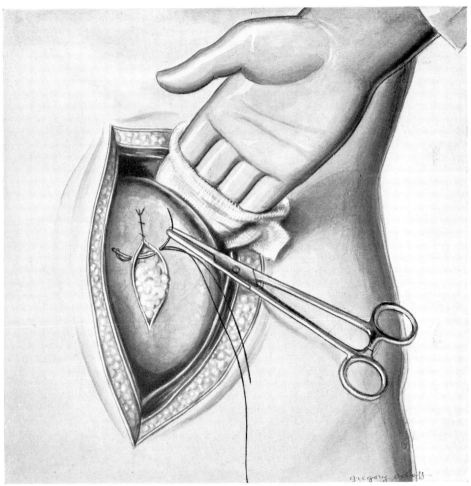

FIG. 294. SPLENORRHAPHY.

coagulant. The edges of the capsule of the spleen are sutured to each other with heavy catgut over the piece of omentum (Fig. 294).

IV. SPLENOPEXY.

Definition.

The term consists of two Greek words: σπλήν, spleen and πῆξις, to fasten. It signifies "fixation of the spleen". The fixation may be either intraperitoneal or extraperitoneal, or combined intra- and extraperitoneal.

Indications.

a. **Movable spleen,** when this condition is the cause of symptoms, mostly pressure on the adjacent structures and particularly on the colon.

b. As one of the methods of treatment of ascites due to **cirrhosis of the liver.** Tuffier was the first who performed a splenopexy, in 1882. The next who performed it was Kouwer, of Haarlem, Netherland, in 1891. How-

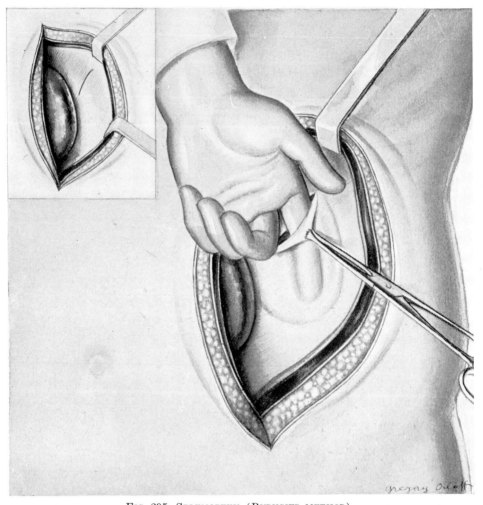

FIG. 295. SPLENOPEXY (RYDYGIER METHOD).
INSERT. Incision of the parietal peritoneum on the posterior abdominal wall.
MAIN PICTURE. Formation of a pocket.

ever, interest in this operation was revived by Rydygier, who performed his first case in 1895. Since that time this operation has been used by many surgeons.

1. KOUWER METHOD.

Step 1. The abdomen is opened.

Step 2. Between the upper and lower surfaces of the spleen and the corresponding surfaces of the diaphragm are placed gauze tampons which are brought outside the abdominal cavity. The spleen is placed back in its normal position. A few days later, the tampons are removed. By this time adhesions will be formed between the spleen and the diaphragm.

Some surgeons are even yet using this method. They only supplement this technic by vigorously rubbing the diaphragmatic surface of the spleen and the diaphragm with gauze in order to facilitate the formation of adhesions before they place the gauze-tampons.

2. RYDYGIER METHOD.

This method was reported to the XXIV Congress of the Deutsche Gesellschaft für Chirurgie, in April, 1895.

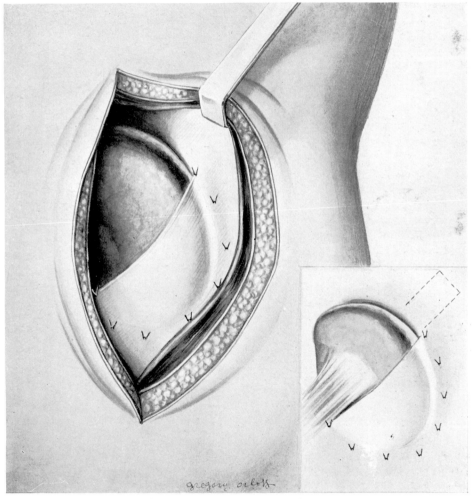

FIG. 296. SPLENOPEXY (RYDYGIER METHOD).
INSERT. Formation of a peritoneal flap to cover a portion of the spleen.
MAIN PICTURE. The lower pole of the spleen is placed in the pocket.

Step 1. The abdomen is opened in the left hypochondrium.

Step 2. A slightly convex incision running somewhat upward (Fig. 295, insert), the length of which should be equal to the width of the spleen, is made on the inner surface of the thoraco-abdominal wall from below upward extending from the eleventh to the ninth ribs. The peritoneum of the lower lip which is thus formed is separated bluntly from

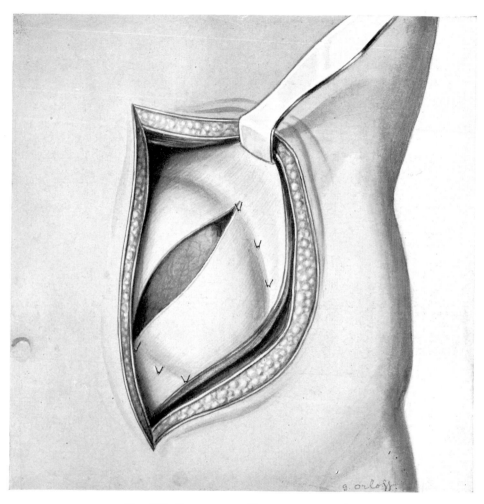

FIG. 297. SPLENOPEXY (RYDYGIER METHOD).
Placing the upper pole of the spleen in the upper pocket.

the superimposed soft tissues, so that a pocket is formed with its bottom directed downward (Fig. 295). The lower pole of the spleen is placed in this pocket (Fig. 296). In order to prevent further separation of the peritoneum from the superimposed structures of the pocket by the lower pole of the spleen, the peritoneum is sutured to the superficially lying structures by a series of interrupted sutures approximately half an inch away from the distal end of the bottom of the pocket (Fig 296).

Step 3. The upper lip of the peritoneum is separated from the muscle of the diaphragm so as to form an upper pocket into which the upper pole of the spleen is placed (Fig. 297).

[Whereas **Step 2** is an essential part of the Rydygier method, **Step 3**

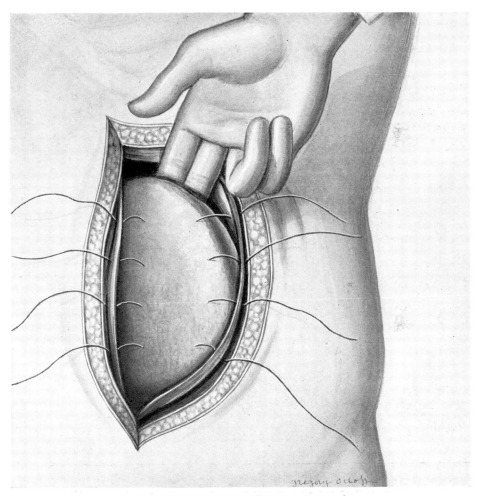

FIG. 298. SPLENOPEXY (TUFFIER METHOD).

is done only in case it is possible to form an upper pocket, since in many cases it is difficult to separate the peritoneum from the muscle of the diaphragm.]

In order to reinforce the new position of the spleen in those cases in which only the lower pocket was made, Rydygier made a ⌐ -shaped peritoneal flap laterally to the spleen and reflected this medially, so that it covered the anterior surface of the spleen, and then sutured the free border of the flap to the gastro-splenic ligament (Fig. 296, insert). However, this step is not essential. The true **characteristic feature of the Rydygier method is the formation of a lower pocket into which is placed the lower pole of the spleen.**

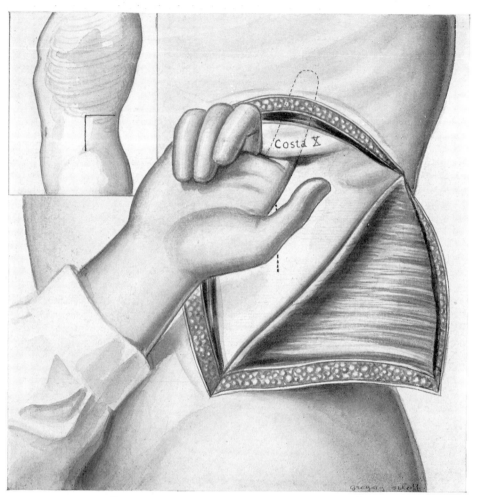

FIG. 299. SPLENOPEXY (BARDENHEUER METHOD).
Separation of the peritoneum from the superimposed structures.

3. TUFFIER METHOD. (FIG. 298).

This method consists in suturing the spleen to the abdominal parieties. A bite is taken through the entire thickness of the abdominal wall, except the skin, of one lip. Then one is taken through the spleen, penetrating not only the capsule but also a thick layer of the parenchyma of the spleen, then again through the entire thickness of the abdominal wall, except the skin, of the other lip. The number of sutures depends upon the

size of the spleen. These sutures are not tied at this time. This is postponed until all the layers of the abdomen (except the skin) have been
sutured. Then the splenopexy sutures are tied. After this the skin is
closed.

Although the name of Greifenhagen has been attached to this method,
it is, however, the method which was used first by Tuffier and later by
Kouwer in his very first case of splenopexy, but which he (Kouwer) did
not subsequently use on account of the danger of hemorrhage.

4. BARDENHEUER METHOD.

This method was described by Plücker, one of Bardenheuer's asso-
ciates, in October, 1895.

Step 1. The abdominal cavity is opened by an incision running along

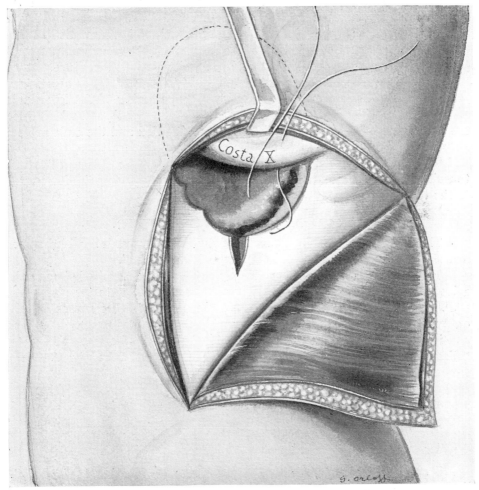

FIG. 300. SPLENOPEXY (BARDENHEUER METHOD).
Fixing the lower pole of the spleen to the tenth rib.

the left midaxillary line, starting immediately above the crest of the ilium and extending for four inches upward until the tenth left rib is almost reached (Fig. 299, insert). Then it turns laterally nearly perpendicularly to the vertical incision and runs for another four inches. The entire thickness of the flap thus formed is cut down to the peritoneum, which is not yet opened. This musculo-cutaneous flap is reflected (Fig. 299).

Step 2. The exposed peritoneum is separated from the superimposed soft tissues as far as possible upward and downward (Fig. 299). A small incision is made through the peritoneum, just large enough to draw the spleen outside of the abdominal cavity (Fig. 300). The spleen is placed extraperitoneally in the sac thus formed, precisely in the same position as it lies normally intraperitoneally (Fig. 300). The slit in the peritoneum is sutured to the gastro-splenic ligament.

Step 3. A thread of silkworm-gut is passed around the tenth rib (which is freely exposed for this purpose), and then through the lower pole of the spleen (Fig. 300). The ends of this thread are not tied at this time. A series of interrupted sutures are inserted between the lowermost part of the separated peritoneum and the superimposed structures, so as to prevent separation of the peritoneum from these structures in a downward direction, thereby preventing a downward slipping of the lower pole of the spleen. Then the long ends of the silkworm-gut thread which fixed the lower pole of the spleen to the tenth rib are tied and the ends are cut short. The wound is closed in layers.

Thus, this method is characterized by **placing the spleen extraperitoneally, attaching the hilum to the peritoneum, and fixing the lower pole to the tenth rib.**

5.   SCHIASSI METHOD (SPLENOCLEISIS).

The term splenocleisis consists of two Greek words: σπλήν, spleen and κλείσις closure. It signifies "closure of the spleen".

This method consists in producing extensive adhesions between the spleen and all the surrounding tissues, including the anterior abdominal wall. A thick capsule is formed around the spleen which compresses that organ, thus diminishing the amount of blood passing through the spleen and increasing the degree of anastomosis of the veins between the portal and systemic venous systems. This method was published in 1906 and again suggested in 1934.

Indications.

The method is used as a substitute for splenectomy in cases of blood-diseases in which splenectomy, for some reason, is hazardous. **It is practically the substitution of a physiological for a mechanical splenectomy.**

Technic.

Step 1. The abdomen is opened by an incision starting at the middle line and running parallel to and two fingers below the left costal arch until the left midaxillary line is reached.

Step 2. A roll of gauze is placed behind and below the lower pole of the spleen, another medially to the hilum, a third laterally to the lateral border, a fourth above and behind the upper pole, and a fifth and a sixth between the antero-lateral and antero-medial surfaces of the spleen and the anterior abdominal wall. The ends of all these rolls are brought outside the abdominal wound through its upper and lower angles. The anterior surface of the spleen is scarified.

Step 3. The abdominal wall is sutured in layers.

On the fifth day the roll is removed from the upper pole, and each following day another roll of gauze is removed. **The last roll is removed from the lower pole.**

As already mentioned, this operation produces a large amount of connective tissue around the spleen, which compresses the organ.

V. LIGATION OF THE ENTIRE SPLENIC PEDICLE OR OF THE SPLENIC ARTERY ALONE.

a. The ligation of the entire pedicle has been performed as a substitute for splenectomy. It may be advisable to do this in cases in which extensive adhesions between the spleen and the diaphragm make splenectomy a very difficult procedure. However, in some cases gangrene of the spleen may follow this procedure. For this reason it is very seldom used now.

b. Ligation of the **artery only** was done first by Clément Lucas, in 1882, as a substitute for splenectomy. It was performed also by Stubenrauch for thrombopenia, as a substitute for splenectomy, **since, if the vein is not injured, ligation of the artery may produce the desired atrophy of the spleen.**

Ligation of the artery, as a therapeutic measure for the treatment of ascites due to cirrhosis of the liver, was advocated by E. Holman, in 1933. However, further observations are necessary to show whether or not this procedure should be recommended.

VI. SPLENECTOMY.

Historical.

Splenectomy was first performed by Zacarelli, of Palermo, in 1549, for an enlarged spleen. The patient recovered. To Viard is given the credit of being the first, in 1581, to remove the spleen, which prolapsed through the wounded anterior abdominal wall. This patient also recovered. Since that time, due to technical difficulties, this operation has been used very infrequently. The first deliberately planned splenectomy on a human, with preliminary practice on animals for this purpose, was made by Quittenbaum, in 1826. The patient died after the operation. In the middle of the Nineteenth Century interest in this operation was again revived. Küchler, of Darmstadt, performed it in 1855 for the removal of an enlarged malarial spleen (the patient died from hemorrhage a few hours after the operation), and G. Volney Dorsey, of Piqua, Ohio, performed it in the same year for the same condition. His patient recovered. **This case may be considered as the first successfully performed splenectomy for malaria in modern times.** Péan, in 1864, was the first to perform a splenectomy for unilocular cyst of the spleen (the patient recovered). Koeberlé was the first who performed splenectomy for echinococcus, in 1873. For Banti's disease the first splenectomy was performed in 1881. Picou and Ramond were the first to perform splenectomy for Gaucher disease, in 1896. Micheli was the first to perform splenectomy for hemolytic icterus, in 1906, and Schloffer was the first to perform it for thrombopenia, in 1917.

Definition.

The term splenectomy consists of two Greek words: σπλήν, spleen and ἐκτομή, excision. It means "excision of the spleen".

Indications.

There are many indications for the performance of this operation.

1. **Rupture of the Spleen.**

In some cases it may be advisable to suture the torn edges, but usually splenectomy is indicated for this condition.

2. **Wandering Spleen.**

The majority of surgeons prefer to perform splenopexy for this condition. However, if torsion of the pedicle occurs, splenectomy is the only remedy.

3. **Abscess of the Spleen.**

Splenectomy is advisable only in cases in which there is no thrombophlebitis, the presence of which strongly suggests the existence of abscesses in the liver, which makes the operation useless.

4. **Non-parasitic Cysts.**

5. **Parasitic Cysts (echinococcus).**

6. **Isolated Primary Tuberculosis of the Spleen.**

In case this is of the secondary form, splenectomy is contraindicated.

7. Greatly enlarged **Malarial Spleens,** if their size produces distressing symptoms. Splenectomy will not alleviate the disease itself.

8. **Leukemia.**

Splenectomy does not alleviate this disease. It is indicated only when the greatly enlarged spleen produces mechanical difficulties, or threatens to rupture. Lately, many give preference to X-ray therapy.

9. **Malignant Tumors.**

Splenectomy is indicated only in those cases which are primary, and when no metastases are present.

10. **Hemolytic Jaundice.**

Splenectomy gives a symptomatic cure in the majority of the cases.

11. **Anemia Splenica Infantum (Jaksch-Hayem Anemia).**

Splenectomy should be preceded by medical treatment, which frequently gives good results. In obstinate cases which do not yield to medical treatment, splenectomy combined with a few repeated blood-transfusions gives excellent results.

12. Gaucher Disease (Large-cell Splenomegaly).

Splenectomy does not cure this condition. It gives only mechanical relief. However, cases have been observed in which a long continued remission has followed the operation.

13. Splenic Anemia (including Banti Disease).

Splenectomy gives excellent results in the **first stage** of this disease. In the **second stage** (which is characterized by anemia, leukopenia and gastro-intestinal manifestations), the results are not so good. In the **third stage** (Banti disease proper), the results are unsatisfactory. Many believe that at this stage splenectomy should not be performed at all. Even the followers of splenectomy believe that it should be supplemented by some type of the Talma operation.

14. Essential Thrombopenia.

Splenectomy gives good results in early cases. Some (Stubenrauch) had good results following ligation of the splenic artery only.

15. Splenomegaly of Unknown Origin.

Splenectomy is done only when mechanical difficulties arise, due to the size of the spleen.

16. Thrombosis of the Splenic Vein.

Splenectomy should be done, since gangrene of the spleen may occur.

17. Infarct of the Spleen.

This condition arises occasionally as a complication of typhus fever.

18. Kala-Azar (Leishman Disease).

Splenectomy should be done only in those cases which have responded to a previous treatment with antimony (tartar emetic) and in which the spleen is not enlarged. Otherwise, splenectomy is of no avail.

19. Cirrhosis of the Liver with Ascites.

Splenectomy is used by some surgeons with the object of removing a very important tributary of the portal vein. However, the majority of surgeons give preference to splenopexy, and we are in complete accord with them.

Technic.

The operation may be very simple, when the pedicle is long, the spleen movable, and no adhesions are present. In cases in which the spleen is very much enlarged, the pedicle short, and many adhesions are present, the operation may offer insurmountable difficulties, so that many experienced surgeons under circumstances prefer not to perform the splenectomy.

There are two methods used in removing the spleen, namely, either to start with separation of the spleen from the diaphragm, with ligation of the pedicle as the last step of the operation, or to start the operation with ligation of the pedicle, and separation of the spleen from the diaphragm as the last step. Both operative types have many followers.

Step 1. The abdomen is opened.

Step 2. The spleen is separated from the diaphragm by the hand (Fig. 301). If strong adhesions are present, they are cut by scissors between clamps. As soon as the spleen is lifted from the diaphragm, large packs, moistened in hot normal salt-solution, are introduced and placed upon the exposed bed of the spleen. Two things are thus accomplished:

a. Checking of the venous oozing from the diaphragm.

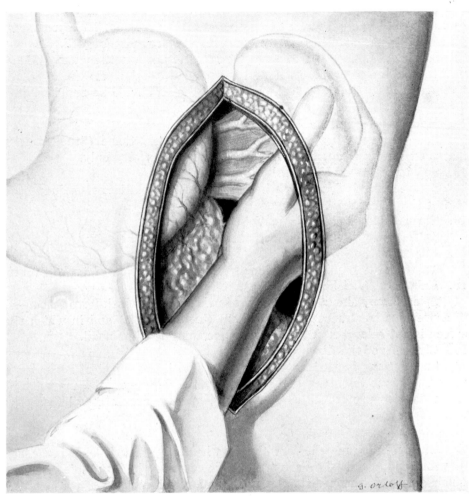

FIG. 301. SPLENECTOMY.
Manual separation of the spleen from its bed.

b. The facilitation of further manipulation of the spleen, such as clamping of the pedicle, etc.

Step 3. The gastro-splenic ligament above the pedicle is divided between clamps, care being taken not to injure the fundus of the stomach which lies very close to the spleen (Fig. 302).

Step 4. Ligation of the Splenic Pedicle.

This can be done either "en masse" or in sections. The latter should be given preference.

If the ligation is done in sections, the artery should be ligated first so as to give the vein a short time to carry away the blood from the spleen. [We should remember that the splenic artery runs either as a single trunk

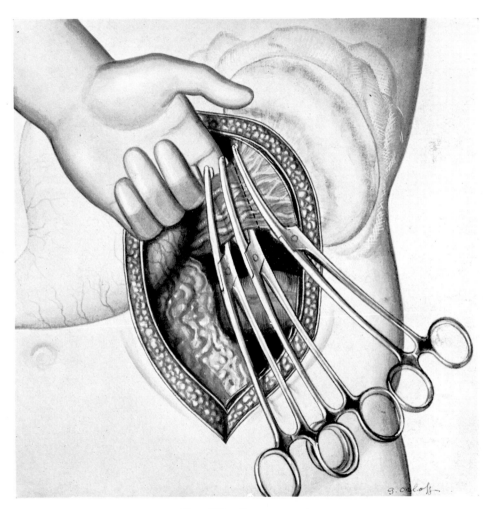

FIG. 302. SPLENECTOMY.
Cutting of the splenic pedicle between clamps.

or is already divided into two branches. The vein is still composed of two or three branches and runs below the artery.] If the stump is ligated "en masse", three large curved arterial forceps clamp the pedicle, which is cut between the clamp closest to the spleen and the middle one. In this manner, two clamps will safeguard against hemorrhage from the splenic artery and one from the splenic vein. The stump is ligated twice with a double strand of No. 2 plain catgut.

Before clamping the splenic pedicle the surgeon should obtain a clear view of it posteriorly, since not infrequently the tail of the pancreas reaches nearly to the hilum of the spleen, and in such cases may actually be adherent to the splenic pedicle posteriorly. By clamping the pedicle

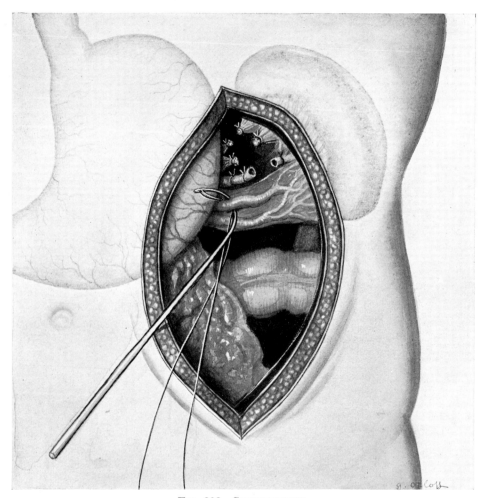

FIG. 303. SPLENECTOMY.
Ligation of the blood-vessels of the splenic pedicle.

without a previous separation of the tail, part of the pancreas may be caught in the clamp.

Step 5. All additional ligaments connecting the spleen with surrounding structures should be cut between two clamps and carefully ligated.

Step 6. The moist pack is removed from the bed of the spleen.

Step 7. The abdomen is closed in layers.

Alternate Method in which the Pedicle is Ligated first (Fig. 303).

Step 1. The abdomen is opened.

Step 2. The spleen is pushed laterally, so as to expose clearly the gastro-splenic omentum above the pedicle, which is then divided between the clamps. The finger is introduced through the opening thus formed and slipped behind the pedicle. The tail of the pancreas lies behind and the pedicle in front of the finger. The pedicle is ligated either sectionally or "en masse".

Step 3. The spleen is separated from the diaphragm and removed.

Step 4. The abdomen is closed in layers.

BIBLIOGRAPHY.

I. Abell. Wandering spleen with torsion of the pedicle.
Ann. of Surg. 98:722-735; y. 1933.

M. Acuña. La esplenectomía en las anemias graves de la infancia.
Arch. argent. de pediatr. II:627-638; y. 1931.

E. Aievoli. Tra la spleno-cleisi e la spleno-ectomia.
Gazz. internaz. med.-chir. 44:225-229; y. 1934.

H. Bailey. Traumatic rupture of the normal spleen.
Brit. Journ. of Surg. 15:40-46; y. 1927-1928.

D. Balfour. The technique of splenectomy.
Surg. Gyn. & Obst. 23:1-6; y. 1916.

D. Balfour. Indications for splenectomy in certain chronic blood disorders. Technic of operation.
Journ. Am. Med. Ass. 67:790-793; y. 1916.

D. Balfour. Splenectomy for repeated gastro-intestinal hemorrhages.
Ann. of Surg. 65:89-94; y. 1917.

G. Banti. La splénomegalie hémolitique.
La Semaine Méd. 265-268; y. 1912.

E. Beer. Essential thrombocytopenic purpura—Purpura hæmorrhagica and its treatment by splenectomy.
Ann. of Surg. 84:549-560; y. 1926.

E. Behr. Case of agenesis of the spleen.
Nederl. tijdschr. v. geneesk. 76:1490-1493; y. 1932.

W. Bergemann. Operationserfolg nach Entfernung der Milz im dritten Stadium der Bantischen Krankheit.
Bruns Beitr. z. klin. Chir. 137:748-750; y. 1926.

C. Bertone. Occlusione e turbe funzionali dello stomaco e dell' intestino da ectopia splenica o da tumor di milza.
Riforma med. 50:765-770; y. 1934.

A. Biondo. Su un caso di torsione della milza sul peduncolo con sindrome appendicolare acuta.
Policlinico (sez. prat.), 41:650-656; y. 1934.

L. Bischof. Ueber das Unterbinden der Gefässe bei Exstirpation der Milz.
Deutsche Zeitschr. f. Chir. 183:396-399; y. 1923.

A. Blalock. Transpleural splenectomy for ruptured spleen; case report.
South. Surgeon, 3:37-38; y. 1934.

E. Bray. Grandezze ponderali di alcuni visceri umani in rapporto alle dimensioni esterne dei corrispondenti segmenti corporei. Elaborazione statistica del materiale raccolto a Firenze da Castaldi e Vannucci. Milza, reni, utero.
Arch. ital. di anat. e di embriol. 30:198-214; y. 1932.

H. Bremer. Über die Früh-und Spätfolgen der wegen Verletzung ausgeführten Milzexstirpationen.
Deutsche Zeitschr. f. Chir. 239:433-443; y. 1933.

E. A. Bullard. Pelvic spleen with the torsion of the pedicle.
Am. Journ. of Obst. & Gyn. 25:599-600; y. 1933.

M. B. Clopton. Splenectomy for Purpura hemorrhagica.
Ann. of Surg. 82:413-420; y. 1925.

W. Coleman & J. A. Hartwell. Splenectomy for pernicious anemia.
Med. Rec. 85:1160-1162; y. 1914.

J. P. Collier. Some of the common indications for splenectomy, with case reports.
Journ. Med. Ass. of Alabama, 4:301-309; y. 1935.

T. B. Cooley. Indications for splenectomy in childhood.
Journal-Lancet, 54:673-676; y. 1934.

C. Currado. Rottura spontanea della milza in corso di malarioterapía.
Minerva med. I:859-862; y. 1933.

E. C. Cutler. Abscess of the spleen.
Journ. Am. Med. Ass. 75:1712-1715; y. 1920.

J. B. Deaver & S. P. Reimann. Splenic enlargement with cirrhosis of the liver.
Ann. of Surg. 88:355-360; y. 1928.

P. Decary. Deux cas de rupture de la rate consécutive à la malariathérapie.
Union méd. du Canada, 63:1015-1017; y. 1934.

M. Delhougne. Beitrag zur Frage der Splenektomie bei myeloischer Leukämie.
Bruns Beitr. z. klin. Chir. 104:153-166; y. 1917.

R. Desjacques, F. Bérard & H. Lathuraz-Viollet. Les ruptures associées de la rate et du rein gauche.
Revue de Chir. 68:296-317; y. 1930.

F. Dinand. Riesige epitheliale Solitärcyste der Milz.
Arch. f. klin. Chir. 158:485-499; y. 1930.

C. A. Elliot & A. B. Kanavel. Splenectomy for hemolytic icterus.
A discussion of the familial and acquired types with a report of splenectomized cases.
Surg. Gyn. & Obst. 21:152-153; y. 1915.

J. F. Erdmann & J. J. Moorhead. Splenectomy for splenomegaly (Gaucher type).
Am. Journ. of the Med. Sc. 147:213-224; y. 1914.

E. Eulenburg. Anzeigen und Ergebnisse der Milzexstirpation.
Fol. hæmat. 26:176-202; y. 1919-1920.

E. Finochietto & J. J. Beretervide. Bazo ectópico a pedículo retroperitoneal.
Prensa méd. argent. 20:1285-1292; y. 1933.

R. H. Fowler. The surgery of the splenic anemia.
Amer. Journ. of Surg. 37:153-157; y. 1923.

F. Franke. Ueber die Annähung der Wandermilz.
Deutsche Zeitschr. f. Chir. 47:580-589; y. 1898.

C. Friesdorf. Milzexstirpation bei hämolytischen Ikterus.
Mitteilung aus dem Grenzgeb. der Med. und Chir. 41:127-130; y. 1928.

R. Gardiner. Delayed hæmorrhage from ruptured spleen.
Brit. Med. Journ. I:416; y. 1935.

P. Geiger. Ein Fall von stielgedrehter Nebenmilz.
Zbl. f. Chir. 58:1772-1774; y. 1931.

J. C. A. Gerster. Ligation of the splenic and gastro-epiploica sinistra arteries in the surgery of the spleen.
Journ. Am. Med. Ass. 65:527; y. 1915.

H. Z. Giffin & T. L. Szlapka. The treatment of pernicious anemia by splenectomy.
Journ. Am. Med. Ass. 76:290-295; y. 1921.

H. Z. Giffin & J. K. Halloway. A review of twenty-eight cases of Purpura hæmorrhagica, in which splenectomy was performed.
Am. Journ. of Med. Sc. 170:186-204; y. 1925.

W. Greifenhagen. Zur Technic der Splenopexis und Aetiologie der Wandermilz.
Zbl. f. Chir. 24:124-128; y. 1897.

Grekow. Zur Frage der Freilegung der Milz bei Verletzungen derselben.
St. Petersb. Med. Wchnschr. 35: 613-615; y. 1910.

R. M. Gurevich. Splenectomy for extensive echinococcosis of the spleen.
Vestnik Khir. 36:42-45; y. 1934.

A. Gutiérrez. Esplenectomia. Sus Indicaciones.
Revist. de cirugía de Buenos Aires, 12:801-828; y. 1933.

H. Harttung. Beiträge zur Milzexstirpation bei Purpura thrombopenica in akuten Stadium.
Deutsch. Zeitschr. f. Chir. 191:91-94; y. 1925.

A. P. Heineck. Rupture traumatique de la rate normale. Trois observations personnelles; revue rapide de la literature.
Union méd. du Canada, 58:740-750; y. 1929.

H. Herfarth. Beiträge zur Chirurgie der Milz.
Bruns Beitr. z. klin. Chir. 128:284-309; y. 1923.

H. Hirschfeld & R. Mühsam. Chirurgie der Milz.
Neue Deutsche Chirurgie, 46; y. 1930.

J. M. Hitzrot. The surgical treatment of pernicious anemia.
Ann. of Surg. 75:31-37; y. 1922.

H. Hoffmann. Zur Chirurgie der Milz.
Bruns Beitr. z. klin. Chir. 92:396-436; y. 1914.

P. Huard & M. Montagné. Recherches sur la technique de la splénectomie pour splénomegalie (Utilisation de l'espace infrapleural et de la zone muette de la plèvre; abord postérieur du pédicule).
Journ. de Chir. 41:698-726; y. 1933.

O. Ivanissevich. Quistes hidaticos del bazo. Su tratamiento quirúrgico.
Bol. Inst. de clin. quir. 5:209-214; y. 1929.

E. Jacobi & H. Herholz. Spontanruptur der Milz bei Impfmalaria.
Klin. Wchnschr. XI:599-602; y. 1932.

M. Jaffé. Ueber den Wert der Milzexstirpation bei Bantischer Krankheit.
Zbl. f. Chir. 33:112-113; y. 1906.

R. H. Jaffé. Die Sichelzellenanämie.
Virch. Arch. 265:457-471; y. 1927.

B. Jutz & A. Jacobi. Spontanruptur der Milz bei Impfmalaria.
Münch med. Wchnschr. 78:395-396; y. 1931.

M. M. Kasakoff. Methods of arresting hemorrhage in injuries of the spleen.
Voyen. med. journ. (No. 1); I:11-23; y. 1930.

W. Keuenhof. Über angeborenen Milzmangel.
Frankfurt. Ztschr. f. Path. 46:446-452; y. 1934.

H. Kment. Ueber die sogenannte zweizeitige Milzruptur.
Zbl. f. Chir. 57:2176-2178; y. 1930.

D. Kokories. Ueber die Splenektomie bei Kala-Azar.
Münch. Med. Wchnschr. 62:1008-1009; y. 1915.

Kouwer. Behandeling der wandelende Milt door splenopexis.
Neder. Tijdschr. v. Geneeskunde, 31:669-673; y. 1895.

H. Kreckel. Über Abscesse der Milz und ihre Behandlung.
Zeitsch. f. Chir. 54:970-971; y. 1927.

L. P. Kuhn & J. D. Willems. Rupture of spleen with splenectomy.
Intern. Journ. of Med. & Surg. 47:5-8; y. 1934.

W. Langston. Indications and contraindications for splenectomy.
Oklahoma Med. Ass. Journ. 27:319-323; y. 1934.

R. Levy. Zur Operation grosser Milztumoren. Mit einem Beitrag zur chronischen Tuberkulose der Milz.
Arch. f. klin. Chir. 170:180-197; y. 1932.

P. Lombard. Note sur Procédé de Splénectomie. La Splénectomie Sous-Capsulaire.
Bull. et mém. Soc. de chir. de Paris, 47:826-828; y. 1921.

P. Lombard. Note sur l'ablation de la rate anatomiquement adhérente. Le Decollement Spléno-parietal.
Presse Méd. 31:132; y. 1923.

Lucas. A case of splenic hypertrophy.
Med. Times and Gaz. II:605; y. 1882.

G. Lundell. Über spontane Milzruptur.
Acta chir. Scandin. 75:547-569; y. 1934.

E. M. Margorin. Der Plexus lienalis und sein Verbreitungsgebiet beim Menschen.
Ztschr. f. d. ges. Anat. (Abt. I), 97:356-375; y. 1932.

M. Mauro. Contributo allo studio delle cosi dette cisti ematiche della milza.
Ann. ital. di chir. 12:1547-1580; y. 1933.

M. Mauro. La sindrome emorragica tardiva nelle rotture della milza da contusioni.
Ann. ital. di chir. 13:933-950; y. 1934.

W. Mayo. Surgery of the spleen.
Surg. Gyn. & Obst. 16:233-239; y. 1913.

W. Mayo. Surgical considerations of splenectomy.
Ann. of Surg. 62:172; y. 1915.

W. Mayo. Splenectomy in splenic anemia and Banti's disease.
Journ. Am. Med. Ass. 77:34-37; y. 1921.

J. C. McCoy. Splenectomy for rupture of the spleen.
Ann. of Surg. 54:597-611; y. 1911.

A. H. McIndoe. Delayed hemorrhage following traumatic rupture of the spleen.
Brit. Journ. of Surg. 20:249-268; y. 1932.

Monnier. Eine seltene Komplikation der Appendicitis. Ein Fall von Milzabszess.
Schweiz. med. Wchnschr. 61:687-688; y. 1931.

R. Mühsam. Die operative Behandlung des Morbus Gaucher.
Arch. f. klin. Chir. 153:215-234; y. 1928.

R. Mühsam. Indikation und Technik der Milzexstirpation.
Med. Welt, 6:803; 844; y. 1932.

G. Nyström. Beitrag zur Kenntnis der traumatischen Milzrupturen.
Zbl. f. Chir. 44:1055; y. 1917.

G. Oulié. Sur le traitement chirurgical des kystes hydatiques de la rate à propos de huit observations personelles.
Bull. et mém. Soc. nat. de chir. 56:888-893; y. 1930.

G. Oulié. Rate ectopique dans la fosse iliaque droite; torsion du pédicule avec occlusion intestinale.
Annal. d'anat. pathol. 9:85-86; y. 1932.

N. M. Percy. Twisted pedicle of a wandering spleen in a boy ten years of age.
Surg. Clin. of North Amer. 14:971-975; y. 1934.

M. G. Peterman. Congenital absence of spleen and left kidney.
Journ. Am. Med. Ass. 99:1252; y. 1932.

Plücker. Ueber Splenopexis bei Wandermilz.
Zbl. f. Chir. 22:905-907; y. 1895.
(Description of Bardenheuer method).

E. H. Pool. Transfusion and splenectomy for Von Jacksch's anemia.
Ann. of Surg. 61:349-351; y. 1915.

E. H. Pool & R. G. Stillman. Surgery of the spleen.
Appleton & Co., Publishers; y. 1923.

Rydygier. Die Behandlung der Wandermilz durch Splenopexis.
Wien. klin. Wchnschr. 8:431-433; y. 1895.
Also in Arch. f. klin. Chir. 50:880-886; y. 1895.

L. Sabadini. Les kystes hydatiques de la rate: étude anatomoclinique et thérapeutique.
Journ. de chir. 45:534-560; y. 1935.

B. Schiassi. La splénocleisis contre l'anémie splenique et la maladie de Banti.
La Semaine Méd. 26:73-76; y. 1906.

B. Schiassi. Le nuove indicazioni della splenocleisi nel trattamento di taluni patimenti del sangue.
Arch. ital. di chir. 36:489-527; y. 1934.

E. F. Schmid. Zum Problem der zweizeitigen Milzerreissung.
Zbl. f. Chir. 62:857-859; y. 1935.

Schoemaker. Milzexstirpation bei Blutungen aus dem Magen-Darmkanal.
Zbl. f. Chir. 55:2349; y. 1928.

W. Schultz. Therapie und Prognose des Morbus Werlhof.
Deutsch. Med. Wchnschr. 51:1355-1358; y. 1925.

N. W. Schwarz. Zur Diagnostik und operativen Behandlung der Splenomegalie.
Arch. f. klin. Chir. 149:356-369; y. 1928.

V. A. Shaak. Dangers and complications of splenectomy for blood-diseases.
Sovetskaia Khirurgia, 5:280-284; y. 1933.

V. A. Shaak. Errors, hazards and unexpected complications of splenectomy
especially when indicated by various blood-diseases.
Sovet. vrach. gazz. pp. 821-829; y. 1934.

H. R. Shands. Surgical diseases of the spleen.
New Orleans Med. & Surg. Journ. 83:156-159; y. 1930.

L. Silvestrini. Asportazione graduale della milza ipertrofica ed aderente.
Arch. ital. di chir. 24:690-711; y. 1929.

H. Steindl. Das Fassungsvermögen der Milz an Blut nach Unterbindung
der Vena lienalis.
Zbl. f. Chir. 62:197-203; y. 1935.

V. Stubenrauch. Zur Milzchirurgie. Die Ligatur der Arteria Lienalis.
Deutsch. Zeitschr. f. Chir. 172:374-384; y. 1922.

C. A. Traver. Cyst of pancreas associated with ectopic splenic island.
Ann. of Surg. 95:127-133; y. 1932.

M. Trincas. Abscesso acuto della milza.
Annal. ital. di chir. 13:951-970; y. 1934.

A. Troell. Über die Unterbindung der Milzgefässe als Ersatzoperation für
die Splenektomie bei Blutkrankheiten.
Ref. in Zbl. f. Chir. 43:481; y. 1916.

A. Troell. Die Erkrankungen der Milz vom chirurgischen Standpunkt.
Arch. f. klin. Chir. 171:734-743; y. 1932.

Tuffier. Fixation de la rate.
IX Cong. franç. de chir. 9:505-506; y. 1895.

C. C. Ungley. Pernicious anæmia following gastrectomy and splenectomy.
Lancet, II:1426-1427; y. 1932.

P. W. Vestal. What patients are benefited by splenectomy?
Surg Clin. of North America, II:321-328; y. 1931.

R. Vogel. Milzexstirpation bei Blutkrankheiten.
Deutsche Zeitschr. f. Chir. 180:37-106; y. 1923.

A. J. Walton. Indications for and results of removal of the spleen.
Ann. of Surg. 98:379-384; y. 1933.

S. Warren & A. H. Davis. Studies on tumor metastasis; metastases of
carcinoma to the spleen.
Am. Journ. of Cancer. 21:517-533; y. 1934.

P. E. Weil & R. Gregior. Indications opératoires dans les splénomégalies
primitives.
Presse Méd. 35:937-939; y. 1927.

Whipple. Splenectomy as a therapeutic measure in thrombocytopenic purpura hæmorrhagica.
Surg. Gyn. & Obst. 42:329-341; y. 1926.

D. P. D. Wilkie. Splenectomy; its indications and technique.
Am. Journ. of Surg. 14:340-355; y. 1931.

W. D. Wise. Hemostasis during splenectomy.
Ann. of Surg. 99:875; y. 1934.

A. Zell. Milzexstirpation aus vitaler Indikation in einem Fall von hepato-
lienaler Erkrankung.
Zbl. f. Chir. 62:90-94; y. 1935.

S. N. Zhdanovich. Case of volvulus of stomach caused by torsion of dis-
located spleen.
Vestnik Khir. 34:157-158; y. 1934.

CHAPTER XXIII.

SURGERY OF THE PANCREAS.

I. SURGICAL ANATOMY OF THE PANCREAS.

The pancreas is an elongated, narrow viscus, the length of which is from 15 to 26 cm., the width from 4 to 9 cm., and the thickness from 2 to 3 cm. It extends from the second portion of the duodenum nearly to the hilum of the spleen. It is subdivided into four parts: **head, neck, body,** and **tail.**

a. Holotopic Relations.

The pancreas starts in the right hypochondrium, traverses the epigastric region and ends in the left hypochondrium.

b. Skeletotopic Relations.

The head of the pancreas is situated to the right of the first, second and, occasionally, the third lumbar vertebra. **The body** runs in a slightly upward direction across the body of the first lumbar vertebra, and the **tail** ends in the left hypochondrium at the level of the eleventh or twelfth thoracic vertebra.

c. Syntopic Relations.

The pancreas lies between the posterior wall of the stomach in front and the posterior abdominal wall, including the great blood-vessels, behind. It is covered in front by the parietal peritoneum of the posterior abdominal wall. It is separated from the posterior wall of the stomach by the bursa omentalis.

Behind the body of the pancreas lies the solar plexus. This is the reason why the pain in tumor or swelling of the pancreas is almost unbearable.

The blood-supply of the pancreas is derived from one of the terminal branches of the gastro-duodenal branch of the hepatic artery (arteria pancreatico-duodenalis superioris), from the inferior pancreatico-duodenal artery, which is a branch of the superior mesenteric artery, and from small branches of the splenic artery. The veins are tributaries either of the superior mesenteric or of the splenic vein.

The **Wirsung's duct** was described by the German anatomist Wirsung, in 1642, although he did not know its exact purpose. The accessory pancreatic duct, although known as the **duct of Santorini,** was described before him by Graaf and by Haller. The further syntopic relations of the different portions of the pancreas are as follows:

1. The Head.

Behind the head are the right renal artery and vein, the common bile-duct, which quite frequently is incorporated into its substance, the pancreatic duct, the vena cava inferior, the superior mesenteric vein and the abdominal aorta. Some believe that most frequently the portion of the pancreas lying in front of the superior mesenteric vein and artery is the **neck** of the pancreas.

In front of the head are the anastomosis between the superior and inferior pancreatico-duodenal arteries (which runs in the groove between the head and the concavity of the duodenum), and the parietal peritoneum of the posterior abdominal wall. At the upper border of the head, the portal vein, formed by the merging of the splenic and superior mesenteric veins appears. [However, quite often the splenic and the superior mesenteric veins unite below the upper border of the pancreas. In such cases a portion of the portal vein lies behind the pancreas].

2. **The Body.**

The structures lying **behind** the body are the superior mesenteric artery, the splenic vein, the inferior mesenteric vein, and, occasionally, the splenic artery [which in most cases runs in front of the pancreas]. **In front** are the parietal peritoneum of the posterior abdominal wall (which separates it from the anteriorly situated stomach) and, usually, also the splenic artery. On the lower border are the superior mesenteric artery and vein and the duodeno-jejunal junction of the bowel.

3. **Tail.**

Behind this portion of the pancreas are the splenic vein and occasionally the splenic artery, the upper pole of the left kidney and, occasionally, the left renal artery and vein. **In front,** are the parietal peritoneum of the posterior abdominal wall (which separates it from the stomach) and the splenic artery. The tail reaches occasionally as far as the hilum of the spleen.

DIFFERENT ROUTES FOR EXPOSURE OF THE PANCREAS.

The pancreas may be reached either through the anterior or posterior abdominal wall.

A. **Anterior Route.**

This can be accomplished in six different ways:

a.   Through the gastro-hepatic ligament.

b.   Through the anterior and posterior walls of the stomach.

c.   Through the gastro-colic ligament.

d.   Through the transverse mesocolon.

e.   Through the mobilization of the duodenum in order to reach the posterior surface of the head of the pancreas.

f.   Retro-omental.

a.   **Approach through the gastro-hepatic ligament** (Fig. 230).

This route is advisable only in cases in which either there is a marked gastroptosis, or if the pancreas is situated higher than normally. The latter is a rare condition.

b. Through the anterior and posterior gastric walls.

This approach is unusual and not advisable. However, a case is recorded (Hagen) in which this approach was the only one possible.

c. Through the gastro-colic ligament (Figs. 232 and 304).

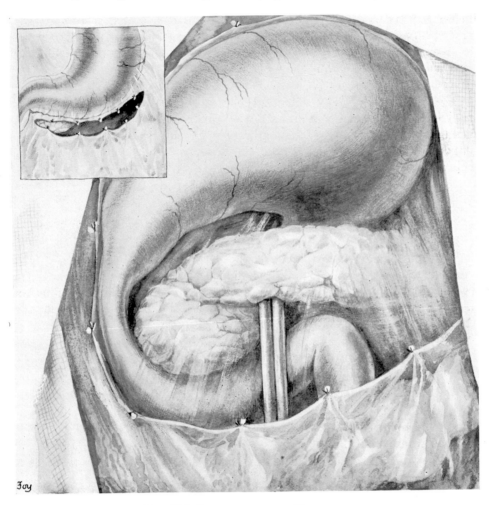

FIG. 304. EXPOSURE OF THE PANCREAS.
The gastrocolic ligament is cut and the stomach is reflected upward.

This is the best approach, and it is employed more frequently than any other.

d. Through the transverse mesocolon (Fig. 201).

This approach is not advisable, particularly if drainage through the anterior abdominal wall is contemplated.

e. Approach through the mobilization of the second portion of the duodenum.

This is an excellent approach to the posterior surface of the head of the pancreas (Fig. 221).

f. Retro-omental route of approach.

The omentum is lifted and put on the stretch. The serosa of the transverse colon is incised along the line of junction with the omentum. A finger is introduced into the opening thus formed, and the bowel is separated bluntly from the omentum. Thus, a large opening is made which exposes the posterior wall of the stomach, the pancreas, and also the third portion of the duodenum.

B. Posterior Route.

This is possible only when surgery of the tail is contemplated. The body of the pancreas is not accessible by this route, since the spinal column lies behind it. This route is not advisable for the head, on account of the important structures lying behind the head, and the poor accessibility of this region.

II.   OPERATIONS FOR ACUTE PANCREATITIS.

If the patient is in a state of profound shock, operation is hardly advisable. However, if there is no shock, then the patient should always be operated upon, and the sooner the better. The aim of the operation is to incise the capsule (so as to relieve the intracapsular pressure and to prevent any further compression of the blood-vessels, and thus increase the resistance of the gland), and to prevent the escape of exudate into the free peritoneal cavity by "walling off" the gland from the rest of this cavity. The operation then is as follows:

Step 1. The abdomen is opened by a midline incision extending from the ensiform process down to the umbilicus.

Step 2. The gastrocolic ligament is cut (as described in Chapter VIII), and the stomach is turned upward, thereby exposing the pancreas.

Step 3. The lesser peritoneal cavity is packed with rolls of gauze, which surround the pancreas, and the ends of which are brought outside the abdominal cavity.

Step 4. The capsule of the pancreas is incised in several places **in a direction parallel** to the pancreatic ducts, and a gauze-drain is placed over the incised capsule.

Step 5. Cholecystostomy is done (or choledochostomy, if the cystic duct is blocked by a stone).

Cholecystostomy is just as an important step of the operation as the others, since the external drainage of bile will prevent it from running into Wirsung's duct and reinfecting the pancreas, which is the most important etiological factor in producing pancreatitis. **No attempt should be made at this stage to do any radical biliary surgery. This should be deferred to some future time when the condition of the patient is improved.**

III. OPERATIONS FOR CHRONIC PANCREATITIS.

The most commonly used procedure consists of cholecystectomy, after which the sphincter of Oddi becomes paralyzed and does not offer any resistance to the passage of bile into the duodenum. [Of course, it is understood that before closing the abdomen the surgeon should be certain that no stones are left in the common bile-duct.] The next most common method employed consists in making numerous incisions in the pancreatic capsule alone, or even of cutting into the parenchyma of the pancreas in order to diminish the intracapsular pressure. However, many surgeons, quite justly, are opposed to cutting the pancreatic substance for fear of a possible hemorrhage, and are content with cutting the capsule alone. Next in frequency is drainage of the bile, **externally** by a cholecystostomy, or **internally** by cholecysto-gastrostomy or cholecysto-enterostomy. **We believe that the safest of all procedures is to produce internal drainage of bile by means of a cholecysto-gastrostomy.**

IV. OPERATIONS FOR STONES IN THE PANCREATIC DUCT. (Fig. 305).

The occurrence of stones in the pancreatic duct was recorded by Graaf, in 1667, when he mentioned the observations of Panarol and Gæia. Bonetus, in 1700, Galeati, in 1757, Morgagni, in 1765, Greding, in 1769, and Cowley, in 1788, reported cases in which pancreatic stones were found. Cowley's case is the first of pancreatic stones published in England. However, these cases are very infrequent. Johnston, in 1883, was able to collect from the literature only 35 cases of pancreatic stones, and Giudiceandrea, in 1896, only 48 cases. However, Opitz, in 1901, was able to collect 97 cases of pancreatic stones. This number includes all the cases found in operation and on the dissecting-table. Guleke, in 1924, was able to collect 25 cases in which operation had been performed, and Schmieden, in 1927, twenty cases more, thus making a total of 45 cases up to the year 1927.

The stones, which were found, were most frequently single. However, two, three or more stones have been found, and a case is reported in which 54 stones were found. The size of the stone varies from a grain of sand to $2\frac{1}{2}$ inches by half-an-inch (case of Schupman). In Matani's case, the weight of the stone was two ounces. Most frequently the stones are met with in the head, then in the body, and finally in the tail.

The presence of pancreatic stones is associated with changes in the pancreatic tissue, such as cystic degeneration and acute and chronic pancreatitis. Whether the stones are the cause or sequela of these changes or just a concomitant manifestation is unsettled.

Treatment.

This is surgical only. The prognosis of cases of untreated stones is bad, whereas, if they are removed it is excellent. The approach depends on whether the stones are in the head, body or tail of the pancreas. If the stone is located in the head (and this is true in the majority of cases), then the approach is either transduodenal or retroduodenal. If, however, the stone is located in the body or in the tail, the approach is made either by cutting the gastrocolic ligament, or, less frequently, by cutting the gastro-hepatic ligament, thus exposing the pancreas, and then cutting through the pancreatic tissue and the duct. **We should never fail after opening the duct to probe it in order to ascertain whether all the stones have been removed.**

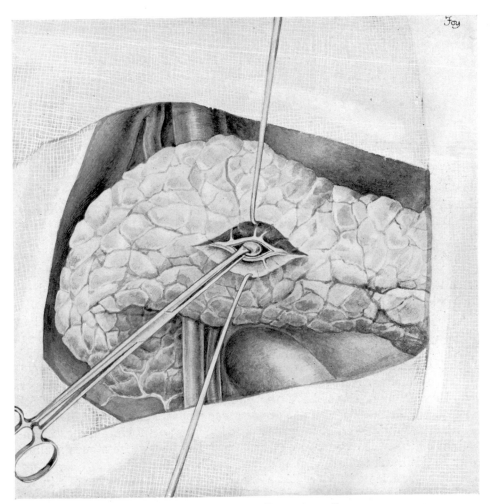

FIG. 305. REMOVAL OF A PANCREATIC STONE.

Before the pancreatic tissue is cut, the line of intended incision is surrounded by gauze the ends of which are brought outside the abdominal cavity. The gland and the duct are opened, the stone removed, the gland with the duct resutured, and the gauze-drain left for several days. Moynihan was the first who made a transduodenal extraction of a stone after a preliminary correct diagnosis.

V. OPERATIONS FOR PANCREATIC CYSTS.

Kőrte divides all varieties of cysts into the following sub-groups:

1. Retention cysts;
2. Proliferation cysts;
3. Degeneration cysts;
4. Pseudo-cysts;
5. Echinococcus cysts.

The common site of pancreatic cysts is shown in Figs. 306 and 307.

Three methods of treatment are used:

a. Incision and drainage of the cyst-cavity.

b. Extirpation of the cyst.

c. Partial removal of the cyst and implantation of its remnants into the stomach, duodenum, or gall-bladder.

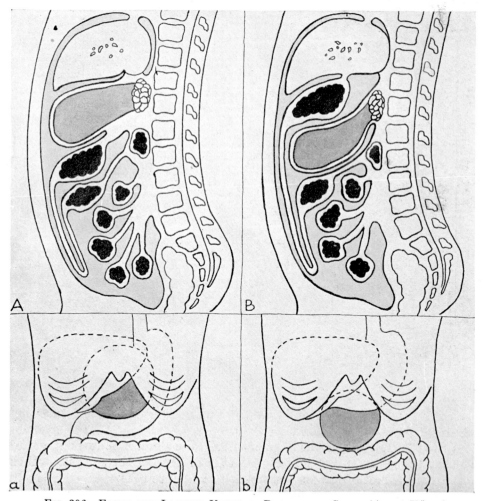

FIG. 306. FRONT AND LATERAL VIEWS OF PANCREATIC CYSTS (AFTER KŐRTE).

a. INCISION AND DRAINAGE OF THE CYST-CAVITY.

This is done by the majority of surgeons as a one-stage operation, although some surgeons perform it by the two-stage technic.

Technic.

Step 1. The abdomen is opened by a midline incision extending from the ensiform process to the umbilicus.

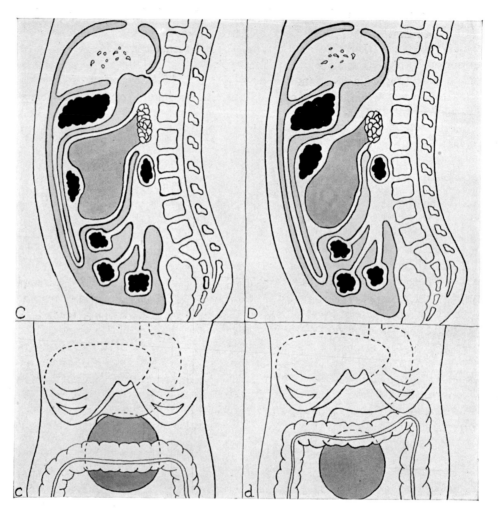

FIG. 307. FRONT AND LATERAL VIEWS OF PANCREATIC CYSTS (AFTER KŐRTE).

Step 2. The gastrocolic ligament is cut, the stomach is turned upward so that the pancreas is well exposed (Fig. 304), and the cyst is "walled off" from the rest of the peritoneal cavity by gauze rolls.

Step 3. A needle is thrust into the cystic cavity and the fluid is aspirated. Then the opening is enlarged and the cavity is immediately packed with gauze the ends of which are brought outside the abdominal cavity.

Step 4. The gauze surrounding the pancreas is removed. The wall of the pancreatic cyst is sutured to the parietal peritoneum of the anterior abdominal wall (marsupialization of the cyst).

This is a good method for all types of cysts except the malignant variety of adenocystoma, which should be treated by extirpation only.

b. EXTIRPATION OF THE CYST.

This method is technically difficult, since the wall of the cyst is usually strongly adherent to the pancreatic tissue and is surrounded by numerous blood-vessels. For this reason, this method should be employed only for the malignant type of cysts.

In the early days of surgery of the pancreas some treated the cysts by aspirating its contents by a trocar passed through the cyst. **This should never be employed, since it is dangerous and the results are very unsatisfactory.**

The results of treatment of cysts by excision and drainage or by extirpation are good. A cure follows in more than ninety per cent.

c. IMPLANTATION OF THE REMNANT OF THE CYST INTO THE DUODENUM, STOMACH OR GALL-BLADDER (PANCREATO-DUODENOSTOMY; PANCREATO-GASTROSTOMY; PANCREATO-CHOLECYSTOSTOMY).

In order to prevent the occurrence of a pancreatic fistula in cases in which the cyst cannot be entirely removed, R. Jedlicka, in 1921, advised implanting the remnant of the cyst connected with the pancreas into the posterior wall of the stomach. He suggested doing this not as a **secondary** operation, when a fistula is already formed, **but as one of the steps of the primary operation.** As a secondary operation it was used many years previously by Kehr and Michon. Moreover, the implantation of the remnant of the cyst into the duodenum as a primary operation was performed much earlier than was done by Jedlicka, namely by Ombrédanne, in 1911. Hammesfahr, in 1923, implanted the remnants of the pancreatic cyst into the gall-bladder.

VI. OPERATIONS FOR INJURY OF THE PANCREAS (FIG. 308).

An exploratory abdominal section for injuries of the upper abdomen is not complete unless the pancreas is examined. Time and again cases have been reported in which injury to other organs have been repaired, in which the patient died soon afterward, and autopsy showed a torn or badly damaged pancreas. The danger in pancreatic injuries lies in hemorrhage and in the escape of pancreatic juice.

Technic.

Step 1. The abdomen is opened by a midline incision extending from the ensiform process down to the umbilicus.

Step 2. The gastro-hepatic ligament is opened for inspection of the pancreas. If it is found to be injured it should immediately be packed around with gauze, the ends of which are brought outside. [If there is not a good exposure through this ligament, then the gastrocolic ligament should be cut and the stomach reflected upward. This will insure an excellent exposure.]

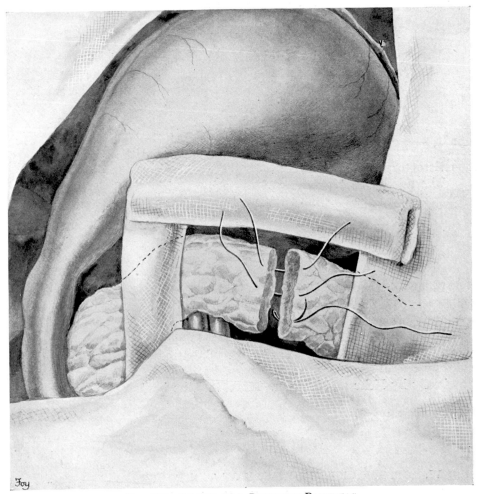

FIG. 308. SUTURE OF A RUPTURED PANCREAS.

Step 3. A heavy catgut-suture penetrates the thickness of the pancreatic tissues and of the capsule on each side of the pancreatic wound. The ends are tied and cut short. This will arrest profuse hemorrhage. If the length of the torn portion is considerable, two or three such deep sutures are inserted. If necessary, a few superficial sutures of fine catgut may be inserted between the deeper sutures. This will stop the superficial hemorrhage.

In placing the deep sutures care should be taken not to injure or to occlude Wirsung's or the Santorini's pancreatic duct.

Step 4. A rubber drain (wrapped with gauze) is laid over the sutured portion of the pancreas and its free end is brought outside the abdominal cavity through the abdominal incision. Some surgeons close the anterior abdominal wall and prefer to drain the pancreas through a posterior incision.

VII.   OPERATIONS FOR PANCREATIC TUMORS.

Pancreatic tumors are subdivided into:

> A.   Benign tumors.
> B.   Malignant tumors.

A.   Benign Tumors.

The benign type was formerly considered as an extremely rare variety. Haberer, up to 1927, was able to collect from the literature only ten cases, which were either fibroma, fibro-adenoma or cystadenoma. However, during the last few years several cases have been reported. These are of particular interest, since some were associated with symptoms of hyper-insulinism. The treatment consists in their removal. The operative risk is small. They usually give one complication, namely a pancreatic fistula of long standing.

B.   Malignant Tumors.

Malignant tumors are most commonly encountered among the tumors of the pancreas. They are most frequently located in the head (60%), then almost as frequently in the body as in the tail (about 8 per cent. in each variety). They occur as a generalized growth involving the entire pancreas in 24 per cent.

The incidence of cancer of the pancreas is approximately two per cent. of the entire number of cancer cases met in the human.

Treatment.

This is:

> a.   Palliative.
> b.   Radical.

a.   Palliative Treatment.

This consists in relieving the obstruction of the bile-flow by performing some kind of side-tracking operation, such as cholecysto-gastrostomy or cholecysto-enterostomy. [Cholecystostomy is not advisable, since it will permanently drain the bile outside the body.] Although it is only a palliative procedure, nevertheless it is advisable to perform it, since it relieves such symptoms as itching, which greatly aggravates the suffering of the patient.

b.   Radical Treatment.

This consists in removing the tumor with the surrounding portion of the pancreas, or in the performance of a partial or subtotal pancreatectomy with or without the removal of the second and third portions of the duodenum. In the case of carcinoma of the tail or of the body, partial pancreatectomy is feasible, whereas in the case of carcinoma of the head the operation is extremely difficult [since it is necessary, in order to remove the head of the pancreas, to remove the second and part of the third portion of the duodenum, to cut the common bile-duct, the pancreatic and the accessory pancreatic ducts, to perform gastro-jejunostomy, to implant the bile-duct and the pancreatic ducts into the bowel with the possible dangers resulting from leakage of biliary, intestinal and pancreatic juices.] However, several cases of nearly total (subtotal) pancreatectomy have been reported, which shows that as difficult as the technic is, it is still possible, and that a very small portion of the pancreas will produce enough external and internal secretion to satisfy the needs of the body.

During the last few years several cases of adenoma of the islands of Langerhans have been reported, which have been clinically manifested by symptoms of hyperinsulinism. Removal of the adenoma with a small portion of the surrounding tissue in some cases alleviated, and in others entirely cured, the condition.

TECHNIC OF PANCREO-DUODENECTOMY

Step 1. The abdomen is opened by a midline incision.

Step 2. Mobilization of the duodenum by the Kocher method, with the difference only that the separation of the duodenum from behind is continued until this bowel is detached from the vena cava and the superior mesenteric vessels are reached.

Step 3. Ligation of the right gastric and of the gastroduodenal arteries and also of the gastrocolic ligament.

Step 4. The pylorus is cut between two clamps and the pyloric end of the stomach is closed. The common bile-duct is divided **close** to the pancreas, if we wish to use this duct for reëstablishing the communication between the biliary and the intestinal passages, and **far away** from the pancreas if the gall-bladder is used for this purpose.

Step 5. The duodenum is now attached only to the upper leaflet of the transverse mesocolon from which it must now be carefully separated. Then the duodenum is carefully and gently separated from the superior mesenteric artery and vein, which lie in front of the duodenum between the pars uncinatum of the pancreas and the duodeno-jejunal junction.

Step 6. The duodenum is cut at the duodeno-jejunal junction between two clamps placed immediately to the left of the superior mesenteric vessels.

Step 7. The pancreas is cut between two clamps. The duodenum and the head of the pancreas are thus entirely free and are removed from the abdomen.

Step 8. The common bile-duct is implanted into the stomach or jejunum.

Step 9. The hemorrhage from the cut surface of the pancreas is checked by sutures. Wirsung's duct is separated from the pancreatic tissue for at least 2 to 3 cm., and is then implanted into the duodeno-jejunal junction. If it is impossible to implant it separately, then the entire stump of the pancreas is invaginated into the duodeno-jejunal opening. Otherwise, the open duodeno-jejunal end is closed.

Step 10. Posterior gastro-jejunostomy is performed.

Due to the magnitude of this operation it is best to perform it in two or even in three stages.

In case of a three-stage method, the steps of the operation are:

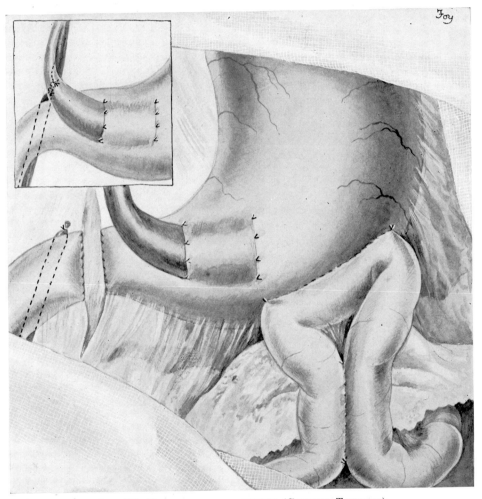

FIG. 309. PANCREO-DUODENECTOMY (SPIVACK TECHNIC).

INSERT. Subserous cholecystogastrostomy was done; the common bile-duct is cut and two ends of it are ligated.

MAIN PICTURE. Anterior gastroenterostomy with entero-anastomosis is made. Pyloro-duodenal junction is cut and two ends closed.

SPIVACK TECHNIC.

Stage 1.

Step 1. The abdomen is opened by a transverse bilateral transrectus incision at a level of one inch above the umbilicus, and this is supplemented by an oblique incision in the right upper quadrant.

Step 2. A subserous cholecysto-gastrostomy is performed in the manner described above (Figs. 274, 275, 276). The supra-duodenal portion of the common bile-duct is ligated just above the duodenum and cut between the ligatures (Fig. 309). The abdomen is closed.

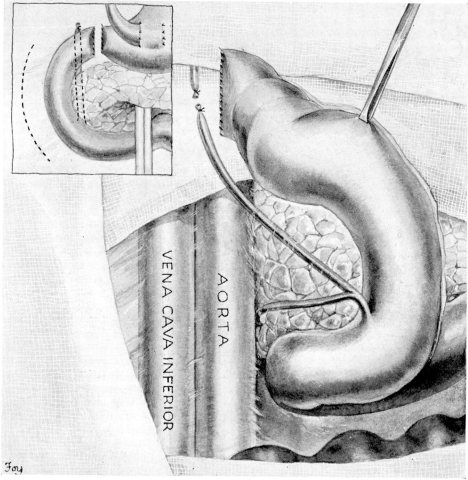

FIG. 310. PANCREO-DUODENECTOMY (SPIVACK TECHNIC).
INSERT. Mobilization of the second portion of the duodenum.
MAIN PICTURE. The second portion of the duodenum is reflected.

One week later, the second stage is performed.

Stage II.

Step 1. The abdomen is reopened.

Step 2. The right gastric and the right gastro-epiploic arteries are ligated in the manner already described.

Step 3. The pyloro-duodenal junction is cut. The duodental and the stomach ends are closed (Fig. 309). An anterior gastro-jejunostomy is performed, supplemented by an entero-anastomosis (Fig. 309).

One week later, the third stage is performed.

Stage III.

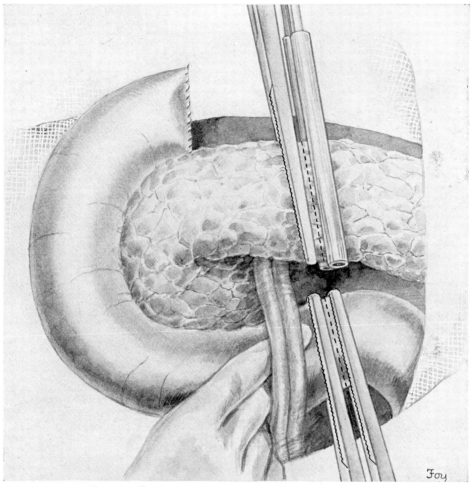

FIG. 311. PANCREO-DUODENECTOMY (SPIVACK TECHNIC).
The duodenum is separated from the superior mesenteric vessels; the third portion of the duodenum is clamped by a pair of arterial forceps and the duodenum is cut between them. The body of the pancreas is clamped by two intestinal clamps and the pancreas is cut between them.

Step 1. The abdomen is reopened.

Step 2. The gastrocolic ligament is divided and the colon transversus drawn downward. The duodenum is mobilized by the Kocher method. However, this mobilization affects not only the second portion but also the third portion of the duodenum, that is, it reaches the duodeno-jejunal junction (Fig. 310). The duodenum should be carefully separated from the superior mesenteric artery and vein, which lie in front of the duodenum between the pars uncinatum of the pancreas and the duodeno-jejunal junction.

Step 3. The duodenum is cut at the duodeno-jejunal junction between two crushing-clamps.

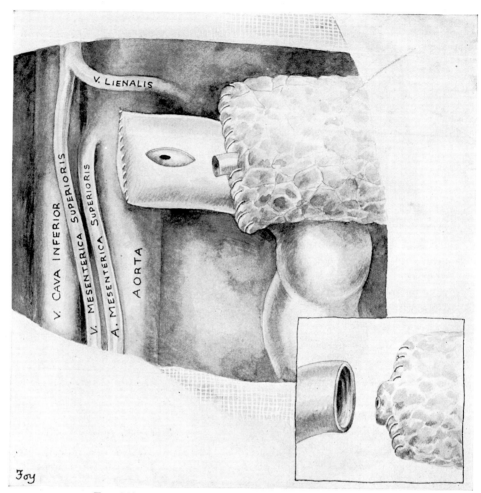

FIG. 312. PANCREO-DUODENECTOMY (SPIVACK TECHNIC).
MAIN PICTURE. Implantation of the pancreatic duct into the wall of the third portion of the duodenum.
INSERT. Alternate method of inserting the stump of the remaining portion of the pancreas into the third portion of the duodenum.

Step 4. The pancreas is cut between two clamps (Fig. 311). Thus, the duodenum and the head of the pancreas are entirely separated from the other abdominal viscera.

Step 5. The hemorrhage from the cut surface of the pancreas is checked by sutures. Wirsung's duct is separated from the pancreatic tissue for at least 2 or 3 cm. and is then **subserously** implanted into the jejunum close to the point of the former duodeno-jejunal junction (Fig. 312). However, if it is impossible to isolate Wirsung's duct or to implant the isolated duct, then the entire stump of the pancreas is invaginated into the duodeno-jejunal opening, which up to this time was not sutured (Fig. 312, insert).

Step 6. The clamped end of the jejunum at the duodeno-jejunal junction is now closed (unless it was closed already in Step 5).

Step 7. The abdomen is closed.

BIBLIOGRAPHY.

F. D. Ackman & A. Ross. Pancreatic lithiasis.
Surg. Gyn. & Obst. 55:90-95; y. 1932.

E. W. Archibald & M. Kaufmann. Surgical diseases of the pancreas.
In Dean Lewis "Practice of Surgery", 7:1-65; y. 1932.

N. Berglund. Fälle traumatischer subcutaner isolierter Pancreasruptur.
Acta chir. Scandinav. 70:287-298; y. 1931.

F. Bernhard. Die Beziehungen zwischen den Erkrankungen der Gallenwege und dem Auftreten der akuten Pankreasnekrose und Beobachtungen über die diagnostischen Hilfsmittel zur Erkennung der akuten Pankreasveränderungen.
Deutsche Zeitschr. f. Chir. 231:1-30; y. 1931.

K. Blond. Ueber Duodenektomie und eine neue Methode zur Transplantation des Ductus choledochus und pancreaticus.
Arch. f. klin. Chir. 156:736-757; y. 1930.

A. Bodart. Modes de production et evolution des fistules pancreatiques.
Arch. franco-belges de chir. 32:545-575; y. 1930.

Brugeas. Pancréatite œdemateuse.
Bull. et mém. Soc. nat. de chir. 58:1365-1367; y. 1932.

A. Ceballos. Elección de método en el tratamiento de las úlceras del estómago y del duodeno penetrantes en el páncreas.
Bol. y trab. de la Soc. de cir. de Buenos Aires, 17:881-893; y. 1933.

B. Chlyvitch. Trajet prépancréatique anormal du cholédoque (Contribution au développement exceptionnel d'un pancreas humain).
Ann. d'anat. path. 9:1047-1053; y. 1932.

J. Cottalorda & Escarras. Epithelioma langerhansien. Extirpation, guérison.
Lyon chir. 30:248-253; y. 1933.

G. H. Cowen. Case of subcutaneous injury of the pancreas: Operation: Recovery.
Brit. Med. Journ. I:1048-1049; y. 1907.

D. Dedes. Ueber einen Fall von Pankreasechinococcus.
Zbl. f. Chir. 60:698-700; y. 1933.

A. Desjardins. Technique de la Pancréatectomie.
Rev. de Chir. 35:945-973; y. 1907.

B. Desplas. Formes cliniques des pancréatites aiguës chirurgicales.
Journ. de méd. et chir. prat. 103:809-822; y. 1932.

L. R. Dragstedt, H. E. Haymond & J. C. Ellis. Pathogenesis of acute
pancreatitis (acute pancreatic necrosis).
Arch. of Surg. 28:232-291; y. 1934.

C. E. Farr. Aberrant pancreas.
Surg. Clin. of North Amer. 10:483-488; y. 1930.

F. Felsenreich. Klinik der akuten und subakuten Pankreasnekrose.
Arch. f. klin. Chir. 168:307-348; y. 1931.

J. Finney. Resection of the pancreas.
Ann. of Surg. 51:818-829; y. 1910.

J. Finney & J. Finney Jr. Resection of the pancreas.
Ann. of Surg. 88:584-592; y. 1928.

J. Finney Pancreatic emergencies.
Ann. of Surg. 98: 750-759; y. 1933.

R. D. Forbes. Abdominal signs in acute pancreatic disease.
West. Journ. of Surg. 40:425-428; y. 1932.

F. Franke. Ueber die Exstirpation der Krebsigen Bauchspeicheldrüse.
Arch. f. klin. Chir. 64:364-392; y. 1901.

J. Friedenwald & T. S. Cullen. Carcinoma of the pancreas: Clinical observations.
Amer. Journ of Med. Science, 176:31-41; y. 1928.

I. M. Gage. Surgical diseases of pancreas.
New Orleans Med. & Surg. Journ. 82:795-805; y. 1930.

R. W. Garis & W. C. Merkel. Symptom-complex of complete external pancreatic fistula; report of a case.
Surg. Gyn. & Obst. 59:590-597; y. 1934.

C. Garré. Totaler Querriss des Pankreas durch Naht geheilt.
Bruns Beiträge zur klin. Chir. 46:233-240; y. 1905.

E. Gold. Spätergebnisse nach Pankreatozystanastomosen.
Mitt. a. d. Grenzgeb. d. Med. u. Chir. 43:591-598; y. 1934.

G. Gordon-Taylor. The radical surgery of cancer of the pancreas.
Ann. of Surg. 100:206-214; y. 1934.

E. A. Graham & N. A. Womack. Application of surgery to hypoglycæmic
state due to islet tumors of pancreas and to other conditions.
Surg. Gyn. & Obst. 56:728-742; y. 1933.

E. Graham & A. F. Hartmann. Subtotal resection of the pancreas for hypoglycemia.
Surg. Gyn. Obst. 59:474-479; y. 1934.

I. I. Grekow. Surgery of the pancreas. The diagnosis and treatment of primary carcinoma of the pancreas, particularly of the body and tail of the gland.
Abstract in Surg. Gyn. & Obst. 36:327; y. 1923.

O. Gross & N. Guleke. Die Erkrankungen des Pancreas.
Julius Springer, Publishers, Berlin, y. 1924.

N. Guleke. Die neueren Ergebnisse in der Lehre der akuten und chronischen Erkrankungen des Pancreas, mit besonderer Berücksichtigung der entzündlichen Veränderungen.
Ergebn. d. Chir. u. Orthop. 4:408-507; y. 1912.

F. B. Hagen. Zur operativen Behandlung der Pankreas-Cysten.
Arch. f. klin. Chir. 62:157-178; y. 1900.

C. Hammesfahr. Zur Behandlung von Pancreasfisteln.
Zbl. f. Chir. 50:1758-1760; y. 1923.

S. Harris. Hyperinsulinism and dysinsulinism.
Journ. Am. Med. Ass. 83:729-733; y. 1924.

G. Hartlieb. Neuere Arbeiten über die operative Behandlung der akuten Pankreasnekrose bzw. akuten Pankreatitis.
Bruns Beitr. z. klin. Chir. 157:539-557; y. 1933.

H. H. Haynes. A new surgical procedure for acute pancreatitis.
Arch. Surg. 26:288-294; y. 1933.

N. v. Hedry. Beitrag zur Klinik der Accessorischen Pankreas.
Bruns Beitr. z. klin. Chir. 130:349-352; y. 1924.

E. Heller. Fortschritte der Pankreaschirurgie.
Zbl. f. Chir. 57:1667-1685; y. 1930.

L. G. Heyn. Hyperinsulinism.
Journ. Amer. Med. Ass. 98:1441-1443; y. 1932.

E. Holman. Partial pancreatectomy for hyperinsulinism.
Surg. Clin. North Amer. 13:71-76; y. 1933.

E. Holman & O. C. Railsback. Partial pancreatectomy in chronic spontaneous hypoglycæmia, with review of cases of hypoglycæmia surgically treated.
Surg. Gyn. & Obst. 56:591-600; y. 1933.

R. Holzapfel. Die Mündung von Gallen- und Pankreasgang bei Menschen.
Anat. Anz. 69:449-453; y. 1930.

G. Howland, W. R. Campbell, E. J. Maltby & W. L. Robinson. Dysinsulinism. Convulsions and coma due to islet cell tumor of the pancreas with operation and cure.
Journ. Amer. Med. Ass. 93:674-679; y. 1929.

N. J. Howard. Annular pancreas.
   Surg. Gyn. & Obst. 50:533-540; y. 1930.

N. L. Isnardi & J. Zanardo. Tratamiento de una fístula pancreática. Su abocamiento gástrico: consideraciones.
   La Seman. Med. 32:1166-1169; y. 1925.

R. M. Janes. Pancreatic fistula; report of a case cured by pancreato-gastrostomy.
   Brit. Journ. of Surg. 22:296-300; y. 1934.

R. Jedlicka. Eine neue Operationsmethode der Pankreascysten (Pancreato-gastrostomie).
   Abstr. in Zbl. f. Chir. 50:132; y. 1923.

E. S. Judd & F. N. Allan & E. H. Rynearson. Hyperinsulinism. Its surgical treatment.
   Journ. Amer. Med. Ass. 101:99-102; y. 1933.

A. Jung & J. Henriet. Traitement d'une fistule pancréatique par implantation du trajet fistuleux dans l'intestin.
   Rev. de chir. 53:804-806; y. 1934.

A. Jurasz. Zur Frage der operativen Behandlung der Pankreascysten.
   Arch. f. klin. Chir. 164:272-279; y. 1931.

W. Kausch. Das Carcinom der Papilla duodeni und seine radikale Entfernung.
   Bruns Beitr. z. klin. Chir. 78:439-486; y. 1912.

O. Kleinschmidt. Die Behandlung der Fisteln des Pankreas und des Ductus pancreaticus.
   Arch f. klin. Chir. 135:363-372; y. 1925.

W. Kőrte. Die Chirurgischen Krankheiten und die Verletzungen des Pancreas.
   Deutsch. Chirurgie, Lief. 45d, y. 1898.   F. Enke, Publishers, Stuttgart.

G. E. Konjetzny. Pankreasfistel nach Magenresektion und ihre Behandlung.
   Zbl. f. Chir. 60:2375-2377; y. 1933.

M. Krabbel. Operative Heilung der chronischen interstitiellen Pankreatitis.
   Bruns Beitr. z. klin. Chir. 151:672-676; y. 1931.

F. Krause. Hyperinsulinismus mit hypoglykämischen Symptomenkomplex.
   Klinisch. Wchnschr. 9:2346-2349; y. 1930.

K. Laqua. Experimentelle Untersuchungen über die vollkommene äussere Pankreasdauerfistel.
   Bruns Beitr. z. klin. Chir. 150:507-516; y. 1930.

A. Lefort. Kyste de la tête du Pancreas. Ablation. Guérison.
   Bull. et mém. Soc. de chirurg. de Paris, 24:363-372; y. 1932.

A. Lehrnbecher. Ueber isolierte subkutane Pankreasruptur.
   Bruns Beitr. z. klin. Chir. 132:560-569; y. 1924.

R. Leriche. Pancréatotomie pour pancréatite scléreuse de la tête non suppurée sans ictère. Résultat au bout de vingt ans.
Lyon Chir. 31:306-312; y. 1934.

G. Loewy. Dérivation totale du sac pancréatique par anastomose pancréatico-urétérale.
Compt. rend. Soc. de biol. III:583-585; y. 1932.

G. Mansfeld. Versuche zu einer operativen Behandlung des Diabetes.
Klin. Wchnschr. 6:195-198; y. 1927.

P. Mariconda. Calcolosi pancreatica generalizzata del dutto di Wirsung e delle sue diramazioni.
Policlinico (sez. med.), 42:37-42; y. 1935.

H. E. Marsh. Hyperinsulinism with report of a case.
Wiscon. Med. Journ. 30:339-343; y. 1931.

A. Mayo Robson. The pathology and surgery of certain diseases of the pancreas.
Lancet, I:911-916; y. 1904.

J. B. McNaught. Annular pancreas; a compilation of forty cases, with report of a new case.
Am. Journ. of Med. Science, 185:249-260; y. 1933.

E. Melchior. Beiträge zur chirurgischen Duodenalpathologie.
Arch. f. klin. Chir. 128:1-19; y. 1924.

Mikulicz. Surgery of the pancreas.
Annals of Surg. 38:1-29; y. 1903.

H. Mondor, P. Gauthier-Villars & A. Sicard. Sarcome du pancréas.
Presse méd. 41:1201-1205; y. 1933.

B. Moynihan. Some cases of chronic pancreatitis.
Lancet, II:856-859; y. 1902.

B. Moynihan. Abdominal operations. 4th Ed. y. 1926.

C. D. Muspratt. Acute haemorrhagic pancreatitis: Operation: Recovery.
Brit. Med. Journ. I:304; y. 1904.

H. Nicolaus. Akute Pankreatitis, ihre Behandlung und Dauererfolge.
Bruns Beitr. z. klin. Chir. 152:351-368; y. 1931.

F. Ody. La transfixion abdomino-lombaire dans la pancréatite aiguë.
Presse méd. 38:1628-1630; y. 1930.

Ombrédanne. Sur les kystes du pancréas.
Bull. et mém. de la Soc. de Chir. de Paris, 37:977-983; y. 1911.

Ch. Perrier. Pseudo-kyste traumatique du Pancreas. Marsupialisation. Guérison.
Bull. et mém. de la Soc. de Chirurg. de Paris. 24:483-489; y. 1932.

I. Philipowicz. Radikaloperation eines Duodenalgeschwürs mit Resektion des Pankreas und der Papille.
Zbl. f. Chir. 60:2188-2189; y. 1933.

A. W. Phillips. Hypoglycemia associated with hypertrophy of the islands of Langerhans.
Journ. Americ. Med. Ass. 96:1195-1198; y. 1931.

L. Pollak. Symptomatologie der Pankreaserkrankungen.
Wien. med. Wchnschr. 80:334-340; y. 1930.

H. L. Popper. Die paravertebrale Nervenausschaltung bei Pankreatitis.
Wien. klin. Wchnschr. 44:998-999; y. 1931.

H. K. Ransom. Carcinoma of the body and tail of the pancreas.
Arch. of Surg. 30:584-606; y. 1935.

W. F. Reinhoff Jr. & Dean Lewis. Surgical affections of the pancreas met with in the Johns Hopkins Hospital from 1889 to 1932, including a report of a case of an adenoma of the islands of Langerhans, and a case of pancreatolithiasis.
Bull. of Johns Hopkins Hospital, 54:386-429; y. 1934.

L. I. Ross & J. M. Tomasch. Hyperinsulinemia secondary to adenoma of the pancreas; report of a case with operative cure.
Arch. of Surg. 28:223-231; y. 1934.

P. Santy, P. Mallet-Guy & V. Pasquier. Du traitement des pancréatites chroniques avec ictère; le drainage transvésiculaire du choledoque.
Rev. de Chir. 68:85-104; y. 1930.

P. J. Sarma. Surgical exposure of the pancreas.
Am. Journ. of Surg. 21:390-392; y. 1933.

L. Sauvé. Des pancréatectomies et specialment de la pancréatectomie cephalique.
Rev. de Chir. 37:113-152 and 335-386; y. 1908.

G. Scherk. Diagnostische Schwierigkeiten bei Erkrankungen der Bauchorgane. Cholelithiasis und akute Pankreatitis.
Med. Klin. 26:1564-1565; y. 1930.

V. Schmieden & W. Sebening. Chirurgie des Pankreas.
Arch. f. klin. Chir. 148:319-387; y. 1927.

S. J. Seeger. Pancreatic lithiasis.
Surg. Gyn. & Obst. 40:841-846; y. 1925.

S. N. Sennett. Pancreatic lithiasis.
Brit. Med. Journ. II:3-5; y. 1933.

S. Simkins. Variations in pancreatic ducts and minor duodenal papilla.
Amer. Journ. of Med. Sc. 182:626-639; y. 1931.

W. E. Sistrunk. The surgical removal of pancreatic stones.
Ann. of Surg. 74:380-385; y. 1921.

F. Smoler. Schlauchüberbrückung bei operativem Defekt des Ductus Wirsungianus.
Zbl. f. Chir. 59:413-415; y. 1932.

F. Stein. Ueber einen wenig beachteten Weg der Pancreas freilegung bei akuter Pankreatitis.
Zbl. f. Chir. 53:2844-2850; y. 1926.

A. Steinbock. Subcutaneous rupture of the pancreas.
Duodecim, 50:467-489; y. 1934.

H. Stocker. Ein Beitrag zur Statistik und Klinik der akuten Pankreasnekrosen.
Arch. f. klin. Chir. 156:84-95; y. 1929.

E. Streissler. Zur chirurgischen Behandlung der akuten Pankreatitis von rückwärts.
Arch. f. klin. Chir. 131:327-357; y. 1924.

G. de Takats. Chirurgische Massnahmen zur Hebung der Zuckertoleranz.
Klin. Wochenschr. 12:623-625; y. 1933.

G. de Tarnowsky & P. J. Sarma. Surgical treatment of chronic pancreatitis.
Ann. of Surg. 101:1342-1352; y. 1935.

W. Thalhimer & F. D. Murphy. Carcinoma of the islands of the pancreas.
Journ. Americ. Med. Ass. 91:89-91; y. 1928.

E. Thoenes. Multiple Venenthrombosen, ein bisher unbekannten Frühsymptom bei Pankreaskarzinomen.
Műnch. med. Wchnschr. 79:1677-1678; y. 1932.

G. Thomason. Hyperinsulinism, hypoglycemia, subtotal pancreatectomy.
West. Journ. of Surg. 43:185-192; y. 1935.

L. Ugelli. I pancreas accessori e loro importanza chirurgica.
Policlinico (sez. chir.), 41:424-452; y. 1934.

G. Vecchi. Innere Drainage einer grossen Pankreaszyste mittels Pankreatogastrostomie.
Wien. klin. Wchnschr. 48:45-48; y. 1935.

C. S. Venable. Rupture of the pancreas.
Surg. Gyn. & Obst. 56:652-658; y. 1932.

F. Wohlwill. Ulcus pylori und akzessorischer Pankreaskeim.
Klin. Wchnschr. 8:2137-2138; y. 1929.

E. Wolff. Pankreascysten und pseudocysten.
Bruns Beitr. z. klin. Chir. 74:487-514; y. 1911.

A. Yódice. Estudio anátomo-quirúrgico del duodeno y conductos pancreáticos en relación con la cirugía del estómago, páncreas, duodeno y vías biliares, basado en 70 disecciones.
Bol. y trab. de la Soc. de cir. de Buenos Aires. 16:1477-1480; y. 1932.

W. Zahn. Pankreasfistel und pathologische Funktion des Pankreas.
Zbl. f. Chir. 59:328-335; y. 1932.

PART V.

CHAPTER XXIV.

HERNIA.

Definition.

The word "hernia" as used in modern surgical literature, is derived from the Greek "εϱνος", which means "a projection". It signifies a protrusion of a viscus through a congenital or an acquired opening of the wall surrounding the corresponding cavity.

In former times authors preferred to use the word "cele", which is a latinized Greek word "kele" (κήλη), "a swelling", and which was used as a suffix of the word designating the contents of the hernia, as enterocele (intestinal hernia), omphalocele (umbilical hernia), etc.

Nomenclature.

The name given to a definite type of hernia either designates its contents, its location, its etiology, or its condition.

1. According to its contents, herniæ are designated as hernia of the small bowel, hernia of the large bowel, etc.

2. According to its location, herniæ are inguinal, femoral, umbilical, diaphragmatic, ventral, perineal, etc.

3. According to the etiology, herniæ are congenital, acquired and post-operative.

4. According to their condition, herniæ are reducible or irreducible, strangulated, etc.

A. INGUINAL HERNIA.

I. SURGICAL ANATOMY OF INGUINAL HERNIA.

The inguinal canal is approximately one and one-half inches long. It begins at the abdominal (internal) inguinal ring and ends at the subcutaneous (external) inguinal ring. The abdominal inguinal ring lies about one-fourth of an inch above the middle of Poupart's ligament, and the subcutaneous inguinal ring lies in front of the lateral portion of the pubic bone. When the individual is in the erect posture, the boundaries of the inguinal canal are:

Anterior Wall.

The skin, superficial fascia (Camper's layer, Scarpa's layer), deep fascia (a very thin layer), and the aponeurosis of the external oblique muscle. These layers lie in front of the entire length of the inguinal canal, whereas the next layer, namely, the internal oblique muscle, lies in front of the lateral third of the inguinal canal only. Thus, we may say, that

610

the **strength of the anterior wall of the inguinal canal diminishes from its lateral to its medial portion.**

Posterior Wall.

The posterior wall of the inguinal canal is formed by the transversalis fascia through the entire length of the canal, by the conjoined tendon in the medial half of the canal, and by the triangular ligament in its most medial portion. Thus, we may say, that **the posterior wall of the inguinal canal also is not of the same strength in its entire length. It is weakest in the lateral portion and strongest in the medial portion.** The strength of the posterior wall is reverse to that of the anterior wall of the inguinal canal. It can be stated that **the mutual relationship of the walls of the inguinal canal is such that where it is the strongest anteriorly, it is weakest posteriorly, and vice vêrsa.**

The roof of the canal is composed of the arched fibers of the internal oblique muscle (which forms also the antero-lateral wall of the inguinal canal) and of the lower border of the transversus abdominis muscle (which usually stops immediately above the abdominal inguinal ring).

The floor consists of the inguinal (Poupart) ligament, and at its inner end, the lacunare ligament (Gimbernat's ligament).

The contents of the inguinal canal are:

In the male: The spermatic cord, the ilio-inguinal nerve and the genital branch of the genitocrural nerve.

In the female: The round ligament of the uterus, the ilio-inguinal nerve and the genital branch of the genitocrural nerve.

The abdominal inguinal ring (Internal ring O.T.) is an opening in the transversalis fascia. Its radius is about 1 cm. It lies midway between the anterior superior iliac spine and the symphysis pubis, and about one-half to one-fourth of an inch above the inguinal ligament. Its boundaries are the arched fibers of the transversus abdominis muscle—above and laterally, and the inferior epigastric artery and vein—medially. It transmits the spermatic cord in the male and the round ligament of the uterus in the female. From the circumference of the ring a thin funnel-shaped membrane, the internal spermatic fascia (processus infundibuliformis, O.T.), which is a portion of the transversalis fascia, is prolonged on the cord around its entire circumference.

Subcutaneous inguinal ring (External ring, O.T.). This actually is not a ring but a triangular space, the base of which is formed by the crest of the pubis and the two sides (which are called the crura of the ring) by the split aponeurosis of the external oblique muscle. The crus medially is called crus superior, and that which lies more laterally, crus inferior. The crura join each other at a point which forms the apex of the external inguinal ring. In order that the crura should not separate from each other above the apex of the subcutaneous ring, there are fibers which run in a semicircular manner transversely and which are called the intercolumnar fibers.

The superior crus is broad and flat and is attached to the body of the pubic bone. The inferior crus is attached to the tubercle of the pubic bone. **Therefore the subcutaneous inguinal ring lies in front of and medially to the inguinal ligament.** Consequently, the contents of an inguinal hernia after they pass through the inguinal canal **lie in front of the inguinal (Poupart) ligament.**

The inferior epigastric artery takes its origin from the external iliac artery just above the inguinal (Poupart) ligament, and runs in an upward and medial direction until it reaches the rectus abdominis muscle to which it furnishes its blood-supply. This artery forms with the lateral border of the rectus muscle and with the inner half of the inguinal ligament a triangle—**Hesselbach's triangle.** This triangle lies chiefly behind that portion of the posterior wall of the inguinal canal which is formed by the falx inguinalis (conjoined tendon, O.T.).

II. SUBDIVISIONS OF INGUINAL HERNIA.

The inguinal herniæ are of two varieties:

A. **Indirect Inguinal Hernia,** in which the sac enters the inguinal canal through the abdominal inguinal ring, traverses the entire length of the inguinal canal and leaves this canal through the subcutaneous inguinal ring. **In this variety, the hernial sac lies laterally to the inferior epigastric vessels.**

B. **Direct Inguinal Hernia.**

In this variety, the sac bulges through Hesselbach's triangle into the lower portion of the inguinal canal and makes its exit through the subcutaneous inguinal ring. **The inferior epigastric artery lies lateral to the sac.** This type usually has a small sac with a large neck. It occurs generally in adults. It rarely descends into the scrotum.

III. OPERATIVE TREATMENT OF INDIRECT INGUINAL HERNIA.

a. BASSINI OPERATION.

This was described by E. Bassini in 1883, and modified by him in 1888. **The characteristic feature of his technic consists in a high ligation of the sac, reconstruction of the posterior wall of the inguinal canal, and transplantation of the cord.**

Technic.

Step 1. The skin-incision is three or four inches long in adults and two to three inches in children. Lying half an inch above the Poupart ligament, it begins one inch lateral to the middle point of this ligament and runs downward parallel to this ligament until the subcutaneous ring is reached (Fig. 313, insert). After the skin is incised, the superficial circumflex iliac and the superficial epigastric vessels are seen traversing the superficial fascia. They are clamped and cut between the clamps. The opening thus made in the fascia is prolonged by cutting with scissors upward and by a knife downward. The aponeurosis of the external oblique muscle is now exposed. The superficial epigastric and circumflex iliac vessels are ligated and the ends of the ligature cut short (Fig. 313). Skin-towels are now attached to the lips of the wound.

Step 2. The aponeurosis of the external oblique muscle is incised along the entire length of the skin-incision. This can be done either by cutting

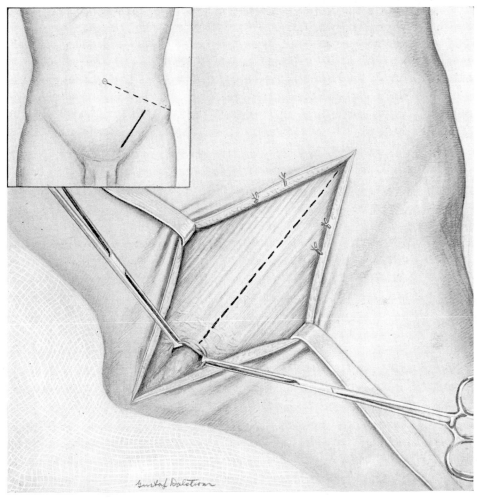

FIG. 313. INGUINAL HERNIOTOMY BY THE BASSINI METHOD.
MAIN PICTURE. Allis clamps are placed at the upper portion of the external inguinal ring.
INSERT. Skin-incision.

it on a grooved director introduced behind the aponeurosis through the external inguinal ring, or by dividing it in the direction from the internal to the external ring. In either case, care should be taken not to injure the ilio-inguinal nerve and not to cut the aponeurosis close to Poupart's ligament, since it is desirable to have the lower flap rather wide. Three Allis forceps grasp each aponeurotic lip. One is placed at the upper third of each lip, another at the middle, and the third at the point which forms the arched border of the subcutaneous ring. **These lower forceps are used as landmarks for resuturing the external oblique aponeurosis at the end of the operation** (Fig. 314, a).

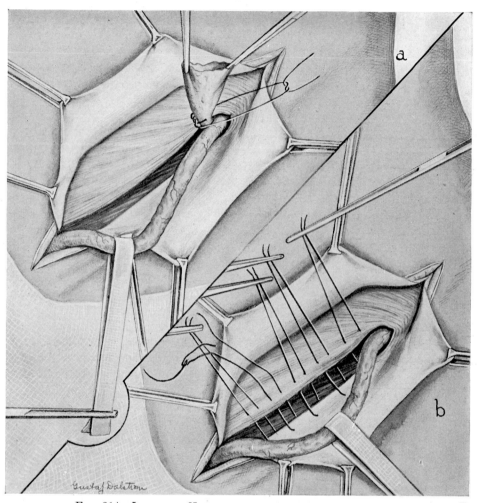

FIG. 314. INGUINAL HERNIOTOMY BY THE BASSINI METHOD.
a. The aponeurosis of the external oblique muscle is cut and reflected; the cord is lifted; the hernial sac is ligated;
b. The stump of the sac is dropped into the peritoneal cavity. Reconstruction of the posterior wall of the canal begun.

Each lip of the incised aponeurosis is retracted. The inner (or upper) lip is retracted for about half an inch, and the lower lip until the shelving portion of the inguinal ligament is exposed down to the spine of the pubic bone

Step 3. Lifting of the cord (round ligament).

The external spermatic fascia is divided along the side of the cord which is then lifted by the finger. A tape is placed around the cord [care should be taken not to twist the cord]. The free ends of the tape are clamped and held by the assistant (Fig. 314, a).

Step 4. Management of the hernial sac.

The sac is situated in front of and to the inner side of the cord. At this stage of the operation the entire length of the sac is not yet exposed, since the portion of it adjoining the abdominal ring is covered by the lower edge of the internal oblique muscle. Exposure of the sac becomes possible by making two movements with an ordinary toothed tissue-forceps, one, in an upward direction, penetrating the cremasteric muscle (which is a downward prolongation of the internal oblique muscle) and lifting the arcuate fibers of the internal oblique muscle (until the abdominal inguinal ring is reached), and another, by penetrating through the internal spermatic fascia (or infundibuliform fascia, which is a continuation of the transversalis fascia on the cord) in a downward direction. The sac is thus exposed, and can be easily recognized by the opaque white convex border of the fundus.

The fundus of the sac is now grasped by an artery-forceps and the sac is separated from the cord until its neck is reached. It is now opened (care being taken not to injure its contents, if there are any), and its contents are reduced into the peritoneal cavity. A transfixing ligature passes through the neck (Fig. 314, a). The ligature is tied and the sac excised, leaving a large stump which is allowed to drop behind the abdominal ring into the free peritoneal cavity.

Step 5. Reconstruction of the inguinal canal.

The cord is retracted laterally. The internal oblique muscle and the conjoined tendon are sutured to the shelving part of the Poupart ligament. It is very important to insert the stitch closest to the exit of the cord from the abdominal ring at the right place. It should be neither too close to the ring, so as not to compress the cord, nor too far from the ring, so as to leave a large open ring through which a new hernia may develop. A round full curved needle, threaded with chromic catgut No. 2, passes through the internal oblique muscle, and, if possible, **through the edge of the transversalis fascia which forms the border of the internal ring,** care being taken not to injure the inferior epigastric vessels. Then the needle passes outward through the shelving portion of the Poupart ligament; the direction of the needle is then reversed and is inserted into the internal oblique muscle; thus, this suture, just the same as the rest, is of a mattress type. [Care should be taken when making the bite through the shelving portion of the Poupart ligament not to injure the femoral or the external iliac artery, which passes behind the ligament at this point—the "femoral point."] **Before tying this particular suture we should be certain that it does not compress the cord.** This can be ascertained on palpation of the cord by noting the pulsation of the internal spermatic artery.

However, this suture is not tied until the remainder of these deep sutures are inserted. These sutures, similarly constructed and four to five in number, are placed one-third of an inch apart (Fig. 314, b). The lowermost suture grasps the conjoined tendon in front of the pubic crest, Gimbernat's ligament (particularly in large herniæ), and Poupart's ligament. The sutures are now tied and the ends are cut short (Fig. 315, a).

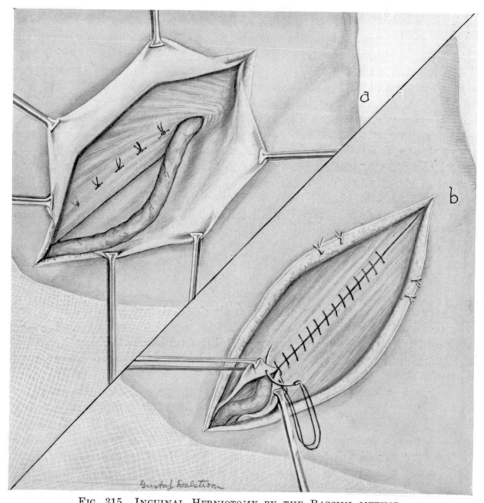

FIG. 315. INGUINAL HERNIOTOMY BY THE BASSINI METHOD.
a. The posterior wall is reconstructed.
b. The cord is laid on the newly formed floor and the anterior wall of the canal is reconstructed.

Step 6. The cord is now placed on the newly formed posterior wall of the canal, and the anterior wall is reconstructed by suturing the anterior lips of the aponeurosis of the external oblique muscle to each other with plain catgut No. 1. The lower end of this anterior wall is readily recognized, since two clamps were placed there at the beginning of the operation (one at each side), when the aponeurosis of the external oblique muscle was incised (Fig. 315, b). **[Care should be taken when inserting the lowermost suture in the anterior wall not to compress the cord.]** The skin is closed by interrupted suture of horse-hair or dermol.

b. ANDREWS IMBRICATION OR "LAP-JOINT" METHOD.

This method was described by E. Wyllys Andrews, of Chicago, in 1895.

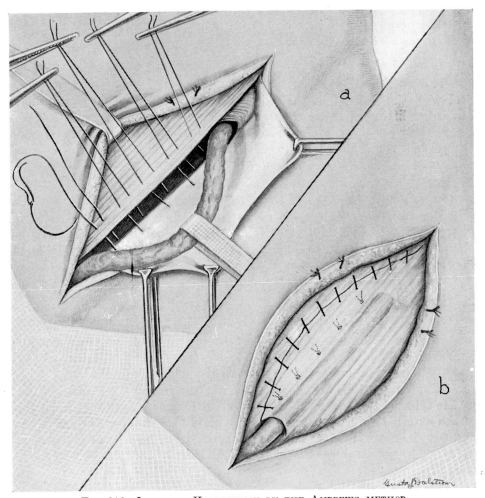

FIG. 316. INGUINAL HERNIOTOMY BY THE ANDREWS METHOD.
a. Reconstruction of the posterior wall of the canal.
b. The lower flap is sutured over the cord to the anterior surface of the upper flap.

It carries the essential elements of the Bassini operation (high ligation of the sac, reconstruction of the posterior wall of the inguinal canal, preservation of the obliquity of the canal), and, as an additional feature, it gives **a reinforcement of the anterior wall of the canal by overlapping** the upper flap by the lower flap of the aponeurosis of the external oblique muscle.

Technic.

Steps 1 to 4 are precisely the same as in the Bassini method.

Step 5 is the same as in the Bassini method, with this difference, that not only the internal oblique muscle and the conjoined tendon but also the aponeurosis of the external oblique muscle are sutured to the shelving portion of the Poupart ligament (Fig. 316, a).

Step 6. The lower lip of the aponeurosis of the external oblique muscle is sutured over the cord to the anterior surface of the upper lip of this aponeurosis (Fig. 316, b).

c. FERGUSON METHOD.

This operation is similar to the Bassini operation in the steps which deal with the making of the skin-incision, the opening of the inguinal canal, the lifting of the cord, and the management of the sac. **The difference between these two methods is, that whereas in the Bassini method the cord is transplanted, in the Ferguson method it lies in its original position.**

Technic.

Steps 1 to 4. As steps 1 to 4 in the Bassini operation.

Step 5. The cord is replaced in its original position. A series of interrupted sutures half an inch apart are inserted, uniting the internal oblique muscle and the conjoined tendon to the shelving portion of the Poupart ligament.

Step 6. The edges of the aponeurosis of the external oblique muscle are sutured to each other.

d. POSTEMPSKI'S MODIFICATION OF THE BASSINI OPERATION.

This method was employed by Postempski, of Rome, in 1884, and published in 1890.

The operation is a typical Bassini operation up to the point when the hernial sac is ligated. Then the cord is lifted, and the inner lip (that is, the internal oblique muscle, the conjoined tendon and the aponeurosis of the external oblique muscle) is sutured to the shelving portion of the Poupart ligament. **Postempski closes the external ring, thus obliterating entirely the inguinal canal. The cord is laid behind the skin and the superficial fascia.**

IV. OPERATIVE TREATMENT OF DIRECT INGUINAL HERNIA.

This type of hernia gives a high percentage of recurrence variously estimated by different surgeons as between 5 and 20 per cent. The reason for this high percentage of recurrence lies in the fact, that whereas in indirect inguinal hernia the trouble is the weakening of the fascia at the place where the blood-vessels (internal spermatic) pass through it while the surrounding structures (transversalis fascia and the muscles) are not altered, in this variety that is not the case. **The entire transversalis fascia in this region is weakened,** and sewing it will not make it any stronger. The only hope for preventing a recurrence of this type of hernia is to reinforce the weakened structures lying in front of the hernial protrusion by the strong muscles in the immediate vicinity. And as a strong muscle is only one factor (and not the most important) in the prevention of hernia-formation, **the other being a strong fascia (which in this case is weak and cannot be replaced by a strong transversalis fascia),** it is evident that recurrences may occur quite frequently in the treatment of a direct hernia.

a. DOWNES TECHNIC.

This was described in 1911. It is a further improvement of the Bloodgood method, which was described in 1898.

Step 1. The skin-incision is the same as in the Bassini operation.

Step 2. The incising of the aponeurosis of the external oblique muscle, the retracting of the arcuate fibers of the internal oblique muscle, the cutting of the cremasteric muscle and fascia, and the exposure of the sac are the same as in the Bassini operation. The sac is incised at its upper end (in order to keep away as far as possible from the urinary bladder), a finger is introduced into its lumen, the sac is isolated from the surrounding structures, and is ligated by a transfixion-suture flush with the opening in the transversalis fascia, and then is cut off. The lips of the transversalis fascia are sutured, if possible, to each other as in an ordinary laparotomy closure.

Step 3. Reconstruction of the posterior wall.

The sheath of the rectus abdominis muscle is cut along its lateral margin from the level of the abdominal inguinal ring down to its attachment to the pubic bone. Three or four chromic or kangaroo sutures, inserted at a distance of one-half to three-fourths of an inch from each other, unite the lateral margin of the rectus muscle with the shelving portion of Poupart's ligament. [If the transversalis fascia was not sutured as a separate layer, it is now caught in the bites of the rectus muscle.] The internal oblique muscle and the conjoined tendon are sutured to Poupart's ligament superficial to the previously inserted deep sutures, precisely as in the Bassini operation. The cord is laid on this newly formed posterior wall.

Step 4. The lips of the aponeurosis of the external oblique muscle are sutured to each other either as in the Bassini operation or as in the Andrews imbrication method.

b. McNEALY TECHNIC.

Step 1. The incision of the skin, fascia and aponeurosis of the external oblique muscle, and the lifting of the spermatic cord, are the same as in the Bassini operation.

Step 2. The transversalis fascia is incised, the sac is isolated, and its neck is closed by a transfixion-suture (Fig. 317, a). The sac is cut off distal to the ligature, and the stump is held by an Allis forceps in order to facilitate its invagination in the next step of the operation (Fig. 317, b).

Step 3. A number of mattress-sutures are inserted uniting on the inner lip the internal oblique muscle with the transversalis fascia (in the

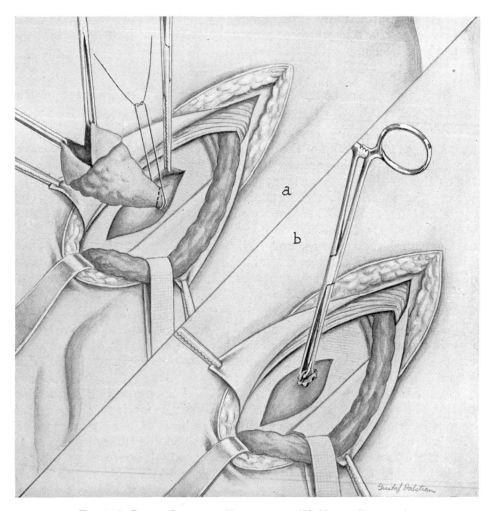

FIG. 317. DIRECT INGUINAL HERNIOTOMY (McNEALY TECHNIC).
a. The neck of the sac is ligated by a transfixing suture.
b. The stump of the sac is held by an Allis forceps in order to facilitate its invagination.

upper portion of the wound) and the conjoined tendon with the transversalis fascia (in the lower portion of the wound) with the shelving portion of Poupart's ligament of the outer lip (Fig. 318, c). The ends of each thread are tied to each other (Fig. 318, d).

Step 4. The reconstructed wall is reinforced by suturing the edges of the lower (lateral) flap of the aponeurosis of the external oblique muscle to the anterior surface of the internal oblique muscle (Fig. 319, e). The cord is placed on the newly formed floor. The upper lip of the aponeurosis of the external oblique muscle is sutured over the cord to the anterior

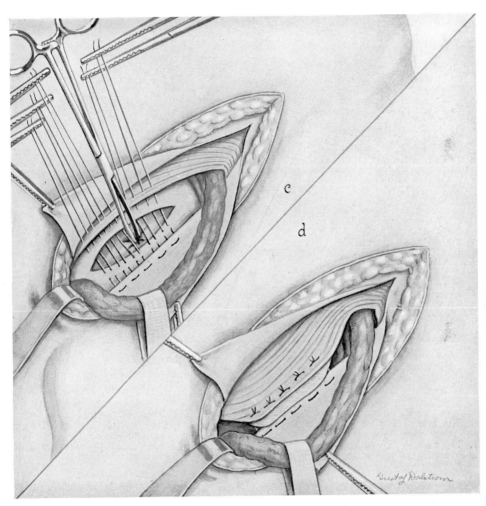

FIG. 318. DIRECT INGUINAL HERNIOTOMY (McNEALY TECHNIC).

c. Mattress-sutures are inserted;

d. The mattress-sutures are tied, thus bringing the internal oblique muscle and the transversalis fascia to the shelving portion of the Poupart ligament.

surface of the lower lip of the aponeurosis of the external oblique muscle (Fig. 319, f).

Step 5. The skin is closed.

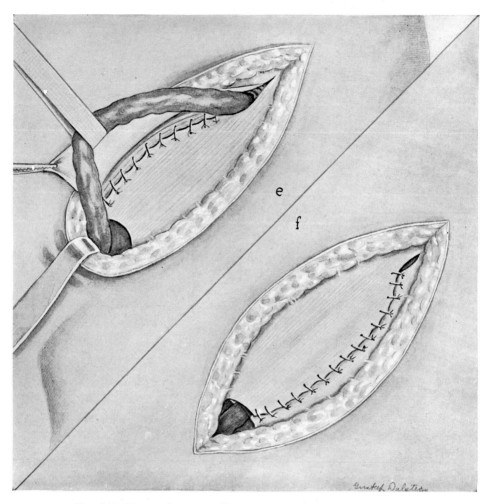

FIG. 319. DIRECT INGUINAL HERNIOTOMY (McNEALY TECHNIC).
e. The lateral flap of the aponeurosis of the external oblique muscle is sutured over
the anterior surface of the internal oblique muscle and conjoined tendon.
f. The medial flap of the aponeurosis of the external oblique muscle covers the cord
and is sutured to the anterior surface of the Poupart ligament.

V. OPERATIVE TREATMENT OF CO-EXISTANT DIRECT AND INDIRECT HERNIA (PANTALOON HERNIA).

Hoguet Method.

This was described in 1920. The characteristic features of this
operation consist in:

a. Pulling the portion of the sac which forms the direct inguinal hernia
lateral to the deep epigastric vessels, thus transforming **the direct and
indirect portions of the sac into one sac lying lateral to these vessels.**

b. Suturing a duplicated portion of the aponeurosis of the external oblique muscle to the shelving portion of the Poupart ligament.

Technic.

Steps 1 to 3. The incision of the skin and of the aponeurosis of the external oblique muscle and the lifting of the cord are precisely the same as in Steps 1 to 3 of the Bassini operation.

Step 4. The management of the sac.

The sac is exposed. That portion of it lying lateral to the deep epigastric vessels is grasped and pulled laterally. This will draw laterally the direct portion of the sac, thus transforming a pantaloon hernia into an oblique inguinal hernia. [If the blood-vessels are in the way, it is best to divide them between ligatures, although in the majority of cases this is not necessary.] The sac is now handled as in the Bassini operation.

Step 5. Reconstruction of the floor of the inguinal canal.

The inner lip of the aponeurosis of the external oblique muscle is reflected in such a manner that along the line of reflection a duplication is formed half an inch wide. This duplicated aponeurosis together with the internal oblique muscle and conjoined tendon are sutured to the shelving portion of the Poupart ligament by a series of interrupted mattress-sutures lying half an inch apart.

Step 6. As in the Bassini operation.

VI. TRANSVERSE INCISION FOR DOUBLE INGUINAL HERNIA OPERATION.

a. Edmunds Incision (Fig. 320, e).

This was suggested in 1908.

The incision starts at a point midway between the abdominal and subcutaneous inguinal rings on one side and extends in a slightly curved manner to the symmetrical point of the opposite side. It runs within the pubic hair approximately one inch above the symphysis pubis. This incision gives a good exposure for the management either of a direct or of an indirect inguinal hernia. It leaves a scarcely noticeable scar, and for this reason is particularly suitable for operations on unmarried women.

b. Judd Transverse Incision (Fig. 320, d).

This was described in 1913.

This incision starts at a point midway between the abdominal and subcutaneous inguinal rings on one side and runs straight across the anterior abdominal wall until it reaches the symmetrical point of the opposite side.

VII. OPERATIVE TREATMENT OF INGUINAL HERNIA AND UNDESCENDED TESTIS.

The undescended testis may be found either in the abdominal cavity, in the inguinal canal, or below the external ring. If it is found at the internal ring, it may be difficult to bring it down and for this reason it is advisable either to slip it back into the abdominal cavity (which is done by the majority of surgeons) or to remove it entirely (which is not recommended). In case it is decided to place it in the abdominal cavity, some surgeons advise making a pocket in the wall of the small

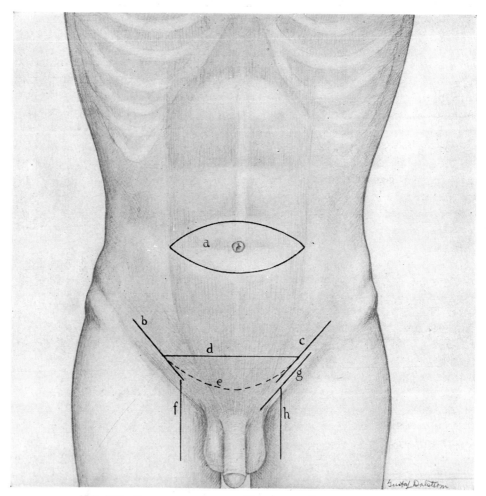

FIG. 320. SKIN-INCISIONS FOR DIFFERENT TYPES OF HERNIA.
a. Umbilical herniotomy by the Mayo method;   b. and c. Inguinal herniotomy; d. Judd incision for bilateral inguinal herniotomy;   e. Edmunds' incision for bilateral inguinal herniotomy;   f. and h. Skin-incision for femoral herniotomy;   g. Inguinal approach for femoral herniotomy.

pelvis and placing it there. **However, an attempt should always be made to lodge it in the scrotum, since in the majority of cases this is feasible.**

As this condition usually comes to the attention of the surgeon while the patient is very young, it becomes a problem at what age to operate. The majority of surgeons still think that the best time to operate is about the age of fifteen, that is, immediately following puberty. **However, in the recent work of many investigators it was definitely proved that if we wait until puberty the patients remain sterile, whereas in case of early operation the testicle is preserved as a reproductive organ, and for this reason we believe the best time to operate is between the ages of six and nine years.** Of the numerous methods suggested the most commonly used is that of A. D. Bevan, described in 1899.

a. BEVAN METHOD.

If the undescended testicle has not reached the inguinal canal, the occurrence of a coëxisting hernia is a rare coincidence. However, if the testicle lies in the inguinal canal, a coëxisting hernia is present in 50 per cent. of the cases. Therefore, at least in 50 per cent. the operation consists not only of making a new domicile for the testicle but also in performing a herniotomy.

The principle of this operation is based on the fact that if the spermatic cord is freed from its coverings so that the testis hangs only on the vas deferens and the spermatic vessels, the cord becomes elongated and the testicle can be placed several inches below the previous lowermost position.

Technic.

Step 1. The skin is incised as in inguinal herniotomy. The aponeurosis of the external oblique muscle is split. The testicle is lifted from the bed of the inguinal canal. The vaginal process (the sac) is carefully separated from the cord, ligated high, cut distal to the ligature, and the stump dropped into the peritoneal cavity. All the coverings of the cord are now removed, leaving the testicle hanging only on the vas and spermatic vessels. Now the testis can readily be brought down for a distance of from two to three inches.

Step 2. A pocket is made in the scrotum for the reception of the testis, care being taken to make it just as large as is necessary for it to retain the testis. The testis is not sutured to the scrotum in order to avoid any complications.

Step 3. The walls of the inguinal canal are reconstructed according to any of the recognized methods of treatment of an inguinal hernia.

b. KEETLEY-McKENNA METHOD.

Keetley, in 1894, suggested keeping the undescended testicle attached to the thigh after the cord has been elongated. In his earliest work, he sutured the tunica albuginea of the testicle to the fascia lata and kept it there for from three to six months, after which he detached it, and let it remain in the scrotum. Later, he discarded this method, and suggested (in 1905) another method in which he sutured the gubernaculum Hunteri to the fascia lata, leaving the testicle in the scrotum. Six months after the operation, he cut the bridge between the scrotum and the thigh (which consists of skin and gubernaculum) and closed each opening (that is, that on the thigh and that in the scrotum). This operation was long forgotten, but interest in it was recently revived by C. M. McKenna, of Chicago, who elaborated the technic.

Technic.

Step 1. Skin-incision as in inguinal herniotomy (Fig. 321, insert).

Step 2. The testicle and the cord are lifted from their bed. They

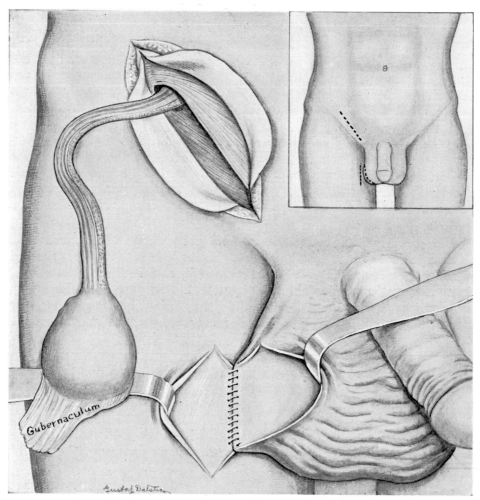

FIG. 321. ORCHIDOPEXY BY THE KEETLEY-McKENNA METHOD.
INSERT. Skin-incision in the inguinal region, scrotum and thigh.
MAIN PICTURE. The inner lips of the scrotal and femoral incisions are sutured together.

are freed from everything but the musculo-fibrous bands forming the gubernaculum. The gubernaculum is cut as far as possible from the testicle [Lucas Championnière showed that by freeing the cord from all connective tissue and leaving it hanging only on the vas deferens and the spermatic vessels, the cord becomes elongated to such an extent that the testicle can be brought from two to three inches lower than before, an observation which was utilized by Bevan in his method of treatment of undescended testis and by Keetley in his method of orchidopexy] (Fig. 321).

Step 3. The scrotum is stretched by two fingers introduced into it, in order to give sufficient room in which to lodge the testicle. A small

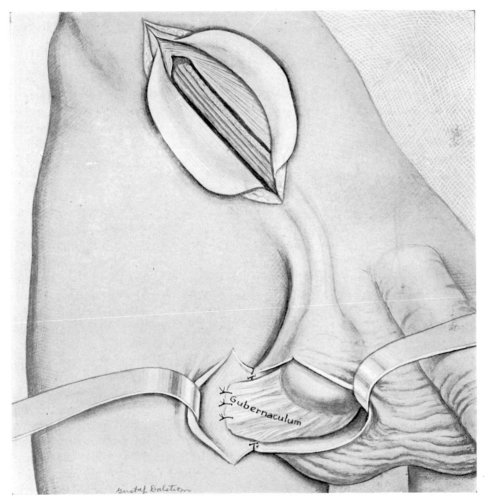

FIG. 322. ORCHIDOPEXY BY THE KEETLEY-McKENNA METHOD.
The testicle is lodged in the scrotum and the gubernaculum is sutured to the fascia lata.

incision, one and one-half inches long, is made on the bottom of the scrotum and another incision of the same length is made on the thigh at the same level (Fig. 321, insert).

Step 4. The adjoining inner lips of the incisions made on the scrotum and the thigh are sutured to each other (Fig. 321).

Step 5. An artery forceps, passing through the scrotum from below upward, grasps the gubernaculum and carries it with the testis through the scrotum until the gubernaculum is lodged on the fascia lata of the thigh. The testicle remains in the scrotum. The gubernaculum is now sutured to the fascia lata (Fig. 322).

Step 6. The lateral cutaneous lip on the thigh is sutured to the lip of the scrotum, thus closing both openings (on the thigh and on the scrotum).

Six months later, the cutaneous bridge which connects the thigh with the scrotum is cut under local anesthesia. The two lips of the skin of the thigh are sutured to each other. The same is done with the edges on the scrotum.

Franz Torek, of New York, in 1909, suggested suturing the testicle to the fascia lata. He considered this an improvement in the method of suturing the gubernaculum. However, as mentioned already, this method of Torek is actually one of the oldest variations used by Keetley, which he later discarded for his "gubernaculum-method".

VIII.   SLIDING HERNIA.

This variety of hernia of the large bowel was first described by Scarpa. However, it did not attract the attention of the profession until the beginning of this century, when the French surgeons again called attention to it.

Not every hernia of the large bowel is a "sliding hernia". The conditions are not synonymous by any means. However, in some cases, hernia of the large bowel may become a "sliding hernia". It is difficult to give the definition of the term in a few words. For this reason, it will be necessary to define it in a more descriptive manner.

When a structure such as the small bowel, the transverse colon, or the sigmoid leaves the abdominal cavity and enters the inguinal (or the femoral) canal, it becomes the content of an ordinary hernial sac. However, if the ascending or the descending colon, which is not completely invested by visceral peritoneum, becomes dislodged and begins to move in a downward direction in such a manner **that its peritoneum, which covers it in front and at the sides, remains immobile, while the bowel itself slides down until it appears in the inguinal (or femoral) canal, then it becomes a "sliding hernia".** This bowel may be the entire content of the canal, and in such a case, there is no sac present; this is a **sacless type** of hernia. Or, the protruded part of the bowel may be only a part of the contents of the inguinal canal, the rest consisting of the usual peritoneal sac, the contents of which are any abdominal viscera which ordinarily may be in the hernial sac. In this variety the "sliding" bowel **lies behind the posterior wall of the sac.**

From this description it is clear that any of the abdominal viscera which are **completely surrounded by peritoneum,** cannot become **(under** ordinary **circumstances)** a part of the sliding hernia. **Only structures which are invested by the peritoneum in front, or in front and at the sides, can become the contents of the sliding hernia.**

An abdominal viscus completely surrounded by peritoneum which forms a mesentery may become a part of a sliding hernia only under such an unusual circumstance as when the two leaflets of the mesentery begin to separate from each other, and the mesenteric border of the bowel loosens from its attachment to the mesentery. Then the bowel begins to slide, **whereas the leaflets of the mesentery remain immobile.**

The operative technic varies, depending on whether we deal with the small **sacless hernia** ("pushing" variety of Moschcowitz) or with sliding hernia with a sac ("pulling" variety of Moschcowitz).

The technic of operation in the "pushing" variety is as follows:

Step 1. The skin-incision is made as in ordinary inguinal herniotomy. The skin, the fascia, the aponeurosis of the external oblique muscle are incised. The cord is lifted, and the cremasteric muscle and the lower edge of the internal oblique muscle are retracted upward. The projecting portion of the bowel is pushed back into the **retroperitoneal space.** If there is difficulty in doing this, some blunt dissection will help.

Step 2. Deep sutures are placed connecting the internal oblique muscle and the transversalis fascia of the inner lip to the shelving portion of the Poupart ligament, care being taken to hold the replaced bowel in position until the deep sutures are tied. The rest of the operation is the same as described in inguinal herniotomy.

The technic of operation in the "pulling" variety is as follows:

Step 1. The incision through the skin, superficial fascia and aponeurosis of the external oblique muscle, the retraction of the aponeurotic lip, and exposure of the hernial sac, are precisely the same as in the Bassini operation.

Step 2. The sac is opened and its contents reduced into the free peritoneal cavity. All but the sliding portion of the bowel is easily reduced. This portion of the bowel refuses to budge [**this itself should make the surgeon suspect that it is probably a "sliding hernia".** If he sees appendices epiploicæ or tænia longitudinalis coli, then he will be sure that he is dealing with a piece of large bowel, *i.e.* he is confronted with a "sliding hernia".] The sac is carefully separated from the cord until the internal ring is reached. The sac together with the herniated bowel are lifted from the posterior wall of the hernial space. The liberation of the sac should start and continue from the outer side. This will minimize the possibility of injury to the blood-vessels of the bowel.

Step 3. The intestines and the sac (the invaginated posterior wall thereof) are lifted so as to put the bowel-attachment to the posterior wall on a moderate stretch. Then it will be seen that the posterior wall of the sac drops down over the nutrient blood-vessels of the bowel. The posterior wall of the sac is now incised longitudinally in two places, and the flap thus formed is sutured here and there to the stretched peritoneum, so that some sort of a mesentery is formed. The bowel now is entirely liberated from the sac and is reduced without any difficulty. The remnants of the sac are ligated at the internal ring and cut off.

Step 4. The canal is repaired by any of the methods hitherto described.

ALTERNATIVE METHOD OF TREATING A SLIDING HERNIA (LARDENNOIS METHOD).

Step 1. As Step 1 in the previous operation.

Step 2. The abdomen is opened, the hernia contents of the sac are reduced, the sliding portion of the bowel is corrected. Colopexy is done by suturing the wall of the bowel to the parietal peritoneum of the posterior abdominal wall. The sac is dislodged from its bed in the hernial canal from within the abdominal cavity and extirpated.

Step 3. The abdomen is closed in layers.

Step 4. The inguinal canal is repaired in the usual manner.

ADDITIONAL REMARKS.

As suture-material the majority of surgeons use chromic catgut No. 2 for reconstruction of the posterior wall of the inguinal canal and No. 1 for the anterior wall. Very few now use kangaroo-tendon. Recently there has been revived an interest in "living-sutures" as suture-material. This was suggested by L. L. McArthur as long ago as 1901, and was used quite extensively for some time. With the improved methods of sterilization of suture-material this method was employed less and less frequently. The reason for the revival of the interest in it in recent times is that it is claimed by some investigators that the strips of aponeurosis of the external oblique muscle connected with the mother-ground will live indefinitely, so that no foreign-body is present and no absorption of suture-material takes place. However, very few surgeons use "living sutures" for repair of inguinal or femoral hernia.

In recent years, several clinics reported a series of cases of inguinal hernia successfully treated by the **injection method.** The sclerosing material is injected along the course of the inguinal canal starting at the internal ring and gradually approaching the external ring with each subsequent injection. **This method certainly should be condemned.** As a matter of fact the method is not new. It was used quite extensively in pre-antiseptic days, and as the irritant material tincture of iodine, infusion of oak bark, zinc chlorid and alcohol were used.

Many disastrous reports were then recorded, as peritonitis, sloughing of the abdominal wall, wounding of the intestine, and injection into the femoral artery or vein. But whereas there was some excuse in using the injection method in pre-antiseptic days, when opening of the sac was dangerous and when the etiology of hernia was not clear, there is no excuse for its use today. It is generally accepted that for radical cure of an inguinal hernia **two facts are essential,** namely, high ligation of the sac (which means obliteration of the sac) and reinforcement of the inguinal canal (which is considerably less important than high ligation of the sac). In the injection method the sac is not removed. The entire hope lies in the expectation of making a barrier against the downward movement of the abdominal contents. **For these reasons, we believe that the injection method aside from being dangerous, does not offer any hope for permanent cure and certainly should not be employed.**

B. FEMORAL HERNIA.
Definition.

A femoral hernia is the protrusion of one or more abdominal viscera through the femoral ring into the femoral canal.

It occurs more frequently in women than in men, employing the percentage basis of the number of femoral herniæ to the number of inguinal herniæ occuring in each sex. However, in absolute numbers it is met more frequently in men than in women since men suffer from hernia more frequently than women.

Surgical anatomy.

The femoral canal is a short, narrow channel, the length of which is about one-half to three-fourths of an inch, and which is situated between the femoral vein and the inner wall of the femoral sheath. It communicates with the abdominal cavity through **the femoral ring.**

The boundaries of the femoral ring are Poupart's ligament **in front,** the femoral vein **laterally,** Gimbernat's ligament (ligamentum lacunare) **medially,** and the horizontal ramus of the pubic bone, covered by Cooper's ligament and the origin of the pectineus muscle, **posteriorly.**

The contents of the femoral canal are a few lymph-glands and some fatty tissue. The coverings of the femoral hernia are: The skin, the superficial fascia, the cribriform fascia, the transversalis fascia (femoral sheath), the properitoneal fat and the peritoneum.

Operative treatment.

Numerous operative procedures have been suggested for the cure of a femoral hernia. It will probably be safe to say that there are described more than eighty different methods. However, all of these can be classed into a few groups. The reason why so many methods were suggested is that the results are not as satisfactory as in the treatment of an inguinal hernia.

As early as 1879, Socin showed the importance of high ligation of the sac. He believed this to be the only important step necessary for a radical cure of a femoral hernia, and many surgeons even now are of the same opinion. Bassini, DeGarmo, Coley and others **suggested making a high ligation of the sac and obliterating the femoral ring by a crural approach.** The aim is ideal, since these two requirements (high ligation of the sac and relative closure of the femoral ring) is all that is necessary for the radical cure. However, technically it is extremely difficult to close the femoral ring from below or to produce a real high ligation of the sac. This is the reason why many surgeons prefer to expose the femoral ring through the incision for an inguinal herniotomy and to separate the sac, ligate its neck, extirpate it and close the opening from above. There is no question that this method gives a better approach for the radical cure of a femoral hernia. However, such an approach may produce a postoperative direct inguinal hernia. Therefore, the entire question of approach to the femoral hernia hinges on the consideration as to which will occur more frequently, a marked diminution in the recurrence of a femoral hernia after an inguinal approach, or the increased number of direct inguinal herniæ? On theoretical grounds we consider the inguinal approach the better one. But statistics show that recurrences in either method of approach are about the same. **However, in the case of a strangulated femoral hernia the approach from above has many advantages.**

a. FEMORAL APPROACH (BASSINI OPERATION).

Step 1. A skin-incision is begun one-half of an inch above Poupart's ligament and runs downward for 3 or 4 inches over the femoral canal parallel to the femoral vessels. The falciform edge (Margo falciformis) of the fascia lata is well exposed (Fig. 320, f).

Step 2. The cribriform fascia and the transversalis fascia are incised and the sac is grasped and freed from the fat which surrounds it. **It should be kept in mind that the femoral vein lies immediately lateral to the neck of the sac.** The sac is freed from beyond the neck, where it begins to expand again into the peritoneal cavity. It is there transfixed by chromic catgut and ligated. The sac is cut off distal to the ligature.

Step 3. Obliteration of the femoral canal and ring (Fig. 323, a).

Three or four chromic catgut sutures connect the Cooper's ligament with Poupart's ligament, the innermost suture connecting a point of Cooper's ligament near the pubic spine, the other about one-fourth of an inch more laterally, and the third about one-fourth of an inch to the inner side of the femoral vein. These three sutures are not yet tied. Three or four other sutures are now inserted connecting the edge of the falciform process with Cooper's ligament. All the ligatures are now tied, starting first with the upper sutures, connecting Poupart's ligament with Cooper's ligament, and then the lower ones.

Step 4. The skin is closed.

Instead of using several interrupted sutures, Poupart's ligament and the falciform process may be attached to Cooper's ligament by a purse-string suture (Fig. 323, b). This is known as the **Cushing method,** and was described in 1888. The results of this method are identical with that of Bassini.

b. INGUINAL APPROACH.

The inguinal approach for radical cure of a femoral hernia was first carried out by Annandale in 1876. This operation was later described again by Ruggi in 1892, who gave a detailed description of the method. In the United States, Moschcowitz called the attention of the profession to the merits of this approach, hence this method is known in this country as the **Moschcowitz operation.**

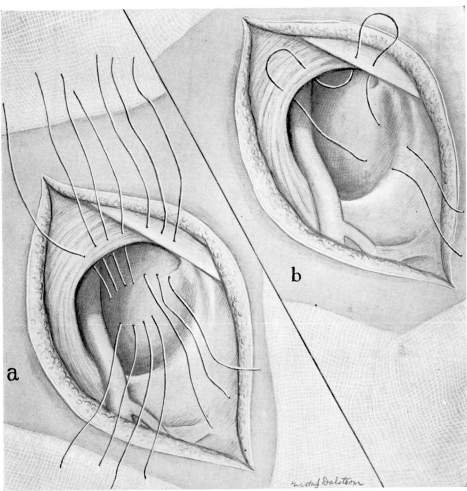

FIG. 323. FEMORAL HERNIOTOMY.
a. Bassini method.
b. Purse-string method.

Technic.

Step 1. The skin-incision, four inches long, is made as for an inguinal herniotomy, with the difference only that the upper end does not reach as high as in the inguinal herniotomy and the lower end reaches further down, even to the spine of the pubic bone (Fig. 320, g). The aponeurosis of the external oblique muscle is divided. The aponeurotic flaps are separated from the underlying structures, and the spermatic cord (or the round ligament) is exposed and lifted. The upper lip of the aponeurosis of the external oblique muscle, the internal oblique muscle, the conjoined tendon, and the spermatic cord are retracted upward and inward. The lower flap of the aponeurosis of the external oblique muscle is retracted downward and laterally (Fig. 324, a). The retraction of these structures will expose the transversalis fascia which is now cut to the inner side and

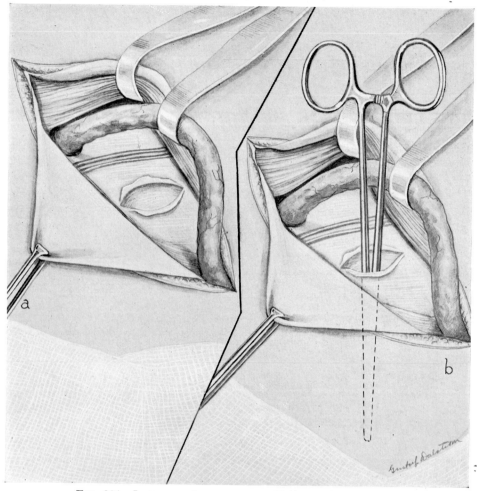

FIG. 324. INGUINAL APPROACH FOR FEMORAL HERNIOTOMY.
a. The transversalis fascia is cut below the deep epigastric vessels;
b. The femoral sac is everted by an artery forceps.

parallel to the deep epigastric vessels which are now retracted outward (Fig. 324, a). (If, however, they are in the way, they should be cut between ligatures.) This will expose the peritoneum and its continuation into the neck of the femoral sac.

Step 2. Management of the sac.

The neck of the sac is opened and its contents withdrawn into the free peritoneal cavity. A clamp is then introduced into the femoral sac, and the fundus of it is caught by the same clamp and pulled out from its bed in an everted position (Fig. 324, b). The neck is ligated by a transfixion-suture of chromic catgut and cut off distal to the ligature. [If, however, the sac cannot be pulled out in the everted position on account of adhesions between it and its bed in the femoral canal, an additional skin-incision should be made along the course of the femoral canal (Fig. 320, h), and the sac exposed and separated from its bed.]

Step 3. Closure of the femoral opening.

A chromic catgut No. 3, or a Pagenstecher celloidin linen thread No. 3, attaches Cooper's ligament to Poupart's ligament immediately medial to the femoral vein. Two or three additional sutures are placed in a similar manner medial to the first, the last one grasping also Gimbernat's ligament (ligamentum lacunare). The lips of the incised transversalis fascia are included in all these bites. The ends are tied only after all the sutures have been inserted. Another layer of sutures is inserted connecting the internal oblique muscle, the conjoined tendon and the aponeurosis of the external oblique muscle with the Poupart ligament in a line just lateral to the previously inserted deep sutures. The cord (or the round ligament) is now laid on the newly formed floor of the inguinal canal. The lower lip of the aponeurosis of the external oblique muscle is then sutured over the cord (round ligament) to the anterior surface of the upper lip of the aponeurosis of the external oblique muscle. The skin is closed by metallic clips or by dermal sutures.

C.   UMBILICAL HERNIA.

Definition.

This is a protrusion of an abdominal viscus through the umbilical ring.

The umbilical hernia is covered by the following structures:

      a.   Skin.
      b.   Superficial fascia.
      c.   Transversalis fascia.
      d.   Peritoneum.

OPERATIVE TREATMENT OF UMBILICAL HERNIA.

There are described various operative methods which differ from each other in the manner of closing the ring after the sac is removed.

a. TRANSVERSE OVERLAPPING METHOD (MAYO METHOD).

Step 1. Skin-incision.

An elliptical transverse incision is made surrounding the umbilicus, the right and the left ends of which reach the semilunar line (linea Spigelii) (Fig. 325, insert). This incision lies at a distance of one inch from the umbilicus, and cuts the skin and fascia, thus exposing the anterior sheaths of the recti muscles. The cutaneo-fascial circular lip around the umbilicus is now reflected centrally until the umbilical ring is reached. The transversalis fascia is cut and the hernial sac is exposed.

Step 2. Management of the sac.

The sac is opened close to the neck. The reason for this is, that the closer the hernial sac is to the umbilical ring the more recent is its origin, and for this reason fewer adhesions are present and there is less

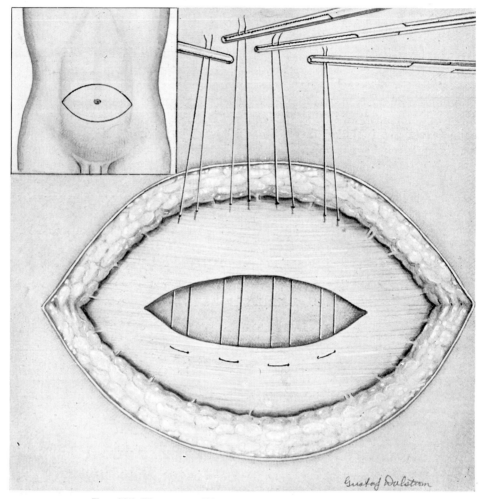

Fig. 325. Umbilical Herniotomy by the Mayo Method.
Insert. Skin-incision.
Main picture. A series of interrupted mattress-sutures are inserted connecting the upper and the lower aponeurotic flaps.

chance of injuring the contents of the sac. The neck is now enlarged sufficiently to admit two fingers into the sac in order to ascertain the nature of its contents and whether they are reducible. If the contents consist of bowel and omentum which can be easily reduced, this is the best thing to do. If the contents consist of omentum only which is firmly adherent to the sac, it is better to cut away the sac with the omentum, presuming, of course, that the omentum has been ligated by a series of transfixion-ligatures. If loops of bowel are present in the sac, they should be separated from each other and from the sac. If it is impossible to separate them from the sac, it is advisable to incise the sac a small distance away from the bowel so as to leave pieces of the sac hanging on the

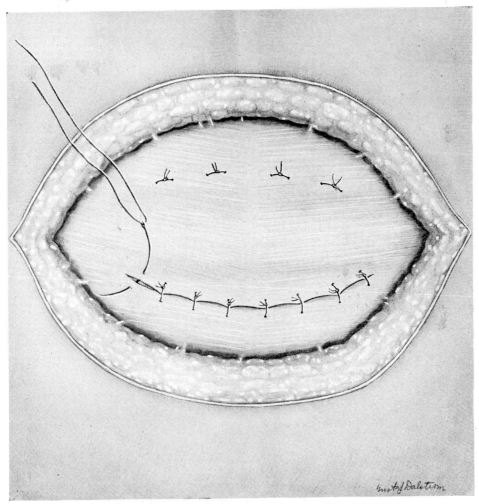

FIG. 326. UMBILICAL HERNIOTOMY BY THE MAYO METHOD.
The lower aponeurotic flap is drawn behind the upper and the mattress-sutures are tied. Suturing of the edge of the upper flap to the lower flap.

bowel. If, however, it seems an impossible procedure to separate the loops of the bowel from the sac without numerous injuries it may be preferable to resect the loop, or loops, of bowel. After the contents of the sac are disposed of, the neck is ligated by a transfixion-suture, and the stump is dropped into the peritoneal cavity.

Step 3. Closure of the ring.

The anterior sheath of the rectus muscle is cleared from overlying fat above and below the wound for a distance of two inches. A series of mattress-sutures, half an inch apart are inserted in such a manner that the loops are situated on the lower flap at a distance of half an inch from its margin, whereas the free ends appear on the upper flap at a distance

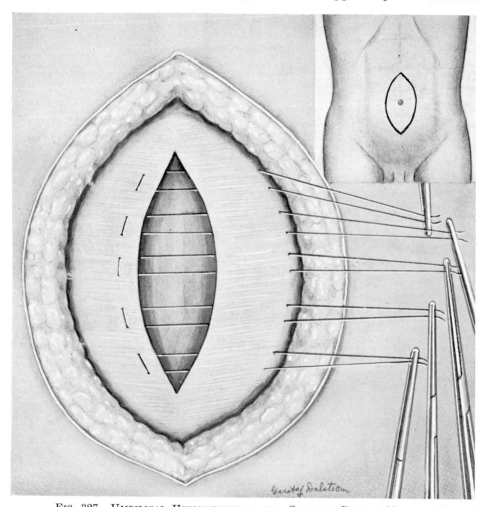

FIG. 327. UMBILICAL HERNIOTOMY BY THE SAPIEJKO-PICCOLI METHOD.
INSERT. Skin-incision.
MAIN PICTURE. A series of interrupted mattress-sutures are inserted connecting the right and left aponeurotic flaps.

of two inches from its free margin (Fig. 325). These sutures do not penetrate the peritoneum. The lower flap is now drawn behind the upper flap for at least a distance of two inches, and the mattress-sutures are tied. The margin of the upper flap is retracted in order to verify whether any gap is left on the suture-line of the two aponeurotic flaps. If a gap is present it should be closed by a buttonhole suture. The upper flap then covers the lower one, and its free margin is sutured to the anterior surface of the lower flap by a few interrupted sutures (Fig. 326). The skin and the superficial fascia are closed by interrupted sutures.

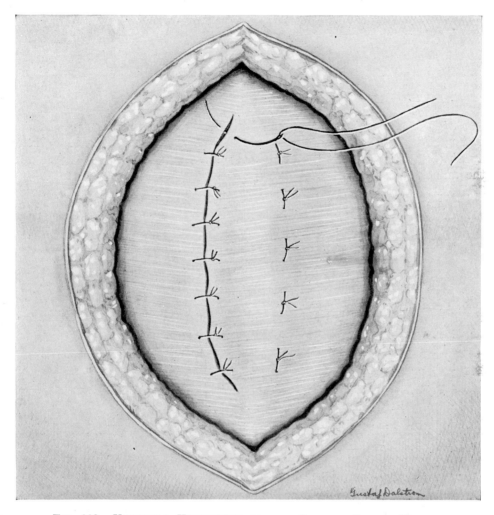

FIG. 328. UMBILICAL HERNIOTOMY BY THE SAPIEJKO-PICCOLI METHOD.
The right aponeurotic flap is drawn behind the left flap; the mattress-sutures are tied; suturing the edge of the left aponeurotic lip to the anterior surface of the right lip.

b. LATERAL OVERLAPPING OF THE FASCIA
(SAPIEJKO-PICCOLI METHOD).

This method has been used by Blake, DeGarmo, Noble and others. It is suitable for very thin subjects. The priority of introducing this method belongs to Sapiejko, who performed it for the first time in 1898, and published it in February, 1900. Independently of Sapiejko, it was described by Piccoli in January, 1900. Thus the priority in reporting belongs to Piccoli and of performing to Sapiejko. In the United States it is known as the **Blake method.**

TECHNIC OF THE SAPIEJKO-PICCOLI METHOD.

Step 1. An elliptical incision is made around the umbilicus with its long axis running longitudinally (Fig. 327, insert). The skin, fascia, anterior sheath of the rectus muscle and the transversalis fascia are cut and the neck of the sac is exposed and freed around the umbilical ring.

Step 2. The management of the sac is the same as in the previous operation.

Step 3. The anterior sheaths of the recti muscles are cleared of fat, and a series of interrupted mattress-sutures are inserted half an inch apart (Fig. 327), so that the anterior sheath on one side is drawn behind the anterior sheath of the other side for a distance of two inches (Fig. 328). Then the free inner margin of the superficially placed sheath is sutured to the anterior surface of the sheath which was drawn behind (Fig. 328).

Step 4. The skin is closed.

c. DuBOSE METHOD.

This method consists in making two horizontal flaps the edges of which are sutured to each other in the median line, and in covering this layer by another layer of sutures made between the upper and lower flaps. It was suggested in 1915.
Technic.
Step 1. Skin-incision.
An elliptical incision is made around the umbilical hernia, the long axis of which runs transversely.

Step 2. The sac is isolated, the contents removed in the usual manner, and the neck of the sac closed by a purse-string suture (Fig. 329, a).

Step 3. Two transverse incisions are made, one immediately above and the other immediately below the umbilical ring, cutting the anterior sheath of both recti muscles (Fig. 329, b). Thus, two lateral flaps are formed, which are sutured to each other in the midline (Fig. 329, c). The upper and the lower lips of the anterior sheath are then sutured to each other, over the previously made suture-line, by a series of interrupted sutures (Fig. 329, c). These vertical sutures are now tied and two figure-of-8 sutures are inserted connecting the skin and the superficial fascia of one lip, then the anterior sheath of the rectus muscle in two places, and then the skin and the superficial fascia of the other lip (Fig. 329, d).

D.   VENTRAL HERNIA.

Definition.

This is a protrusion of the viscera through some point in the anterior abdominal wall. Broadly speaking, the inguinal, femoral and umbilical

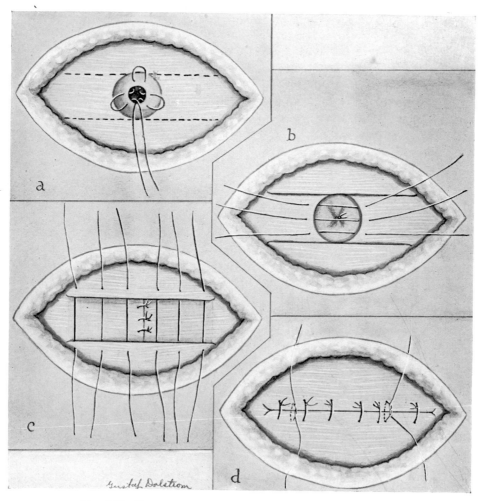

FIG. 329. UMBILICAL HERNIOTOMY BY THE DUBOSE METHOD.

herniæ are varieties of ventral hernia. However, when speaking of a ventral hernia, the inguinal, femoral or umbilical types are excluded.

Ventral hernia may be subdivided, from the topographical standpoint, into:

    a. Hernia lineæ albæ.

    b. Lateral ventral hernia.

From the etiological standpoint it is subdivided into:

    a. Spontaneous hernia.

    b. Acquired hernia.

        1. Traumatic.

        2. Incisional.

a. HERNIA LINEÆ ALBÆ.

This type of hernia constitutes slightly more than one per cent. of all hernia. It occurs in more than 90 per cent. in males and in less than ten per cent. in females. Two types of operation are employed for the radical cure of this type of hernia:

1. **The intraperitoneal operation,** which is used in those cases in which either the abdominal viscera are the contents of the hernia (which is a very rare occurrence), or in which obscure clinical symptoms make it necessary to open the abdomen for exploratory purposes. The closure of the abdomen is made either in the ordinary way, as in any laparotomy, or by a lateral overlapping method as described in the technic of the Sapiejko-Piccoli method of the surgical treatment of an umbilical hernia.

2. **The extraperitoneal operation (Moschcowitz technic).**

Step 1. A small vertical incision is made over the hernial protrusion, cutting the skin and subcutaneous tissue. A lump of fat is then exposed, which is the properitoneal fat (a continuation of the fat on the falciform ligament of the liver). This fat is teased away and its remnants are ligated to prevent a secondary hemorrhage. A search is now made for one of the blood-vessels which penetrates the linea alba from within. It usually lies to the left of the fat. It is ligated. The stump is now pushed downward and the edges of the transversalis fascia are sutured to each other by one or two interrupted sutures. The skin is closed in the usual manner.

b. LATERAL VENTRAL HERNIA.

To this group belong all the cases of protrusion of the abdominal viscera through the anterior abdominal wall with the exception of the inguinal, femoral, umbilical and linea alba herniæ. If they are of the **spontaneous** variety, they usually protrude through the Spigelian line. In cases of the **post-incisional variety,** they are observed at any place where the post-operative scar is present.

1. **Hernia lineæ semilunaris** (Hernia of the Spigelian line).

This hernia is present at the lateral border of the rectus muscle, usually immediately below the place where the posterior sheath of the rectus muscle becomes deficient, that is, immediately below the semicircular line (the fold of Douglas). On the abdomen, it lies at the inner third of the line which connects the anterior superior iliac spine with the umbilicus. The hernia may have one or more openings. The sac may lie either subcutaneously, or still more frequently behind the aponeurosis of the lateral oblique muscles and in front of the transversalis fascia. The hernial sac may lie above the inferior epigastric artery (which is comparatively rare) or below it (which is a frequent variety). The size of these herniæ is usually small. The occurrence of the hernia of the Spigelian line is rare, but it gives a high percentage of strangulation. The operative technic is the same as in a direct inguinal hernia.

2. Post-incisional hernia.

In the surgical treatment of this type of hernia it should be remembered that if adhesions are present they are largely in the region of the fundus of the hernia. For this reason it is always advisable to make the elliptical incision so as to remove the skin close to the fundus together with the sac (if the latter is going to be removed). If the sac is not removed, then the skin close to the fundus is separated very carefully. The sac is incised **at its neck** [the latter can be found by pressing on the abdominal wall with a finger. A sharp edge is then felt which is the place where the neck is situated. The reason for incising the neck of the hernial sac is that there the adhesions are less pronounced. The closer it is to the fundus the more dense and abundant are the adhesions], and the separation of the hernial contents in the direction toward the fundus is begun. After the abdominal contents are returned back into the abdomen, the excess of the sac is excised and its edges sutured to each other. [An alternative method is not to open the sac at all, but to infold it so that it reinforces the closure of the ring by the more superficially lying structures.] Then all the structures (with the exception of the skin) on one side of the opening are sutured to the lip of the other side in an overlapping manner, as in Andrews imbrication method. The edges of the skin are then sutured to each other.

E. DIAPHRAGMATIC HERNIA.

I. ANATOMY (FIG. 330).

The diaphragm is a broad flat structure which serves as a partition between the thoracic and abdominal cavities. Its central portion is tendinous (pars tendinea) and its lateral portion is muscular (pars muscularis). The muscular portion is subdivided into three parts—the lumbar, the costal, and the sternal.

a. Pars lumbalis.—This consists of three crura on each side—medial, intermediate and lateral.

The medial crus takes its origin from the anterior surface of the bodies of the first, second and third lumbar vertebræ on the right side and from the first and second lumbar vertebræ on the left side. In front of the body of the first lumbar vertebra the fibers of the medial crus of one side decussate with the fibers from the other side, forming the aortic opening (hiatus aorticus) for the passage of the aorta. The tendinous band which connects the two medial crura is known as the *middle arcuate ligament*. In its further course, the fibers of the medial crus encircle the esophagus forming an elliptical opening (hiatus esophageus) and still further they join the central portion (centrum tendineum).

The crus intermedium is situated laterally from the medial crus. The splanchnic nerves pass through the opening between the medium and intermedium crura. The lateral crus lies laterally from the previously mentioned crura. It takes its origin chiefly from the medial lumbo-costal arch (which is a fibrous band stretched across the superior end of the psoas muscle and attached to the body of the first or second lumbar vertebra medially and the tip of the transverse process of the first lumbar vertebra laterally), and some of its fibers from the lateral lumbo-costal arch (which is a fibrous band stretched over the upper end of the quadratus lumborum muscle and attached to the transverse process of the first lumbar vertebra

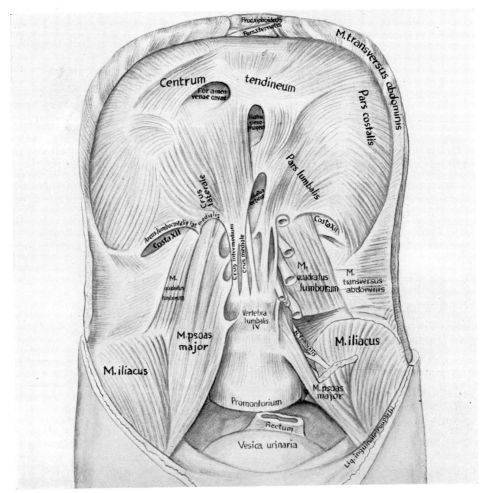

FIG. 330. THE DIAPHRAGM (AFTER RAUBER).

medially and to the twelfth rib laterally). The sympathetic trunk occasionally pierces the diaphragm between the intermediate and lateral crura.

b. Pars costalis.—This takes its origin from the cartilages of the sixth to the twelfth ribs. There its muscular bundles interdigitate with the muscular bundles of the transversus abdominis muscle. After the digits of the costal portion fuse together they join the central part of the diaphragm.

c. Pars sternalis.—This is the smallest subdivision of the diaphragmatic muscle. It arises from the dorsal surface of the ensiform process and of the posterior sheath of the rectus muscle of this vicinity and is directed to the central portion of the diaphragm.

The **central part (centrum tendineum)** has the shape of a three-leafed clover. On the anterior leaf (folium anterius) rests the heart with the pericardium. On each lateral leaf rest the medial portions of the base of each lung. At the posterior border of the anterior leaf lies the opening of the vena cava (foramen venæ cavæ) for the passage of this vein.

THE NERVES AND THE BLOOD-SUPPLY OF THE DIAPHRAGM.

The diaphragm is innervated by the phrenic nerve on each side. This nerve is composed of fibers of the third, fourth and fifth cervical nerves, with occasional branches from the sixth cervical, and still rarer, from the second cervical nerve. In case a branch of the second cervical nerve participates in the formation of the phrenic nerve, it reaches this nerve through the descending branch of the hypoglossal nerve. In case the branch of the sixth cervical participates in the formation of the phrenic nerve it reaches this nerve through the subclavian nerve.

The blood-supply is derived from the branches of the internal mammary artery (aa. pericardiaco-phrenicæ and aa. musculo-phrenicæ) or from the branch of the abdominal aorta (a. phrenicæ inferior) and branches of the lower intercostal arteries.

OPENINGS IN THE DIAPHRAGM.

The diaphragm has two large and several small openings through which different structures are transmitted from the chest into the abdominal cavity and *vice versa*. The third large opening (the aortic) actually lies behind the diaphragm.

a. Aortic opening (Hiatus aorticus).

This opening lies between the crura underneath the middle arcuate ligament. Through it pass the aorta and the thoracic duct. The azygos vein, which is described by some anatomists as passing through this opening, is actually situated postero-laterally from the thoracic duct **behind** the right crus, so that strictly speaking it does not pass through this opening.

b. The vena caval opening (Foramen v. cavæ) lies in the right side of the central tendon. It transmits the vena cava inferior and occasionally the ramus phrenico-abdominalis of the right phrenic nerve.

c. The esophageal opening (Hiatus oesophageus) lies in the muscular portion of the diaphragm posterior to the central tendon. It transmits the esophagus and the two vagi nerves—the left vagus in the anterior part, and the right vagus in the posterior part of the opening.

d. A slit between the crus mediale and crus intermedium through which pass the vena hemiazygos and the splanchnic nerves.

e. A slit between the crus intermedium and crus laterale through which passes the truncus sympathicus.

f. The sternocostal triangle (Larrey space) is situated between the sites of origin of the sternal and costal portions of the diaphragm. Here the internal mammary artery is continued as the superior epigastric artery.

g. The costo-lumbar triangle (trigonum costo-lumbale) is situated between the quadratus lumborum muscle and the costal portion of the diaphragm.

II. CLASSIFICATION AND INCIDENCE

From the etiological standpoint, diaphragmatic herniæ are divided into congenital, acquired and traumatic types.

Congenital hernia is present at birth. A hernial sac may be present **(true hernia)** or absent **(false hernia)**. This type constitutes about 29 per cent. of all diaphragmatic herniæ.

Acquired hernia is the type which develops after birth. It usually develops in those areas which are congenitally weak. They are usually of the true variety (*i.e.* they have a sac). They occur in about 36 per cent. of all cases of diaphragmatic hernia.

Traumatic hernia is the result either of a penetrating injury to the diaphragm or of rupture of the diaphragm due to sudden compression of the thoracic or abdominal walls. It is of the false variety (no hernial sac is present). It occurs in about 35 per cent. of all cases of diaphragmatic herniæ.

About 80 per cent. of non-traumatic hernia are on the left side and about 20 per cent. on the right side. About 95 per cent. of the traumatic type are on the left side and 5 per cent. on the right side.

Herniæ through the esophageal opening comprise about 27 per cent. of all non-traumatic diaphragmatic herniæ on the left side and 9 per cent. of all non-traumatic herniæ on the right side. Herniæ through the central portion of the diaphragm occur in about 20 per cent.

In a few cases two diaphragmatic herniæ not connected with each other have been reported in the same patient.

Contents of the Hernia.

All of the abdominal viscera with the exception of the pelvic organs have been encountered in the hernial sac. In the order of frequency they are: The stomach, the colon, the omentum, the small bowel, the spleen, the liver, the pancreas, the kidney. However, in the greatest majority of cases the contents are not some single organ but a combination of two or more abdominal viscera.

III. OPERATIVE MANAGEMENT.

The approach to the hernia may be from **above** by thoracotomy, or from **below** by celiotomy, or by a combined abdomino-thoracic approach. There is quite a divergence of opinion as to which approach is more advantageous. Each approach has its strong and weak points.

a. Thoracotomy gives a better access to the hernia opening. The contents of the sac can be more readily separated from each other and from the pericardium, pleura and lungs. It is easier to close the rent. The disadvantages of this method are: pneumothorax and greater difficulty in reducing the hernial contents into the abdominal cavity. In case of a repair of a hernia due to an immediately preceding trauma this

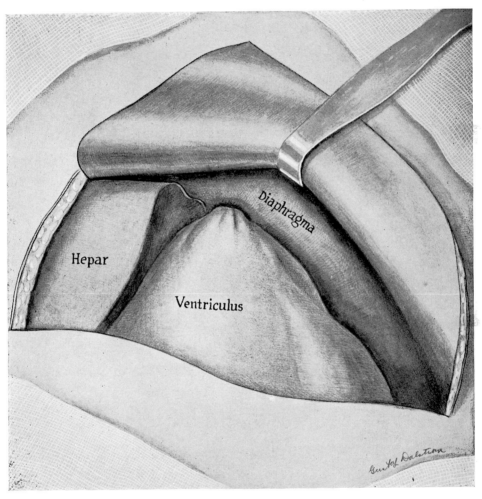

FIG. 331. DIAPHRAGMATIC HERNIA.
The stomach is incarcerated in the diaphragmatic opening.

approach is not good, since no exploration of the abdominal contents is possible.

b. Celiotomy enables a good exploration of the viscera. The objections to this approach are that in many cases the hernial ring lies very deep, and for this reason is inaccessible. The difficulty and the dangers connected with the separation of adhesions which are present on the thoracic side of the hernial opening is greater when working on the abdominal side of the hernia.

c. Combined thoracolaparotomy.

This route of approach is the favorite one with French surgeons.

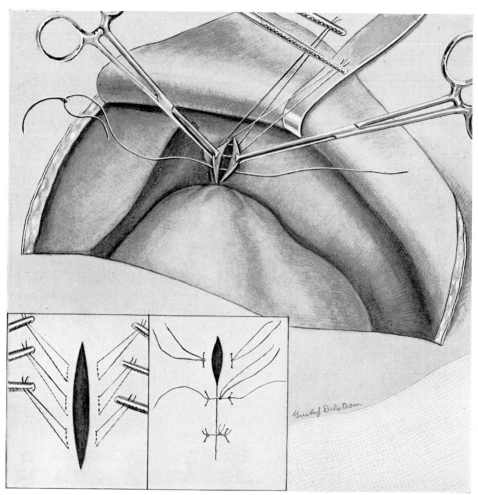

FIG. 332. DIAPHRAGMATIC HERNIA.
Closure of the opening in the diaphragm.
INSERT. The Soresi method of closure.

It has advantages over thoracotomy or celiotomy alone from the standpoint of better exposure. However, it involves greater chances for infection.

Thoracotomy approach.

Different incisions are used by different surgeons. Postempski used a U-shaped flap with the base upward, dividing two to four ribs in two places. The method of Lannelongue, the method of Monod and Vanverts, and the method of Canniot have been already described in Chapter II.

Celiotomy approach.

Different abdominal incisions are used for the approach to a diaphragmatic hernia: Midline, left pararectal, S-incision of Bevan, Fenger incision, left-side Kőnig-Perthes or Czerny-Perthes incision.

Combined Abdomino-Thoracic Approach.

A skin-incision, starting at the anterior axillary line in the seventh intercostal space, runs medially and slightly downward. When it reaches the midline it turns downward until it reaches the umbilicus. The pleural cavity is opened [differential pressure inhalation should be used.] Then the abdominal cavity is opened. The adhesions are separated, and the viscera reduced (Fig. 331). The margins of the opening are sutured to each other. Closure of the diaphragm can be made by a series of interrupted buttonhole sutures, or by mattress-sutures (Fig. 332).

In order to facilitate the closure of the opening in the diaphragm, Soresi takes a series of bites on each lip of the diaphragmatic opening parallel to its margin. He ties the ends of each thread to each other and then to the ends of the other side of the wound (Fig. 332, insert).

BIBLIOGRAPHY.

GENERAL CONSIDERATIONS OF HERNIA.

E. Albert. Die herniologie der Alten.
Beitr. z. Geschichte der Chirurgie, Wien, 1878, II:1-193.

H. Auchincloss. Fascial strip repair of femoral hernia.
Ann. Surg. 81:1009-1010; y. 1925.

K. Berkofsky. Erfahrungen bei der operativen Behandlung des abgeklemmten brandigen Darmes.
Deutsche Ztschr. f. Chir. 109:133-159; y. 1911.

W. G. Carscadden. Aponeurotic suture repair of femoral hernia.
Canad. Med. Ass. Journ. 30:598-601; y. 1934.

W. B. Coley. Hernia. In:Keen's Surgery, 4:17-109; y. 1909.

W. B. DeGarmo. Abdominal hernia, its diagnosis and treatment.
Lippincott, Publishers; y. 1907.

W. E. Gallie & A. B. LeMesurier. The use of living sutures in operative surgery.
Canad. Med. Ass. Journ. II:504-513; y. 1921.

W. E. Gallie & A. B. LeMesurier. The transplant of fibrous tissue in repair of anatomical defects.
Brit. Journ. of Surg. 12:289-320; y. 1924-1925.

W. E. Gallie. Closing very large hernial openings.
Ann. of Surg. 96:551-554; y. 1932.

E. Hesse. Die Behandlung der gangränösen Hernien.
Bruns Beitr. z. klin. Chir. 54:172-203; y. 1907.

Laroyenne. Hernies compliquées d'étranglement retrograde de l'intestin.
Lyon chirurg., 3:698-705; y. 1910.

L. L. McArthur. Autoplastic sutures in hernia and other diastases; final report.
Journ. Am. Med. Ass. 43:1039-1048; y. 1904.

E. A. Printy. An improved needle-forceps.
Surg. Gyn. & Obst. 34:679; y. 1922.

C. O. Rice. The injection treatment of hernia.
Minnesota Medicine, 17:248-252; y. 1934.

F. Sanger. Die Taxisrupturen des eingeklemmten Bruchdarmes.
Bruns Beitr. z. klin. Chir. 68:205-236; y. 1910.

E. Seifert. Anatomische Untersuchungen an Bruchsacken und ihre klinische Bedeutung.
Arch. f. klin. Chir. 171:217-281; y. 1932.

ANATOMY OF INGUINAL HERNIA.

M. Auvray. Hernie inguino-interstitielle chez la femme (Hernie de Goyrand).
Gaz. hebd. de Méd. et de Chir. 47:542-547; y. 1900.

P. Berger. Sur quelques variétés de la hernie inguinale congénitale chez la femme; en particular des hernies compliquées d'un kyste du canal de Nuck et des hernies en bissac.
Bull. et mém. Soc. de chir. de Paris, 17:283-294; y. 1891.

F. Bramann. Der Processus vaginalis und sein Verhalten bei Störungen des Descensus testiculorum.
Arch. f. klin. Chir. 40:137-168; y. 1890

A. M. Fauntleroy. Development of an inguinal hernia through the femoral ring following descent of the testicle by the same route.
Ann. Surg. 72:675; y. 1920.

F. C. Hesselbach. Neueste anatomisch-pathologische Untersuchungen über den Ursprung und das Fortschreiten der Leisten-und Schenkelbruche.
J. Stahel, Publisher, Würzburg; y. 1814.

Jaboulay. La hernie à double sac.
Lyon méd. 83:10-12; y. 1896.

F. Kaiser. Ueber Hernia encystica.
Bruns Beitr. z. klin. Chir. 118:306-317; y. 1920.

J. Langton. The association of inguinal hernia with the descent of testis.
Bradshaw lecture, Royal College of Surgeons.
Lancet, II:1857-1864; y. 1900.

W. W. MacGregor. The demonstration of a true internal inguinal sphincter and its etiologic rôle in hernia.
Surg. Gyn. & Obst. 49:510-515; y. 1929.

R. W. Murray. Hernia, its causes and treatment.
    J. & A. Churchill, Publishers, London; y. 1910.

A. Reich. Die intra-abdominalen Hernien der Foveæ supravesicales:
    Herniæ supravesicales internæ.
    Bruns Beitr. z. klin. Chir. 62:20-77; y. 1909.

R. H. Russell. Inguinal herniæ; their varieties, mode of origin, and classi-
    fication.
    Brit. Journ. Surg. 9:502-508; y. 1921-1922.

V. L. Schrager & J. T. Gault. Fibrous peritonitis of neck and hernial sac.
    Surg. Gyn. & Obst. 52:836-840; y. 1931.

L. F. Watson. Hernia. Pp. 143-170.
    C. V. Mosby Co., Publishers; y. 1924.

E. Zuckerkandl. Ueber den Scheidenforsatz des Bauchfelles und dessen
    Beziehung zur äusseren Leistenherniæ.
    Arch. f. klin. Chir. 20:215-225; y. 1877.

SURGICAL TREATMENT OF INGUINAL HERNIA.

S. Adler. Neues Verfahren zur Verhinderung der Rezidive bei Bruch-
    operationen.
    Zbl. f. Chir. 58:3136-3138; y. 1931.

E. W. Andrews. Imbrication or lap joint method; a plastic operation for
    hernia.
    Chicago Med. Rec. 9:67-77; y. 1895.

T. Annandale. A case in which a reducible oblique and direct inguinal and
    femoral hernia existed on the same side, and were successfully treated
    by operation.
    Edinb. Med. Journ. 21:1087-1091; y. 1875.

W. M. Banks. On the radical cure of hernia, by removal of the sac and
    stitching together the pillars of the ring.
    Brit. Med. Journ. II:985-988; y. 1882.

E. Bassini. Sopra 100 casi di cura radicale dell'ernia inguinale, operata
    con metodo dell'autore.
    Ital. chir. congr. Napoli; y. 1888.

E. Bassini. Ueber die Behandlung des Leistenbruches.
    Arch. f. klin. Chir. 40:429-476; y. 1890.

E. H. Beckman. The repair of hernia from the peritoneal side of the
    abdominal wall.
    Annals of Surg. 55:570; y. 1912.

P. Berger. La hernie inguino-interstitielle et son traitement par la cure
    radicale.
    Rev. de Chir. 25:1-50; y. 1902.

A. D. Bevan. Operation for undescended testicle and congenital inguinal
    hernia.
    Journ. Americ. Med Ass. 33:773-777; y. 1899.

A. D. Bevan. The surgical treatment of undescended testicle.
Journ. Americ. Med. Ass. 41:718-724; y. 1903.

A. D. Bevan. Undescended testes.
Surg. Clin. of Chicago, 2:1101-1117; y. 1918.

W. Birkenfeld. Über die Ursachen der postoperativen Leistenbruchrezidive.
Arch. f. klin. Chir. 174:525-535; y. 1933.

J. A. Blake. The relative bearing of the conjoined tendon and the internal oblique muscle upon the radical cure of inguinal hernia.
Med. Rec. 58:321-324; y. 1900.

W. Block. Bericht über eine Sammlung von 20,199 Leistenbrucnoperationen (Rezidive).
Arch. f. klin. Chir. 175:607-624; y. 1933.   Correction 176:812; y. 1933.

J. C. Bloodgood. The transplantation of the rectus muscle in certain cases of inguinal hernia in which the conjoined tendon is obliterated.
Johns Hopkins Hosp. Bull. 9:96-100; y. 1898.

J. C. Bloodgood. The transplantation of the rectus muscle or its sheath for the cure of inguinal hernia when the conjoined tendon is obliterated. The transplantation of the sartorius muscle for the cure of recurrent hernia when Poupart ligament has been destroyed.
Ann. Surg 70:81-88; y. 1919.

F. R. Brown. Use of strips of hernial sac as fascial (living) sutures.
Brit. Med. Journ. I:858; y. 1930.

A. Catterina. Die Bassini'sche Operation und die Operationen nach Brenner, Hackenbruch-Drüner, Schmieden und Kirschner (Vorläufige Mittheilung).
Zbl. f. Chir. 61:933-944; y. 1934.

M. Cherner. Indirect inguinal hernia in light cf newer interpretation of anatomy.
Ann. of Surg. 99:577-584; y. 1934.

W. B. Coley. Operative treatment of undescended or maldescended testis with especial reference to end-results.
Surg. Gyn. Obst. 28:452-459; y. 1919.

W. B. Coley & J. P. Hoguet. Operative treatment of hernia.
Ann. Surg. 68:255-268; y. 1918.

W. T. F. Davies. A method of operating for radical cure of inguinal hernia.
Brit. Med. Journ. II:727-728; y. 1913.

G. G. Davis. The radical cure of direct inguinal hernia.
Ann. Surg 43:111-113; y. 1906.

W. B. DeGarmo. Abdominal hernia, its diagnosis and treatment.
Lippincott, Publishers, Phila.; y. 1907.

Dengler. Über die Dauerresultate bei Leistenbruchradikaloperationen nach Jaure.
Deutsche Zeitschr. f. Chir. 231:435-438; y. 1931.

C. N. Dowd. Preservation of the iliohypogastric nerve in operation for cure of inguinal hernia.
Ann. Surg. 61:204-208; y. 1915.

W. A. Downes. Management of direct inguinal hernia.
Arch. Surg. 1:53-73; y. 1920.

E. R. Easton. Incidence of femoral hernia following repair of inguinal hernia—ectopic recurrence; proposed operation of external and internal herniorrhaphy.
Journ. Americ. Med. Ass. 100:1741-1744; y. 1933.

A. Edmunds. Double inguinal hernia; operation through a single incision.
Med. Press and Circul. London, 85:348; y. 1908.

A. H. Ferguson. Oblique inguinal hernia; typic operation for its radical cure.
Journ. Americ. Med. Ass. 33:6-14; y. 1899.

A. H. Ferguson. The technic of modern operations for hernia.
Chicago, Cleveland Press; y. 1907.

E. M. Fitch. Some causes of failure in operative treatment of inguinal hernia.
Trans. of New England Surg. Soc. 13:137-154; y. 1930.

E. Forgue. La cure radicale de la hernie inguinale et l'oeuvre initiatrice de Lucas Championnière.
Journ. de méd. et chir. prat. 101:756-769; y. 1930.

G. R. Fowler. A new method for the radical cure of inguinal hernia. Intraperitoneal transplacement of the spermatic cord and typical obliteration of the internal ring and inguinal canal.
Ann. Surg 26:603-623; y. 1897.

S. W. Fowler. Experience with injection treatment of hernia.
Med. Rec. 141:207-209; y. 1935.

S. W. Fowler. Technic of hernial injection treatment.
Med. Rec. 141:387-390; y. 1935.

W. E. Gallie & A. LeMesurier. The use of living sutures in operative surgery.
Canad. Med. Ass. Journ. II:504-513; y. 1921.

W. E. Gallie & A. LeMesurier. Late results of living suture operation in ventral and inguinal hernia.
Canad. Med. Ass. Journ. 23:165-168; y. 1930.

C. L. Gibson & R. K. Felter. End-results of inguinal operations.
Trans. Americ. Surg. Ass. 48:306-315; y. 1930.

W. S. Halsted. The radical cure of inguinal hernia in the male.
Johns Hopkins Hosp. Bull. 4:17-24; y. 1893.

J. C. Hayner. Analysis of mechanism and surgical treatment of inguinal hernia; preliminary report of a new operation.
Journ. Americ. Instit. Homeop. 25:813-825; y. 1932.

K. Henschen. Der interinguinale Querschnitt als Zugangschnitt zur Operation des ein-und beidseitigen Leistenbruches. Zur Frage der Gewebeschäden nach Lokalanästhesie.
Bruns Beitr. z. klin. Chir. 153:630-637; y. 1931.

E. M. Hodgkins. New method of treating the indirect sac in inguinal herniorrhaphy.
New England Journ. of Med. 206:1249-1252; y. 1932.

J. P. Hoguet. Direct inguinal hernia.
Ann. Surg 72:671-674; y. 1920.

P. Huet & S. Blondin. Sur un procédé myoplastique employant le muscle couturier, dans le traitement de certaines hernies inguinales.
Journ. de Chir. 35:22-32; y. 1930.

F. C. Jameson & J. Cantala. Relief of inguinal hernia without operation; successful use of Piña Mestre's method of subcutaneous injection in series of 64 cases.
Med. Journ. & Rec. 131:87-90; y. 1930.

E. S. Judd. A single transverse incision for use in double inguinal herniotomies.
Old Dominion Journ. Med. & Surg., Richmond, 16:153-156; y. 1913.

C. B. Keetley. Temporary fixation of testis to thigh. A series of twenty-five cases operated on for undescended testis.
Lancet II:279-281; y. 1905.

C. B. Keetley. "Exhibition of two cases of retained testis, illustrating a new mode of operating" in the Medical Society of London on April 16, 1894.
Lancet I:1008; y. 1894.

Kirschner. Eine in etwa 4500 Fällen verwendte Abart der Bassinischen Leistenbruchoperation.
Arch. f. klin. Chir. 175-357-366; y. 1933.

T. Kocher. Zur Radicalcur der Hernien.
Corr. Bl. f. Schweiz. Aerzte, 22:561-576; y. 1892.

J. J. Laméris. Zur Behandlung der indirekten Leistenhernie.
Deutsche Zeitschr. f. Chir. 119:569-580; y. 1912.

M. Langer. Über die Hernie und Hydrokele des Kindesalter.
Arch. f. klin. Chir. 181:418-426; y. 1934.

C. Lenormant. L'emploi des greffes aponévrotiques et périostiques dans la cure radicale des hernies volumineuses.
Presse Méd. 20:84-85; y. 1912.

J. Lucas-Championnière. Chirurgie opératoire. Cure radicale des hernies; avec une étude statistique de deux cents soixante-quinze operations.
Paris, Rueff et Cie, Publishers; y. 1892.

J. Lucas-Championnière. Sur la cure radicale des hernies.
Bull. et mém. Soc. de chir. de Paris, 13:737-742; y. 1887.

W. Macewen. On the radical cure of oblique inguinal hernia by internal abdominal peritoneal pad, and the restoration of the valved form of the inguinal canal.
Ann. Surg. 4:89-119; y. 1886.

W. W. MacGregor. Fundamental operative treatment of inguinal hernia.
Surg. Gyn. & Obst. 50:438-440; y. 1930.

H. O. Marcy. The cure of hernia by the antiseptic use of animal ligature.
Trans. VII Internat. Med. Congr. II:446; y. 1881.

P. Mendizabal. Procedimiento para erradicar facilmente el saco de la hernia inguinal.
Gac. méd. de México, 61:278-280; y. 1930.

H. Morestin. La cure esthétique des hernies.
Rev. de gynec. 9:69-84; y. 1905.

A. Moschcowitz & H. Neuhof. The relation of the iliohypogastric nerve to the radical cure of inguinal hernia.
Ann. Surg. 66:79-87; y. 1917.

A. Moschcowitz. Hernia. In Johnson's "Operative Therapeusis", 4:1-79.
Appleton & Co., Publishers; y. 1915.

B. dell'Oro. Un nuevo procedimiento operatorio para la cura de las hernias inguinales.
Rev. méd. del Rosario, 23:449-461; y. 1933.

S. Petrulis. Einige Modificationen in der Radikaloperation der Leisten-hernie.
Arch. f. klin. Chir. 71:937-954; y. 1903.

A. M. Phelps. The Phelps operation for hernia and method of closure of abdominal wounds.
Med. Rec. 58:441-443; y. 1900.

P. Postempski. Nuovo processo operativo per la cura radicale delle ernie inguinale.
Roma, I. Artero; y. 1891.

C. R. Robins. Rectus incision for reduction of strangulated hernia, with report of a case of strangulated hernia in the sac of an undescended testicle.
Old Dominion Journ. Med. & Surg. 8:324-326; y. 1909.

W. Schär. Spätresultate nach Radikaloperation des männlichen Leisten-bruches.
Deutsche Zeitschr. f. Chir. 243:96-117; y. 1934.

F. Schewket. Mein Verfahren bei der inguinalen Herniotomie.
Zbl. f. Chir. 57:649-650; y. 1930.

W. S. Schley. Transposition of the rectus muscle and the utilization of the external oblique aponeurosis in the radical cure of inguinal hernia.
Ann. Surg 77:605-611; y. 1923.

V. Schmieden. Zur Behandlung des Leistenbruches, ein neues Operation-sprinzip.
Arch. f. klin. Chir. 157:615-622; y. 1929.

P. Segond. Cure radicale des hernies.
Thèse de concours, Paris; y. 1883.
(Description of Lucas Championnière method).

R. V. Slattery. An operation for the radical cure of inguinal hernia.
Lancet, II:455; y. 1917.

A. Socin. Ueber Radicaloperation der Hernien.
Arch. f. klin. Chir. 24:391-398; y. 1879.

C. M. Squirru. La hernia inguinal simple.
Tesis, Buenos Aires; y. 1915.

D. Stetten. Further observations on a modified inguinal hernioplasty technic, with completed utilization of the aponeurosis of the external oblique.
Ann. Surg. 78:48-60; y. 1923.

E. L. Swift. A new form of operation for the cure of inguinal hernia.
New York Med. Journ. 66:553-555; y. 1897.

Franz Torek. The technique of orcheopexy.
New York Med. Journ. 90:948-953; y. 1909.

O. H. Wangensteen. Repair of recurrent and difficult hernias and other large defects of abdominal wall employing iliotibial tract of fascia lata as pedicled flap.
Surg. Gyn. & Obst. 59:766-780; y. 1934.

A. Wölfler. Zur Radikaloperation des freien Leistenbruches.
Beiträge z. Chirurgie Festschrift T. Billroth. pp. 552-603.
Stuttgart, f. Enke, Publishers; y. 1892.

G. Woolsey. An operation for the radical cure of inguinal hernia.
New York Med. Journ. 112:21-22; y. 1920.

FEMORAL HERNIA.

T. Annandale. A case in which a reducible oblique and direct inguinal and femoral hernia existed on the same side, and were successfully treated by operation.
Edinb. Med. Journ. 21:1087-1091; y. 1875.

N. Bardescu. Die Leistenmethode in der Operation der Schenkelbruche.
Arch. f. klin. Chir. 85:453-487; y. 1908.

E. Bassini. Nuovo metodo operativo per la cura radicale dell'ernia crurale.
Padova, A. Draghi; y. 1893.

E. H. Beckman. The repair of herniæ from the peritoneal side of the abdominal wall.
Ann. Surg. 55:570; y. 1912.

P. Berger. Hernies. In "Traité de chirurgíe". S. Duplay et P. Reclus.
Masson, Paris, 1892, VI:748-759.

M. Borchardt. Osteoplastischer Verschluss grosser Bruchpforten.
Bruns Beitr. z. klin. Chir. 20:305-314; y. 1898.

P. P. Cole. Radical cure of femoral hernia by the inguinal route.
Brit. Med. Journ. I:763-764; y. 1919.

W. B. Coley. The radical cure of femoral hernia.
Ann. Surg. 44:519-529; y. 1906.

G. P. Coopernail. Femoral hernia; review of operative technique and new method of repair.
Americ. Journ. of Surg. 22:458-460; y. 1933.

W. B. DeGarmo. The cure of femoral hernia; results of one hundred and ten operations by a single method.
Ann. Surg. 42:209-214; y. 1905.

W. B. DeGarmo. Abdominal hernia, its diagnosis and treatment.
Lippincott, Publishers; y. 1907.

G. Desbonnets & H. Desbonnets. La hernie crurale prévasculaire.
Journ. de Chir. 44:691-707; y. 1934.

C. Dujarier. Cure radicale de la hernie crurale par voie inguinale.
Journ. de Chir. 8-9:113-128; y. 1912.

R. Gőbell. Verbesserung der Lotheissen-Főderl'schen radikaloperation der Schenkelhernien durch Anwendung der freien Aponeurosentransplantation.
Zbl. f. Chir. 40:1255-1257; y. 1913.

A. Keith. The "saccular theory" of hernia.
Lancet, II:1398-1399; y. 1906.

G. Keynes. Prevascular femoral hernia.
Brit. Journ. of Surg. 20:55-57; y. 1932.

V. Kofmann. Eine Methode der Schliessung des Canalis femoralis beim Schenkelbruch.
Deutsche Zeitschr. f. Chir. 244:150-155; y. 1934.

Lamazov. Results of radical operation of femoral hernia after the method of Herzen.
Sovetsk. Khir. 4:676-680; y. 1933.

G. P. LaRoque. The intra-abdominal operation for femoral hernia.
Ann. Surg. 75:110-112; y. 1922.

G. P. LaRoque. Intra-abdominal method of removing inguinal and femoral hernia.
Arch. of Surg. 24:189-203; y. 1932.

G. Lotheissen. Zur Radikaloperation der Schenkelhernien.
   Zbl. f. Chir. 25:548-550; y. 1898.

A. V. Moschcowitz. Femoral hernia; a new operation for the radical cure.
   New York State Med. Journ. 7:396-400; y. 1907.

A. V. Moschcowitz. Prevascular femoral hernia.
   Ann. Surg. 55:848-856; y. 1912.

A. V. Moschcowitz. Hernia. In Johnson's "Operative Therapeusis",
   4:79-94; Appleton & Co., Publishers; y. 1915.

S. C. Plummer. Testing the viability of strangulated intestine.
   Surg. Gyn. Obst. 12:528-529; y. 1911.

E. A. Polya. Ein neues Verfahren zur Radikaloperation grosser Schenkelbruch.
   Zbl. f. Chir. 32:489-494; y. 1905.

A. Reich. Ueber die inguinale Radikaloperation der Schenkelbruche.
   Bruns Beitr. z. klin. Chir. 73:104-115; y. 1911.

G. Ruggi. Del metodo inguinale nella cura radicale dell ernia crurale.
   Bologna, N. Zanichelli; y. 1893.

F. A. Salzer. Ein Vorschlag zur Radikalheilung grosser Cruralhernien.
   Zbl. f. Chir. 19:665-669; y. 1892.

M. G. Seelig & L. Tuholske. The inguinal route operation for femoral
   hernia; with a supplementary note on Cooper's ligament.
   Surg. Gyn. & Obst. 18:55-62; y. 1914.

G. Serafini. Sulle varietà dell'ernia crurale e particolarmente sull'ernia
   crurale retro-vascolare intravaginale e sull'ernia pettinea.
   Policlinico (Sez. chir.), 24:230-232; 264-272; 273-283; y. 1917.

P. Sick. Radikaloperation des Schenkelbruchs durch Pektineusplastik.
   Münch. med Wchnschr. 58:1003-1005; y. 1911.

A. Socin. Ueber Radicaloperation der Hernien.
   Arch. f. klin. Chir. 24:391-398; y. 1879.

L. W. Tasche. Etiology of femoral hernia.
   Arch. of Surg. 25:749-782; y. 1932.

E. Tricomi. Nuovo metodo operativo per la cura radicale dell'ernia crurale.
   Riforma med. 7 (Part 2), pp. 556-558; y. 1891.

T. Tuffier. Opération de la hernie crurale par voie inguinale.
   Rev. de chir. 16:240-248; y. 1896.

Vallas & E. Perrin. Cure radicale de la hernie crurale par la voie inguinale,
   sans fermeture de l'anneau crural.
   Lyon Chirurg. I:757-766; y. 1908-1909.

L. F. Watson. Hernia. Pp. 289-326.
   C. V. Mosby Co., Publishers; y. 1924.

Wilms. Radikale Operationen des Schenkelbruches durch Faszienplastik.
   Münch. med. Wchnschr. 58:293; y. 1911.

O. Zuckerkandl. Anatomischer Beitrag zur Operationstechnik bei Schenkelhernien.
Arch. f. klin. Chir. 28:214-216; y. 1883.

UMBILICAL HERNIA.

G. Alder. Ueber Nabelschnurbruche.
Inaug. Diss. Zurich; y. 1904.

A. J. Bengolea. Una nueva técnica para la cura radical de las hernias umbilicales en el adulto.
Prensa méd. argentina, Buenos Aires; IV:365; y. 1917-1918.

J. A. Blake. The operative treatment of umbilical hernia in adults.
Medic. Record, 59:803-807; y. 1901.

R. Condamin. De l'omphalectomie et de la suture à trois étages dans la cure radicale de hernies ombilicales; étude des indications et de quelques procédés opératoires récents.
Arch. prov. de chir. I:193-321; y. 1892.

J. Dauriac. Procédé nouveau pour la cure radicale de la hernie ombilicale (procédé de l'entrecroisement des droits).
Gaz. de hôp. 67:675-676; y. 1894.

W. B. DeGarmo. Abdominal hernia, its diagnosis and treatment.
Lippincott, Publishers; y. 1907.

W. Denk. Zur Operativen Behandlung der Hernia permagna irreponibilis.
Deutsch. Zeitschr. f. Chir. 176:399-401; y. 1922.

F. G. DuBose. A new operation for umbilical hernia.
Surg. Gyn. Obst. 21:771-773; y. 1915.

A. H. Ferguson. Modern operations for hernia.
Chicago, Cleveland Press; y. 1907.

A. Goldspohn. Large ventral and umbilical herniæ in the adult, with three cases of radical cure by an improved technique.
Americ. Gynæc. & Obst. Journ. XI:301-320; y. 1897.

M. A. Gorelow. Zur Anatomie des Nabelkanals.
Arch. f. klin. Chir. 181:395-405; y. 1934.

J. Hahn. Die radical operation der Ueberhernien mit Hülfe der systematischen Dehnung der Bauchdecken.
Arch. f. klin. Chir. 85:718-741; y. 1908.

N. J. MacLean. The extreme pendulous abdomen and its surgical treatment by a new three-flap operation.
Surg. Gyn. Obst. 28:190-194; y. 1919.

J. F. C. H. Macready. A treatise on ruptures.
C. Griffin & Co., Publishers, Lond.; y. 1893.

W. J. Mayo. Remarks on the radical cure of hernia.
Ann. Surg. 29:51-61; y. 1899.

W. J. Mayo. Further experience with the vertical overlapping operation for the radical cure of umbilical hernia.
Journ. Americ. Med. Ass. 41:225-228; y. 1903.

A. V. Moschcowitz. The pathogenesis of umbilical hernia.
Ann. Surg. 61:570-581; y. 1915.

A. V. Moschcowitz. Hernia. In Johnson's "Operative Therapeusis". 4:94-101.
Appleton & Co., Publishers; y. 1915.

N. Niwase. Position of the navel of man.
Am. Journ. Obst. 80:49-52; y. 1919.

C. P. Noble. Overlapping the aponeuroses in the closure of wounds of the abdominal wall—including umbilical, ventral and inguinal herniæ.
Ann. Surg. 43:349-358; y. 1906.

E. Piccoli. Zur Radikalbehandlung der Nabelhernien.
Zbl. f. Chir. 27:36-38; y. 1900.

J. H. Pringle. A method of treating umbilical hernia.
Edinb. Med. Journ. 10:493-496; y. 1913.

J. Ransohoff. The radical cure of umbilical hernia by omphalectomy.
Med. Rec. 51:150-152; y. 1897.

K. Sapiejko. Un nouveau procédé de cure radicale des grandes hernies ombilicales avec diastase des muscles grands droits.
Rev. de Chir. 21:241-261; y. 1900.

G. C. Stewart. Hernia of the umbilical cord.
Brit. Med. Journ. I:247; y. 1905.

H. B. Storer. A new operation for umbilical hernia.
Med. Rec. 1:73-76; y. 1866-1867.

O. Vulpius. Die Radikaloperation der Hernien in der vorderen Bauchwand.
Bruns Beitr. z. klin. Chirurgie, 7:91-134; y. 1890-1891.

L. F. Watson. Hernia; pp. 327-365.
C. V. Mosby Co., Publishers; y. 1924.

J. Wood. On rupture.
J. W. Davies, London, p. 251-257; y. 1863.

VENTRAL HERNIA.

W. S. Bainbridge. Multiple herniæ.
Post-Graduate, N. Y. 20:136-138; y. 1905.

M. Barthélemy. Les hernies abdominales latérales.
Bull. et mém. Soc. de chir. de Paris, 45:1313-1319; y. 1919.

A. D. Bevan. Postoperative ventral hernia.
Surg. Clin. of Chicago, 4:775-781; y. 1920.

C. Blauel. Zur Ætiologie der seitlichen Bauchbruche.
Bruns Beitr. z. klin. Chir. 54:229-237; y. 1907.

W. Capelle. Dauerresultate nach operationen der hernia epigastrica.
Beitr. z. klin. Chir. 63:264-285; y. 1909.

C. Clavel & P. Colson. A propos de la cure opératoire des éventrations post-appendiculaires (contribution à la technique).
Journ. de Chir. 43:677-693; y. 1934.

J. Cloquet. Recherches sur les causes et l'anatomie des hernies abdominales.
Thèse, Paris; y. 1817.

W. Denk. Zur Pathologie und Therapie der Brüche der vorderen Bauchwand.
Arch. f. klin. Chir. 93:711-728; y. 1910.

V. Pérez Fontana. Anatomia quirúrgica de la hernia epigástrica.
Rev. de cir. de Buenos Aires, 13:1-23; y. 1934.

C. L. Gibson. Repair of large incisional ventral herniæ by pedunculated flaps of fascia.
Ann. Surg. 65:761-762; y. 1917.

E. Graser. Zur Technik der Radicaloperation grosser Nabel- und Bauchwandhernien.
Arch. f. klin. Chir. 80:324-349; y. 1906.

I. S. Haynes. The treatment of large ventral hernia by inversion of the hernial sac; with or without opening into the peritoneal cavity.
N. Y. State Journ. Med. 13:630-637; y. 1913.

M. M. Janow. Typen der vorderen Bauchwand und der Abdominalbrüche als Symptom der anatomischen Konstitution.
Arch. f. klin. Chir. 156:533-549; y. 1929.

F. Kőnig. Die Radikaloperation grosser Hernien, besonders der Bauchbruche, unter Verlötung mit frei verpflanzten Periostlappen.
Bruns Beitr. z. klin. Chir. 75:797-811; y. 1911.

J. F. C. H. Macready. A treatise on ruptures.
C. Griffin & Co., Publishers, London; y. 1893.

R. T. Morris. Hernia of the falciform ligament.
West. Med. Times, 39:359:360; y. 1919-1920.

H. B. Robinson. Hernia through the semilunar line.
Brit. Journ. Surg. 2:336-337; y. 1914-1915.

Roth. Ueber die Hernien der linea alba.
Arch. f. klin. Chir. 42:1-45; y. 1891.

E. Rouffart. De la valeur des différentes incisions dans les laparotomies en gynecologie et en obstétrique.
Arch. mens. d'obst. et de gynéc. II:577-622; y. 1919.

A. Stűhmer. Ueber die Hernien der Bauchwand seitlich der Mittellinie unter besonderer Berücksichtigung der Hernien der Linea semilunaris (Spiegelii).
Bruns Beitr. z. klin. Chir. 66:113-135; y. 1910.

L. Thévenot & T. Gabourd. Les hernies spontanées du repli semilunaire de Spiegel.
  Rev. de Chir. 35:568-585; y. 1907.

Villard. Pathogénie des hernies épigastriques.
  Lyon méd. 120:26-29; y. 1913.

T. Voeckler. Ueber eine bisher unbeschriebene Bruchform der Linea alba (Hernia lineæ albæ suprapubica).
  Deutsch. Ztschr. f. Chir. 117:582-598; y. 1912.

O. Vulpius. Die Radikaloperation der Hernien in der vorderen Bauchwand.
  Bruns Beitr. z. klin. Chir. 7:91-134; y. 1890.

L. F. Watson. Hernia. Pp. 336-399.
  C. V. Mosby Co., Publishers; y. 1924.

O. Witzel. Über den medianen Bauchbruch.
  Samml. klin. Vortr. Chir. n. f. (1-25) Leipz.
  y. 1890, pp. 45-68.

DIAPHRAGMATIC HERNIA.

M. Auvray. Hernie diaphragmatique de l'estomac, du côlon transverse et de l'epiploon, consécutive à une plaie thoraco-abdominale ancienne. Intervention. Guérison.
  Bull. et mém. Soc. de chir. de Paris, 45:698-709; y. 1919.

N. R. Barrett & C. E Wheaton. Pathology, diagnosis and treatment of congenital diaphragmatic hernia in infants.
  Brit. Journ. of Surg. 21:420-433; y. 1934.

S. Bayne-Jones. Eventration of the diaphragm.
  Arch. Int. Med. 17:221-237; y. 1916.

A. Blum & L. Ombrédanne. Hernies diaphragmatiques d'origine traumatique.
  Arch. gén. de méd. I:5-23 and 178-196; y. 1896.

V. A. Bochdalek. Einige Betrachtungen über die entstehung des angeborenen zwerchfellbruches. Als Beitrag zur pathologischen Anatomie der Hernien.
  Vrtljschr. f. d. prakt. Heilk. III:89-97; y. 1848.

D. J. Cranwell. Diagnostic et traitement de la hernie diaphragmatique.
  Rev. de Chir. 37:33-54; y. 1908.

T. Dunhill. Diaphragmatic hernia (Arris and Gale lecture).
  Brit. Journ. of Surg. 22:475-499; y. 1935.

A. W. Fischer. Über die Hernien am Hiatus oesophagei.
  Arch. f. klin. Chir. 178:274-287; y. 1933.

C. A. Hedblom. Diagnosis and treatment of diaphragmatic hernia with special reference to selective surgical treatment.
  South. Surgeon, 1:275-286; y. 1933.

E. L. Jenkinson. Absence of half of the diaphragm; thoracic stomach; diaphragmatic hernia.
Americ. Journ. of Roentgenol. 26:899-903; y. 1931.

L. Lacher. Ueber Zwerchfellshernien.
Inaug. Diss. Leipzig; y. 1880.

F. Nord. Phrenic neurectomy as treatment of diaphragmatic hernia.
Acta med. Scandinav. 72:511-526; y. 1919.

G. Paillard. Les variétés anatomiques de la hernie diaphragmatique congénitale.
Thèse, Paris; y. 1903.

L. Prat. Hernies diaphragmatiques.
Journ. de Chir. Paris, 16:43-65; y. 1920.

C. Rauert. Ueber Zwerchfallshernien (Freiburg).
Inaug. Diss. Hanover; y. 1900.

J. Sailer & R. D. Rhein. Eventration of the diaphragm, with a report of a case.
Amer. Journ. Med. Sc. n. s. 129:688-705; y. 1905.

A. Schwartz & J. Quénu. Le traitement des hernies diaphragmatiques (technique opératoire).
Paris méd. 33:162-165; y. 1919.

A. L. Soresi. Diaphragmatic hernia.
Ann. Surg. 69:255-270; y. 1919.

R. Thoma. Vier Fälle von Hernia diaphragmatica.
Virchow Arch. f. pathol. Anat. und Physiologie.
88:515-555; y. 1882.

P. E. Truesdale. Diaphragmatic hernia; the thoracic approach.
Ann. of Surg. 74:347-354; y. 1921.

L. F. Watson. Hernia; pp. 400-425.
C. V. Mosby Co., Publishers; y. 1924.

HERNIA OF THE LARGE INTESTINE.

A. Baumgartner. Les hernies par glissement du gros intestin.
Thése, Paris; y. 1905.

A. Brenner. Radicaloperationen bei Leistenhernien.
Arch. f. klin. Chir. 79:1080-1105; y. 1906.

C. Brunner. Herniologische Beobachtungen.
Beitr. z. klin. Chir. 4:1-39; y. 1888-1889.

J. B. Carnett. Inguinal hernia of the cæcum.
Ann. Surg. 49:491-515; y. 1909.

C. H. Criley. Parasaccular or sliding hernia.
Surg. Gyn. Obst. 31:611-616; y. 1920.

H. Duret. Des variétés rares de la hernie inguinale.
Thèse de concours, Paris; y. 1885.

H. Finsterer. Zur Kenntniss der Gleitbrüche des Dickdarmes.
Beitr. z. klin. Chir. 81:198-239; y. 1912.

Hildebrand. Die Lageverhältniss des Cŏcum und ihre Beziehung zur Entstehung von äusseren Cŏcalbrüchen.
Deutsch. Zeitschr. f. Chir. 33:182-213; y. 1891-1892.

H. Hilgenreiner. Seltene und bemerkenswerte Hernien.
Bruns Beitr. z. klin. Chir. 69:333-430; y. 1910.

L. W. Hotchkiss. Large sliding hernias of the sigmoid.
Ann. of Surg. 50:470-473; y. 1909.

G. S. Huntington. The anatomy of the human peritoneum.
Lea Bros., Publishers, Philadelphia; y. 1903.

W. C. G. Kirchner. The treatment of sliding hernia.
Am. Journ. of Obst. 64:758-768; y. 1911.

G. Labat. Cure radicale de la hernie du colon "par glissement".
Presse méd. 27:182-184; y. 1919.

G. Lardennois & J. Okinczyc. Etude sur les hernies du gros intestin.
Paris, Masson; y. 1910.

C. Lenormant. La colopexie; contribution l'étude thérapeutique du prolapsus du rectum.
Rev. de Chir. 35:191-216; y. 1907.

P. Lesshaft. Die Lumbalgegend in anatomisch-chirurgischer Hinsicht.
Arch. f. Anat. u Physiol. u. Wissensch. Med. Leipzig, pp. 264-299; y. 1870.

H. Morestin. Hernies par glissement de l'Siliaque et de l'iléon.
Bull. et mém. Soc. de chir. de Paris, n. s. 36:709-714; y. 1910.

A. V. Moschcowitz. Hernia of the large intestine with special reference to "sliding hernia".
Ann. of Surg. 59:610-620; y. 1914.

A. V. Moschcowitz. Hernia. In Johnson's "Operative Therapeusis". 4:72-79;
Appleton & Co. Publishers; y. 1915.

J. L. Ransohoff. Adherent hernias of the large intestine.
Ann. Surg. 56:313-327; y. 1912.

E. Rochard. Les hernies.
Paris, O. Doin; y. 1904.

Savariaud. Hernie par glissement de l'Siliaque. Procédé nouveau de cure radicale.
Bull. et mém. Soc. anat. de Paris, 26 (part II):772-777; y. 1900.

F. C. Shulz. Ueber Gleitbruche und über grosse Leistenhernien.
Arch. f. klin. Chir. 98:324-354; y. 1912.

Sprengel. Erfahrungen über den Gleitbruch des Dickdarms.
Arch. f. klin. Chir. 95:702-737; y. 1911.

J. Symington. The relations of the peritoneum to the descending colon
in the human subject.
Journ. Anat. & Physiol. 26:530-537; y. 1891-1892.

F. Treves. Hernia of the cæcum.
Brit. Med. Journ. I:382-385; y. 1887.

A. J. Walton. Extrasaccular hernia.
Ann. Surg 57:86-105; y. 1913.

L. F. Watson. Hernia. Pp. 499-526.
C. V. Mosby Co., Publishers; y. 1924.

CHAPTER XXV.

GYNECOLOGICAL OPERATIONS.

A. SURGICAL ANATOMY OF THE UTERUS AND ADNEXA (FIGS. 333 AND 334).

The **uterus** is a hollow muscular organ lying in the pelvic cavity between the bladder anteriorly and the rectum posteriorly. The normal uterus is 8 cm. in length, 5 cm. in width, (in the widest portion), and its

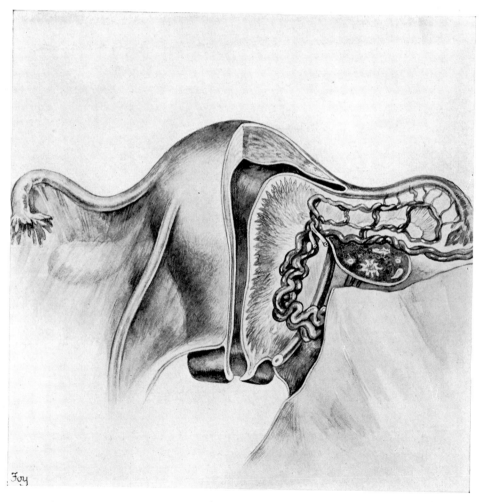

FIG. 333. UTERUS.
Anterior view.
666

maximum thickness is about 2½ cm. The uterus is subdivided into the fundus, corpus and cervix.

The **fundus** is that portion of the uterus which lies above the line connecting the points of entrance of each Fallopian tube into the uterus.

The **corpus** is the portion of the uterus lying below the line connecting

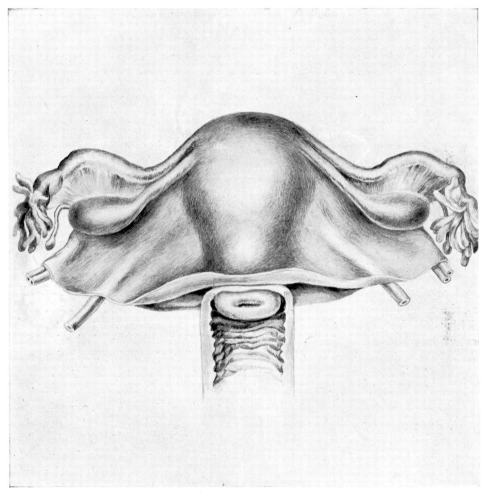

FIG. 334. UTERUS.
Posterior view (After Rauber).

the points of entrance of each tube into the uterus. It has two surfaces: the anterior or the vesical and the posterior or the intestinal.

The **cervix** uteri is cylindrical. It is about one inch long. Its inferior end protrudes into the vagina, so that a portion of the cervix is **supravaginal** and the rest is **intravaginal**. At the point where the supravaginal portion enters the vagina it is attached to its margin. In the vaginal portion of the cervix lies its opening, the **external orifice,** through which the cervical canal and the uterine cavity are connected with the vagina. The opening of the external orifice of the cervix is formed by two lips, the **anterior** and the **posterior.** At the inner end of the cervix lies the opening which connects the cervix with the uterus. It is the **internal orifice** of the cervix and it lies in the supravaginal portion. The peritoneum covers the fundus and the corpus uteri until the bladder is reached. Then it leaves the uterus, being reflected on the bladder to form the **uterovesical fold.** From each side of the upper portion of the uterus extends a **uterine tube** (Fallopian tube, O.T.), which conveys the oöcytes to the cavity of the uterus. Each tube is about four inches long. It opens into the pelvic cavity at one end (abdominal ostium) near the ovary, and into the uterine cavity at the other end (uterine ostium).

The abdominal end of the tube is also called the **fimbriated end** because of numerous irregular small projections which surround this end and which are called fimbriæ. Each tube is subdivided into the **infundibulum** (the lateral portion of which is the fimbriated end), the **ampulla** (which forms the largest portion of the tube), the **isthmus** (which joins the lateral angle of the uterus), and the **uterine portion** (pars uterina), which traverses the thickness of the uterine wall and enters the cavity of the uterus. The abdominal ostium is 2mm. wide and the uterine ostium is only 1mm. wide. Therefore, probing of these openings is not an easy matter.

The **ovaries,** two in number, are almond-shape and they are about one and one-half inches long, and about half an inch in thickness. They lie against the lateral wall of the pelvis. They are connected by peritoneal folds with the pelvic wall and with the broad ligament of the uterus. Each ovary has two extremities—the superior (or the tubal) and the inferior (or the uterine). The tubal extremity adjoins the Fallopian tube, and the uterine extremity is connected with the body of the uterus by a fibrous band—the **ligamentum ovarii proprium.**

The ovary is connected with the lateral pelvic wall by a peritoneal fold, the **suspensory ligament** of the ovary, which becomes the superior and lateral portion of the broad ligament of the uterus. In this place between the leaflets of the broad ligament are situated the ovarian vessels and the sympathetic plexus which traverse them from the lateral pelvic wall until they reach the hilum of the ovary. The ovary is connected with the posterior aspect of the broad ligament by a very short peritoneal fold—the **meso-ovary, so that the ovary lies behind the two leaflets of the broad ligament.**

The **broad ligament** of the uterus is a paired peritoneal fold which extends between the lateral border of the uterus and the pelvic wall on each side. It consists of two leaflets—the anterior and the posterior. It embraces in its upper border the tube, which it invests on all sides. This portion is called the **mesosalpinx.** The portion of the broad ligament below the mesosalpinx is termed the **mesometrium. The ureter and the uterine**

vessels traverse the lower portion of the mesometrium in the region where the mesometrium joins the pelvic floor. Between the layers of the mesometrium, close to the cervix uteri on each side, is a mass of fibrous and muscular tissue which is termed the **lateral cervical ligament.**

The round ligament of the uterus is a paired cord-like structure each of which is attached to the body of the uterus slightly below the opening of the tube into the uterus. It extends in front of the anterior leaflet of the broad ligament in a forward and lateral direction, crosses the brim of the pelvis and enters the inguinal canal. It traverses this through its entire length, leaves it through the subcutaneous inguinal ring, and ends in the skin and the subcutaneous tissue of the labium majus on each side.

B. OPERATIONS FOR RETRODISPLACEMENT OF THE UTERUS.

Numerous operations have been suggested for the correction of uterine retrodisplacement. They differ from each other either by the method of approach (incision of the inguinal canal, celiotomy through a midline incision, vaginal approach), by the structures which serve for fixation (the body of the uterus, the round ligament, the broad ligament), and by the structures to which they are attached (anterior abdominal wall, hammock-like position of the round ligament).

F. F. Simpson groups all the different methods of fixation into the following:

1. Inguinal shortening of the round ligaments.
2. Vaginal shortening of the round ligaments.
3. Intra-abdominal shortening of the round ligaments.
4. Attachment of the round ligaments posterior to the uterus.
5. Attaching the uterus to the anterior abdominal wall firmly, loosely or indirectly.
6. Transperitoneal shortening of the round ligaments.
7. Retroperitoneal shortening of the round ligaments.
8. Shortening of the sacro-uterine ligaments through the abdomen or vagina.
9. Transverse attachment of the base of the broad ligaments in front of the cervix.
10. Intraperitoneal shortening of the round and broad ligaments.

Of the numerous methods suggested only a few are employed today.

1. GILLIAM OPERATION.

This operation consists in grasping the round ligament on each side, bringing it through a perforation made in the anterior abdominal wall, and suturing the protruded portion of the ligament to the anterior sheath of the rectus muscle.

Technic.

Step 1. A temporary ligature is placed around the round ligament of each side at a distance of about one to one and one-half inches from its attachment to the uterus. The thread is clamped by an artery-forceps (Fig. 335).

Step 2. A small incision about one inch long is made through the anterior sheath of the rectus muscle, the rectus muscle itself, and the

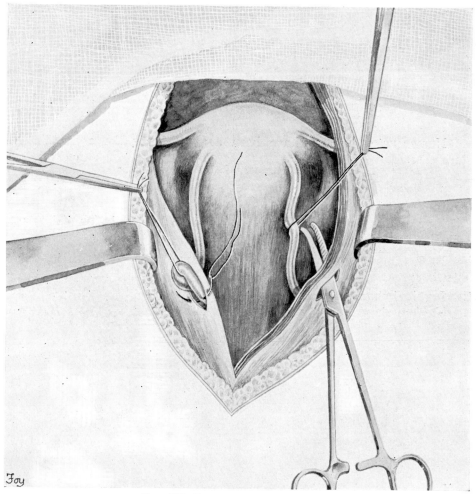

FIG. 335. FIXATION OF THE UTERUS.
Gilliam Method.

transversalis fascia and peritoneum at a distance of one and one-half inches above the pubic bone and one inch lateral from the midline incision. An ordinary forceps is inserted into this opening from without inward, which grasps the thread and brings it and the round ligament outside. The same is done on the other side.

Step 3. The loop of each round ligament is sutured to the aponeurosis of the rectus muscle of the corresponding side.

Step 4. The abdomen is closed in layers.

In this operation the uterus is held forward by strong fibrous round ligaments. This hold is stronger than the normal hold in the healthy

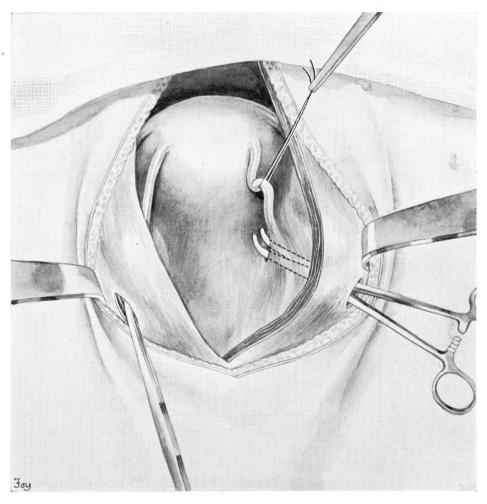

FIG. 336. FIXATION OF THE UTERUS.
Simpson-Montgomery Method.

female, which is a lateral one. The only objection to this method is that the opening between the internal inguinal ring and the round ligament may become the seat into which a loop of bowel may slip and produce internal strangulation. Nevertheless, this is an excellent method and is used more frequently than any other method.

2. SIMPSON-MONTGOMERY METHOD (FIG. 336).

This method, which may be characterized as a **subperitoneal transplantation of the round ligament with a forward pull,** was described by Simpson, of Pittsburg, in 1902, and later modified by Montgomery, of Philadelphia, in 1904, so that the description below is actually Montgomery's modification of the Simpson method.

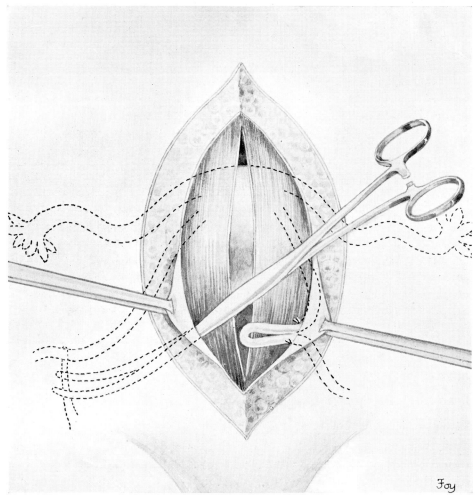

Fig. 337. Fixation of the Uterus.
Barrett Method.

The technic of this modification is as follows:

Step 1. A temporary ligature is passed around the round ligament at a distance of one and a half inches from the uterus.

Step 2. The skin of the abdominal wound is retracted until the outer edge of the anterior sheath of the rectus muscle is reached. The anterior sheath is incised for a length of half an inch at the outer edge of the rectus muscle. A clamp then penetrates a part of the thickness of the anterior abdominal wall down to (but not through) the peritoneum. Then it passes between the leaflets of the broad ligament until the place is reached where the round ligament was ligated. At this point the forceps penetrates the leaflet of the broad ligament, grasps the thread and carries it with the round ligament along the track made by the forceps until the loop of the round ligament appears external to the anterior sheath of the rectus muscle. Here it is fastened to the slit in the anterior sheath. The same is done on the other side.

3.   BARRETT METHOD (FIG. 337).

This technic has several points in common with the Simpson-Montgomery method. The characteristic feature of this method is that **the round ligament is transplanted intramurally with a lateral pull.**

Step 1. A temporary ligature is placed around the round ligament at a distance of two and a half inches from the uterus.

Step 2. A curved artery-forceps enters the abdominal wall at the median incision behind the anterior sheath of the rectus muscle and passes along the wall until the internal inguinal ring is reached. Then the forceps is thrust through the peritoneum, grasps the ligature and carries it together with the round ligament back until it appears in the midline beneath the anterior sheath of the rectus muscle. The same is done on the other side. Each loop of the round ligament is sutured to the under surface of the anterior sheath of its respective side at a distance of about one inch from the median line.

In this method the forward pull is replaced by a lateral pull. It does not offer such a strong hold as a forward pull, but strong enough to keep the uterus in its new position. At the same time there are no rings formed (as in the Gilliam method) in which a loop of bowel may become strangulated. This is an excellent method of fixation of the uterus.

4.   WEBSTER-BALDY OPERATION (FIG. 338).

This operation was described by Webster, of Chicago, in 1901, and by Baldy, of Philadelphia, in 1902. In France it is known as the "Dartigue operation". However, the latter practised this operation only since 1905, and his first report of it appeared in April, 1906 (Presse Médicale, April 7, 1906). Therefore, neither in time of operation nor in time of first publication can the priority be attributed to him.

Technic.

Step 1. A curved artery-forceps penetrates the broad ligament from behind forward immediately below the utero-ovarian ligament. It then grasps the round ligament and draws it through the rent in the broad ligament. The same is done on the other side. The ligaments are grasped one to two inches from the uterus.

Step 2. The round ligament of each side is sutured to the posterior wall of the uterus and to each other in the midline. The round ligament should also be sutured to the broad ligament at the point where it passes through the opening in the ligament.

In this method, the uterus rests as on a hammock and no free bands

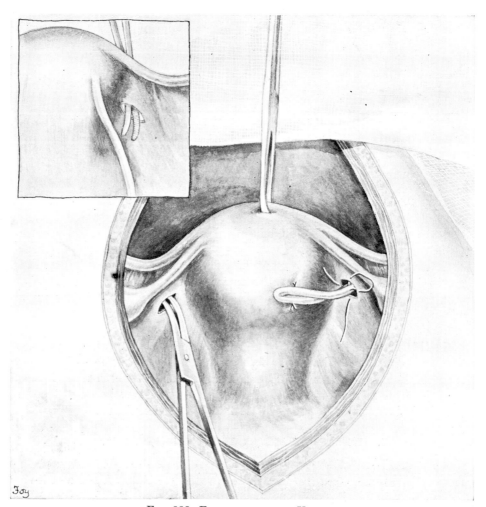

FIG. 338. FIXATION OF THE UTERUS.
Baldy-Webster Method.

are left in the abdominal cavity, so that there is no danger of intestinal obstruction. However, the hold of the uterus is not very strong.

In the following group of operations known as **ventro-fixation,** the uterus is attached to the anterior abdominal wall either by including in the bite only the muscle of the fundus uteri (Leopold technic), the muscle of the anterior surface of the fundus with the round ligament (Olshausen technic), or the muscle of the posterior surface of the fundus with the utero-ovarian ligament (Kelly technic).

5. LEOPOLD TECHNIC (FIG. 339, a).

Step 1. A bite is taken through one lip of the anterior abdominal wall (except the skin), at a distance of two inches above the pubic bone. It then passes through the muscle of the posterior wall of the fundus uteri,

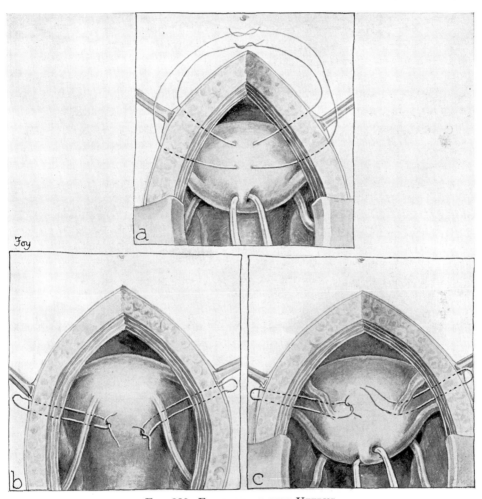

FIG. 339. FIXATION OF THE UTERUS.
a. Leopold Method.
b. Olshausen Method.
c. Kelly Method.

and then through the entire thickness of the other abdominal lip (except the skin). The same procedure is repeated at a distance of one inch below the place in which the first suture was inserted. The ends of the sutures are tied and cut short.

6. OLSHAUSEN TECHNIC (FIG. 339, b).

Step 1. A bite is taken through the anterior surface of the wall of the fundus so as to include the round ligament, then through the entire thickness of one of the lips of the anterior abdominal wall (except the skin), then back through the anterior abdominal wall of the same side, and the ends are tied within the abdominal cavity. The same is done on the other side.

7. KELLY TECHNIC (FIG. 339, c).

Step 1. This is done in a manner analogous to the Olshausen operation with this difference, that the portion of the posterior wall of the uterus with the utero-ovarian ligament is included instead of the anterior wall with the round ligament.

All the methods of ventro-fixation are contra-indicated when future pregnancy is possible.

C. SALPINGECTOMY, OÖPHORECTOMY, SALPINGO-OÖPHORECTOMY.

I. SALPINGECTOMY.

Definition

This term consists of two Greek words: σάλπιγζ, the tube and ἐκτομή, excision. It signifies: the excision of a tube.

Indications.

    a. Pyosalpinx.
    b. Hematosalpinx.
    c. Tuberculosis of the tubes.
    d. Malignancy (carcinoma of the tubes).
    e. Ectopic pregnancy.

Technic.

Step 1. The abdomen is opened by a longitudinal or a transverse (Pfannenstiel) incision. The patient is placed in the Trendelenburg position.

Step 2. The edge of the mesosalpinx is grasped between the fimbriated end of the tube and the ovary. Thus, the tube is placed on a stretch (Fig. 340, insert).

Step 3. An arterial forceps clamps the mesosalpinx along its entire length, which is now cut between the clamp and the tube (Fig. 340).

Step 4. An incision is made around the corner of the fundus of the uterus just beyond the tubo-uterine junction.

Step 5. The mesosalpinx and the open end of the uterus are closed by a continuous suture **starting at the lateral edge of the mesosalpinx.** Thus, the uterine portion is sutured last (Fig. 341).

The suturing line of the angle of the uterus is reinforced by another layer of sutures.

II. OÖPHORECTOMY (FIG. 342).

Definition.

This term consists of 3 Greek words: ῷόν, egg, φέρειν, to bear, and ἐκτομή, excision. It signifies the excision of an ovary.

This operation was first performed by Ephraim McDowell, in 1809.

Indications.

      a. Neoplasm of the ovary.

      b. Infection of the ovary.

      c. Chronic inflammation of the ovary.

      d. Degeneration of the ovary.

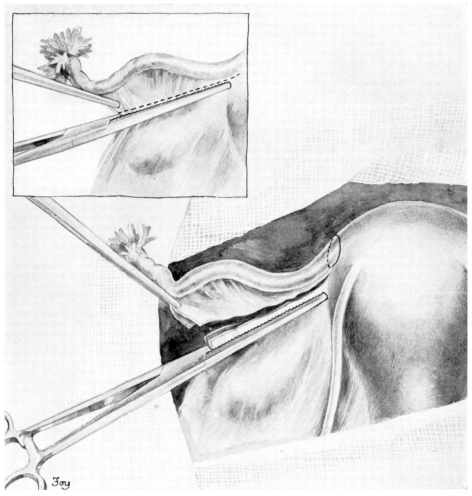

FIG. 340. SALPINGECTOMY.
INSERT. The mesosalpinx is clamped.
MAIN PICTURE. The mesosalpinx is cut. The tube is ready to be cut at the utero-tubal junction.

Technic.

Step 1. The abdomen is opened by a longitudinal or a transverse incision. The patient is placed in the Trendelenburg position.

Step 2. The ovary is lifted. One artery-forceps clamps the ligamentum ovarii proprium with the adjoining portion of the mesovarium (on the uterine side), and another clamps the fimbria ovarica with the adjoining portion of the mesovarium (on the lateral side) (Fig. 342). The mesovarium is cut between the clamps and ovary, and is sutured over the clamps by a running suture (Fig. 342).

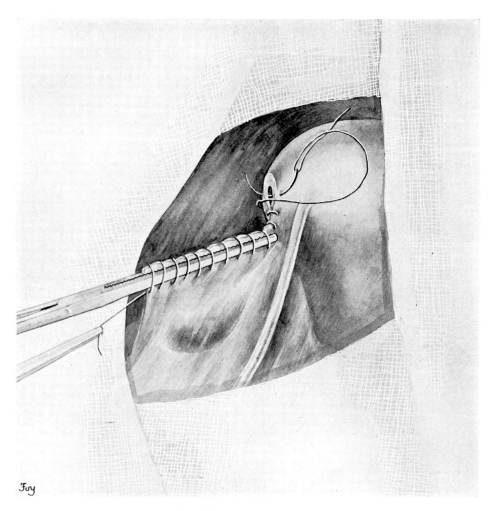

FIG. 341. SALPINGECTOMY.
The mesosalpinx is sutured over the clamp; the cornu uteri is in process of closure.

However, as far as possible an attempt should be made to preserve at least a part of the ovary, and whenever possible to do a resection of the ovary instead of an oöphorectomy.

III. SALPINGO-OÖPHORECTOMY (FIG. 343).

This consists in the removal of both the tube and the ovary (on one or on both sides).

Technic.

Step 1. The abdomen is opened by a midline or transverse incision. The patient is placed in the Trendelenburg position.

Step 2. The fundus uteri is located as a starting point, and from it begins the search for the tube and the ovary, which when found are

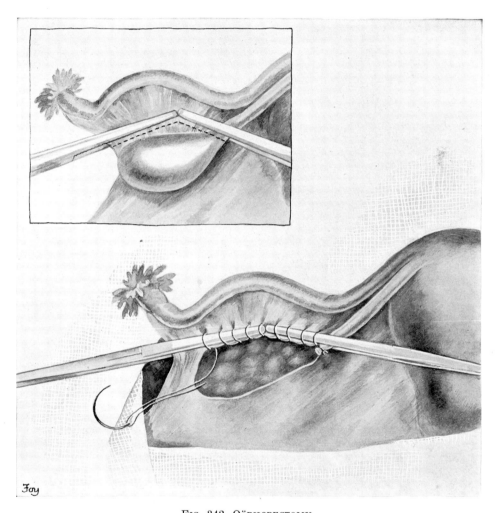

FIG. 342. OÖPHORECTOMY.
INSERT. The mesovarium and the ligamentum ovarii proprium are clamped.
MAIN PICTURE. Suturing the mesovarium over the clamps.

separated from their adhesions. The infundibulopelvic ligament is clamped by two arterial forceps at a point midway between the fimbriated end of the tube and the brim of the pelvis, and is cut between the forceps. The utero-ovarian ligament (ligamentum ovarii proprium) is clamped by two arterial forceps and cut between them. The tube is then removed in the same manner as described under "salpingectomy" (Fig. 340). The infundi-bulo-pelvic ligament is ligated by a transfixing suture. The cornu uteri is sutured in two layers. The ligamentum ovarii proprium is ligated. The two leaflets of the broad ligament are united to each other by a continuous suture.

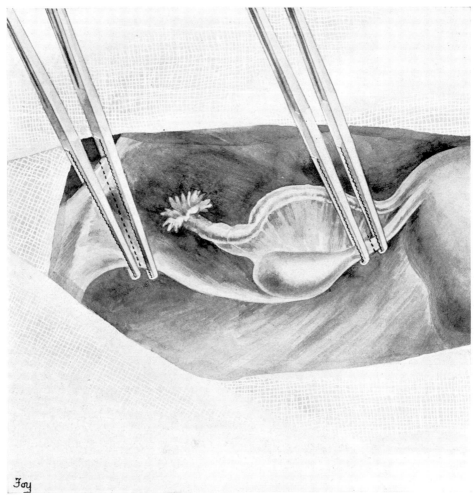

FIG. 343. SALPINGO-OÖPHORECTOMY.
The infundibulopelvic ligament and the ligament. ovarii proprium are clamped each by a pair of arterial forceps.

D.   OPERATIONS DEALING WITH STERILITY.

These include:
    a. Operations for the correction of sterility.
    b. Operations producing sterility.

a. OPERATIONS FOR THE CORRECTION OF STERILITY.

Here we discuss only some of those operative procedures which are employed in the cases in which sterility is due to occlusion of the Fallopian tubes. Occlusion of the fimbriated ends gives the best prognosis from the

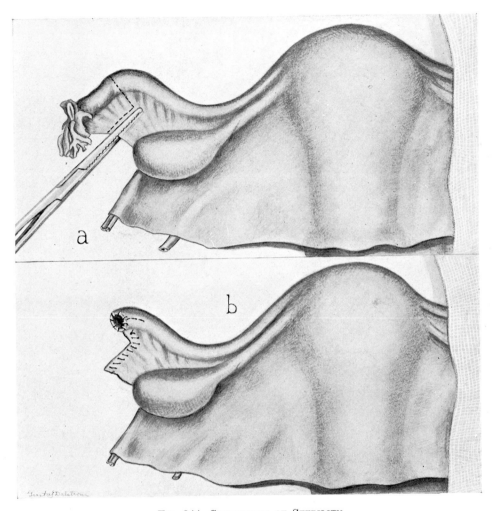

FIG. 344. CORRECTION OF STERILITY.
a. The fimbriated end of the tube is ready to be removed.
b. The fimbriated end is removed; the lumen of the tube is enlarged.

standpoint of overcoming the sterility. Occlusion of the isthmic portions gives a very bad prognosis. In case both tubes are occluded in the isthmus and in which neither can be opened by inflation of air, transplantation of the undamaged portion of the tubes into the fundus uteri may be resorted to with some hope of success.

In case of occlusion of the fimbriated end of the tube the technic is as follows (Fig. 344):

Step 1. The mesosalpinx is grasped by an artery-forceps close to the fimbriated end. The tube is freed from the mesosalpinx along the entire

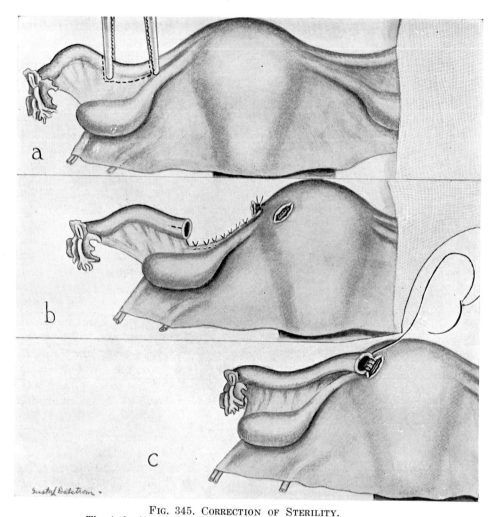

FIG. 345. CORRECTION OF STERILITY.
a. The isthmic portion of the tube is ready to be excised;
b. The isthmic portion of the tube is removed.
c. Implantation of the fimbriated end of the tube into the uterus.

length of its diseased portion. All bleeders are checked. The tube is amputated at the portion where the wall is healthy.

Step 2. A longitudinal incision is made in the tube on its free border (that is on the border opposite to the attachment of the mesosalpinx) for a distance of half an inch, and the angle is rounded. Thus, the lumen of the opening becomes increased. The edges of the wound are whipped over by fine catgut.

In case of occlusion of the isthmus of the tube the technic is as follows:

Step 1. The mesosalpinx is grasped by an artery-forceps close to the fimbriated end. The tube is placed on a stretch and is then clamped by two artery-forceps just lateral to the diseased isthmic portion. It is cut between the clamps. The isthmic portion is ligated (or it may be removed entirely) (Fig. 345, a).

Step 2. The lumen of the open end of the tube is enlarged by making a longitudinal incision on its free border for a distance of half an inch. Then the angles of the flaps thus formed are rounded (Fig. 345, b).

Step 3. A seromuscular incision for the length of one inch is made through the fundus of the uterus. The exposed mucosa is opened for the length of half an inch in its center. The edges of the tube and of the opened mucosa of the uterus are sutured to each other by several interrupted sutures. The lips of the seromuscular layer are now sutured to each other (Fig. 345, c).

b. OPERATIONS PRODUCING STERILITY (FIG. 346).

No surgeon will remove the ovaries in order to sterilize a patient. Different procedures to accomplish sterilization have been suggested, such as a mere ligation of the tube by one ligature, ligation of each tube by two ligatures and cutting the tubes between them, resection of the tubes with or without burying the ligated stumps in the leaflets of the broad ligament, and many others. The reason for this large number of methods is that none of them gives a complete assurance that pregnancy will be eliminated. Of all the methods suggested, the Neumann method seems to be the most reliable. It consists in the removal of a portion of the tube close to the fundus, and also of the interstitial portion of the tube, and then in closure of the opened end of the uterine cornu and the suturing of the closed peripheral end of the tube to the closed cornu uteri. Crossen covers the closed cornu uteri by the round ligament.

Technic.

Step 1. The tube is clamped by two forceps at a distance of one-half an inch from the cornu uteri and is cut between the clamps. The distal end is ligated and buried in the leaflets of the broad ligament (Fig. 346, a and c).

Step 2. The proximal portion of the tube is excised together with the uterine cornu, which is then closed by several interrupted sutures (Fig. 346, a, b).

Step 3. The round ligament is fastened to the sutured cornu of the uterus (Fig. 346, d).

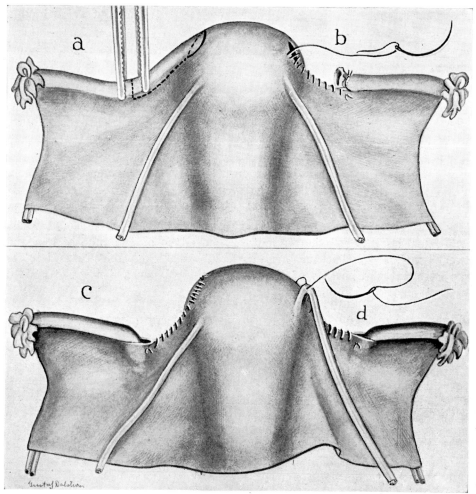

Fig. 346. Producing Sterility.
Neumann Method.

E. HYSTERECTOMY.

This term consists of two Greek words: ὑστέρα, uterus, and ἐκτομή, to excise. It signifies the excision of the uterus. According to the route of approach this operation is subdivided into two groups:

a. Abdominal.
b. Vaginal.

Abdominal hysterectomy is again subdivided into two groups:

a. Supravaginal hysterectomy, in which the fundus and the body are removed but the cervix uteri is left behind.

b. Complete (total) hysterectomy in which the cervix uteri is also removed.

The technic of hysterectomy varies according to whether the adnexa are removed or left, and also whether a preliminary ligation of the blood-vessels is made or the "clamp method" is employed for preventing hemorrhage.

a. SUPRAVAGINAL HYSTERECTOMY.

Indications.

    a. Fibromyoma uteri, particularly when the tumors are large or numerous.

    b. Chronic metritis.

    c. General fibrosis of the uterus.

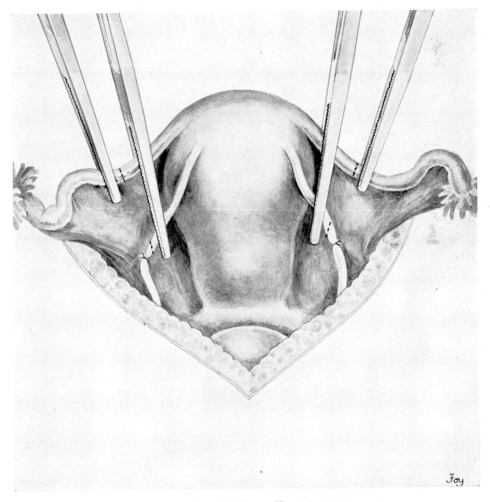

FIG. 347. SUPRAVAGINAL HYSTERECTOMY.
The tube, broad ligament and round ligament are caught on each side by an artery forceps; the tube on each side is clamped by an artery forceps lateral to the previously placed clamps.

d. Myopathic hemorrhages which do not yield to any other method of treatment.

Technic.

Step 1. After the abdomen is opened by a midline or a transverse incision the patient is placed in the Trendelenburg position.   The Fallopian

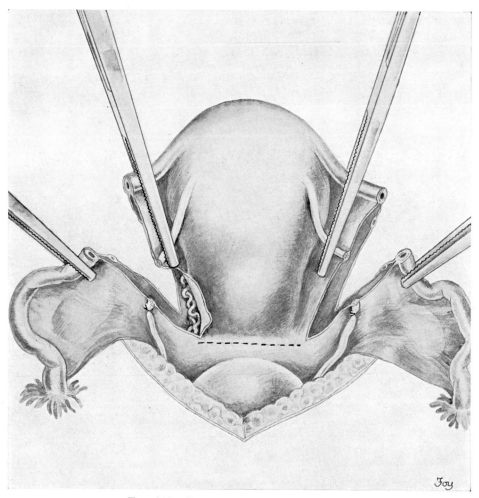

FIG. 348. SUPRAVAGINAL HYSTERECTOMY.
The tubes and adnexa are cut between the clamps. The utero-vesical fold is ready to be cut.

tube, the round ligament, the ligamentum ovarii proprium, and part of the broad ligament are grasped at each side by an artery-forceps which extends along the side of the uterus down to its middle portion (Fig. 347). [This maneuvre eliminates the necessity of employing a uterine grasping-forceps, which occasionally perforates the wall of the uterus.] The body of the uterus is now brought forward and laparotomy pads are placed behind the uterus to cover the loops of small bowel and prevent them from slipping into the operative field. [The thoroughness of covering the bowel is very much facilitated by bringing the uterus forward before the pads are placed in the pelvis behind it.]

Step 2. An artery-forceps clamps each tube at a distance of half an

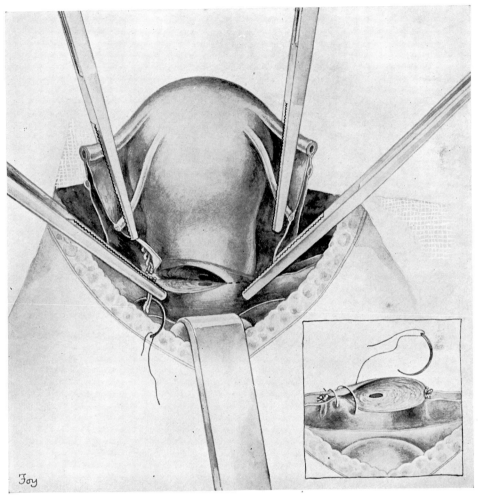

FIG. 349. SUPRAVAGINAL HYSTERECTOMY.
MAIN PICTURE. The uterine arteries are clamped. Beginning to cut through the cervix uteri.
INSERT. The uterine vessels are ligated. Closure of the cervix uteri is begun.

inch from the forceps that clamped the tubo-uterine junction in Step 1. The tube is cut between the clamps on each side, and the stump is ligated by a transfixing-suture. The round ligament is ligated lateral to the body of the uterus and is cut on each side between the ligatures and the clamp placed in Step 1 (Fig. 347).

Step 3. The utero-vesical fold is lifted by two tissue-forceps and cut between them. The opening is enlarged to the right and to the left (Fig. 348). A finger is introduced into the opening and the bladder is pulled upward, separating it from the upper portion of the cervix uteri.

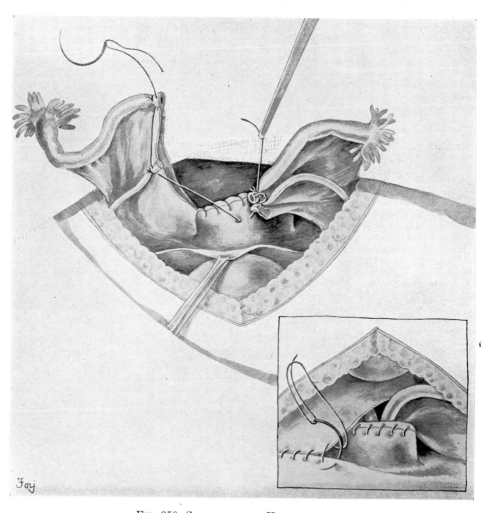

FIG. 350. SUPRAVAGINAL HYSTERECTOMY.
MAIN PICTURE. Suturing of the cervical stump to the stump of the tube and broad ligament of each side.
INSERT. Peritonization of the cervical stump by suturing the vesico-uterine fold to the posterior wall of the cervical stump.

Step 4. The anterior leaflet of the broad ligament of each side is incised along the body of the uterus down to the cervix. A strong artery-forceps clamps on each side the lower portion of the broad ligament in an oblique direction in such a manner that the tip of the blade grasps a portion of the lateral uterine wall in its lower portion, thus clamping the uterine artery on each side (Fig. 349).

Step 5. The uterus is cut transversely at a level of half an inch above the point where the artery-forceps clamps the uterine vessels. The cervical canal is disinfected by tincture of iodine and alcohol (Fig. 349).

Step 6. The uterine vessels are ligated by a transfixion-suture of chromic catgut No. 2 on each side (Fig. 349).

Step 7. The opening leading into the cervical canal is closed by a continuous row of sutures (No. 2 chromic catgut) (Fig. 349, insert).

Step 8. The stump of each tube is sutured to the cervical stump (Fig. 350).

Step 9. The utero-vesical fold which was dissected in Step 3 is brought over the sutured stump of the cervix and sutured to its posterior (intestinal) surface. Thus, the stump is peritonized (Fig. 350, insert).

The omentum is brought over the cervical stump. If, however, the omentum is not long enough, then it is advisable to place the sigmoid over the stump. Otherwise a loop of small bowel may become adherent to the stump and produce an intestinal obstruction.

b. TOTAL HYSTERECTOMY.

In this operation not only the body of the uterus but also the cervix is removed.

Indications.

    a. Malignancy of the uterus.

    b. Myoma of the uterus involving also the cervix.

    c. Any pathology of the uterus requiring supravaginal hysterectomy together with the presence of severe lacerations of the cervix.

Technic.

The vagina is well disinfected by a 5 per cent. solution of tincture of iodine, followed by alcohol. Then:

Steps 1 to 3 are the same as in supravaginal hysterectomy, with this difference that the tubes as a rule are removed, and that separation of the bladder from the uterus and cervix is carried farther than in the case of supravaginal hysterectomy. The bladder is separated from the wall of the vagina as low as possible. Then, with the aid of the thumb placed on the posterior wall of the vagina and of the index-finger placed on the anterior vaginal wall, the cervix uteri is palpated so that the surgeon is able to decide whether the separation of the bladder from the cervix in a downward and lateral direction is sufficient (Fig. 351, insert).

Step 4. Two strong toothed-forceps clamp the broad ligaments and the parametrium lateral to the cervix on each side of the uterus along its entire length down to the wall of the vagina. The clamps are placed obliquely so that the blades lie closer to the midline than the handles. The broad ligaments and the parametrial tissues are cut between each pair of clamps. **[Extreme care should be taken not to catch the ureter in the clamp.]** (Fig. 351).

Step 5. A longitudinal incision is made on the anterior wall of the vagina for the length of one inch (Fig. 352). Each lip of the incised vaginal wall is then grasped by a forceps. The opening into the vagina

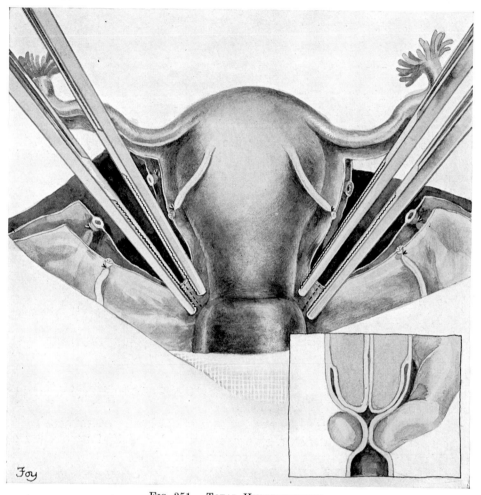

FIG. 351. TOTAL HYSTERECTOMY.

MAIN PICTURE. The infundibulopelvic ligament, the round ligament and the broad ligament on each side are cut; two clamps are clamping the parametrium on each side of the cervix.

INSERT. Palpation of the cervix uteri to be sure that the bladder is separated from the cervix for its entire length.

is disinfected from above by a 2 per cent. solution of iodine. The vagina is now cut circularly **very close to the cervix** [this proximity to the cervix greatly diminishes the possibility of cutting the ureters.] (Fig. 352, upper insert). It is done first on the anterior vaginal wall. Then, after the cervix is pulled out of the vagina and turned laterally, the posterior vaginal wall becomes well exposed and is cut circularly very close to its attachment to the cervix.

Step 6. The vagina is closed with or without drainage of the pelvic cavity (Fig. 352, lower left insert).

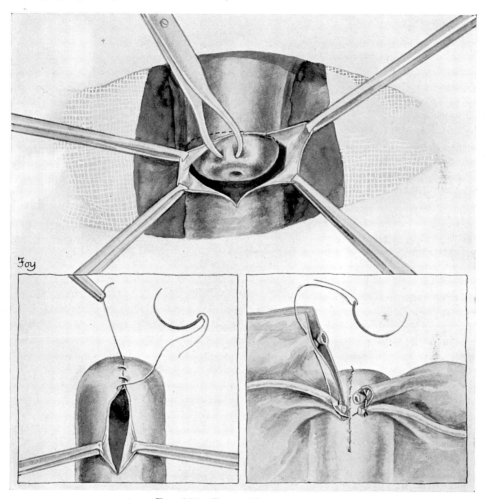

FIG. 352. TOTAL HYSTERECTOMY.
UPPER INSERT. The wall of the vagina is opened and is cut away from the cervix.
LOWER LEFT INSERT. Closure of the vagina after removal of the uterus.
LOWER RIGHT INSERT. The round ligament, broad ligament and infundibulopelvic ligament of each side are attached to the vagina.

Step 7. The stumps of the broad ligament are sutured to the vagina. Thus, prolapse of the vagina is prevented (Fig. 352, lower right insert). The utero-vesical fold covers now the vaginal stump and is sutured to the posterior wall of the vagina. Thus, the stump is peritonized.

Step 8. The abdomen is closed.

F. DEFUNDATION.

This operation consists in the removal of the fundus uteri (together with the tubes). The first who suggested and performed this operation was Dührssen, for the treatment of chronic metritis. However, the operation was not used until Oscar Beuttner suggested it again in 1908. He increased the operative indications and described its technic, and for this reason he is considered as the originator of the operation. W. Blair Bell, in 1914, also described the operation as a new method. The operation is known as the "Beuttner Operation" and as the "Bell-Beuttner operation". However, the priority belongs to Beuttner.

Indications.

    1. In all cases in which salpingectomy or salpingo-oöphorectomy is indicated.

    2. Chronic metritis.

The operation is usually done on comparatively young women in whom it is desirable to preserve menstruation.

BEUTTNER OPERATION.

Technic.

    Step 1. The abdomen is opened by a longitudinal or a transverse (Pfannenstiel) incision. The patient is placed in the Trendelenburg position. The bowels are displaced upward and covered by moist laparotomy pads.

    Step 2. The fundus of the uterus is grasped by a strong uterine forceps. A wedge-incision is made on the fundus cutting first the anterior and then the posterior surface. The size of the wedge depends on whether one or both ovaries are removed, or whether both ovaries are preserved. The fundus is now cut in a sagittal plane, each half of which is grasped by a forceps and cut away, starting at the median line and continuing in a lateral direction. The bleeding point of the uterine artery is caught and ligated. The diseased adnexæ are removed by continued cutting in a lateral direction over a previously placed clamp on the mesosalpinx **(technic of Faure)** until the infundibulopelvic ligament is reached. This ligament is clamped in case the ovary is removed. Otherwise it is not clamped.

    Step 3. The infundibulopelvic ligament is sutured over the clamp by a continuous suture, which when continued closes the broad ligaments. A continuous catgut suture closes the opening in the uterus.

BELL MODIFICATION OF THE BEUTTNER OPERATION.

    Step 1. The same as Step I in the previous operation.

    Step 2. A wedge-shaped incision is made through the fundus starting about half an inch below the point of the tubo-uterine junction. Thus, the attachment of each round ligament to the body of the uterus is severed. The incision is made in a crater form, that is, in such a manner that each deeper lying structure is cut farther away from the fundus than the more superficial. The branch of the uterine artery lying at the lateral side of the body of the uterus is clamped and ligated as soon as the fundus uteri is cut at this point (Fig. 353, a).

Step 3. The tube is separated in a direction beginning medially and extending laterally over a forceps which clamps the mesosalpinx [N.B.

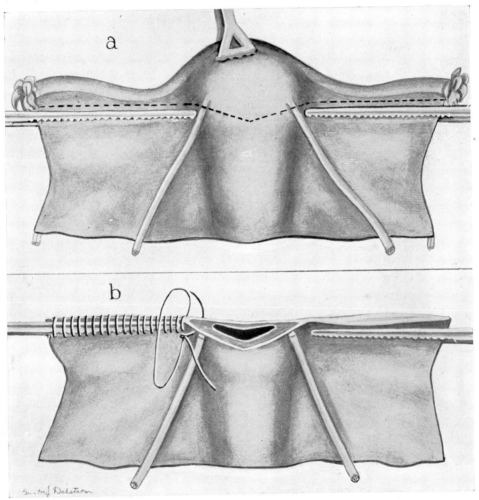

FIG. 353. DEFUNDATION.
a. Arterial forceps clamps each mesosalpinx. Another forceps grasps the fundus uteri. Dotted lines show the line of intended incision.
b. The tubes and fundus are removed. Suturing of the mesosalpinx and the corpus uteri is begun.

The ovaries are not removed unless this is imperative on account of the pathology present.] (Fig. 353, a).

Step 4. The leaflets of the broad ligament are sutured over the clamp, which is then removed. This suture is continued on the uterus, closing its open wound, and then on the broad ligament of the other side (Fig. 353, b).

Step 5. The round ligament on each side is brought over the raw surface of the closed uterus and sutured to its posterior wall (Fig. 354, a, b). This accomplishes two things. It peritonizes the raw surface of the uterus, and by properly adjusting the round ligaments it lifts the remain-

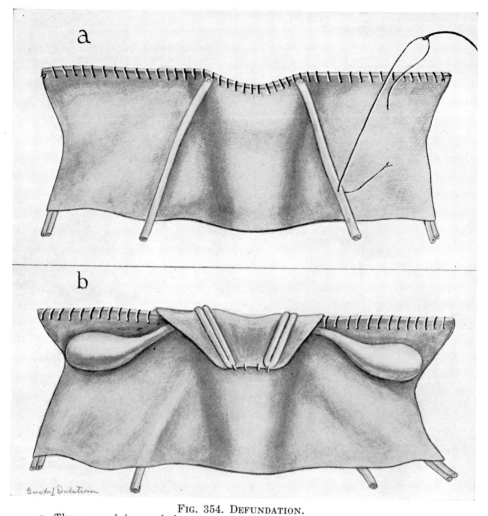

FIG. 354. DEFUNDATION.
a. The mesosalpinx and the corpus uteri are sutured.
b. The round and broad ligaments of each side are covering the raw areas.

ing portion of the uterus, thus preventing the possibility of its retroversion and prolapse.

The advantage of defundation over salpingectomy is that it more thoroughly removes the pathology, since it is a well known fact that salpingitis is quite frequently associated with pathological changes in the fundal endometrium. Its advantage over supravaginal hysterectomy is that menstruation is preserved and there is no interference with the bladder.

G. CESAREAN SECTION.

Definition.

This is the delivery of a child through an incision in the abdominal and uterine walls.

Historical.

The removal of a child through an incision in the abdominal and uterine walls has been known since remote antiquity. In the Hindu Vedas (Súsrutas Agur-Veda) we find the suggestion made to open the abdomen of a pregnant woman immediately after she dies in order to save the child. In the writings of the ancient Greeks and Romans we find allusions to removal of a child by a Cesarean operation. The god Dionys, according to Greek mythology, was born in this way after Zeus had killed his mother Semele by a thunderbolt. Numa Pompilius (715-672 B. C.), the second emperor of ancient Rome, in his "Lex Regia" ("Royal law") makes it imperative to open dead pregnant women immediately in order to save the children. Æsculapius, according to Ovid (Ovid: Metamorphoses, Lib. II, v. 628-630) was born this way. That the word "Cesarian" does not originate from the fact that Julius Cæsar was born in this way is evident, since Scipio Africanus (237-183 B. C.) who lived before Cæsar (100-44 B. C.) was born in this way, as may be seen from the biography of Scipio, written by the great Roman historian Pliny.

This operation was also known in the orient. The great Persian poët Firdouzi (941-1020), in his poem Shahnama (the "Book of Kings", completed in 1010, A. D.) speaks about the birth of Rustam by a Cesarean section performed on his mother Rudabeh. In order to alleviate the pain wine was given to her as an anesthetic. The operation was known to ancient Hebrews, as may be seen from the description in the Talmud of "Jotze Dofan" (birth through the abdomen). In the medieval period Cesarean section was a well known procedure. The Roman Catholic church advised to "remove the child cautiously immediately following the death of the pregnant mother. If the child is alive it should immediately be baptized".

Shakespeare alludes to it at the beginning of the XVIIth century:
"Macduff was from his mother's womb
Untimely ripp'd" (Macbeth, Act. V, Scene VII).

It is frequently mentioned that this operation was performed by Jacob Nufer, a pig-gelder, on his wife, in 1500. However, many believe that this was a case of full term abdominal pregnancy. Today it is generally accepted that Trautmann, of Wittenberg, was the first who in modern times performed a Cesarean operation (in 1610) on a **living** woman with a hernia of the pregnant uterus.

Due to the fact that the uterus at that time was not sutured but was dropped back into the free peritoneal cavity, the mortality was extremely high, the patients dying usually from hemorrhage or peritonitis.

Suturing of the uterine wall was first suggested by Lebas in 1769. However, his work passed unnoticed.

Jőrg, in 1808, suggested using a latero-posterior approach. This operation, **"gastro-elytrotomy"**, consisted in making an abdominal incision above and parallel to Poupart's ligament down to (but not through) the peritoneum. Then, the peritoneum was pushed upward until the uterus was exposed, its wall was incised, and the child was removed. Ritgen, in 1821, carried out the suggestion of Jőrg. Porro, in 1876, suggested a Cesarean operation followed by a supravaginal hysterectomy as a routine procedure (thus eliminating hemorrhage and infection from the escape of lochia into the free peritoneal cavity). Max Sänger, in 1882, gave his classical description of the conservative Cesarean section, and thus this procedure was placed on a safe basis. Since in Sänger's method the uterus is preserved, this method is known as the **conservative** Cesarean operation. In the case of the Porro technic the uterus is removed, and for this reason it is designated as the **radical** Cesarean operation. Frank, of Kőln, introduced in 1907, the **extraperitoneal** method of Cesarean section.

Indications.

1. **Pelvic contraction** of a considerable degree (when the conjugata vera is less than 5.5 cm.) However, if the conjugata vera is less than 7.5 cm. normal delivery is hardly possible, so that many consider a size of the conjugata vera below 7.5 cm. as an indication for the Cesarean operation.

2. **Tumor of the uterus or of the adjacent structures** blocking the delivery of the child.

3. **Eclampsia** (occasionally).

Cesarean section is reserved only for those cases in which quick delivery is necessary and when the cervix is narrow and elongated and the vagina small and rigid, when it would be unsuitable to employ methods of dilatation of the cervix. However, it should be mentioned that there are many obstetricians who believe that in the case of eclampsia the treatment should be medical and no surgery should be applied.

4. **Placenta prævia.**

Although the majority of obstetricians terminate the pregnancy in placenta prævia either by version or by the induction of labor by a dilating bag, nevertheless, some perform a Cesarean section.

5. **Diseases of the Heart.**

Not all heart-lesions are equally dangerous. Patients with mitral stenosis stand labor badly; next come those affected by aortic lesions, and finally those affected by mitral insufficiency. To many obstetricians it seems better to subject the patient to a laparotomy than to a prolonged labor.

6. **Malposition of the fetus, especially in primiparæ.**

7. **Previous Cesarean Section.**

This holds true if the previous Cesarean operation was performed for a permanent indication, such as contracted pelvis with the conjugata vera less than 7.5 cm. If, however, the previous Cesarean operation was performed for temporary reasons, such as placenta prævia, then some obstetricians would permit the patient to have a natural delivery in the hospital, being ready to intervene in case of signs of impending rupture of the uterus. However, the majority of obstetricians believe that "once a Cesarean section, always a Cesarean section".

Contraindications.
  a. Dead fetus.
  b. Presence of uterine infection.
  c. Advanced labor with engagement of the head.

Time of Operation.

The best time to operate is a few days before the estimated date of labor. However, if the labor has started but has not lasted more than a few hours, and if no vaginal examinations have been made, the Cesarean section is just as advisable.

Subdivisions.

Cesarean section is performed either by a **transperitoneal** route or by an **extraperitoneal** route. In the transperitoneal variety it is performed, as a rule, with preservation of the uterus (conservative Cesarean section). Occasionally the uterus has to be removed after the child is delivered (radical Cesarean section—Porro operation, or its modifcations).

I. TRANSPERITONEAL CESAREAN SECTION.

In the transperitoneal variety, the uterus may be cut either in the upper portion of the body (classical Cesarean section) or in the lower uterine segment ("low cervical section"). There is quite a divergence of opinion when to use the classical and when a low cervical Cesarean section. The majority of surgeons still believe that in the case of the elective Cesarean section, the classical operation is the operation of choice, leaving the "low cervical Cesarean section" only for doubtful cases in which infection is not excluded. However, there are many who consider that the "low cervical Cesarean section" should be the operation of choice and replace the classical Cesarean section.

a. CONSERVATIVE CESAREAN SECTION.

Technic.

Step 1. An abdominal incision starts in the midline two inches above the umbilicus and extends downward to the symphysis pubis. It runs semicircularly around the umbilicus to the left and then continues in the midline. [Some prefer to make the incision only in the lower half of the abdominal wall when the uterus is incised while *in situ*. The incision of the uterine wall should be just long enough to permit the delivery of the child. Others prefer to make a midline incision above only. The uterine wall is then incised in the upper portion of the uterus. After the uterus

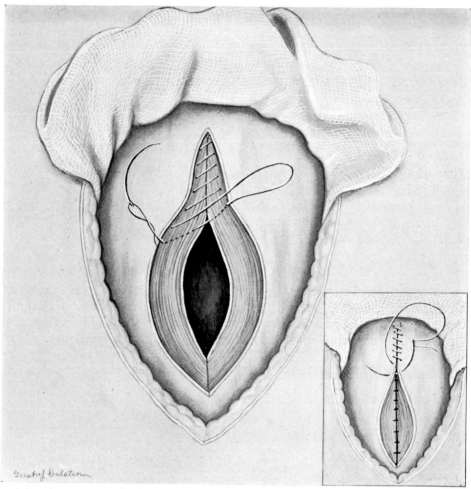

FIG. 355. CONSERVATIVE CESAREAN SECTION.
MAIN PICTURE. Closure of the uterine wall after the child is delivered. Only the muscles are sutured (the decidual lining is not sutured).
INSERT. Suturing of the superficial layer of the muscle and the serosa.

is evacuated it contracts below the level of the umbilicus, and therefore there will be no adhesions between the uterus and the anterior abdominal wall.]

Step 2. The uterus is pushed to the left in order to counteract the normal tilting of the organ to the right. Thus, the midline of the uterus will lie in the middle of the opened wound. Moist laparotomy sponges are introduced to "wall off" the uterus from the rest of the abdominal cavity. One ampule of pituitrin is now injected into the muscle of the uterus or intravenously, thus producing contraction of its musculature. A longitudinal incision is made in the midline of the anterior wall of the uterus, starting at the fundus. The length of this incision varies from 4 to 5

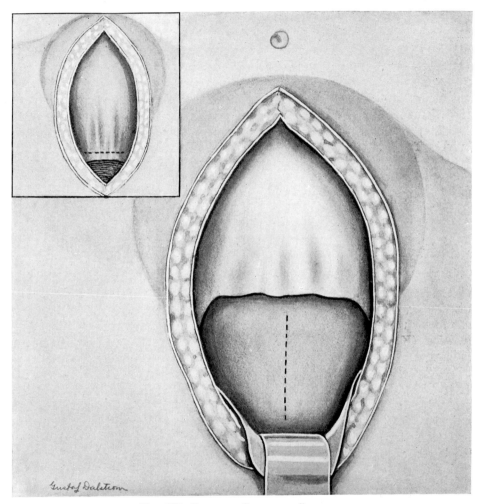

FIG. 356. CERVICAL CESAREAN SECTION.
INSERT. Dotted line shows the intended line of incision of the vesico-uterine fold.
MAIN PICTURE. The bladder is retracted downward and the lower uterine segment is exposed; the dotted line shows the intended line of incision.

inches. Care should be taken not to incise the uterus too low, in order not to injure the bladder accidentally. However, the incision should be long enough to remove the child easily, since fast work is important between the time the uterine incision is made and the extraction of the child.

Step 3. The right hand of the surgeon is introduced into the uterine cavity. One or both feet are caught and the child is extracted. The cord is clamped by two forceps and cut between them.

Step 4. The uterus is now brought outside the peritoneal cavity and the placenta is removed.

Step 5. One of the assistants grasps the uterus close to the cervix and compresses the cervix on each side in the region of the broad ligaments, thus controlling the uterine arteries and diminishing the flow of blood while the uterine wall is being sutured. As the gloved fingers slip, making it a difficult procedure to compress the cervix, this procedure is facilitated by wrapping a moist towel around the lower portion of the uterus and then compressing the cervix. However, many surgeons prefer not to do this, since contraction of the uterus takes place very quickly so that there is little or no hemorrhage.

Step 6. Suturing of the uterine wall is begun. This is done in two layers. The first layer of sutures grasps the deep layer of the muscle only **(the decidual lining is not sutured),** and another penetrates the serosa and the superficial portion of the muscle. The sutures are continuous (though many are using interrupted sutures), and of chromic catgut No. 2 (Fig. 355).

Step 7. The abdomen is closed.

b. LOW CERVICAL CESAREAN SECTION. (FIGS. 356 AND 357).

This consists in opening the abdomen, exposure of the uterus, division of the vesico-uterine fold, and separation of the bladder from the lower uterine segment, then in making either a **longitudinal incision** through the lower uterine segment **(Krőnig method)** or a **transverse** semicircular incision (Kerr incision) (Fig. 356). The child is delivered, the placenta is removed, and the uterus is closed. The upper peritoneal fold is sutured to the lower, thus covering completely the suture-line on the cervix uteri (Fig. 357). However, in order to seal the suture-line on the cervix more securely, some gynecologists suture the upper peritoneal flap to the anterior uterine wall below the line of uterine sutures. Then the lower flap (the utero-vesical) is brought in front of the upper flap, overlapping its lower edge for a distance of one inch, and is sutured to it **(Beck technic).**

c. RADICAL CESAREAN SECTION (PORRO OPERATION).

When the uterus is infected (so that it would be dangerous to leave it in the peritoneal cavity), or when it presents some pathology which requires its removal (multiple myomata and fibromata, extensive hemorrhage into the wall of the uterus in the case of premature separation of the placenta, so that it is evident that the contractile power of the uterus is lost and hemorrhage is highly probable, etc.), the uterus is removed after the child is delivered.

The steps of the operation are the same as in the conservative Cesarean operation up to the point when the child is delivered. Then the technic

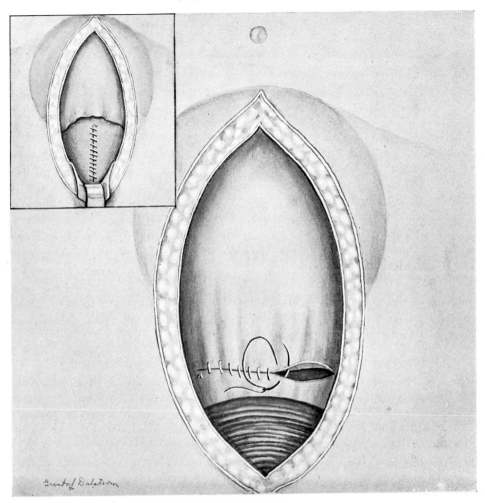

FIG. 357. CERVICAL CESAREAN SECTION.
INSERT. The wall of the uterus is closed after the child is delivered.
MAIN PICTURE. Suturing the upper lip of the vesico-uterine fold to the lower one.

differs. In the original Porro operation (which is rarely used now by any surgeon), an elastic ligature was tied tightly around the cervix. The infundibulopelvic ligament was cut between two clamps and the uterus cut above the elastic ligature and removed. The uterine stump then was transfixed by a knitting needle which was placed on the abdominal wall so as to prevent the stump dropping into the abdominal cavity. The abdomen was closed in layers. In a few days or longer the stump with the ligature sloughed away and the wound healed by granulation.

The original Porro operation is seldom performed now. If the uterus is removed today it is done by the usual method of supravaginal hysterectomy, and as the abdominal wall and the pelvic floor are relaxed it is frequently possible to bring not only the uterus but even the upper portion of the cervix outside the abdominal cavity, so that the performance of the supravaginal hysterectomy does not take more time than the removal of the placenta and suturing the uterine wall in conservative Cesarean section.

d. PORTES METHOD.

Portes, of Paris in 1924, suggested a method of operation in cases of **infected** uterus. The full time pregnant uterus is delivered **unopened** outside of the abdominal cavity and the parietal peritoneum is sutured to the posterior surface of the lower uterine segment. The abdominal wall is closed. Then the uterus is opened, the child delivered, the placenta removed, the uterus sutured and left lying on the abdominal wall, wrapped in moist gauze. Five or six weeks later the abdomen is reopened and the uterus replaced. However, this method, we believe, will hardly appeal to the obstetricians.

II. EXTRAPERITONEAL CESAREAN SECTION.

This method was suggested by Frank, of Köln, in 1907. Since that time many modifications have been suggested. The majority of gynecologists employ this approach only for doubtful cases, that is, when they are not sure that the case is clean (when they perform a classical Cesarean section), or is certainly infected (when the Cesarean section is supplemented by a supravaginal hysterectomy). To this group belong those patients who have been long in labor, or those on whom a manual vaginal examination has been repeatedly made, and also those patients in whom the membranes have been ruptured for a considerable time and unsuccessful attempts for delivery have been tried.

All the varieties of extraperitoneal methods may be classed into two groups:

a. Methods in which the peritoneum is not opened but is pushed upward in front of the lower uterine segment, which segment is incised and the child delivered.

b. Methods in which the lips of the incised parietal peritoneum are sutured to the lips of the incised visceral uterine peritoneum before the uterus is opened (so that extraperitonization of the uterus is effected before it is opened).

Whereas the first group of methods is truly extraperitoneal, the second group is only "extraperitoneal delivery by a transperitoneal route".

a. EXTRAPERITONEAL CESAREAN SECTION.
(LATZKO METHOD).

From 100 to 150 c. cm. of any antiseptic solution is injected into the urinary bladder. This will raise the bladder above the symphysis pubis.

Step 1. A longitudinal incision extending from the umbilicus down to the symphysis pubis (it may be a transverse incision) is carried down to, but not through, the peritoneum. The recti muscles are pulled apart. The parietal peritoneum is drawn upward. Thus the bladder is exposed. The bladder is then separated from the lower uterine segment by gauze-dissection and pushed to the right. The vesico-uterine fold of the peri-

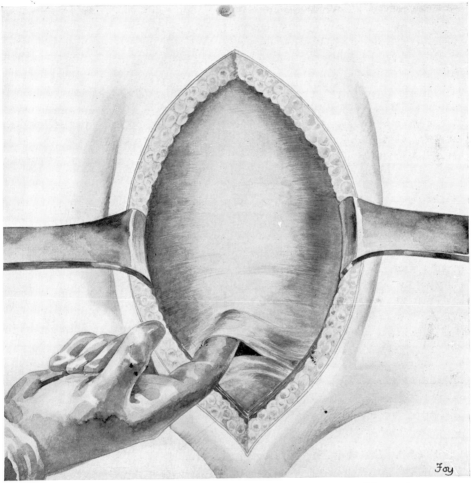

FIG. 358. EXTRAPERITONEAL CESAREAN SECTION (LATZKO METHOD).
Pushing the peritoneal reflection from the uterus onto the bladder upward thus exposing the lower portion of the uterus.

toneum is then bluntly shoved upward until the upper portion of the cervix and the lower segment of the uterus are sufficiently exposed (Fig. 358).

Step 2. A longitudinal incision through the middle of the exposed uterus is made and the child delivered (Fig. 359). The placenta is removed, and the uterine wall is closed by catgut. The urinary bladder is dropped back, thus covering the suture-line.

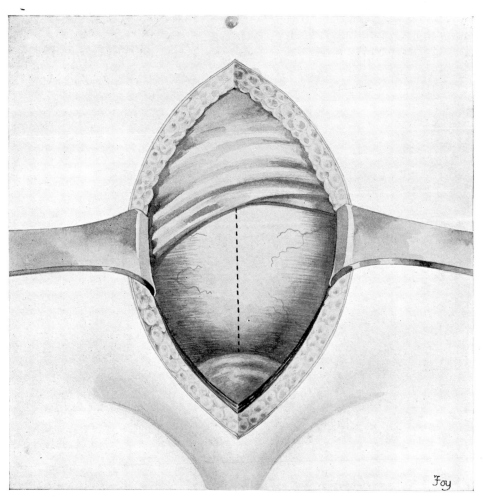

FIG. 359. EXTRAPERITONEAL CESAREAN SECTION (LATZKO METHOD).
The dotted line shows the intended line of the incision on the uterine wall.

Step 3. The abdomen is closed in layers.

Drainage of the abdominal wall is instituted only in cases in which the surgeon believes that the wound has become infected.

b. EXTRAPERITONEAL DELIVERY BY A TRANSPERITONEAL ROUTE. (VEIT-FROMME METHOD).

Step 1. The abdomen is opened by a longitudinal incision extending from the umbilicus to the symphysis pubis.

Step 2. The visceral peritoneum of the uterus is cut longitudinally for the same length as the abdominal wall, and each lip of the visceral peritoneum is sutured to the corresponding lip of the parietal peritoneum.

In their original work the authors clamped the leaflets to each other. Hirst suggested suturing them before the uterus is opened (Fig. 360).

Step 3. The uterus is incised, the child delivered, the placenta removed, and the uterus closed.

Step 4. The abdomen is closed.

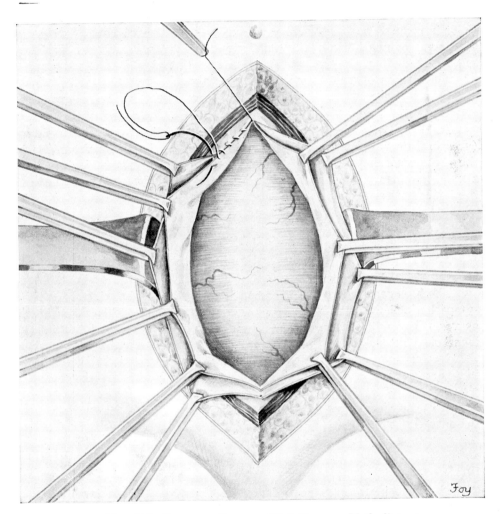

FIG. 360. CESAREAN SECTION (Veit-Fromme Method).

This method of extraperitonel delivery through the transperitoneal route has the advantage over the true extraperitoneal route in this respect, that it gives a better exposure and there is less possibility of injury to the bladder. However, the methods of this group are not as safe (from the point of infection) as the methods of the first group.

H. PELVIC SYMPATHECTOMY.

That severe pain in the pelvic organs not yielding to any gynecological therapeusis, either medical or surgical, can be alleviated by cutting the sympathetic plexuses which represent the efferent pathways going from the genitalia, was known as early as the last quarter of the Nineteenth century. To Jaboulay belongs the credit of being the first, who, in 1898, introduced as a surgical procedure resection of a small portion of the sacral sympathetic chain to eliminate pelvic pain. Ruggi, in 1899, suggested cutting the utero-ovarian plexus (running in the suspensory ligament of the ovary) as a measure for abolishing such pain. Leriche, in 1921, introduced peri-arterial sympathectomy of the internal iliac artery for the relief of intractable pelvic pain.

In 1925, Cotte suggested section of the superior hypogastric plexus (presacral nerve) for the relief of pain in the pelvis. This procedure in the great majority of cases relieves the pain completely, and since it is a much simpler procedure than peri-arterial sympathectomy it replaced the latter entirely.

Anatomy.

a. THE INNERVATION OF THE UTERUS.

The sympathetic fibers of the uterus are derived from the hypogastric and the sacral plexuses.

The **hypogastric** plexus is the continuation of the inferior mesenteric sympathetic plexus. The latter gives origin to the right and left mesenteric nerves, which unite in one common trunk (or plexus) at a point lying one inch below the origin of the inferior mesenteric artery, and this place is the starting point of the hypogastric plexus. This plexus is subdivided into two parts: the superior hypogastric plexus and the inferior hypogastric plexus.

The **superior hypogastric plexus (presacral nerve of Latarjet and Bonnet,** who coined this name) extends from its beginning at the level of the fourth lumbar vertebra downward to the middle of the first sacral vertebra. At this point it subdivides into two portions, the right and the left inferior hypogastric plexuses.

The superior hypogastric plexus, in the greatest number of cases, actually represents a plexus (in about 80 per cent.) and only in about 20 per cent. it runs as a nerve. Latarjet and Bonnet in their anatomical dissections evidently met the latter variety more frequently. That is the reason why they called this the "presacral nerve"; Cotte, in introducing his method of resection, used the name coined by Latarjet. For this reason, this name is retained now. **However, we should bear in mind that resection of the presacral nerve is not a resection of a nerve-trunk but of a nerve-plexus.** The superior hypogastric plexus runs in the midline and is separated from the middle sacral artery by a dense layer of fascia.

The **inferior hypogastric plexus (left** and **right) starts at the middle** of the first sacral vertebra. Its length is between two and three inches. Each plexus runs along the medial side of the internal iliac artery. Each inferior hypogastric nerve terminates in a hypogastric ganglion, which gives off some branches running laterally into the wall of the internal iliac artery, other branches running medially into the wall of the rectum, and some other branches coursing along the utero-sacral ligaments. [This is the anatomical explanation of relief of pain observed in some cases of retroversion of the uterus which were treated by cutting these ligaments. It was believed before that this was due to a mechanical correction. However, in the light of our modern knowledge we know that this was due instead to a division of the branches of the inferior hypogastric sympathetic plexus.]

b. THE INNERVATION OF THE OVARY.

The ovarian sympathetic plexus is derived from the mesenteric and the renal plexuses. It accompanies the ovarian artery. Then it enters the suspensory ligament of the ovary and there it divides into a tubal branch going to the uterine tube and an ovarian branch going to the hilum of the ovary.

Indications for Pelvic Sympathectomy.

1. Severe pain due to inoperable malignant pathological lesions of the uterus or of the adnexa.

2. Pelvic pain due to pathological lesions which do not yield to medical or surgical gynecological therapeusis.

3. Functional dysmenorrhea not yielding to ordinary medical or surgical gynecological therapeusis.

4. As a routine procedure in all pelvic conservative operations in which pain is a prominent pre-operative symptom.

TYPES OF OPERATIONS EMPLOYED FOR
ABOLISHING PELVIC PAIN.

The different procedures employed for the cure of intractable pelvic pain may be subdivided into four groups:

1. Section (or resection) of the superior hypogastric plexus (presacral nerve).

2. Denervation of the ovaries (section of the ovarian nerves).

3. Lower lumbar sympathectomy.

4. Peri-arterial sympathectomy of the internal iliac artery.

Resection of the presacral nerve abolishes the pain in the great majority of cases. As its technic is comparatively simple it should be given preference to any other method of sympathectomy. However, in extensive carcinoma of the pelvic organs accompanied by severe pain, it may be necessary in addition to the resection of the presacral nerve also to resect the lower lumbar chain of sympathetics.

TECHNIC OF THE RESECTION OF THE PRESACRAL NERVE
(FIGS. 361 AND 362).

Step 1. The abdomen is opened by a midline or a transverse incision (Fig. 361, insert).

Step 2. The patient is placed in the Trendelenburg position. The small bowel is pushed upward and packed so as to prevent its slipping into the pelvic cavity. The lower sigmoid is retracted to the left (Fig. 361).

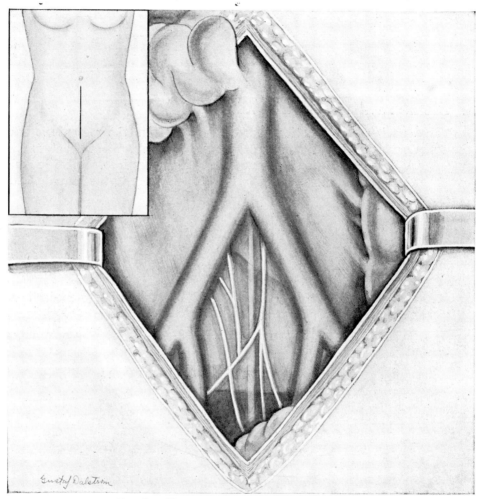

FIG. 361. EXCISION OF THE PRESACRAL NERVE.
INSERT. Skin incision.
MAIN PICTURE. The sympathetic nerves known as the "Presacral nerve" are seen shining through the posterior layer of the parietal peritoneum.

Step 3. The promontory and the right and the left common iliac arteries are identified. The parietal peritoneum covering the anterior surface of the sacrum is incised for three inches in a downward direction in the median line starting from the promontory. Each lip of the incised peritoneum is caught and retracted laterally. Immediately beneath the reflected peritoneum and in front of the midsacral artery are seen numerous nerve-filaments which constitute the superior hypogastric plexus (the presacral nerve). These filaments are isolated and resected for at least one inch so as to preclude any possibility of a nerve-regeneration (Fig. 362).

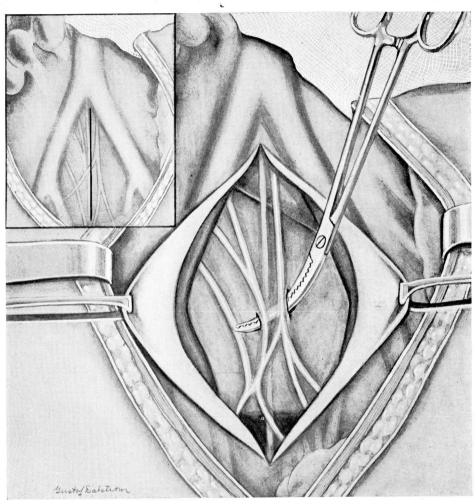

FIG. 362. EXCISION OF THE PRESACRAL NERVE.
INSERT. The parietal peritoneum is incised.
MAIN PICTURE. Some of the fibers of the presacral nerve are separated from the posterior pelvic wall.

Step 4. The lips of the incised parietal peritoneum are sutured.

Step 5. The abdomen is closed in layers.

TECHNIC OF COMPLETE PELVIC SYMPATHECTOMY.

Step 1. The abdomen is opened by a midline incision starting one inch above the umbilicus and extending downward to the symphysis pubis.

Step 2. The patient is placed in the Trendelenburg position. The small bowel is isolated by packs so as to prevent its slipping into the pelvis.

Step 3. The posterior parietal peritoneum is incised in front of the aorta starting immediately below the origin of the inferior mesenteric artery. This incision is carried downward to the promontory and then farther downward in the middle of the concavity of the sacrum. The lips of the peritoneum are reflected laterally. The pre-aortic sympathetic plexus is isolated in front of the aorta and resected. The presacral nerve is isolated and resected. The right and the left lumbar sympathetic chains are isolated and at least two of the lower ganglia on each side are resected. [The right lumbar chain of sympathetics lies at the lateral border of the vena cava inferior. The left lumbar chain lies beneath the left border of the abdominal aorta.]

Step 4. The lips of the incised posterior parietal peritoneum are sutured together.

Step 5. The abdomen is closed.

BIBLIOGRAPHY.

K. V. Bailey. Lower segment section as routine; review of 119 cases.
Lancet, I:672-675; y. 1934.

J. M. Baldy. Retrodisplacements of the uterus and their treatment.
New York Med. Journ. 78:167-169; y. 1903.

J. M. Baldy. The surgical treatment of retroversion of the uterus.
Surg Gyn. & Obst. 20:614-615; y. 1915.

C. W. Barrett. The operative treatment of retrodisplacements, with a new operation; intramural transplantation of the round ligaments.
Surg Gyn. & Obst. I:417-424; y. 1905.

C. W. Barrett. Modifications of Gilliam's operation.
Bost. Med. & Surg. Journ. 161:491; y. 1909.

A. C. Beck. The two-flap low incision caesarean section.
Surg. Gyn. & Obst. 33:290-295; y. 1921.

C. A. Behney. Excision of pelvic autonomic nerves for relief of pain from advanced pelvic carcinoma.
Ann. of Surg. 101:411-417; y. 1935.

W. Blair Bell. A new operative procedure for the treatment of suppurative salpingitis in young women.
Surg. Gyn. Obst. 18:634-637; y. 1914.

R. Bernard & D. Theodoresco. La résection du nerf dit Présacré (Plexus hypogastrique superieur d'Hovelacque).
Journ. de Chir. 31:340-353; y. 1928.

O. Beuttner. Eine neue Methode der Exstirpation doppelseitig erkrankter Adnexe.
Zbl. f. Gynäk. 32:1033-1037; y. 1908.

A. Beyer. Der Kaiserschnitt an der Lebenden.
Stuttgart, J. Fink, Publishers; y. 1889.

R. Bonneau. Technique de la résection du nerf présacré.
Paris chir. 19:115-118; y. 1927.

V. Bonney. The technique and results of myomectomy.
Lancet, I:171-177; y. 1931.

J. G. Clark. The radical abdominal operation for cancer of the uterus.
Surg. Gyn. & Obst. 16:255-265; y. 1913.

R. C. Coffey. Surgical treatment of displacements of the uterus.
Denver Medical Times, 24:339-367; y. 1904.

G. Cotte. La sympathectomie hypogastrique. A-t-elle son place dans la therapeutique gynecologique?
Presse méd. 33:98-99; y. 1925.

G. Cotte. La résection du sympathique pelvien dans les névralgies pelviennes liées au Cancer du col.
Gynecologie, 31:377-385; y. 1932.

Th. S. Cullen. Cancer of the uterus.
D. Appleton and Co., Publishers, New York; y. 1900.

E. P. Davis. The present status of cesarean section.
Americ. Journ. of Obst. 68:12-20; y. 1913.

L. Davis. Carcinoma of the body of the uterus.
Ann. Surg. 82:131-141; y. 1925.

A. Döderlein. Über Extra-peritonealen Kaiserschnitt und Hebosteotomie.
Monatschr. f. Gebh. u. Gyn. 33:1-22; y. 1911.

G. Döderlein. Schnittenbindung nach Gottschalk-Portes.
Zeitschr. f. Geburtsh. u. Gynäk. 108:172-177; y. 1934.

J. A. Dührssen. Zwei weitere Buddhageburten.
Fisher, Publishers, Berlin; y. 1910.

F. Emmert. The recognition of cancer of the uterus in its earlier stages.
Journ. Americ. Med. Ass. 97:1684-1688; y. 1931.

F. Falls. A modification in technic of the Bell-Beuttner operation.
Americ. Journ. of Obst. & Gyn. 27:89-94; y. 1934.

J. L. Faure. L'hystérectomie, indications et technique.
Octave Doin, Editeur, Paris; y. 1906.

F. Fehim. Ueber Stumpfrezidive nach supravaginaler Amputaton des Uterus.
Arch. f. Gynäk. 109:347-357; y. 1918.

A. H. Ferguson. Preliminary report of anterior transplantation of the round ligament for displacements of the uterus.
Journ. Am. Med. Ass. 33:1275-1278; y. 1899.

F. López Fernandez. La Cesárea baja. Su concepto actual.
Vida nueva, 34:305-315; y. 1934.

Firdouzi. Livre de Rois, 1:349-353. French translation: Paris; y. 1838.

R. Fontaine & L. G. Herrmann. Clinical and experimental basis for surgery of the pelvic sympathetic nerves in gynecology.
Surg. Gyn. & Obst. 54:131-163; y. 1932.

F. Frank. Über den subkutanen Symphysenschnitt und die suprasymphysäre Entbindung.
Monatschr. f. Geb. & Gyn. 32:680-692; y. 1910.

F. Fromme. Studien zum klinischen und pathologisch-anatomischen Verhalten der Lymphdrüsen bei malignen Erkrankungen, hauptsächlich dem Carcinoma colli uteri.
Arch. f. Gynäk. 79:197-271; y. 1906.

H. Fuchs. Der Längs—, Inner — und Bogenschnitt bei der Sectio Cæsarea Inferior.
Zbl. f. Gynäk. 57:2549-2555; y. 1933.

T. Gilliam. Round-ligament ventrosuspension of the uterus. A new method.
Americ. Journ. of Obst. 41:299-303; y. 1900.

W. P. Graves. Uterine myomata. In A. H. Curtis "Obstetrics and Gynecology", II:745-921; y. 1933.
W. B. Saunders, Publishers.

P. Guéniot. Quelle place doit encore occuper la césarienne haute classique?
Gynécologie, 33:761-770; y. 1934.

Hafeman. Ein Kaiserschnitt in Alter Zeit.
Med. Welt. 8:1037-1038; y. 1934.

R. E. Haughton. That first hysterectomy.
Americ. Journ. of Surg. & Gynec. 12:233-235; y. 1899.

W. P. Healy & M. Cutler. Radiation and surgical treatment of carcinoma of the body of the uterus.
Americ. Journ. Obst. & Gyn. 19:457-489; y. 1930.

M. Henkel. Der Transperitoneale Cervikale Kaiserschnitt (33 Fälle).
Verhandl. des VI Internat. Kongr. f. Geburtsh. u. Gynäk. pp. 434-437; y. 1912.

A. Hovelacque. Anatomie des nerfs craniens et rachidiens et du système grand sympatique chez l'homme.
G. Doin & Co., Publishers, Paris; y. 1926.

Jaboulay. Le traitement de la névralgie pelvienne par la paralysie du sympathique sacré.
Lyon méd. 90:102-104; y. 1899.

F. Jayle. L'idée de la conservation dans les operations utero-salpingo-
ovariennes.
Rev. franç. de gynéc. et d'obst. 29:837-843; y. 1934.

M. I. Jury. Simpaticectomias pelvianas especialmente en relacion con
ginecologia.
Thesis de doct. Santiago; y. 1929.

G. Kaboth. Die Technik des extraperitonealen Entbindungsschnittes.
Zbl. f. Gynäk. 58:310-325; y. 1934.

H. A. Kelly. On hysterorrhaphy.
Johns Hopkins Hospital Bulletin, 1: 17-19; y. 1890.

F. Kermauner. Zur Behandlung der Gebärmutterkrebse durch abdominale
Operation.
Wien Klin. Wchnschr. 42:1097-1098; y. 1929.

J. M. Munro Kerr. The lower uterine segment incision in conservative
Cæsarean section.
Journ. Obst. & Gyn. of Brit. Empire, 28:475-487; y. 1921.

Koblanck. Ætiologie, Symptomatologie, Diagnostik und Radikalbehand-
lung des Gebärmutterkrebses.
Veit's Handbuch der Gynäk. 3 (second half) :647-805; J. F. Bergmann,
Publishers, Wiesbaden; y. 1908.

B. Krőnig. Transperitonealer cervicaler Kaiserschnitt.
In Dőderlein und Krőnig: "Operative Gynäkologie"; y. 1912.

Laignel-Lavastine & Abbas Maficy. Opération césarienne avec emploi du
vin comme anesthesique d'après "Livre de rois" de Firdouzi.
Bull. Soc. franç. d'hist. de la méd. 28:42-44; y. 1934.

A. Latarjet & P. Bonnet. Le plexus hypogastrique chez l'homme.
Lyon chir. 9:619-644; y. 1913.

M. M. Latta. Hysterectomy priority in America.
Americ. Med.-Surg. Bull. New York, 7:591-592; y. 1894.

W. Latzko. Eine neue Methode der intraperitonealen Ligamentverkűrzung.
Zbl. f. Gynäk. 32:1278-1280; y. 1908.

W. Latzko. Úber den extraperitonealen Kaiserschnitt.
Zbl. f. Gyn. 33:275-283; y. 1909.

W. Latzko & J Schiffmann. Klinisches und Anatomisches zur Radikaloperation des Gebärmutterkrebses.
Zbl. f. Gynäk. 43:689-705; y. 1919.

C. G. Leopold. Ueber die Annähung der retroflektirten aufgerichteten
Gebärmutter an der vorderen Bauchwand.
Volkmann's Sammlung Klinischer Vorträge, Gynäkologie, IV, Heft
333; pp. 2401-2418; y. 1890.

A. E. Mahle. The morphological histology of adenocarcinoma of the body of the uterus in relation to longevity.
Surg. Gyn. & Obst. 36:385-395; y. 1923.

J. C. Masson. Total versus subtotal abdominal hysterectomy.
Americ. Journ. Obst. & Gyn. 14:486-492; y. 1927.

A. F. Maxwell. Review of Cesarean sections.
West. Journ. of Surg. 42:14-28; y. 1934.

G. Meinhold. Die moderne Kaiserschnittstechnik besonders mit Rűcksicht auf die Behandlung der Atonia uteri durch Tamponade mit Jodoformgaze.
Inaug. Dissertation, Berlin; y. 1893.

P. Meyer. Quelques reflexions sur la section césarienne au XVIII siècle.
Gynécologie, 33:733-742; y. 1934.

E. E. Montgomery. A new modification of operative procedure for retroflexion of the uterus.
Therapeut. Gazette, Detroit; 28:371-374; y. 1904.

F. S. Newell. Cesarean Section.
D. Appleton & Co., Publishers; y. 1920.

R. Olshausen. Űber Ventrale Operation bei Prolapsus und Retroversio uteri.
Zbl. f. Gynäk. 10:698-701; y. 1886.

E. Opitz. Zur Technik des Kaiserschnittes.
Zbl. f. Gynäk. 35:970-974; y. 1911.

F. A. Pemberton. The relation between the treatment of cancer of the cervix and the cell type.
Americ. Journ. Obst. & Gyn. 12:536-543; y. 1926.

A. Péradon. Contribution a l'étude de l'opération césarienne moderne: indications; technique opératoire; résultats; suites opératoires; statistique. Paris; y. 1913.

L. E. Phaneuf. The cervical cesarean section; analysis based on the study of 515 personal operations.
New England Journ. of Med. 210:245-251; y. 1934.

A. Plaut. The relation of prognosis to the histological findings in carcinoma of the cervix.
Surg. Gyn. & Obst. 43:450-458; y. 1926.

E. Porro. Della amputazione utero-ovarica come complemento di taglio cesareo.
Milano, Rechiedei, Publishers; y. 1876.

L. Portes. La cæsarienne suivie d'exteriorisation temporaire de l'uterus.
Gynéc. et Obst. 10:225-259; y. 1924.

E. Ries. Eine neue Operationsmethode des Uteruscarcinoms.
Zeitschr. f. Geburtsh. u. Gynäk. 32:266-274; y. 1895.

M. Sänger. Der Kaiserschnitt bei Uterusfibromen nebst vergleichender Methodik der Sectio Cæsarea und der Porro-Operation. Kritiken Studien und Vorschlage zur Verbesserung des Kaiserschnitts.
W. Engelmann, Publishers, Leipzig; y. 1882.

V. Schrattenbach. Beitrag zur operativen Behandlung von Gebärmutterblutungen.
Zbl. f. Gynäk. 58:2958-2961; y. 1934.

H. Sellheim. Der extraperitoneale Uterusschnitt.
Zbl. f. Gyn. 32:133-142; y. 1908.

F. F. Simpson. Intraabdominal but retroperitoneal shortening and anterior fixation of the round ligaments for posterior uterine displacement.
Trans. South Surg. & Gyn. Soc. 15:223-239; y. 1902.

F. F. Simpson. Retroperitoneal shortening of the round ligaments.
Journ. Americ. Med. Assn. 56:553-559; y. 1911.

L. J. Stacy. Carcinoma of the fundus of the uterus.
Surg. Gyn. & Obst. 49:43-47; y. 1929.

J. Stur. Die erste gynäkologische Laparotomie zu Wien im Jahre 1549.
Arch. f. Gynäk. 157:472-481; y. 1934.

P. Trillat. Les conséquences eloignées de la césarienne basse.
Gynécologie, 33:743-760; y. 1934.

J. C. Webster. A satisfactory operation for certain cases of retroversion of the uterus.
Journ. Americ. Med. Assn. 37:913; y. 1901.

INDEX OF NAMES.

717

SUBJECT INDEX.